Critical de
in en

Volume 36 Number 1: **January 2022**

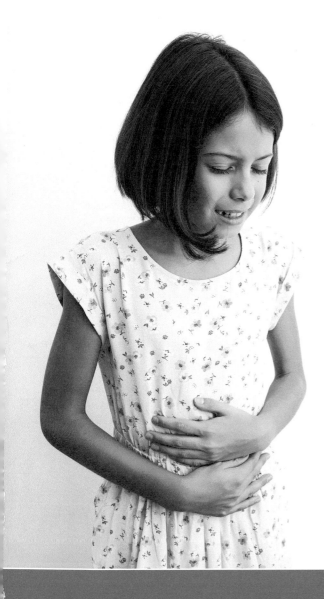

Bellyaching

The differential diagnosis for unexplained vomiting in pediatric patients is broad and red flags are easy to miss in children. It is imperative for emergency physicians to have a stepwise and age-based approach to these patients to ensure that critical diagnoses are recognized and both low- and high-risk causes are appropriately managed.

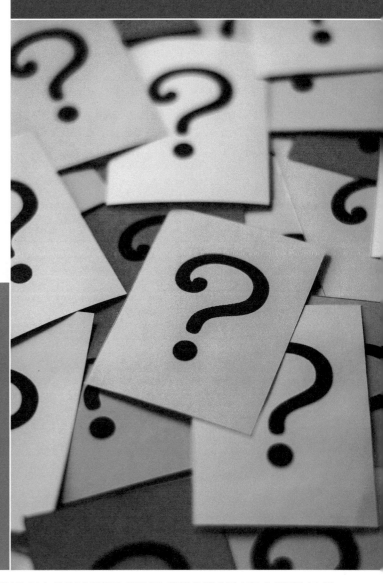

FYI

Medical disinformation regarding COVID-19 vaccination and treatment options has become an important topic in emergency departments across the country. Emergency physicians need to know how to address these issues with patients and understand how disinformation can negatively impact their patient outcomes and practice.

THE OFFICIAL CME PUBLICATION OF THE AMERICAN COLLEGE OF EMERGENCY PHYSICIANS

Individuals in Control of Content

1. Zachary Aust, MD – Faculty
2. Robert Barnes, MD – Faculty
3. Lacey L. Floyd, DO – Faculty
4. Zackary Funk, MD – Faculty
5. Matthew P. Hanley, MD – Faculty
6. John Hurley, MD – Faculty
7. Jedidiah Leaf, MD – Faculty
8. Laila LoVecchio — Faculty
9. Nicholas G. Maldonado, MD, FACEP – Faculty
10. Katherine Stewart, MD – Faculty
11. Gowri S. Stevens, MD, FAAP – Faculty
12. Michael S. Beeson, MD, MBA, FACEP – Faculty/Planner
13. Joshua S. Broder, MD, FACEP – Faculty/Planner
14. Ann M. Dietrich, MD, FAAP, FACEP – Faculty/Planner
15. Andrew J. Eyre, MD, MS-HPEd – Faculty/Planner
16. John Kiel, DO, MPH – Faculty/Planner
17. Frank LoVecchio, DO, MPH, FACEP – Faculty/Planner
18. Sharon E. Mace, MD, FACEP – Faculty/Planner
19. Amal Mattu, MD, FACEP – Faculty/Planner
20. Christian A. Tomaszewski, MD, MS, MBA, FACEP – Faculty/Planner
21. Steven J. Warrington, MD, MEd, MS – Faculty/Planner
22. Tareq Al-Salamah, MBBS, MPH, FACEP – Planner
23. Wan-Tsu Chang, MD – Planner
24. Kelsey Drake, MD, MPH, FACEP – Planner
25. Walter L. Green, MD, FACEP – Planner
26. John C. Greenwood, MD – Planner
27. Danya Khoujah, MBBS, MEHP, FACEP – Planner
28. Nathaniel Mann, MD – Planner
29. George Sternbach, MD, FACEP – Planner
30. Joseph F. Waeckerle, MD, FACEP — Planner
31. Mark Paglia – Planner/Reviewer

Contributor Disclosures. In accordance with the ACCME Standards for Commercial Support and policy of the American College of Emergency Physicians, all individuals with control over CME content (including but not limited to staff, planners, reviewers, and authors) must disclose whether or not they have any relevant financial relationship(s) to learners prior to the start of the activity. These individuals have indicated that they have a relationship which, in the context of their involvement in the CME activity, could be perceived by some as a real or apparent conflict of interest (eg, ownership of stock, grants, honoraria, or consulting fees), but these individuals do not consider that it will influence the CME activity. Joshua S. Broder, MD, FACEP, is a founder and CEO of OmniSono Inc, an ultrasound technology company. Sharon E. Mace, MD, FACEP, performs contracted research that is funded by Biofire Corporation, Genetesis, Quidel, and IBSA Pharma. All remaining individuals with control over CME content have no significant financial interests or relationships to disclose.

This educational activity consists of two lessons, a post-test, and evaluation questions; as designed, the activity should take approximately 2 hours to complete. The participant should, in order, review the learning objectives, read the lessons as published in the print or online version, and complete the online post-test (a minimum score of 75% is required) and evaluation questions. Release date January 1, 2022. Expiration date December 31, 2024.

Accreditation Statement. The American College of Emergency Physicians is accredited by the Accreditation Council for Continuing Medical Education to provide continuing medical education for physicians.

The American College of Emergency Physicians designates this enduring material for a maximum of 2 AMA PRA Category 1 Credits™. Physicians should claim only the credit commensurate with the extent of their participation in the activity.

Each issue of *Critical Decisions in Emergency Medicine* is approved by ACEP for 2 ACEP Category I credits. Approved by the AOA for 2 Category 2-B credits.

Commercial Support. There was no commercial support for this CME activity.

Target Audience. This educational activity has been developed for emergency physicians.

Critical Decisions in Emergency Medicine is a trademark owned and published monthly by the American College of Emergency Physicians, PO Box 619911, Dallas, TX 75261-9911. Send address changes and comments to Critical Decisions in Emergency Medicine, PO Box 619911, Dallas, TX 75261-9911, or to cdem@acep.org; call 844-381-0911, or 972-550-0911.

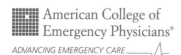
American College of Emergency Physicians®
ADVANCING EMERGENCY CARE

Critical decisions
in emergency medicine

Critical Decisions in Emergency Medicine is the official CME publication of the American College of Emergency Physicians. Additional volumes are available.

EDITOR-IN-CHIEF
Michael S. Beeson, MD, MBA, FACEP
Northeastern Ohio Universities, Rootstown, OH

SECTION EDITORS
Joshua S. Broder, MD, FACEP
Duke University, Durham, NC

Andrew J. Eyre, MD, MHPEd
Brigham & Women's Hospital/
Harvard Medical School, Boston, MA

John Kiel, DO, MPH
University of Florida College of Medicine, Jacksonville, FL

Frank LoVecchio, DO, MPH, FACEP
Maricopa Medical Center/Banner Phoenix Poison and Drug Information Center, Phoenix, AZ

Amal Mattu, MD, FACEP
University of Maryland, Baltimore, MD

Christian A. Tomaszewski, MD, MS, MBA, FACEP
University of California Health Sciences, San Diego, CA

Steven J. Warrington, MD, MEd
MercyOne Siouxland, Sioux City, IA

ASSOCIATE EDITORS
Tareq Al-Salamah, MBBS, MPH, FACEP
King Saud University, Riyadh, Saudi Arabia/
University of Maryland, Baltimore, MD

Wan-Tsu W. Chang, MD
University of Maryland, Baltimore, MD

Ann M. Dietrich, MD, FAAP, FACEP
University of South Carolina College of Medicine, Greenville, SC

Kelsey Drake, MD, MPH, FACEP
St. Anthony Hospital, Lakewood CO

Walter L. Green, MD, FACEP
UT Southwestern Medical Center, Dallas, TX

John C. Greenwood, MD
University of Pennsylvania, Philadelphia, PA

Danya Khoujah, MBBS
University of Maryland, Baltimore, MD

Sharon E. Mace, MD, FACEP
Cleveland Clinic Lerner College of Medicine/
Case Western Reserve University, Cleveland, OH

Nathaniel Mann, MD
Greenville Health System, Greenville, SC

George Sternbach, MD, FACEP
Stanford University Medical Center, Stanford, CA

Joseph F. Waeckerle, MD, FACEP
University of Missouri-Kansas City School of Medicine, Kansas City, MO

EDITORIAL STAFF
Mark Paglia, Senior Manager
mpaglia@acep.org

Melissa Mills, Associate Editor

ISSN2325-0186 (Print)   ISSN2325-8365 (Online)

Contents

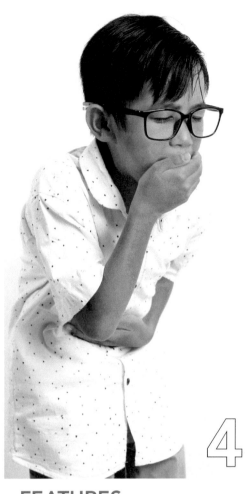

Lesson 1 4
Bellyaching
Unexplained Vomiting in Pediatric Patients
By Gowri S. Stevens, MD, FAAP; and Lacey L. Floyd, DO
Reviewed by Ann M. Dietrich, MD, FAAP, FACEP

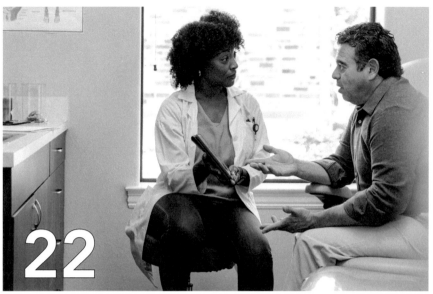

22

Lesson 2 22
FYI
Handling Medical Disinformation at the Bedside
By Robert Barnes, MD; Zachary Aust, MD; and Jedidiah Leaf, MD

4

FEATURES

Clinical Pediatrics — A Misdiagnosis of Pediatric Rash:
Staphylococcal Scalded Skin Syndrome...12
    By Katherine Stewart, MD
    Reviewed by Sharon E. Mace, MD, FACEP

The Critical ECG — Multifocal Atrial Tachycardia 14
    By Amal Mattu, MD, FACEP

The LLSA Literature Review — Cardiac Syncope 15
    By Matthew P. Hanley, MD; and Nicholas G. Maldonado, MD, FACEP
    Reviewed by Andrew J. Eyre, MD, MS-HPEd

Critical Cases in Orthopedics and Trauma — Septic Prepatellar Bursitis 16
    By Zackary Funk, MD; and John Hurley, MD
    Reviewed by John Kiel, DO, MPH

The Critical Procedure — Subcutaneous Single-Injection Digital Nerve Block 19
    By Steven J. Warrington, MD, MEd, MS

The Critical Image — A Boy With Abdominal Pain 20
    By Joshua S. Broder, MD, FACEP

CME Questions 26
    Reviewed by Michael S. Beeson, MD, MBA, FACEP

Drug Box — Nirmatrelvir/Ritonavir 28
    By Frank LoVecchio, DO, MPH, FACEP; and Laila LoVecchio

Tox Box — Vitamin D Toxicity..28
    By Christian A. Tomaszewski, MD, MS, MBA, FACEP

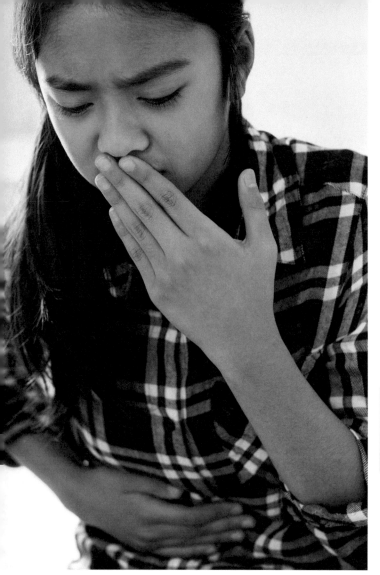

Bellyaching

Unexplained Vomiting in Pediatric Patients

LESSON 1

By Dr. Gowri S. Stevens, MD, FAAP; and Dr. Lacey L. Floyd, DO
Dr. Stevens is an assistant professor and assistant residency program director, and Dr. Floyd is a resident physician in the Department of Emergency Medicine at the McGovern Medical School at UTHealth, Houston, Texas.

Reviewed by Ann M. Dietrich, MD, FAAP, FACEP

Objectives

On completion of this lesson, you should be able to:

1. Describe the initial approach to pediatric patients with unexplained vomiting.
2. List warning signs for emergent causes of unexplained vomiting.
3. Determine an age-based differential diagnosis for unexplained vomiting.
4. Describe the appropriate assessment of a pediatric patient with unexplained vomiting.

From the EM Model

1.0 Signs, Symptoms, and Presentations
    1.3   General
          1.3.12 Dehydration
                1.3.32   Nausea/Vomiting

■ CRITICAL DECISIONS

- How should unexplained vomiting be approached and assessed in the emergency department?

- What is the differential diagnosis of unexplained vomiting in pediatric patients?

- How should low-risk causes of vomiting be managed?

- How should unexplained vomiting with red flags be managed?

The differential diagnosis for unexplained vomiting in pediatric patients is broad, and red flags are easy to miss in children. Emergency physicians must have a stepwise and age-based approach with these patients to ensure that critical diagnoses are recognized and both low- and high-risk causes are appropriately managed.

CASE ONE

A 6 year old without a medical history presents with vomiting for the third time in 2 weeks. The parents report that the child has woken up at night with headaches and is walking differently. The child continues to have episodes of nonbilious emesis despite using a previously prescribed antiemetic.

CASE TWO

A 10 year old without a medical history presents with abdominal pain and vomiting. She states that the pain has been intermittent for a few days but suddenly worsened today. Her pain is located in the periumbilical area. She has had a decreased appetite and sometimes feels nauseous. She had one episode of nonbilious emesis just prior to arrival. When asked, the child states that she has not had a bowel movement in 1 week and that the last one was hard and painful.

CASE THREE

A 3-week-old full-term infant is brought to the emergency department for vomiting. The infant is breastfed and has been taking 10 minutes per side every 2 hours. For the last 2 days, he has vomited 10 minutes after every feed with increasing severity. Prior to this, he had no spit-up and had been otherwise well. He has had one wet diaper in the last 24 hours. On examination, the infant has dry mucous membranes and a sunken fontanelle; he seems hungry and fussy.

Introduction

Unexplained vomiting is a common pediatric complaint in the emergency department and can be as simple as a symptom of a viral infection or as serious as a surgical emergency. The insidious nature of this chief complaint can make it easy to miss life-threatening pediatric illnesses that need further workup or transfer to a children's hospital. Although vomiting is usually a sign of problems within the GI tract, it can also be a presenting sign of severe, life-threatening endocrine or neurologic problems. Emergency physicians must have a stepwise and age-based approach to pediatric vomiting to discern low-risk from high-risk conditions.

CRITICAL DECISION

How should unexplained vomiting be approached and assessed in the emergency department?

Performing the airway, breathing, and circulation steps and obtaining vitals are initial assessments to stabilize patients with vomiting. After stabilization, pediatric patients should undergo a thorough history and physical examination, with inquiry into the contents of emesis and whether it is bilious, nonbilious, or bloody. Timing of the emesis can also be helpful — bilious vomiting is most likely to occur in the morning. Bilious vomiting is considered a surgical emergency until proven otherwise and warrants pediatric surgery consultation.[1,2] The chronicity of the vomiting is also important to determine and can be elicited by asking about its onset and frequency as well as any events associated with it, such as aggravation from food.[1] Specific symptoms to inquire about include abdominal pain, fever, diarrhea, urinary symptoms, polyphagia and polydipsia, headache, and any neurologic symptoms. The history should also include details regarding any recent exposure to similarly sick contacts, recent trauma, urinary output and hydration status, the opportunity for potential ingestion of toxins, history of congenital abnormalities, and any surgical history, particularly abdominal surgeries.[1,3]

The physical examination in a child should always start with subtle observation, including looking to see if the child is interactive, obviously uncomfortable, or consolable when with a parent. In an 8- to 18-month-old pediatric patient with stranger anxiety, consider having the parent palpate the abdomen and watch for voluntary guarding or pain. In children with vomiting, the examination should focus on overall appearance, evaluation of the abdomen, volume and perfusion status, and a neurologic assessment.[1] A comprehensive neurologic examination must be age-appropriate and should assess for gait, if possible, and bulging or fullness at the fontanelle. All areas of the skin should be inspected for jaundice, rash, or signs of trauma. Examine the abdomen for distention, and palpate all quadrants for tenderness with special attention to the right upper and lower quadrants. Assess for peritoneal signs and costovertebral angle tenderness. Assess for peritoneal signs, costovertebral angle tenderness, work of breathing, and signs of dehydration. Signs of dehydration can include a sunken fontanelle, decreased tear production, dry mucous membranes, decreased skin turgor, poor capillary refill, an increased heart rate, lethargy, and no wet diapers in 12 hours or less than half the normal number of wet diapers in 24 hours.[1,3] A complete examination of the genitalia and groin should be performed in boys of all ages and girls when neonates and infants. Evaluate the groin for swelling, tenderness, and overlying skin-color changes. If an inguinal hernia is present, an attempt at manual reduction can be made if there are no signs of strangulation. Vomiting in girls with ambiguous genitalia can indicate congenital adrenal hyperplasia, the most common cause of infantile adrenal insufficiency.[3] Boys should be carefully evaluated for testicular torsion and girls for ovarian torsion. Doppler ultrasound may be needed to better evaluate for these conditions, especially for ovarian torsion.[4]

Red flags in the history and physical examination can signal serious and life-threatening etiologies that require prompt consultations and symptom management. If at any point a child with bilious vomiting is unstable or has peritonitis, a pediatric surgeon should be consulted immediately while resuscitation efforts are performed. Bilious vomiting, projectile vomiting, severe pain, peritoneal signs, and marked abdominal distension are suggestive of GI obstruction. A bulging or full fontanelle in a neonate with decreased activity or altered sensorium is concerning for increased intracranial pressure.[1] Altered level of consciousness, focal neurologic deficits, seizures, vomiting upon waking, headaches, recent head trauma, ataxic gait, and visual neglect in children of any age are all alarms for intracranial pathology.[3]

This stepwise method of performing a thorough history and physical examination and watching for red flags of life-threatening etiologies can help develop a thorough and accurate differential diagnosis.

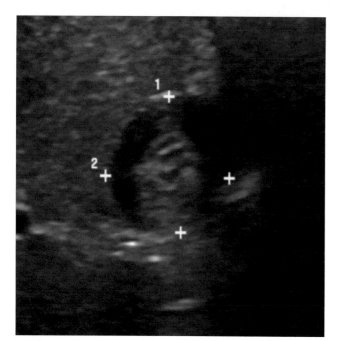

FIGURE 1. A transverse view of the pylorus measuring more than 13 mm[2]

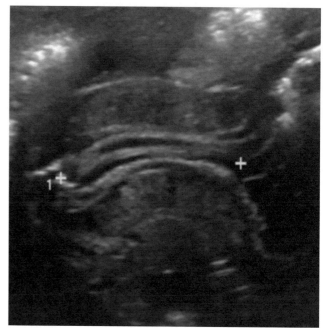

FIGURE 2. A longitudinal view of the pylorus measuring more than 15 to 17 mm[2]

CRITICAL DECISION

What is the differential diagnosis of unexplained vomiting in pediatric patients?

The differential diagnosis for vomiting in pediatric patients is broad. Emergency physicians need a systematic approach to promptly decipher between the etiologies. A good start is to consider age and separate causes of vomiting that are most likely to occur in children younger than 2 years from those most likely in children older than 2 years.

Causes of Vomiting in Children Younger Than 2 Years

Obstructive Causes

If vomiting is bilious or projectile, the most likely pathology is an intestinal obstruction. Obstructive pathologies include malrotation with volvulus, intestinal atresia, Hirschsprung disease, pyloric stenosis, incarcerated hernia, and intussusception. Intestinal obstructions can present with either bilious or nonbilious vomiting, depending on the exact location of the blockage; presentations of either bilious or projectile vomiting are concerning for surgical emergencies.[2]

Malrotation is a developmental abnormality of the intestines that can lead to intestinal twisting, volvulus obstruction, and irreversible intestinal necrosis. Malrotation with volvulus typically presents with bilious emesis. The onset of bilious vomiting may be sudden, and an acute abdomen may be present on examination. Although volvulus typically occurs in infancy, it can occur later in childhood as well.[5] Duodenal obstructions and other intestinal atresias present similarly to a midgut volvulus and are usually diagnosed in the hospital nursery when a newborn cannot tolerate oral intake and eventually vomits bile.[3]

Hirschsprung disease, or congenital aganglionic megacolon, is usually diagnosed shortly after birth when passage of the meconium is delayed; however, the condition can sometimes occur later in life and present more severely. Signs and symptoms include vomiting, abdominal distention, lethargy, and decreased oral intake. Children with Hirshsprung disease, including those who have had the condition treated with anal pull-through surgery, are at risk of developing Hirschsprung-associated enterocolitis (HAEC). HAEC remains the greatest cause of morbidity and mortality in children with Hirschsprung disease and can present with acute-onset vomiting, severe diarrhea, lethargy, and signs of sepsis. Abdominal x-ray findings can include dilated loops of bowel with air-fluid levels, a rectosigmoid cutoff sign, pneumatosis intestinalis, and even signs of perforation. Because of the risk of developing HAEC, any child with a history of Hirschsprung disease, even when well appearing, usually requires admission to the hospital for serial abdominal examinations and broad-spectrum antibiotics.[6,7]

Hypertrophic pyloric stenosis typically presents between 3 weeks and 3 months of age with progressively worsening nonbilious vomiting. It predominantly occurs in boys.[1] The pylorus undergoes hypertrophy and hyperplasia, leading to gastric outlet obstruction and postprandial, projectile, and nonbilious vomiting. When patients present a while after symptom onset, laboratory tests will show a hypochloremic metabolic alkalosis, but most cases are diagnosed earlier and may not show any electrolyte disturbance or other signs of dehydration.[3] An ultrasound will show a pylorus greater than 15 to 17 mm in length on longitudinal views and greater than 13 mm in diameter on transverse views (*Figures 1* and *2*).[8]

Inguinal hernias can cause vomiting in infants, especially if incarcerated or strangulated. An incarcerated or strangulated inguinal hernia should be suspected in an infant presenting with vomiting and a swollen or tender unilateral groin. In addition to the intestines, the gonads can also become entrapped; an associated ovarian torsion must be ruled out in any girl with an incarcerated inguinal hernia. A doppler ultrasound should be performed to determine the contents of the hernia and to evaluate for decreased blood flow to the ovary or testis.[4] Inguinal hernias may also be complicated by small-bowel obstructions in infants, in which case an abdominal plain x-rays will show multiple air-fluid levels.[9]

Intussusception is the most common cause of intestinal obstruction in children ages 6 months to 3 years and peaks during infancy.[3] In intussusception, a portion of the intestine telescopes onto itself, which causes intermittent severe abdominal pain associated with inconsolable fussiness, nonbilious vomiting, and a drawing up of the legs to the abdomen. Symptoms intermittently resolve with temporary resolution of the invagination. An abdominal ultrasound can detect an active intussusception but can miss the condition if conducted when the intussusception is temporarily resolved. Enemas can be diagnostic, as well as therapeutic, in children who are highly suspected of having intussusception.

Nonobstructive Causes

The most common cause of vomiting in any neonate or infant is gastroesophageal reflux. Gastroesophageal reflux is a normal physiologic response and is best described as effortless spit-up or regurgitation, which some parents may call "vomiting." Pathologic gastroesophageal reflux disease (GERD) occurs less commonly and is characterized by recurrent fussiness, food aversion, and less body growth.[3]

Nasal congestion is a source of vomiting in young children. Children younger than 12 months are obligate nose breathers, so they can vomit or get strangled when they have moderate to severe nasal congestion during a viral infection. Many parents are hesitant to suction their children's secretions because they are unsure of how to use a suctioning device and afraid of hurting their child. Nasal congestion should be considered a potential cause if no red flags are present and if consistent with the history and physical examination.

Urinary tract infections (UTIs) may can also cause unexplained vomiting. A urinalysis and urine culture (catheter sample) may need to be obtained.

Other nonobstructive causes of vomiting in children are inborn errors of metabolism and congenital adrenal hyperplasia. In most states, these disorders will have already been identified in newborn screens.

Causes of Vomiting in Children Older Than 2 Years

Past infancy, gastroenteritis is the most common cause of vomiting in children. Although usually caused by viruses, gastroenteritis can also be caused by bacteria or parasites. It generally manifests suddenly but with quick resolution of both vomiting and diarrhea with crampy abdominal pain.[3,10] Other associated symptoms such as fever, mental status change, and rashes may indicate a more serious disorder. Symptoms range from mild to severe and history may reveal similarly sick contacts, day care exposure, or recent travel.[10]

Another cause of vomiting, appendicitis occurs most commonly in the second decade of life, with a familial and boy-to-girl predominance. It is frequently caused by appendiceal lumen obstruction and classically presents as initial vague and periumbilical abdominal pain with migration of pain to the right lower quadrant of the abdomen approximately 12 hours after initial onset.[10,11] The migration of pain occurs as luminal inflammation, which causes vague pain and progresses to serosal inflammation, which causes localized, sharp pain.[2,10] Common associated symptoms include anorexia, nausea, vomiting, and fever. Examination findings concerning for appendicitis include maximal tenderness location at McBurney point; a positive Rovsing, obturator, or psoas sign; and peritoneal signs such as pain with jumping.[2]

Diabetic ketoacidosis (DKA) is, unfortunately, still a frequent complication of newly diagnosed type 1 diabetes. DKA is a state of insulin deficiency associated with hyperglycemia, acidosis, and ketosis. In patients with no known history of diabetes, DKA should still be considered a probable diagnosis because type 1 diabetes can first present as ketoacidosis. Risk factors for DKA in new-onset diabetes include younger age (<4 years), low socioeconomic status, limited access to health care, and parents with lower education levels. DKA can occur in patients with established type 1 diabetes when insulin injections are missed or if blood glucose or urine ketones are not commonly checked, so inquiring about compliance in the history is essential. Presenting symptoms include abdominal pain, vomiting, weight loss, polyuria, polydipsia, and polyphagia. Children may develop tachycardia, hypotension, and Kussmaul breathing. Signs of dehydration, lethargy, altered mental status, and irritability can also be present.[10,12]

Other disorders like cyclic vomiting syndrome (CVS), migraines, and gastroparesis may explain repetitive or chronic vomiting. Cyclic vomiting syndrome (CVS), a condition of uncertain cause, is characterized as recurrent and stereotypical episodes of vomiting that can last hours to days, with a return to baseline health between each episode. CVS often starts in school-aged children and presents with profound nausea and vomiting. It is commonly associated with migraine headaches, and migraine-specific therapies have proven effective for treating CVS.[13] Migraines are typically unilateral headaches with episodic throbbing and associated nausea, vomiting, photophobia, phonophobia, and occasionally abdominal pain. In patients who present with migraine-like headaches but have no history of migraines, intracranial pathology should be considered a possible etiology before assuming a diagnosis of migraine.

Gastroparesis is a chronic neuromuscular disorder of the upper GI tract that causes a delayed emptying of the stomach in the absence of mechanical obstruction. Symptoms include recurrent nausea, postprandial vomiting, bloating, early satiety, and upper abdominal pain.[13] Gastroparesis can occur after an acute viral illness (most commonly rotavirus); after opioid or anticholinergic drug use; and alongside other neuromuscular disorders, such as cerebral palsy, diabetes, and muscular dystrophy.[3] Depending on the severity, vomiting associated with CVS, migraines, and gastroparesis can cause electrolyte alterations and volume depletion but is not associated with red-flag signs or symptoms.

Like infants, toddlers and older children can also present with intussusception, but they are also at risk of other obstructive conditions not encountered in infants — small bowel obstruction (SBO) and superior mesenteric artery syndrome (SMAS). With SBO, a disruption in bowel patency leads to a disruption in bowel motility. Increased intraluminal pressure leads to decreased absorption, decreased lymphatic drainage, and increased risk of ischemia and bowel wall necrosis. The major risk factor for a mechanical SBO in the

United States is adhesions from prior abdominal surgeries, so any child with a history of abdominal surgery who presents with vomiting and abdominal pain should be evaluated for SBO. The pain is often crampy, episodic, and located periumbilically or diffusely. The vomiting may be bilious if the obstruction is proximal or feculent if distal. Constipation, decreased flatus, abdominal distension, and increased bowel sounds are other associated signs and symptoms.[13] SMAS is an unusual form of GI obstruction that can occur in children of slender build or after a period of acute weight loss, including from anorexia nervosa or recent gastroenteritis. SMAS is the compression of the duodenum by the superior mesenteric artery anteriorly and the abdominal aorta posteriorly. It presents with symptoms similar to SBO, including vomiting (can be bilious), early satiety, and abdominal pain.[14]

Although less likely, pancreatitis, cholelithiasis, and cholecystitis can present in adolescence. Gallbladder pathology should be suspected in cases of epigastric or right upper quadrant pain that is associated with nausea and vomiting and worsens after eating fatty food. Pediatric risk factors for gallstones include hemolytic disease, prolonged parenteral nutrition, and celiac disease. Pancreatitis from children is most likely from drugs, infection (eg, mumps or mycoplasma), trauma, or anatomic abnormalities.

Pregnancy should be considered in any girl of reproductive age. Menstruation typically presents around the age of 12 but can occur much younger; age of menarche should be asked about as part of the history. In some cases, girls who give vague complaints may be attempting to conceal their pregnancies, so physicians who suspect a pregnancy should not hesitate to order a urine pregnancy test.[3] Physicians must also be aware of the age of consent for the state they practice in, in case child protective services or law enforcement needs to be notified.

Although more common in adults, peptic ulcer disease, gastritis, and esophagitis are also causes of vomiting in children. Mucosal inflammation and damage associated with these diseases can also cause epigastric pain, nausea, and decreased appetite. Symptoms can be exacerbated by eating or lying flat. Unless complicated by mucosal perforation or GI bleed, patients with these conditions should not present with red-flag signs or symptoms.

Causes of Vomiting in Pediatric Patients of Any Age

Regardless of age, other reasons for vomiting include infections, child abuse or trauma, increased intracranial pressure, or ingestion of foreign bodies or toxicologic agents. Swallowed foreign bodies are a frequent cause of pediatric emergency department visits, usually for toddlers. Although foreign body ingestions can be asymptomatic, symptoms can include dysphagia, drooling, nausea and vomiting, cough, stridor, wheezing, or post-tussive emesis. Even if the foreign body is in the esophagus, persistent esophageal obstruction can block oral secretions from passing through the esophagus, which can eventually cause respiratory symptoms. In cases of a suspected swallowed foreign body, knowing the type of object potentially swallowed is critical because sharp objects, magnets, and batteries require emergent and careful removal.[15] For cases of suspected foreign body ingestion, a two-view chest and abdominal x-ray can rule out radiopaque foreign bodies.

Ingestion of toxic agents or medication overdoses can cause a variety of symptoms, including nausea, vomiting, abdominal pain, altered mental status, respiratory depression, and coma. A thorough history includes obtaining information on what was potentially ingested, the amount ingested, and the timing. Vital sign abnormalities and examination findings will vary depending on the substance consumed. Poison control should be contacted as soon as ingestion is suspected.

Sepsis and various infections can cause nausea and vomiting; careful history taking and physical examination can yield the potential source of infection. Meningitis can present with vomiting, headache, fever, neck stiffness, a decreased level of consciousness, and photophobia; whereas, fever in addition to nausea, vomiting, abdominal pain, and urinary symptoms can indicate a UTI. UTIs are common in children but can be difficult to diagnose based on history alone when children cannot vocalize their symptoms, especially prior to potty training. Typical presenting symptoms in children are fever, decreased appetite, vomiting, fussiness, and vague abdominal pain. For boys younger than 12 months and girls of any age with these symptoms, clinical suspicion should be high. UTIs can progress to pyelonephritis and even urosepsis, both of which present with more severe signs and symptoms.

Other infectious causes of vomiting that can specifically cause post-tussive emesis are upper and lower respiratory infections, viral illnesses, and asthma exacerbations. Some young children also have vomiting from ear pain with otitis media. Strep pharyngitis usually causes symptoms of a sore throat and abdominal pain, but it can also cause nausea.

Intermittent and colicky unilateral flank pain with nausea and vomiting should raise concern for an obstructing ureteral stone. Although ureterolithiasis is more common in adults, obstructive uropathies can occur in pediatric patients with unexplained vomiting and flank pain or urinary complaints. There is usually a family history of kidney stones to help narrow the diagnosis.

✔ Pearls

- Not all causes of vomiting originate from the abdomen. Emergency physicians must do a thorough history and physical examination that includes a complete neurologic examination, checking glucose levels, and assessing for developmental milestones.

- Major red flags in vomiting children are altered mental status, bilious emesis, weight loss, downward-crossing growth curve percentiles, and dehydration with an inability to hydrate orally.

- For cases of suspected foreign body ingestion, a two-view chest and abdominal x-ray can rule out radiopaque foreign bodies.

- The majority of a pediatric physical examination can be done through observation and parental assistance with palpating.

Head traumas, both abusive and accidental, are causes of vomiting to consider in every pediatric patient but especially in nonverbal children younger than 2 years who present with an altered level of consciousness or visible signs of injury. Early recognition of sentinel injuries including bruising, subconjunctival hemorrhages, and intraoral injuries can help identify children prior to the occurence of a life-threatening injury. Distinguishing abusive from nonabusive trauma can be difficult but is crucial because abused children with a history of head trauma are at a high risk of more traumatic injuries. In addition, head trauma is the most common cause of death in abused children.[16] Clinical features that are more suggestive of abusive head trauma include a lack of adequate history to explain the observed injury; the presence of retinal hemorrhages; concomitant rib, long bone, or metaphyseal fractures; seizures within 24 hours; and the presence of cerebral ischemia. By contrast, epidural hemorrhages, scalp swelling, and isolated skull fractures are more frequently associated with nonabusive head trauma.[17] If there is any concern for possible abusive trauma, further investigation with a skeletal survey as well as the involvement of child protective services is essential. Many children's hospitals have child abuse teams on call that can be consulted if the situation is unclear.

Increased intracranial pressure can be caused by space-occupying lesions such as abscesses, tumors, hemorrhages, CNS infections, hydrocephalus, trauma, and metabolic encephalopathy–induced pathology. Idiopathic intracranial hypertension, also known as benign intracranial hypertension or pseudotumor cerebri, is another cause of increased intracranial pressure, but one that is associated with normal results on neuroimaging. It typically occurs in obese young women but can occur in adolescents. It presents with headaches, nausea, and vomiting. Any increase in intracranial pressure causes vomiting because it increases pressure at the area postrema, the vomiting center in the brainstem. Vomiting caused by increased intracranial pressure can occur in the morning on awakening or with an abrupt change in position. It may also occur alongside neurologic deficits and altered mentation. This type of vomiting warrants further workup in the emergency department.[3]

✖ Pitfalls

- Relying on laboratory tests instead of clinical examination (eg, heart rate, mucous membranes, capillary refill, and urine output) to assess hydration status in children. Hydration status is best determined by clinical examination.

- Treating vomiting in children with liquid oral ondansetron instead of the dissolving tablet, which is easier to place back into children's mouths should they spit it out.

- Failing to thoroughly instruct parents on return precautions and the importance of pediatric follow-up prior to discharge.

- Overlooking subtle signs of sentinel injuries in young children who are victims of nonaccidental trauma. trauma.

Mnemonic VOMITING	
Vestibular	Otitis media
Obstruction	Pyloric stenosis, malrotation, volvulus, intussusception, incarcerated hernia, SBO, or SMAS
Metabolic	Diabetic ketoacidosis, inborn errors of metabolism, or congenital adrenal hyperplasia
Infection	Gastroenteritis, enterocolitis, appendicitis, pancreatitis, cholecystitis, UTI, upper or lower respiratory infection, sepsis, or meningitis
Toxins	Various poisons, chemotherapy, iron, organophosphates, theophylline, salicylates, alcohol, or lead
Intracranial	Intracranial abscesses, tumors, or hemorrhages; CNS infections; hydrocephalus; trauma; migraines; or idiopathic intracranial hypertension
Nephrology	Pyelonephritis, UTI, or obstructive uropathy
Gastrointestinal or Genitourinary	Gastroesophageal reflux, formula intolerance, peptic ulcer disease, CVC, gastroparesis, testicular torsion, ovarian torsion, or pregnancy

TABLE 1. The mnemonic VOMITING can be used to develop a differential diagnosis for pediatric vomiting[1]

CRITICAL DECISON

How should low-risk causes of vomiting be managed?

Low-risk causes of vomiting include those that do not require surgery, are not associated with red-flag signs or symptoms, and can continue to be managed at home after discharge from the emergency department. Examples of low-risk causes of vomiting are viral gastroenteritis, UTIs, gastroesophageal reflux, and migraines. Laboratory testing is unnecessary in most of these patients unless required to diagnose the condition, such as in the case of UTIs or suspected pregnancies. For UTIs in young, febrile patients in particular, a urine sample should be obtained using straight catheterization. Alternatively, the "two-step process" can be used. It includes obtaining a urine sample in a bag and reserving catheterization for patients whose bagged sample is positive for moderate or large leukocyte esterase or nitrites. However, this alternative approach requires patients remain in the emergency department for a longer time.[18] To screen for new-onset diabetes, a simple urine point-of-care test for glucose can be obtained, with further testing for diabetes ordered if urine results are positive. Even when red flags are absent, patients with known diabetes who present with vomiting should complete a point-of-care glucose screen and tests for diabetic ketoacidosis if the screen is positive. Patients with a history of chronic vomiting — for instance, from CVC — may need laboratory tests to check for dehydration and then may need fluid replacement if they are experiencing prolonged episodes of vomiting. Although most low-risk causes of vomiting do not require laboratory tests, physicians should consider testing on a case-by-case basis depending on which abnormalities are suspected.[10]

If vomiting is secondary to nasal congestion in a child younger than 12 months, physicians should teach families how to use a bulb syringe or other home suctioning device with nasal saline for clearing secretions. Suctioning secretions in the emergency department is both diagnostic and therapeutic if the child can swallow without vomiting after the intervention.

For hydration therapy in uncomplicated cases of pediatric vomiting with mild to moderate dehydration, oral trials of rehydration should be tried before considering intravenous fluids. The American Academy of Pediatrics defines mild dehydration as a fluid deficit of less than 5%, moderate dehydration as a deficit from 6% to 9%, and severe dehydration as a deficit of greater than 10%. For mild dehydration, administer oral rehydration in a 50-mL/kg solution over 4 hours; for moderate dehydration, administer 100-mL/kg solution over 4 hours. If unable to tolerate either of these amounts, intravenous hydration with an isotonic solution may be necessary.[2,19]

To treat vomiting, the serotonin receptor antagonist ondansetron is considered the most useful antiemetic. A single oral dose of 0.15 mg/kg can be given every 4 hours as needed or, alternatively, 2 mg if patients weigh less than 15 kg and 4 mg if they weigh more than 15 kg. An oral dissolving tablet of ondansetron is preferred over liquid because it is easier to place back in children's mouths should they spit it out and can be cut in half for smaller children.[2,10] For pain or fever control, alternate between acetaminophen and ibuprofen as needed, giving 15 mg/kg of oral acetaminophen every 6 hours and 10 mg/kg of oral ibuprofen every 6 hours. If bacterial infections are the cause of vomiting, oral antibiotics should be initiated. Regarding disease-specific treatment, migraine cocktails—a combination of NSAIDs, antiemetics, and oral diphenhydramine with or without a 20-mL/kg normal saline bolus — provide effective pain relief; Pyridoxine (vitamin B6) is the first-line therapy for morning sickness.[3]

Before discharging patients, make sure their vital signs are at baseline and that they are in no apparent distress. Dehydrated patients must also be tolerating oral fluids and producing urine before leaving the emergency department. Additionally, parents should have close and reliable follow-up care with a pediatrician. Admission should be considered for patients who do not meet these criteria for discharge.[10] Parents of patients ready for discharge from the emergency department should be instructed on return precautions for new or worsening symptoms and to follow-up with a pediatrician 24 to 48 hours after discharge.

CRITICAL DECISION

How should unexplained vomiting with red flags be managed?

Any red-flag signs or symptoms, as well as findings that suggest the need for surgery, should undergo prompt evaluation in the emergency department. If the patient is ill appearing, the first step is to establish rapid intravenous access with two large-bore intravenous catheters, and if intravenous access cannot be obtained, intraosseous placement should be considered. Point-of-care or serum glucose testing should be performed immediately in any child with changes in mental status, signs of severe dehydration, or with a known history of diabetes.[1,10] In patients who are severely dehydrated or have signs of shock, aggressively treat them with a 20-mL/kg bolus of isotonic solution for hemodynamic stabilization. The 20-mL/

kg bolus can be repeated up to three times in the first hour, with reassessments in between each bolus. Prevent rapid infusion and unnecessary fluid administration to avoid complications of cardiac insufficiency and pulmonary edema. Once vital signs are stabilized, continue hydration to replace existing and ongoing losses.[2,19]

Unlike with low-risk causes of vomiting, laboratory tests and imaging are usually necessary in patients presenting with red flags or concerns for a surgical emergency. However, these tests should only be performed if patients are stable. In any unstable patient, immediately consult pediatric surgery, who can obtain additional diagnostic studies as needed.

In stable patients with bilious emesis that is concerning for an obstruction, obtain abdominal x-rays. If no signs of obstruction are found, consider nonsurgical causes of vomiting and plan for likely admission or transfer to a pediatric hospital for observation. In cases of suspected malrotation, obtain an upper GI series, and if there is concern for a distal obstruction, such as with Hirschsprung disease, a contrast enema may be needed for diagnosis.[1,3] In nonbilious, projectile vomiting that is concerning for hypertrophic pyloric stenosis, obtain an ultrasound and consult pediatric surgery if the ultrasound is positive. Ultrasounds of the abdomen should also be obtained urgently if there is concern for appendicitis; intussusception; or gallbladder, ovarian, or renal pathology.[1] In patients with neurologic deficits, CT or rapid MRI of the brain can evaluate for causes of increased intracranial pressure. Pediatric neurosurgery should be contacted immediately if the patient is unstable.

Regarding laboratory studies, obtain a CBC, urinalysis, urine culture, and blood cultures if concerned for sepsis. A lumbar puncture with CSF analysis should be performed in all febrile neonates 28 days or younger, in febrile infants 29 to 60 days old suspected of having serious bacterial infections, and in febrile children with altered sensorium.[10,20] Obtain laboratory tests if there are signs of severe dehydration. In patients with suspected gastroenteritis who present with bloody or prolonged diarrhea, stool cultures can rule out bacterial and parasitic causes. Associated hematemesis in pediatric patients should prompt liver function tests and coagulation studies. Additional laboratory testing and imaging should be tailored to the specific diagnosis of concern.[10]

In all patients with vomiting, consider treatment with antiemetics, antipyretics, pain medication, and rehydration solutions, as needed. In patients with high-risk causes of vomiting, admission should be the disposition. If results are equivocal or if pain persists or oral intake is not tolerated, admission for observation is recommended.

Summary

The vomiting child is one of the most difficult diagnostic challenges because of a vast differential diagnosis and challenges with obtaining an accurate history. Obtaining as thorough of a history as possible along with a comprehensive physical examination and age-based differential can help distinguish benign from more serious causes that need further workup. Immediate stabilization measures and transfer for pediatric surgical evaluation are necessary for any child with red flags. For those without red flags, oral-hydration challenge, observation in the emergency department, explicit return precautions, and pediatrician follow-up are essential for discharge planning.

CASE RESOLUTIONS

CASE ONE

The continued emesis and gait change were concerning for a neurologic rather than a GI or infectious cause. A CT of the brain was performed, and a posterior fossa tumor was identified. CT of the brain was performed, and a posterior fossa tumor was identified. The child was immediately transferred to the nearest children's hospital for emergent pediatric neurosurgical evaluation.

CASE TWO

The physical examination was reassuring, and the child otherwise appeared well. Because the child was vomiting, the physician decided to obtain an abdominal x-ray to determine if an inpatient bowel cleanout was warranted. The x-ray showed a large stool burden. An enema was administered, but the child continued to have crampy pain after a bowel movement. The patient was admitted for an inpatient cleanout.

CASE THREE

Recognizing the signs of dehydration, the physician asked for intravenous access, a point-of-care glucose test, and an electrolyte panel. The physician also gave the patient a 20-mL/kg isotonic fluid bolus for rehydration when the glucose was 70 g/dL. An ultrasound was also ordered to evaluate for pyloric stenosis. The ultrasound showed a muscle length of 16 mm and width of 5 mm, a positive result. The child was given 5% dextrose and sodium chloride at a maintenance rate and was transferred to the closest children's hospital for a pediatric surgery consultation.

REFERENCES

1. Singhi SC, Shah R, Bansal A, Jayashree M. Management of a child with vomiting. *Indian J of Pediatr.* 2013 Apr;80(4):318-325.

2. Tintinalli JE, Ma OJ, Yealy DM, et al, eds. *Tintinalli's Emergency Medicine: A Comprehensive Study Guide*, 9th ed. McGraw-Hill Education; 2020.

3. Lorenzo CD. Approach to the infant or child with nausea and vomiting. UpToDate. Updated February 1, 2023. https://www.uptodate.com/contents/approach-to-the-infant-or-child-with-nausea-and-vomiting

4. Mathison DJ. Evaluation of inguinal swelling in children. UpToDate. Updated May 21, 2021. https://www.uptodate.com/contents/evaluation-of-inguinal-swelling-in-children

5. Heidsma CM, Hulsker CC, van der Zee D, Kramer WH. Malrotation with or without volvulus. *Ned Tijdschr Geneeskd.* 2015;159:A8859.

6. Frykman PK, Short SS. Hirschsprung-associated enterocolitis: prevention and therapy. *Semin Pediatr Surg.* 2012 Nov;21(4):328-335.

7. Hirschsprung-associated enterocolitis. Winchester Hospital. https://www.winchesterhospital.org/health-library/article?id=626205

8. Amini B, Kearns C, Worsley C, et al. Pyloric stenosis. Radiopaedia.org. Revised January 4, 2023. www.radiopaedia.org/cases/74392

9. Dawes L. Pediatric small bowel obstruction from incarcerated inguinal hernia. Radiopaedia.org. March 1, 2021. www.radiopaedia.org/cases/35965

10. Hoffman RJ, Wang VJ, Scarfone RJ, Godambe SA, Nagler J, eds. *Fleisher & Ludwig's 5-Minute Pediatric Emergency Medicine Consult.* 2nd ed. Wolters Kluwer; 2020.

11. Jacobs DO. Acute appendicitis and peritonitis. In: Jameson J, Fauci AS, Kasper DL, Hauser SL, Longo DL, Loscalzo J, eds. *Harrison's Principles of Internal Medicine.* 20th ed. McGraw-Hill Education; 2018.

12. Chase P, Frohnert BI, Rewers M. Diabetes mellitus. In: Hay WW Jr, Levin MJ, Abzug MJ, Bunik M, eds. *Current Diagnosis & Treatment: Pediatrics.* 26th ed. McGraw-Hill Education; 2022.

13. Nagarwala J, Dev S, Markin A. The vomiting patient: small bowel obstruction, cyclic vomiting, and gastroparesis. *Emerg Med Clin North Am.* 2016 May;34(2):271-291.

14. Biank V, Werlin S. Superior mesenteric artery syndrome in children: a 20-year experience. *J of Pediatr Gastroenterol Nutr.* 2006 May;42(5):522-525.

15. Hackam DJ, Upperman J, Grikscheit T, Wang K, Ford HR. Pediatric surgery. In: Brunicardi F, Andersen DK, Billiar TR, et al, eds. *Schwartz's Principles of Surgery.* 11th ed. McGraw-Hill Education; 2019.

16. Jenny C, Hymel KP, Ritzen A, Reinert SE, Hay TC. Analysis of missed cases of abusive head trauma. *JAMA.* 1999 Feb 17;281(7):621-626.

17. Richardson NC, Rappaport DI. Pediatric head trauma: abuse or not? *Hosp Pediatr.* 2012 Oct;2(4)247-248.

18. Lavelle JM, Blackstone MM, Funari MK, et al. Two-step process for ED UTI screening in febrile young children: reducing catheterization rates. *Pediatrics.* 2016 Jul;138(1):o20153023.

19. Vega RM, Avva U. *Pediatric Dehydration. StatPearls [Internet].* StatPearls Publishing;2022. https://pubmed.ncbi.nlm.nih.gov/28613793/

20. Fever in infants 0 to 60 days. Children's Hospital Colorado. https://www.childrenscolorado.org/health-professionals/clinical-resources/clinical-pathways/fever-in-infants-0-to-60-days/

A Misdiagnosis of Pediatric Rash: Staphylococcal Scalded Skin Syndrome

By Katherine Stewart, MD

Brown Emergency Medicine Residency, Hasbro Children's Hospital, Providence, Rhode Island

Reviewed by Sharon E. Mace, MD, FACEP

Objective

On completion of this article, you should be able to:

■ State the presentation and management of scalded skin syndrome.

CASE PRESENTATION

A 6-month-old boy presents with a progressive rash. The patient's mother states that his itchy rash began 3 days ago on his ears and then spread to his face, trunk, and extremities. Two days prior to this visit, the boy was seen at an outside urgent care center where he was given diphenhydramine and cetirizine for a suspected urticarial reaction, but this did not improve his rash. He was then seen one day prior to this visit at another emergency department where he was thought to have an eczematous rash and so was given steroids and acetaminophen. The patient's symptoms improved for a few hours but then promptly returned.

The infant is afebrile and without GI symptoms. He has had no exposure to new soaps, foods, or other identifiable irritants. His vaccines are current. When asked about prior rashes, his parents report that he had a skin infection under his nose 2 weeks ago that resolved with topical mupirocin.

On examination, his vital signs, including temperature, are within normal limits. The patient is irritable but consolable. His ears are scaling and excoriated bilaterally. His lips and perioral area are red and cracked, but he has no intraoral or tongue changes. There is diffuse erythroderma and desquamation across the upper back and buttocks but no palm or sole involvement (*Figures 1* and *2*).

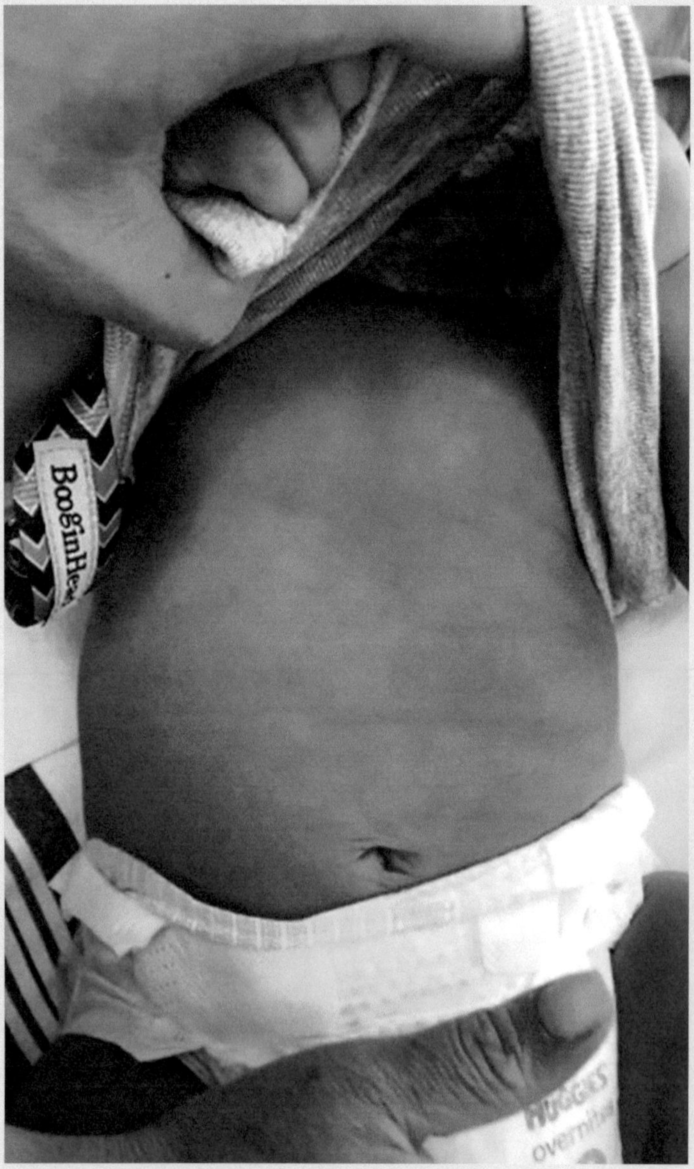

FIGURE 1. Front view of the patient's rash

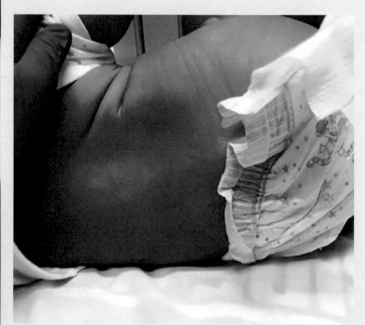

FIGURE 2. Back view of the patient's rash

Discussion

Staphylococcal scalded skin syndrome (SSSS) with a recent history of a rash, likely impetigo, is this patient's diagnosis. The differential diagnosis includes scarlet fever, multisystem inflammatory syndrome in children (MIS-C), drug reaction with eosinophilia and systemic symptoms (DRESS) (although there is no recent drug use), and toxic epidermal necrolysis (TEN) or skin immune system (SIS) (although there is no mucosal involvement).

Management

Basic laboratory tests, blood cultures, antistreptolysin (ASO) titers, and a viral panel were obtained. The patient was started on intravenous clindamycin for SSSS. He was continued on intravenous cefazolin and clindamycin for 2 days, with marked improvement in erythema and regression in desquamation. Blood cultures were negative.

Pathophysiology

SSSS is a rare cause of rash with an incidence of 0.09 to 0.56 per 1,000,000 people.[1] It is most common in children younger than 5 years. The rash is caused by group II coagulase-positive staphylococci that express an exfoliative toxin, epidermolysis, that damages desmoglein-1 in the epidermal layer of skin.[2] The toxin typically originates from a primary infection site — most commonly the diaper region, umbilicus, or face in newborns and infants — and disseminates through the circulation to the rest of the skin, causing an exfoliating, sandpaper-like rash. The rash is often worse along the perioral area and skin creases of the extremities, neck, and groin but spares the mucosal surfaces.[3] Other symptoms that can develop with the classic rash are fluid-filled blisters, fever, irritability, and fatigue. The rash is most often diagnosed clinically, but wound and blood cultures. Biopsies can be used when the diagnosis is uncertain. Antibiotics are the mainstay of treatment, including nafcillin, oxacillin, or cephalosporins — more than 95% of cases are caused by methicillin-sensitive *Staphylococcus aureus* (MSSA).[3] With antibiotics and wound care, the rash typically resolves in 5 to 7 days after initiating antibiotic treatment.[2]

— CASE RESOLUTION

After admission to the hospital, the patient was treated with intravenous cefazolin and clindamycin along with emollient cream for 48 hours. His rash improved, and his redness resolved with treatment. While in the hospital, he continued to be afebrile, with normal vital signs and negative blood cultures. He was discharged home with 3 additional days of oral cephalexin to complete an antibiotic course for a total of 5 days. Close pediatrician follow-up was also recommended.

REFERENCES

1. Staphylococcal scalded skin syndrome. Johns Hopkins Medicine. https://www.hopkinsmedicine.org/health/conditions-and-diseases/staphylococcal-scalded-skin-syndrome
2. Rehmus WE. Staphylococcal scalded skin syndrome (Ritter disease). Merck Manual Professional Version. Modified September 2022. https://www.merckmanuals.com/professional/dermatologic-disorders/bacterial-skin-infections/staphylococcal-scalded-skin-syndrome
3. Staphylococcal scalded skin syndrome. National Organization for Rare Disorders. Updated October 18, 2018. https://rarediseases.org/rare-diseases/staphylococcal-scalded-skin-syndrome

The Critical ECG
Multifocal Atrial Tachycardia

By Amal Mattu, MD, FACEP
Dr. Mattu is a professor, vice chair, and director of the Emergency Cardiology Fellowship in the Department of Emergency Medicine at the University of Maryland School of Medicine in Baltimore.

Objective

On completion of this article, you should be able to:
- Recognize ECG findings consistent with MAT.

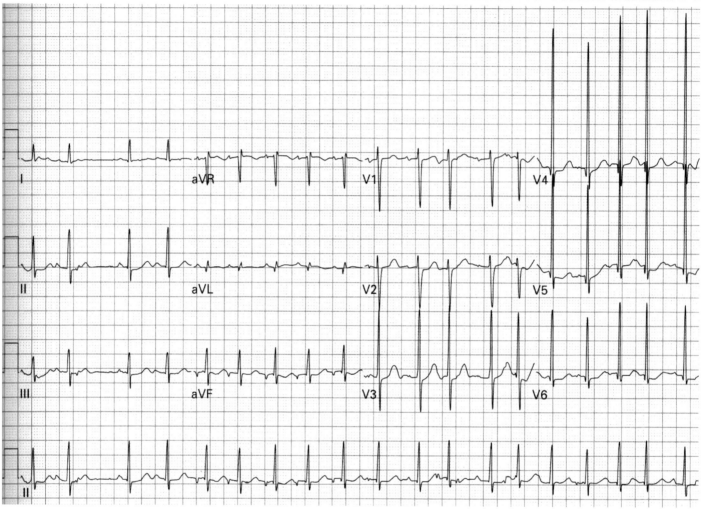

FIGURE 1. A 61-year-old woman with dyspnea and hypoxia

Multifocal atrial tachycardia (MAT), rate 115, left ventricular hypertrophy (LVH), diffuse ischemia. When the rhythm is an irregularly irregular tachycardia, the main diagnostic considerations are atrial fibrillation, atrial flutter with variable atrioventricular conduction, and MAT. The presence of distinct P waves excludes the diagnosis of atrial fibrillation. By contrast, P waves are present with at least three different morphologies and occur at irregular intervals, confirming the diagnosis of MAT and excluding the diagnosis of atrial flutter. MAT is often associated with pulmonary disease — this patient was suffering from an acute exacerbation of emphysema. Slight ST-segment depression is noted in multiple leads and resolved with treatment of the patient's hypoxia.

Cardiac Syncope

By Elmira Andreeva, MD; and Laura Welsh MD
Department of Emergency Medicine,
Boston University, Massachussetts

Reviewed by Andrew J. Eyre, MD, MS-HPEd

Objective

On completion of this article, you should be able to:

- State the factors associated with cardiac syncope for improved diagnosis.

Albassam OT, Redelmeier RJ, Shadowitz S, Husain AM, Simel D, Etchells EE. **Did this patient have cardiac syncope? The rational clinical examination systematic review.** *JAMA.* 2019;321(24):2448-2457.

KEY POINTS

- Cardiac syncope is a common and dangerous cause of syncope that must not be missed in the emergency department.

- Syncope in patients older than 35 years and with a history of CAD or other cardiac conditions significantly increases the likelihood of cardiac syncope.

- A normal ECG and no history of heart disease significantly decrease the likelihood of cardiac syncope.

- Biomarkers such as troponin and NT-proBNP, while helpful, should not be used to definitively diagnose cardiac syncope.

Syncope is defined as a transient loss of consciousness because of decreased cerebral perfusion, followed by a return to baseline. The various causes of syncope range from benign to serious. A dangerous cause is cardiac syncope, which is responsible for 5% to 21% of all cases of syncope presenting to the emergency department.

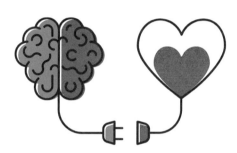

Cardiac syncope results from decreased cardiac output because of cardiopulmonary issues such as arrhythmias, structural heart disease, or pulmonary emboli. It can often be challenging to distinguish cardiac conditions from other causes of syncope, and the increased morbidity and mortality of cardiac syncope make it a diagnosis that cannot be missed. This article is a systematic review that explores the accuracy of the history, examination, and laboratory findings to identify cardiac syncope. Eleven studies of cardiac syncope were included with a total of 4,137 patients. The studied population represented adult patients presenting with syncope to primary care, emergency department, or specialty clinics.

In terms of historical factors, both a history of coronary artery disease (CAD) and onset of the first syncopal event at 35 years or older were associated with a greater likelihood of cardiac syncope. Additionally, a history of atrial fibrillation or flutter, heart failure, or known severe structural heart disease was associated with an increased likelihood of cardiac syncope. However, these factors all had relatively low sensitivities. Certain precipitating factors such as pain or a medical procedure were less likely to be associated with cardiac syncope.

Prodromal symptoms of dyspnea or chest pain were associated with a higher likelihood of cardiac syncope, while the sensation of palpitations rendered inconclusive results in this review. Absence of a prodrome was not associated with either a high or low likelihood of cardiac syncope. Cyanosis during the syncopal event was associated with a higher likelihood of cardiac syncope, while an inability to recall events leading up to the syncopal event was associated with a lower likelihood. However, both elements had low sensitivity. Traumatic injury from the syncopal event was not associated with either a high or low likelihood of cardiac syncope.

Diagnostically, cardiac syncope was significantly less likely if there was a normal ECG and no history of heart disease. Elevated biomarkers, including troponin T or I and NT-proBNP, were associated with a higher likelihood of cardiac syncope; however, high cutoffs for troponin and NT-proBNP were required to achieve a predetermined specificity of 95%.

In summary, while certain factors such as age and presence of known cardiac disease can increase the likelihood of cardiac syncope, there is no single variable that can make this diagnosis. Classically taught findings such as palpitations or absence of prodrome lack accuracy in differentiating causes of syncope. In agreement with both the European Society of Cardiology and American College of Cardiology guidelines, the authors advise against the routine use of troponin or NT-proBNP when evaluating syncope.

Limitations of this study include misclassification bias because there is no gold standard to definitively identify cardiac syncope, which may lead to increases in specificity and sensitivity. Moreover, patients with a diagnosis of unexplained syncope were excluded from some of the studies, which could have also altered the sensitivity and specificity of the reported findings.

Critical Decisions in Emergency Medicine's LLSA literature reviews features articles from ABEM's 2022 Lifelong Learning and Self-Assessment Reading List. Available online at acep.org/moc/llsa and on the ABEM website.

Volume 36 Number 1: **January 2022** 15

Septic Prepatellar Bursitis

By Zackary Funk, MD; and John Hurley, MD
University of Florida College of Medicine — Jacksonville

Reviewed by John Kiel, DO, MPH

Objective

On completion of this article, you should be able to:

■ State how to diagnose septic prepatellar bursitis.

CASE PRESENTATION

A 29-year-old man presents after 2 weeks of gradually progressive pain and swelling over the left anterior knee. He has a history of left prepatellar bursectomy following a wrestling injury in 2011. There are no recent inciting injuries, but the patient states he was surfing just prior to symptom onset. His pain did not respond to ibuprofen or to a steroid taper that was prescribed at an urgent care clinic. He decided to come to the emergency department after redness and warmth spread on the anterolateral aspect of his knee and leg. There are no associated fevers, chills, malaise, or other systemic symptoms.

Initial examination is significant for erythema on the anterior and lateral aspects of the patella that extends down the anterior and lateral shin and lateral knee joint, with fluctuance along the inferomedial and inferolateral aspects of the joint. There is a well-healed midline incision over the anterior patella. The patient can ambulate and bear weight without difficulty. No pain occurs with active or passive range of motion, and no tenderness is noted on palpation. Ultrasound shows cobblestoning of the subcutaneous tissue, without fluid collection in the prepatellar bursa; no joint effusion is detected. The patient is discharged on clindamycin for suspected cellulitis given the cobblestoning and absence of joint effusion on the initial ultrasound. He returns 4 days later with a subjective fever, an increase in existing swelling, tender left inguinal lymphadenopathy, decreased range of motion, and worsening pain with weight-bearing (*Figure 1*). At this visit, plain x-rays show marked prepatellar swelling, and ultrasound identifies a discrete fluid collection in the prepatellar space (*Figure 2*).

The fluid collection is aspirated for analysis and to attempt symptomatic relief. An ultrasound with a linear probe is used to initially characterize the fluid collection. An approach from the lateral aspect of the collection is planned (*Figures 3, 4,* and *5*). The site is then prepped with a chlorhexidine swab and a wheal of local anesthetic overlying the approach vector is raised. Sterile gloves are donned, and a sterile probe cover is applied to the ultrasound probe. His skin is again cleansed with a sterile chlorhexidine swab, and using an ultrasound for guidance, an 18-gauge × 3.8-cm needle is advanced into the fluid collection for aspiration on entry. The proceduralist aspirates a total of 4 mL of serosanguinous fluid from the collection. The patient tolerates the procedure well without any immediate postprocedural complications.

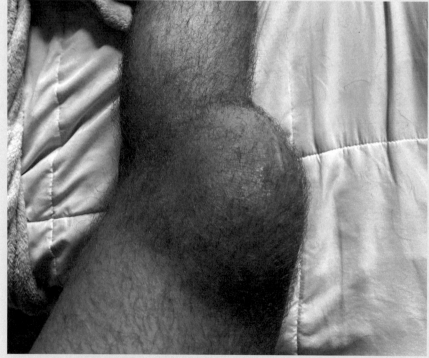

FIGURE 1. Left lower extremity showing significant prepatellar soft-tissue swelling

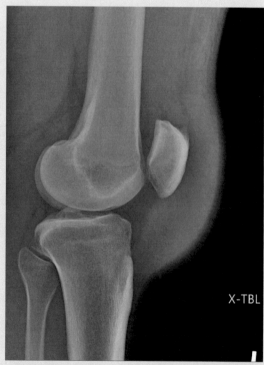

FIGURE 2. Knee x-ray showing significant prepatellar soft-tissue swelling

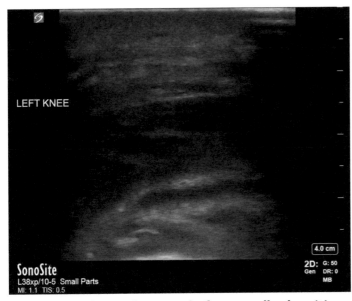

FIGURE 3. A knee ultrasound of prepatellar bursitis

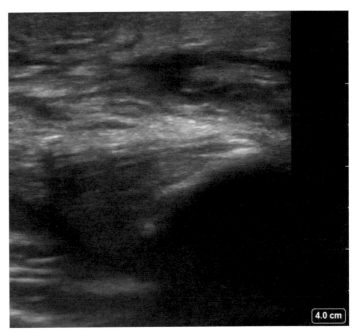

FIGURE 4. A long-axis view of prepatellar bursitis on a knee ultrasound

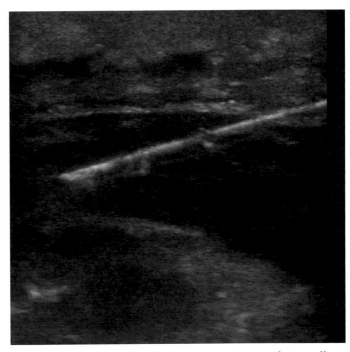

FIGURE 5. Prepatellar Bursa Aspiration with Needle in Plane

Discussion

Approximately one-third of bursitis presentations are from septic bursitis; *Staphylococcus aureus* is the most commonly isolated organism in the condition and is thought to be introduced through direct inoculation from microtrauma in most cases.[1] Risk factors are more prevalent in men and include trauma, inflammation of the bursa from other causes (eg, gout or rheumatologic diseases), disruptions to skin integrity (eg, eczema or psoriasis), immunosuppression (eg, HIV and AIDS, diabetes mellitus, chronic steroid therapy, or alcohol use disorder), and recent procedures involving the presenting joint such as arthrocentesis.[1] Erythema, warmth, and swelling over the joint are common presentations of both septic and aseptic bursitis, with fever exclusive to septic bursitis according to recent literature reviews.[2] Unlike septic arthritis, range of motion is relatively unaffected in septic bursitis; however, movements that stretch the overlying bursa (eg, knee flexion) will often elicit pain. Extension into surrounding tissues, abscess formation, draining sinus formation, structural complications of mass effect, and systemic infections are possible complications of septic bursitis. Aseptic sympathetic joint effusion can also occur from the local effect of inflammatory mediators involved.[3]

Plain x-rays should be obtained to evaluate for other possible causes of pain and swelling (eg, fracture, foreign bodies, crystallopathies, or arthritic processes). Ultrasound can be a useful adjunct in both the diagnosis and management of septic bursitis. Bursae on ultrasound are typically either not visualized or consist of a very thin, linear, hypoechoic stripe that represents physiologic bursal fluid. The soft tissue surrounding the area shows either typical tissue septations (eg, in dermal or subcutaneous tissue) or muscle and tendon fibers of normal fibrillation patterns and anisotropy. In cases of bursitis, there may be an increase in hypoechoic fluid, possibly with a heterogeneous echotexture that represents complex collection. Signs of surrounding tissue edema include cobblestoning, thickening of the dermal tissue, or other fluid collections (possibly representing abscesses or sympathetic effusion).

Fluid analysis will likely show a WBC count greater than 2×10^9 cells/L with a neutrophil predominance. A Gram stain and culture of the aspirate are considered the gold standard for diagnosis; however, diagnostic accuracy with this method varies — the lowest reported accuracy was 67% in one study, although most of these patients had already received antibiotic therapy when samples were collected.[1,4] Surgical resection (ie, bursectomy) may be indicated for chronic or recurrent bursitis. Reported recurrence rates after bursectomy vary, but a recurrence rate as high as 20% has been reported.[5] Because septic bursitis often occurs after trauma, tetanus immunization status should be assessed and updated as appropriate.

REFERENCES

1. Baumbach SF, Lobo CM, Badyine I, Mutschler W, Kanz KG. Prepatellar and olecranon bursitis: literature review and development of a treatment algorithm. *Arch Orthop Trauma Surg*. 2014 Mar;134(3):359-370.
2. Ho G Jr, Tice AD. Comparison of nonseptic and septic bursitis. Further observations on the treatment of septic bursitis. *Arch Intern Med*. 1979 Nov;139(11):1269-1273.
3. Tan IJ, Barlow JL. Sympathetic joint effusion in an urban hospital. *ACR Open Rheumatol*. 2019 Mar 15;1(1):37-42.
4. Martinez-Taboada VM, Cabeza R, Cacho PM, Blanco R, Rodriguez-Valverde V. Cloxacillin-based therapy in severe septic bursitis: retrospective study of 82 cases. *Joint Bone Spine*. 2009 Dec;76(6):665-669.
5. Degreef I, De Smet L. Complications following resection of the olecranon bursa. *Acta Orthop Belg*. 2006 Aug;72(4):400-403.

CASE RESOLUTION

Aspirate obtained under ultrasound guidance showed a WBC count of 13×10^9 cells/L with polymorphonuclear neutrophil predominance, numerous RBCs, and no isolated organisms on an initial Gram stain. Serum studies showed no leukocytosis but profound elevations in the erythrocyte sedimentation rate and C-reactive protein levels. Gonorrhea and chlamydia nucleic acid amplification tests were negative, as were hepatitis B and C serologies. The patient was started on vancomycin and underwent debridement and irrigation with drain placement in the orthopedic surgery department. Initial aspirate cultures returned positive for *S. aureus*. Intraoperative cultures were consistent with the bedside arthrocentesis culture. The drain was removed on postoperative day 2, and the patient was discharged on a 2-week course of trimethoprim-sulfamethoxazole and to date has not returned for follow-up.

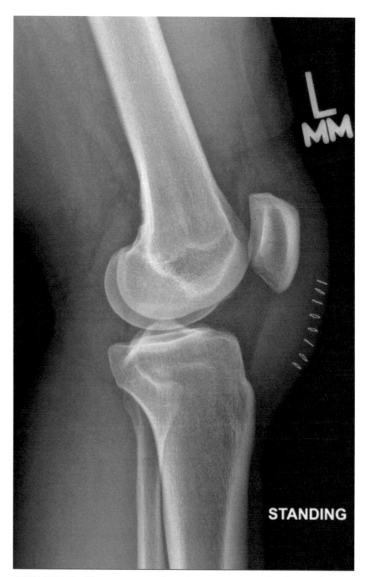

FIGURE 6. Knee x-ray showing postsurgical staples after a washout in the operating room

The Critical Procedure
Subcutaneous Single-Injection Digital Nerve Block

By Steven J. Warrington, MD, MEd, MS
MercyOne Siouxland, Sioux City, Iowa

Objective

On completion of this article, you should be able to:

- Describe how to administer a subcutaneous single-injection digital nerve block.

Introduction

There are multiple options for digital anesthesia depending on the situation. Subcutaneous single-injection digital nerve block (SDNB) is a lesser-known technique that provides multiple benefits. When using this technique, however, the dorsal surface will be anesthetized only at the portion approximately distal to the distal interphalangeal joint.

Contraindications

- Allergy to a component of the medication
- Infection overlying the injection site

Benefits and Risks

The primary benefit of the SDNB technique is that it provides anesthesia to the affected digit, primarily on the volar surface but with some coverage of the dorsal surface as well. Other benefits of the SDNB technique compared to other techniques such as a transthecal injection or double dorsal injection digital nerve block include: 1) No entry into the tendon sheath (like with the transthecal approach); 2) A theoretically decreased risk of damage to the neurovascular bundle because the injection is farther from it; and 3) Less local anesthetic in the proximal digit and, thus, less compression on the venous system and swelling of the affected digit.

A primary risk of SDNB is failure of the block to adequately anesthetize for the required procedure. Aside from that, the risks of the procedure are similar to other injections, such as infection, allergic reaction to the medication, and damage to nearby structures (eg, tendon sheath or neurovascular bundle).

Alternatives

Digital nerve blocks can instead be performed using a double dorsal injection or the transthecal (ie, tendon sheath) approach. A more proximal approach to regional anesthesia (eg, wrist) can also be used. There are also situations when moderate sedation or repair in the operating room is more appropriate. The technique or approach chosen depends on the individual situation, taking into account factors such as the age of the patient, procedures required, and capabilities of the physician and institution.

Reducing Side Effects

Attention to the injection site and injection depth help reduce the risk of injury to associated structures. Injections should be made superficially to the flexor tendon or sheath proximal to the affected digit.

Ensuring the injection site is cleaned and properly prepared can reduce the risk of infection. Pretreatment with vapocoolant, an anxiolytic, or an analgesic can reduce pain and anxiety.

Special Considerations

When selecting a specific technique or approach, the physician must consider the area to be anesthetized. The SDNB technique provides good anesthesia to the volar surface of the digit and generally provides coverage distal to the distal interphalangeal joint. If the rest of the dorsal finger needs to be anesthetized, an additional single dorsal injection may be needed at the level of the distal metacarpal.

TECHNIQUE

1. **Obtain** consent from the patient and explain the technique.
2. **Gather** supplies and consider if pretreatment is beneficial.
3. **Identify** and clean the intended injection site.
4. **Insert** the needle. If concerned insertion is too deep (into the tendon sheath), have the patient gently flex and extend the affected digit. If inserted into the tendon sheath, the needle will move in response to this gesture.
5. **Inject** 2 to 3 mL of the anesthetic.
6. **Have** the patient gently massage the area for approximately 5 to 10 minutes. Other tasks can be accomplished during this time.
7. **Check** for effectiveness of the anesthesia and determine if additional time, anesthetics, or alternative approaches are needed.

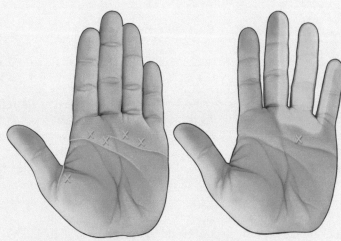

FIGURE 1. Examples of injection sites. Avoid injecting into creases.

FIGURE 2. Example of the injection site and the anesthetized area

The Critical Image

A Boy With Abdominal Pain

By Joshua S. Broder, MD, FACEP
Dr. Broder is a professor and the residency program director in the Department of Emergency Medicine at Duke University Medical Center in Durham, North Carolina.

Objective

On completion of this article, you should be able to:

■ Recognize less common presentations of pneumonia in children.

CASE PRESENTATION

A 4-year-old boy presents with right lower abdominal pain, poor oral intake, and a fever that has lasted 4 days. He was also evaluated yesterday in this emergency department. At that time, the patient had a WBC count of 17×10^9 cells/L, with 72% neutrophils and 18% bands. An ultrasound had been performed to evaluate for appendicitis but was equivocal. CT showed a normal appendix, so the patient was discharged. His fever continues, and his mother reports that he is urinating less. His vital signs are BP 151/85, P 160, R 24, T 38.8°C (101.8°F); SpO_2 is 97% on room air.

The patient is awake but ill appearing, with tachypnea and shallow breathing. He is tachycardic and has diminished breath sounds on his right side. His abdomen is tender in the right upper quadrant. The patient has a normal pulse and capillary refill time.

The emergency physician obtains chest x-ray (*Figure 1*).

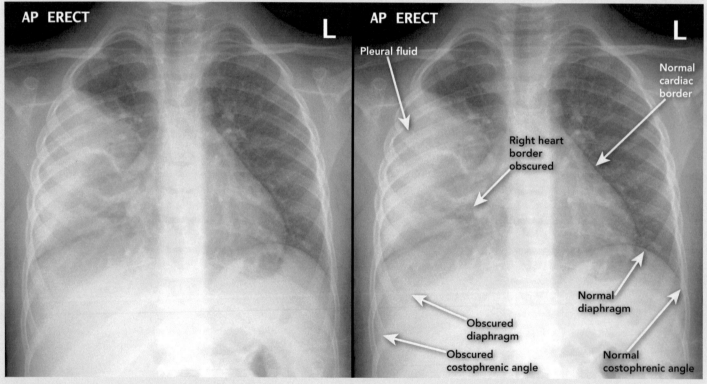

FIGURE 1. **Chest x-ray on the second emergency department visit, without and with labels.** In the labeled image, normal findings are marked on the patient's left side. On the patient's right, an infiltrate obscures the right heart border, diaphragm, and costophrenic angle. Normally, low-density lung tissue ("air density") is readily distinguished from solid organs ("fluid density" because they are mostly water). The normal boundaries between these tissues are called the "silhouette sign." Loss of the silhouette sign is pathologic.

In patients of any age, chest pathology can present with abdominal pain. Physicians should consider this possibility in their differential diagnosis for patients with abdominal pain, particularly when other explanations for pain have not been identified. In one study of children ages 3 to 14 years who were admitted with pneumonia, acute abdominal pain was the chief complaint in 8.5% of cases.[1] Vomiting or diarrhea are seen in 27% of children with pneumonia, perhaps distracting physicians toward an abdominal etiology.[2]

Ultrasound demonstrates a high sensitivity and specificity for pneumonia in multiple studies.[3] A meta-analysis showed a pooled sensitivity of 96% (95% CI, 94%-97%) and specificity of 93% (95% CI, 90%-96%).[4] Point-of-care ultrasound may be somewhat less accurate (sensitivity 86%; 95% CI, 71%-94% and specificity 89%; 95% CI, 83%-93%).[5] Physicians should consider their own ultrasound experience in applying results to clinical care.

If CT is performed to evaluate abdominal pain, lung windows can be reviewed to evaluate chest pathology. This patient's CT scan appears normal, but the upper chest is excluded from the field of view. Lung pathology can rapidly evolve, and repeat imaging may be necessary if a patient's clinical condition deteriorates.

CASE RESOLUTION

The patient was admitted and treated for community-acquired pneumonia complicated by parapneumonic effusion. He received intravenous antibiotics and underwent pigtail chest tube placement. The patient improved clinically over the course of 5 days, and the chest tube was removed. He was discharged on oral antibiotics.

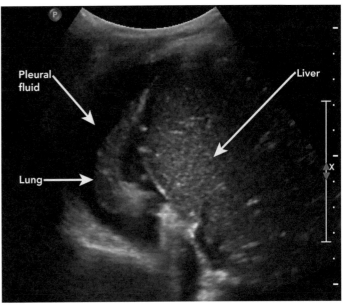

FIGURE 2. **An ultrasound of the right lower chest, transverse position, from the second visit.** Pleural fluid is visible. The consolidated lung is echogenic and called "hepatization" for its similarity to the sonographic appearance of the liver, which is also visible in this image. Bright echoes within the consolidated lung represent air bronchograms.

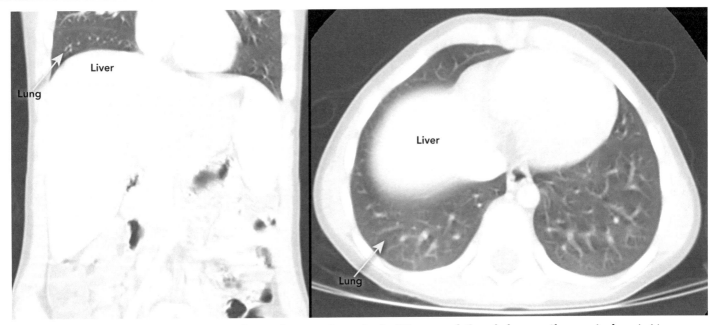

FIGURE 3. **Coronal and axial images from the previous day's CT scan of the abdomen (*lung windows*).** No evidence of lung pathology is visible, although the upper chest is not included within the field of view.

REFERENCES

1. Kirovski I, Micevska V, Seckova L, Nikolovski L. Abdominal pain as a predictor of pneumonia in children. *Eur Resp J.* 2011;38:1152.
2. Shah SN, Bachur RG, Simel DL, Neuman MI. Does this child have pneumonia? The rational clinical examination systematic review. *JAMA.* 2017 Aug;318(5):462-471.
3. Stadler JAM, Andronikou S, Zar HJ. Lung ultrasound for the diagnosis of community-acquired pneumonia in children. *Pediatr Radiol.* 2017 Oct;47(11):1412-1419.
4. Pereda MA, Chavez MA, Hooper-Miele CC, et al. Lung ultrasound for the diagnosis of pneumonia in children: a meta-analysis. *Pediatrics.* 2015;135(4):714-722.
5. Shah VP, Tunik MG, Tsung JW. Prospective evaluation of point-of-care ultrasonography for the diagnosis of pneumonia in children and young adults. *JAMA Pediatr.* 2013;167(2):119-125.

Feature Editor: Joshua S. Broder, MD, FACEP. See also *Diagnostic Imaging for the Emergency Physician* (Winner of the 2011 Prose Award in Clinical Medicine, the American Publishers Award for Professional and Scholarly Excellence) and *Critical Images in Emergency Medicine* by Dr. Broder.

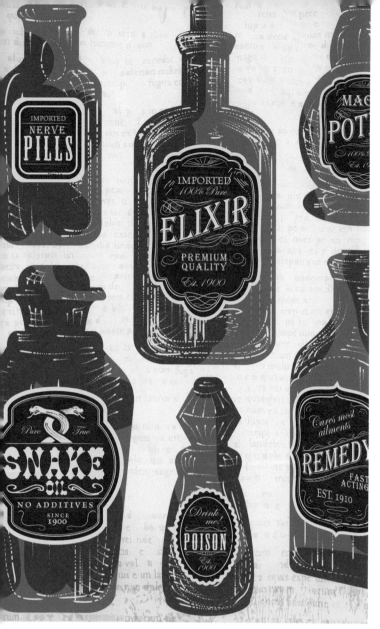

FYI

Handling Medical Disinformation at the Bedside

LESSON 2

By Robert Barnes, MD; Zachary Aust, MD; and Jedidiah Leaf, MD

Dr. Barnes, Dr. Aust, and Dr. Leaf are assistant professors in the Department of Emergency Medicine at the University of Texas Southwestern Medical Center in Dallas.

Objectives

On completion of this lesson, you should be able to:

1. Differentiate between medical misinformation and disinformation.
2. Understand why both misinformation and disinformation spread.
3. Explain strategies to insulate against misinformation and disinformation.
4. Recognize and be able to report misinformation and disinformation.
5. Use several strategies to correct misconceptions.

From the EM Model

20.0 Other Core Competencies of the Practice of Emergency Medicine

     20.1   Interpersonal and Communication Skills

▬ CRITICAL DECISIONS ▬

- What is COVID-19 disinformation?

- What are the consequences of spreading misinformation?

- How is the spread of disinformation and misinformation managed?

- What strategies combat disinformation?

Medical disinformation on COVID-19 vaccinations and treatment has become an important topic in emergency departments across the country. From dangerous therapeutics to ill-informed ideas about vaccines, emergency physicians need to know how to address these issues with patients and how to keep disinformation from worsening patient outcomes.

CASE ONE

A 38-year-old man presents for evaluation of a mild upper respiratory infection. As part of his workup, a COVID-19 PCR test is obtained but is negative for COVID-19 infection. When the patient asks if he should receive a COVID-19 vaccination, his nurse responds that the vaccine carries significant risks and is not highly effective. She also states that COVID-19 infection is not serious and carries no more risk than the yearly influenza virus.

CASE TWO

A 40-year-old woman presents with congestion. She is nontoxic, hemodynamically stable, and has no signs of pneumonia. Her COVID-19 PCR test is negative, and no other life-threatening causes are found in her workup or examination. She appears to have a viral upper respiratory infection. The patient is requesting a prescription for antibiotics because she states that these symptoms occur around this time every year and are always treated with antibiotics.

CASE THREE

A 62-year-old woman presents with a distal radius fracture after walking and falling in the dark. She has a history of COPD, diabetes, and hypertension. While having a sugar-tong splint placed for her fracture, she tells the physician she is considering getting the COVID-19 vaccine but wants to know more about its safety.

Introduction

Misinformation is not a new problem in medicine. It affects everyone from physicians to patients. It influences the type of care physicians provide and the type of care patients are willing to receive. The medical topics most plagued by disinformation include cancer treatments, vaccinations, and antibiotic therapies.[1] At the individual level, misinformation can lead to worse patient outcomes; at the community level, it can influence public health policy.

Since early 2020, COVID-19 has changed the landscape of medicine. One of the more difficult aspects of managing this pandemic has been the misinformation and disinformation surrounding it. The age of social media gives people numerous platforms to tout themselves as experts in the field. Even within medicine, inconsistencies in evidence and expert opinion exist. Unsurprisingly, patients have a difficult time deciding which information to trust. The burden is placed on emergency physicians to dispel false information and misguided beliefs to provide better patient care.

CRITICAL DECISION

What is COVID-19 disinformation?

Misinformation is generally defined as "[i]nformation that is false but not created with the intention of causing harm."[2] This is different from disinformation, which is false information that is deliberately created to deceive.[1,2,3] For example, some of the information on social media is considered part of a deliberate effort to promote vaccine disinformation and has effectively decreased the overall vaccination rate.[4] Misinformation, by contrast, can be due to a fundamental misunderstanding of the facts, such as when patients believe that an antibiotic will help cure their viral upper respiratory infection because they have been prescribed this treatment in the past. In cases of misinformation and disinformation, physicians and patients may have a fundamentally flawed understanding of a situation.

The COVID-19 "infodemic" showed that identifying something as misinformation or disinformation is not so straightforward.[5] Physicians and patients have been barraged with rapidly changing health guidance, research, misinformation, and disinformation, which has degraded patients' trust in health care. The WHO has unequivocally stated, "Misinformation costs lives."[5] The US Surgeon General's advisory panel redefines misinformation as anything that goes against the "best available evidence."[6] They also note that severely misleading information, such as anecdotes taken without context or extreme outlier cases, may fall into this category. Patients and physicians have their own biases based on their perception of the truth. These perceptions are affected by the type and quality of information they consume.

CRITICAL DECISION

What are the consequences of spreading misinformation?

Throughout the pandemic, many physicians have had varying stances on COVID-19 therapeutics and vaccinations, including when little to no evidence was available on them. Over the past several months, many professional organizations have taken strong stances against the spread of misinformation, threatening licensure and certification.

The American Board of Emergency Medicine (ABEM) stated that any emergency medicine–boarded physician who is found to be spreading COVID-19 misinformation — information that is contrary to prevailing medical advice — may be subject to ABEM review and, if found guilty, may have their certification revoked.[7]

✔ Pearls

- Patient disinformation and misinformation are dangerous to public health. ABEM and FSMB take strong stances against disinformation.
- Patient concerns regarding misinformation and disinformation should not be dismissed.
- Physicians should let data and statistics inform their position on an issue and should relate verified information to patients in a story-based, personal approach.

The Federation of State Medical Boards (FSMB) has also stated that the spread of misinformation and disinformation may result in the revocation of state medical licensure.[8]

The American College of Emergency Physicians (ACEP) and the American Academy of Emergency Medicine (AAEM) have also discouraged physicians from propagating medical disinformation.

Patients have a significant amount of trust in physicians, and physicians have a significant amount of power in terms of relaying medical news. In an effort to protect public health, physicians who spread medical disinformation and misinformation may face strict consequences.

CRITICAL DECISION

How is the spread of misinformation and disinformation managed?

Disinformation and misinformation from health care professionals are dangerous. When encountered, the best first approach is to discuss the source of this information or the evidence for the claim. Often, the evidence is purely anecdotal or the source is the media or social media. Reminding health care professionals of their oath to provide patient care that is backed by evidence-based medicine can help.

The next approach is to address the spread of misinformation and disinformation with a medical director or the facility's administration department, especially considering misinformation and disinformation threaten the health care organization's public image. Furthermore, not addressing the spread of misinformation or disinformation internally could draw the attention of medical and state licensing boards.

CRITICAL DECISION

What strategies combat disinformation and misinformation?

Much has been written about fighting disinformation and misinformation at a public health level. However, addressing disinformation and misinformation at the bedside with individual patients is just as important. Because of shorter patient interaction times in the emergency department, effectively addressing disinformation and misinformation is a challenge. Conversations on the subject that follow a general framework can make the process more successful.

Although the COVID-19 vaccine magnifies the issues, disinformation, misinformation, and vaccine hesitancy have existed through history. Prior studies provide approaches for addressing these topics with patients. Physicians must also understand their patients' views on these issues. Believing disinformation or misinformation does not stem from a lack of intelligence, and physicians should not be so insensitive as to quickly invalidate or dismiss patients' concerns. Physicians should also expect incremental gains in educating their patients against disinformation and misinformation. Although vaccination may be the end goal, getting a patient from a mindset of "I am absolutely not getting the vaccine," to "I am going to consider it," should be considered a success in the fight against disinformation and misinformation .[8,9] The goal of the conversation is not to be correct; it is to provide patients with the best information possible so that they can make a properly informed decision.

The recommended general framework for conversations:
1. Build rapport and trust;
2. Use empathy and open-ended questions to elicit reasoning, and listen for and acknowledge concerns;
3. Give advice from a compassionate stance rather than a prescriptive one;
4. Give information in small bits and assess understanding in the process known as "chunking"[8,10]; and
5. Direct patients to appropriate resources.

Patients' trust in their physicians is most influential in getting patients to follow accurate medical advice. Building a good rapport is an important first step to developing trust.[8,9] Doing so means physicians must be mindful of their body language and give full attention to patients during their interactions. Sitting, rather than standing, has been shown to make patients feel that their physician is spending more time attending to them.[11] Asking open-ended questions and having nonjudgmental conversations can encourage patients to vocalize their concerns.

Patients' autonomy in decision-making should be acknowledged by helping them decide on a treatment rather than telling them what to do. Responses to their concerns should also be empathetic, and physicians should maintain their composure, especially when there is disagreement.[9,10] Evidence and data must be presented in a truthful manner and not in absolutes. For example, physicians should never say false statements like there are no possible side effects to a vaccine. Vaccines are associated with mild and serious side effects, with mild side effects being common and serious side effects being rare enough for the benefits to outweigh the risks most of the time. During conversation, physcians can use the technique of chunking to guide patients and their expectations.[10] Chunking is the practice of breaking information down into smaller parts and frequently checking patients' understanding so that they are not overloaded with information. Data also suggest that physicians build trust when they disclose more personal stories to patients since people tend to remember stories better than facts.[12] Use good judgment with every situation, but examples from personal clinical experience may be more effective evidence than reciting facts.

At the end of discussions with their physicians, patients may not reach a definitive conclusion in one visit. Physicians should attempt to give patients trusted information sources that they can investigate after the interaction. If patients already established a relationship with a primary care physician,

---

✖ Pitfalls

- Ignoring disinformation and misinformation from health care professionals instead of addressing these issues when they arise.

- Regarding only incremental changes in patients' acceptance of new information as failure.

- Taking a confrontational or pejorative approach to correcting misinformation instead of listening with empathy and providing true information to patients.

CASE RESOLUTIONS

■ CASE ONE

After overhearing the misinformation provided by the nurse, the physician decided to address the patient and nurse separately.

In the patient's room, the physcian explained that the patient should have the vaccine because he has no contraindications. The physician cited the evidence of the vaccine's safety and the risks associated with it and explained the potential implications of COVID-19 infection. The patient agreed to get vaccinated.

The physician then addressed the nurse about the overheard misinformation. After the nurse cited social media as the source for this information, the physician discussed the lack of evidence behind these claims and how such misinformation could significantly impact public health. The nurse did not take this response well. The physician told the nurse that this issue would be taken to the emergency department nursing management team over concern that this misinformation could be dangerous to patient safety.

■ CASE TWO

After sitting and listening to the patient's concern, the physician refrained from immediately responding, "This is a viral infection, and you don't need antibiotics." The patient has had these symptoms before, and around week 3 of her infection, she usually received a prescription for antibiotics that made the symptoms go away. The physician acknowledged the unpleasantness of having symptoms for so long and explained the typical course of a viral infection. The possible negative side effects of antibiotics in situations when they are not needed were discussed. The patient was appreciative of the information from this interaction and verbalized that she understood why antibiotics were not needed.

■ CASE THREE

The physcian told the patient that the vaccine is a good idea for most people but asked her to elaborate on her thoughts. The patient said that she heard on social media that the virus is not any worse than the flu and that she is afraid of the vaccine's side effects. In a HIPAA-compliant manner, the physician told a story about a COVID-19 patients that required intubation and was in the ICU for 2 weeks. The physician also discussed encouraginh family members to get vaccinated and that they feel much safer now going out in public. At discharge, the patient is given a link to the hospital's website that has more information about COVID-19 and vaccine locations.

coordinating with them to continue the conversation can be beneficial. Although the fight against misinformation and disinformation will continue to require larger public health initiatives, physicians can make a difference at the bedside.

Summary

Misinformation and disinformation have plagued the landscape of medicine, becoming more prevalent in the recent past because of COVID-19. Whether related to vaccinations, therapeutics, or the epidemiology and impact of a disease, numerous opinions and beliefs are not backed by evidence. Emergency physicians have the responsibility to educate and protect their patients by combating misinformation and disinformation at the bedside, as appropriate. Employing strategies of listening, empathizing, chunking information, and using personal narratives can help patients make a more informed decision.

REFERENCES

1. Grimes DR. Medical disinformation and the unviable nature of COVID-19 conspiracy theories. *PLoS One.* 2021 Mar 12;16(3):e0245900.
2. Journalism, "fake news" and disinformation: a handbook for journalism education and training. UNESCO. https://en.unesco.org/fightfakenews
3. O'Connor C, Murphy M. Going viral: doctors must tackle fake news in the covid-19 pandemic. *BMJ.* 2020 Apr 24;369:m1587.
4. Wilson SL, Wiysonge C. Social media and vaccine hesitancy. *BMJ Global Health.* 2020 Oct;5(10):e004206.
5. WHO; UN; UNICEF; UNDP; UNESCO; UNAIDS; ITU; UN Global Pulse; IFRC. Managing the COVID-19 infodemic: promoting healthy behaviours and mitigating the harm from misinformation and disinformation. World Health Organization. 2020 Sep 23. https://www.who.int/news/item/23-09-2020-managing-the-covid-19-infodemic-promoting-healthy-behaviours-and-mitigating-the-harm-from-misinformation-and-disinformation
6. Confronting health misinformation: the U.S. surgeon general's advisory on building a healthy information environment. US Department of Health and Human Services; 2021. https://www.hhs.gov/sites/default/files/surgeon-general-misinformation-advisory.pdf
7. ABEM statement about ABEM-certified physicians providing misleading and inaccurate information to the public. American Board of Emergency Medicine. 2021 Aug 26. https://www.abem.org/public/news-events/news/2021/08/27/abem-statement-about-abem-certified-physicians-providing-misleading-and-inaccurate-information-to-the-public
8. FSMB: spreading COVID-19 vaccine misinformation may put medical license at risk. Federation of State Medical Boards. 2021 Jul 29. https://www.fsmb.org/advocacy/news-releases/fsmb-spreading-covid-19-vaccine-misinformation-may-put-medical-license-at-risk
9. Southwell BG, Wood JL, Navar AM. Roles for health care professionals in addressing patient-held misinformation beyond fact correction. *Am J Public Health.* 2020 Oct;110(suppl 3):S288-S289.
10. Leask J, Kinnersley P, Jackson C, Cheater F, Bedford H, Rowles G. Communicating with parents about vaccination: a framework for health professionals. *BMC Pediatr.* 2012 Sep 21;12:154.
11. Swayden KJ, Anderson KK, Connelly LM, Moran JS, McMahon JK, Arnold PM. Effect of sitting vs. standing on perception of provider time at bedside: a pilot study. *Patient Educ Couns.* 2012 Feb;86(2):166-171.
12. Zink KL, Perry M, London K, et al. "Let me tell you about my…" provider self-disclosure in the emergency department builds patient rapport. *West J Emerg Med.* 2017 Jan;18(1):43-49.

ADDITIONAL READING

Wood S, Schulman K. Beyond politics — promoting COVID-19 vaccination in the United States. *N Engl J Med.* 2021 Feb 18;384:e23.

CME Questions

Reviewed by **Michael S. Beeson, MD, MBA, FACEP**

Qualified, paid subscribers to *Critical Decisions in Emergency Medicine* may receive CME certificates for up to 5 ACEP Category I credits, 5 *AMA PRA Category 1 Credits*™, and 5 AOA Category 2-B credits for completing this activity in its entirety. Submit your answers online at acep.org/cdem; a score of 75% or better is required. You may receive credit for completing the CME activity any time within 3 years of its publication date. Answers to this month's questions will be published in next month's issue.

1 **What is the most likely age for a patient with pyloric stenosis?**
   - A.   3 weeks to 9 weeks
   - B.   6 months to 8 months
   - C.   6 months to 2 years
   - D.   12 months to 15 months

2 **Which are not red flags that indicate a vomiting child may need further evaluation?**
   - A.   3-week-old infant who recently started vomiting after every feed and has had one wet diaper in 24 hours
   - B.   6-month-old child with six wet diapers in 24 hours who turns red when trying to pass stool
   - C.   2-year-old child who sometimes falls with attempts at walking and has to hold on to something for balance
   - D.   10-year-old child with dry, cracked lips who has been drinking liquids all day and breathing faster than usual

3 **A 5-year-old girl had a temperature of 39.4°C (103°F) at home. She has had two episodes of nonbloody and nonbilious emesis and a diminished appetite for 2 days; she has had no dysuria but has recently struggled to pass very hard stools. Which additional symptoms would warrant imaging?**
   - A.   One episode of watery, nonbloody diarrhea in the waiting room
   - B.   Two siblings have similar symptoms at home
   - C.   Right lower quadrant pain to palpation and refusal to jump secondary to pain
   - D.   Runny nose, nasal congestion, and cough are positive on review of systems

4 **An 18-month-old boy presents in the middle of the night for fussiness and irritability. His parents gave him acetaminophen just prior to arrival, which settled him down slightly. Which step is likely needed?**
   - A.   CT of the abdomen and pelvis with contrast
   - B.   Liver function tests
   - C.   Ondansetron oral dissolving pill
   - D.   Ultrasound of the abdomen

5 **A toddler presents with vomiting, diarrhea, and refusal to drink water. Oral rehydration is attempted, but 30 minutes later the toddler is unable to keep fluids down. What is the best next step?**
   - A.   Two-view abdominal x-ray
   - B.   Admission to the pediatric inpatient unit
   - C.   CBC with differential
   - D.   Peripheral line placement and a 20-mL/kg normal saline bolus

6 **A 15-month-old girl presents with fever and vomiting. She has had four episodes of nonbilious and nonbloody vomiting in the last 24 hours and 5 days of watery, nonbloody diarrhea, approximately four to six episodes per day. The child is fussy but consolable by her mother. On examination, the child has dry mucous membranes; a 3-second peripheral capillary refill time; a normal oropharynx; normal work of breathing and lung sounds; and no lymphadenopathy, abdominal pain to palpation, or hepatosplenomegaly. The patient has a diaper rash on her bottom that spares the inguinal folds; no other rashes are noted. What laboratory study is most likely to yield a diagnosis?**
   - A.   Basic metabolic panel
   - B.   Blood culture
   - C.   C-reactive protein
   - D.   Urinalysis and urine culture

7 **A 3-year-old boy presents with vomiting and diarrhea. The child has refused to drink despite his parents' efforts. His mother does not believe he used the restroom to urinate this morning when he woke up. He does not have a fever and has a normal oropharynx, mucous membranes, and pupillary response. His tympanic membranes are clear bilaterally and no rashes, cervical lymphadenopathy, hepatosplenomegaly, or abdominal pain to palpation is noted. His penis and testicles are normal with no pain to palpation. His capillary refill time is 3 seconds. What is the most appropriate next step?**
   - A.   Two-view abdominal x-ray
   - B.   Abdominal ultrasound
   - C.   Basic metabolic panel and an intravenous 20-mL/kg normal saline bolus
   - D.   Ondansetron and oral rehydration attempt

8 **An 8-year-old girl with abdominal pain and vomiting is brought in after her mother noticed that she appeared very tired and was breathing fast. Upon further questioning, the physician learns the child has had a 10-lb weight loss in the last week, with frequent water consumption and urination. Her lungs are clear on auscultation; she is tachycardic but has normal S1/S2 heart sounds. Her capillary refill time is 4 seconds. She has no rashes. A glucose test taken during triage read greater than 500 g/dL. What is the best initial step?**
   - A.   Chest x-ray
   - B.   Subcutaneous insulin
   - C.   Pediatric endocrinology consultation
   - D.   Peripheral line placement and a normal saline bolus

9 A 14-year-old girl presents with no appetite for the last week and vomiting for the last 2 days. She denies dysuria, fever, and abdominal pain. During a private discussion with the teenager, she discloses that she has been having unprotected sex with her mother's live-in boyfriend. What is the course of action?

A. All of these
B. Child protective services consultation
C. Law enforcement consultation
D. Urine pregnancy test

10 A 2-week-old infant presents with vomiting. The emesis looks like milk and is not green. The infant has not been waking up to feed at night and has had one wet diaper in 24 hours. On examination, she has a sunken fontanelle, has dry mucous membranes, and is arousable to painful stimuli but goes back to sleep. Her respiratory examination and S1/S2 heart sounds are normal. She has no hepatosplenomegaly, but her labia appear dark for her age. What is the best first step?

A. Glucose point-of-care test
B. Basic metabolic panel
C. Chest x-ray
D. Abdominal ultrasound

11 What is misinformation?

A. False information created deliberately to deceive
B. False information not made with malicious intent
C. Information believed to be false
D. Information that is not clearly true or false

12 What is disinformation?

A. False information created deliberately to deceive
B. False information not made with malicious intent
C. Information believed to be false
D. Information that is not clearly true or false

13 What must be avoided when discussing misinformation at the bedside?

A. Immediately dismissing obviously false beliefs
B. Giving trusted follow-up resources
C. Respecting the patient's autonomy
D. Using open-ended questions

14 What is good practice when discussing misinformation at the bedside?

A. Chunking information
B. Illustrating facts with true stories from clinical experience
C. Responding empathetically
D. All of these

15 What are the consequences of physicians propagating medical disinformation or misinformation?

A. They may lose their state licensure
B. They may lose their specialty certification
C. They may lose their current job
D. A and B

16 A physician spreads disinformation by repeatedly telling patients that the COVID-19 vaccine is ineffective and that it is safer to "take your chances" with exposure and infection. How should a colleague who overhears the physician handle this situation?

A. Do nothing and let the behavior continue
C. Report the physician to the state medical licensing board
B. Report the physician to the medical director
D. Talk with the physician and change their mind

17 Which factor most influences patients' willingness to accept medical advice?

A. Compatibility between patients' and physicians' political views
B. Patients' trust in their physicians
C. The international reputation of the journal cited
D. The number of times patients hear the information

18 Which are sources of possible misinformation and disinformation?

A. Close personal contacts
B. News platforms
C. Social media platforms
D. All of these .

19 A patient becomes angry when the physician tries to clarify the patient's cited disinformation. What is the best course of action?

A. Agree with them to improve the patient-physician relationship
B. Continue to disprove their citations with scientific evidence
C. Acknowledge their belief and inquire to understand where the misinformation is coming from
D. Point out their lack of expertise

20 A coworker is spotted posting disinformation on social media. What should be done?

A. Comment on the inaccuracy
B. Directly discuss the matter with the coworker
D. File a report with the American Board of Emergency Medicine
C. Repost the information

ANSWER KEY FOR NOVEMBER 2022, VOLUME 36, NUMBER 11

1	2	3	4	5	6	7	8	9	10	11	12	13	14	15	16	17	18	19	20
B	A	D	C	A	B	B	A	B	B	A	B	A	A	C	B	C	A	A	C

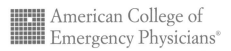

American College of
Emergency Physicians®

ADVANCING EMERGENCY CARE ─────√\─

Post Office Box 619911
Dallas, Texas 75261-9911

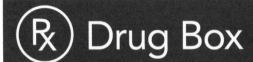

Nirmatrelvir/Ritonavir

By Frank LoVecchio, DO, MPH, FACEP; and Laila LoVecchio
Valleywise Health and ASU, CHS, and University of Arizona, Tucson

Objective
On reading this column you should be able to
■ State the indications and contraindications for nirmatrelvir/ritonavir.

Nirmatrelvir/ritonavir is the first oral antiviral SARS-CoV-2-3CL protease inhibitor that received emergency use authorization (EUA) from the FDA. Nirmatrelvir blocks the activity of the SARS-CoV-2-3CL protease, an enzyme required for viral replication. Coadministration with ritonavir slows nirmatrelvir's metabolism, which allows for longer and higher drug concentrations. Nirmatrelvir/ritonavir is prescribed for adults and children 12 years or older (weighing at least 40 kg) with mild to moderate COVID-19 who are at risk of severe disease or hospitalization. In an unpublished randomized trial of 2,246 unvaccinated adult outpatients with at least one risk factor for severe disease, administration of nirmatrelvir/ritonavir within 3 days of symptom onset reduced the risk of hospitalization or death at 28 days by 89%.

Dosing
Nirmatrelvir tablets are copackaged with ritonavir tablets, and both must be administered together. Treatment should be initiated as soon as possible after COVID-19 diagnosis and within 5 days of symptom onset. Nirmatrelvir/ritonavir can be administered with or without food.

Dosage is 300 mg nirmatrelvir (two 150-mg tablets) with 100 mg ritonavir (one 100-mg tablet). All 3 tablets are taken together twice daily for 5 days (30 pills total).

Limitations (to Date)
Nirmatrelvir/ritonavir is not authorized for patients with severe or critical COVID-19 who require hospitalization. It is not authorized for pre- or postexposure prophylaxis for COVID-19. It should not be used for more than 5 consecutive days.

Adverse Events
■ Dysgeusia
■ Diarrhea
■ Hypertension
■ Myalgia

Precautions
Nirmatrelvir/ritonavir is not recommended in patients with severe renal impairment (estimated glomerular filtration rate <30 mL/min) or severe hepatic impairment until more data are available.

Nirmatrelvir/ritonavir is contraindicated if allergic, with drugs that are highly dependent on CYP3A for clearance, and with drugs that are associated with serious and life-threatening reactions at elevated concentrations. Nirmatrelvir/ritonavir is also contraindicated with drugs that are potent CYP3A inducers, which can significantly reduce nirmatrelvir or ritonavir plasma concentrations to weaken their virologic response and possibly promote viral resistance.

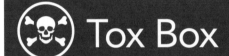

Vitamin D Toxicity

By Christian A. Tomaszewski, MD, MS, MBA, FACEP
University of California, San Diego Health

Objective
On reading this column you should be able to
■ Discuss manifestations and treatment of vitamin d toxicity

Vitamin D — D2 ergocalciferol or D3 cholecalciferol — is a fat-soluble vitamin used to treat rickets, osteomalacia, and hypoparathyroidism. Most recently, it has been proffered as an unproven treatment for COVID-19. Mild toxicity can occur after acute overdose, but chronic ingestion of large amounts can cause severe toxicity; hence use of D3 as a rodenticide.

Pharmacology
■ Vitamin D is metabolized into 25-hydroxyvitamin D [25(OH)D] by vitamin D-25-hydroxylase.
■ Promotes hypercalcemia via effect on intestine and bones
■ Most inadvertent ingestions can be monitored at home.
■ Acute ingestion > 100 times RDA (2.5 million units in toddler; 4.0 million units in adults) may lead to toxicity
■ Chronic daily ingestions > 2000 units in children or 75,000 units in adults may produce toxicity

Clinical Manifestations
■ *GI:* nausea, vomiting, and abdominal cramps
■ *CNS:* headache, dizziness, irritability, fatigue, and seizures
■ *Cardiac:* hypertension and dysrhythmias (prolonged PR and QRS, shortened QT)
■ *Metabolic:* renal failure and hypercalcemia

Diagnostics
■ Electrolytes, calcium, and phosphorus
■ Urinalysis
■ ECG/cardiac monitoring if symptomatic
■ Plasma 25-hydroxyvitamin [25(OH)D] may be elevated

Treatment
■ May give activated charcoal oral if <1 hour post ingestion of excessive amounts (>100 times RDA or 17 pellets of rodenticide bait)
■ Fluids and forced diuresis (furosemide) may promote calcium excretion
■ Benzodiazepines for seizures
■ Dialysis (with calcium-free dialysate) for refractory hypercalcemia
■ Prednisone or bisphosphonates have also been used for refractory hypercalcemia

Disposition
■ Observe acute overdoses for 4-6 hours post ingestion
■ Admit if severe hypercalcemia or neurological findings

Critical decisions
in emergency medicine

Volume 36 Number 2: **February 2022**

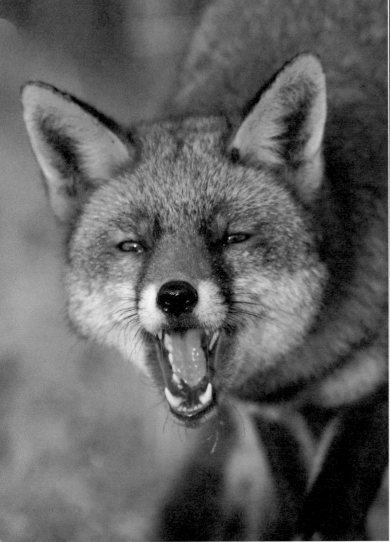

Once Bitten, Twice Shy

All mammals are capable of biting – and they do. Emergency physicians will inevitably be asked to evaluate patients that are victims of such bites. Familiarity with the proper management, including patient disposition, of these injuries is critical to the emergency physician and the patient.

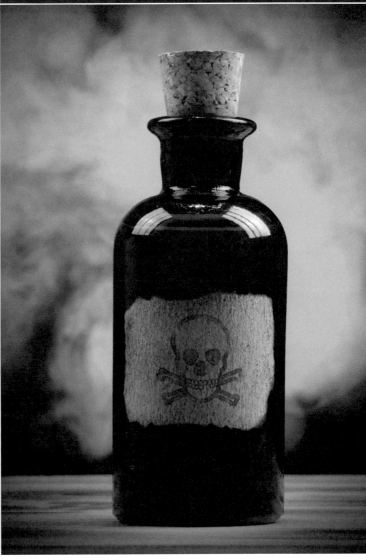

Seek and You Shall Find

Sherlock Holmes always enjoyed a good mystery, and so too shall the emergency physician seeing presentations for pediatric toxic ingestions. Overlapping intricacies of their pathologic presentations challenge the physician to identify and manage a massive array of sedative or hypnotics, anticholinergics, and sympathomimetics.

THE OFFICIAL CME PUBLICATION OF THE AMERICAN COLLEGE OF EMERGENCY PHYSICIANS

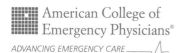
American College of Emergency Physicians®
ADVANCING EMERGENCY CARE

Critical decisions
in emergency medicine

Critical Decisions in Emergency Medicine is the official CME publication of the American College of Emergency Physicians. Additional volumes are available.

EDITOR-IN-CHIEF
Michael S. Beeson, MD, MBA, FACEP
Northeastern Ohio Universities, Rootstown, OH

SECTION EDITORS
Joshua S. Broder, MD, FACEP
Duke University, Durham, NC

Andrew J. Eyre, MD, MHPEd
Brigham & Women's Hospital/
Harvard Medical School, Boston, MA

John Kiel, DO, MPH
University of Florida College of Medicine, Jacksonville, FL

Frank LoVecchio, DO, MPH, FACEP
Maricopa Medical Center/Banner Phoenix Poison and Drug Information Center, Phoenix, AZ

Amal Mattu, MD, FACEP
University of Maryland, Baltimore, MD

Christian A. Tomaszewski, MD, MS, MBA, FACEP
University of California Health Sciences, San Diego, CA

Steven J. Warrington, MD, MEd
MercyOne Siouxland, Sioux City, IA

ASSOCIATE EDITORS
Tareq Al-Salamah, MBBS, MPH, FACEP
King Saud University, Riyadh, Saudi Arabia/
University of Maryland, Baltimore, MD

Wan-Tsu W. Chang, MD
University of Maryland, Baltimore, MD

Ann M. Dietrich, MD, FAAP, FACEP
University of South Carolina College of Medicine, Greenville, SC

Kelsey Drake, MD, MPH, FACEP
St. Anthony Hospital, Lakewood CO

Walter L. Green, MD, FACEP
UT Southwestern Medical Center, Dallas, TX

John C. Greenwood, MD
University of Pennsylvania, Philadelphia, PA

Danya Khoujah, MBBS
University of Maryland, Baltimore, MD

Sharon E. Mace, MD, FACEP
Cleveland Clinic Lerner College of Medicine/
Case Western Reserve University, Cleveland, OH

Nathaniel Mann, MD
Greenville Health System, Greenville, SC

George Sternbach, MD, FACEP
Stanford University Medical Center, Stanford, CA

Joseph F. Waeckerle, MD, FACEP
University of Missouri-Kansas City School of Medicine, Kansas City, MO

EDITORIAL STAFF
Mark Paglia, Senior Manager
mpaglia@acep.org

Melissa Mills, Associate Editor

ISSN2325-0186 (Print)   ISSN2325-8365 (Online)

Contents

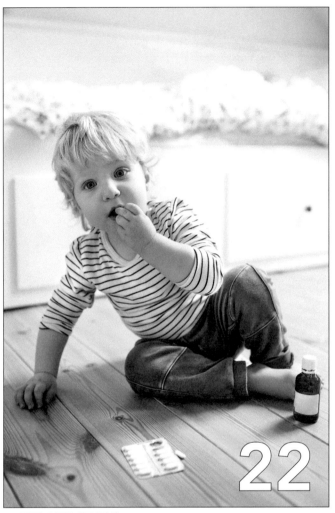

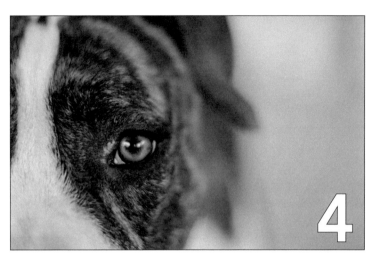

Lesson 3 . . . . **4**
Once Bitten, Twice Shy
Mammalian Bites
By Nanditha Shivaprakash, MD; and
Robert Vezzetti, MD, FAAP, FACEP
Reviewed by Kelsey Drake, MD; and Nathaniel Mann, MD

Lesson 4 . . . . **22**
Seek and You Shall Find
Pediatric Toxic Ingestions
By Vandana Thapar, MD; Cynthia Orantes, MD, FAAP; and
Latonia Miller, MD, MS
Reviewed by Ann Dietrich, MD, FAAP, FACEP

FEATURES

The Critical ECG — Atrial Bigeminy 11
   By Amal Mattu, MD, FACEP

Clinical Pediatrics — Twisting Intestines: Bilious Emesis 12
   By Heather Jones, DO, Zachary Burroughs, MD; and Ann Dietrich, MD
   Reviewed by Sharon E. Mace, MD, FACEP

The LLSA Literature Review — Established Status Epilepticus Treatment Trial (ESETT) 14
   By Mallori Wilson, MD, LT, MC, USN; and Daphne P. Morrison Ponce, MD, CDR, MC, USN
   Reviewed by Andrew J. Eyre, MD, MS-HPEd

The Critical Procedure — Closed Thoracic Lavage Rewarming 16
   By Steven J. Warrington, MD, MEd, MS

Critical Cases in Orthopedics and Trauma — Inferior Shoulder Dislocation 18
   By William Chan, MD; and Victor Huang, MD
   Reviewed by John Kiel, DO, MPH

The Critical Image — Headache and Blurred Vision 20
   By Joshua S. Broder, MD, FACEP

CME Questions 28
   Reviewed by Kelsey Drake, MD; Nathaniel Mann, MD; and Ann Dietrich, MD, FAAP, FACEP

Drug Box — Fluvoxamine in Outpatient COVID-19 30
   By Frank LoVecchio, DO, MPH, FACEP

Tox Box — Pediatric Cannabis (THC) Ingestions 30
   By Christian A. Tomaszewski, MD, MS, MBA, FACEP

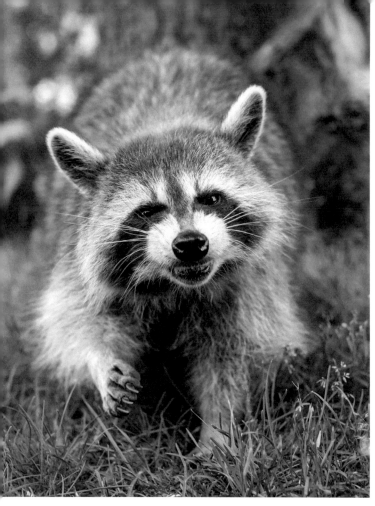

Once Bitten, Twice Shy

Mammalian Bites

LESSON 3

By Nanditha Shivaprakash, MD; and
Robert Vezzetti, MD, FAAP, FACEP

Reviewed by Kelsey Drake, MD; and Nathaniel Mann, MD

Objectives

On completion of this lesson, you should be able to:

1. State the most common sources of mammalian bites.
2. Describe the common pathogens and complications from infections associated with mammalian bites.
3. Discuss the important historical and physical examination findings critical to managing mammalian bites.
4. Explain how to manage mammalian bites, including selecting the appropriate closure type and the appropriate antibiotics for prophylaxis and management of infectious complications.
5. Recognize when rabies prophylaxis is indicated and when tetanus immunization is required.

From the EM Model

6.0 Environmental Disorders
    6.1 Bites and Envenomation
        6.1.2 Mammals
18.0 Traumatic Disorders
    18.1 Trauma
        18.1.3 Cutaneous Trauma

■ CRITICAL DECISIONS ■

- What are the common sources of mammalian bites?

- Which pathogens are associated with mammalian bites?

- What are the important clinical manifestations and complications of mammalian bites?

- What is the appropriate course of action for wound management in the emergency department?

- When is it appropriate to provide prophylaxis for rabies and tetanus?

- What factors determine appropriate patient disposition?

Mammalian bites are common causes of visits to the emergency department. An estimated 250,000 human bites, 400,000 cat bites, and 4.5 million dog bites occur yearly in the United States, with an estimated annual cost of more than $50 million.[1,2] These injuries can be trying on pediatric patients and their families, with the literature reporting children younger than 5 years as the most affected pediatric group.[3] A careful history and physical examination are essential when evaluating patients who have been bitten, as are familiarity with local rabies surveillance patterns, proper wound care, appropriate antibiotic selection, and timely follow-up.

CASE PRESENTATIONS

■ CASE ONE

A 10-year-old boy is brought in after his best friend's pit bull bit his right hand. He states that he was "playing around" with the animal and "may have teased him." He has several puncture wounds to the dorsal aspect of his hand. He is neurovascularly intact and his pain is well controlled with ibuprofen. There is minimal swelling. His immunizations are up to date.

■ CASE TWO

The parents of a 10-month-old girl are referred to the emergency department by their primary care physician after the girl was exposed to a bat. Earlier in the morning the father discovered a bat in the child's room that flew away through an open window as he approached it. The child is discovered to have several unexplained small scratches on her face but is otherwise at her baseline with normal vital signs and a normal physical examination.

■ CASE THREE

A 23-year-old man arrives after being bitten in the face by a dog he encountered while at the park. He states that the dog "just ran up and bit him." He denies any factors that would indicate a provoked bite. He has a significant full-thickness left facial laceration that extends from the posterior cheek to the left corner of the mouth. The dog reportedly ran away after biting the man.

CRITICAL DECISION

What are the common sources of mammalian bites?

Canine Bites

Canine bites are the majority of bites seen in the emergency department, and pediatric patients are more likely than adults to sustain these injuries. For all reported bites, extremity wounds are the most common; facial wounds are more often seen in young children.[4] Pit bulls and Rottweilers are the most common breeds associated with fatalities, although no one breed can be linked to the majority of bite injuries.[2,5] Most victims know the dog that bit them, and the majority of bites are reported as unprovoked.[2] Tissue damage and crush injuries are common with dog bites: Dogs can produce as much as 450 psi of pressure when biting.[4] Wounds should be carefully explored for complications, such as fractures, associated with such injuries, especially in younger patients.

Feline Bites

Feline bites account for up to 10% of mammalian bite wounds evaluated in the emergency department. Most of these bites involve the extremities and are reported as provoked.[2] The extent of damage from feline bites is often misjudged — the puncture wound created by the bite may actually be deeper than what is initially apparent. Thus, prompt evaluation and treatment of these injuries are essential. Signs of infection have been reported in as little as 3 hours post injury.[4]

Human Bites

The true incidence of human bite injuries is unknown. These injuries are more commonly seen among boys and men, especially those in their late teens and early twenties. Most bites occur as a result of an altercation involving punching.[4,6] This mechanism of injury results in a closed-fist bite — the hand is injured by the teeth of the participant receiving the punch. Another form of human bite injury is an occlusion bite, in which the teeth penetrate the skin directly. These bites, unlike closed-fist bites, tend to occur more in women than in men and often involve the extremities.[4]

Bats

Bats are important for the ecology of many locations, but they pose a particular risk of subtle injury because their small teeth and claws can make a bite or scratch difficult to detect. Thus, caregivers for child or adult victims may not seek medical evaluation and treatment. Bats pose a risk for rabies transmission in every state in the United States, except for Hawaii.

Other Mammals

An estimated 28 million households keep exotic pets, totaling around 45 million animals.[7] The extent of bite injuries from these pets depends on the animal involved and the location of the injury.

Prevention

Prevention is a critical first step in reducing the incidence of injury. Because dog bites account for 80% to 90% of mammalian bites, several studies have shown the benefit of counseling parents and children on dog safety. Recommendations include[2,8]:
- Socializing puppies
- Keeping a distance from unfamiliar dogs
- Visiting a veterinarian regularly
- Leaving dogs alone when they are are eating, sick, in pain, or caring for puppies
- Monitoring children when they are with dogs

CRITICAL DECISION

Which pathogens are associated with mammalian bites?

Mammalian bites are commonly polymicrobial. The bacteria that are most commonly associated with mammalian bites reflect the oral flora of the biting animal, which typically include naturally present organisms, organisms from ingested prey, and organisms from surrounding environments such as water sources or contact surfaces. In the United States, some pathogens from mammalian bites are more likely to be encountered (*Table 1*). Of note, when managing an immunocompromised patient, rarer pathogens should also be considered, such as a *Capnocytophaga* infection, which poses a significant risk of sepsis in asplenic patients and those with hepatic disease.

Other organisms are not as common but should be considered when patients present with systemic illness after a bite event. Tularemia, cat-scratch disease due to *Bartonella* species, and sporotrichosis due to *Sporothrix* species can be caused by cat bites. Cytomegalovirus, herpes simplex virus, and syphilis can all be transmitted by human bites.

Common Mammalian Mouth Flora			
	Dog Bites	Cat Bites	Human Bites
Most Common Pathogen	*Pasteurella canis*	*Pasteurella multocida*	*Streptococcus pyogenes* and *Eikenella corrodens*
Most Common Aerobic Species	*Pasteurella, Staphylococcus,* and *Streptococcus*	*Pasteurella, Staphylococcus,* and *Streptococcus*	*Staphylococcus, Streptococcus,* and *Eikenella*
Most Common Anaerobic Species	*Fusobacterium, Bacteroides, Prevotella, Porphyromonas,* and *Propionibacterium*	*Fusobacterium, Bacteroides, Prevotella, Porphyromonas,* and *Propionibacterium*	*Fusobacterium, Prevotella,* and *Peptostreptococcus*
Special Considerations	Tetanus and rabies	Rabies	Bloodborne viruses: HBV, HCV, and HIV

TABLE 1. Common mammalian mouth flora

CRITICAL DECISION

What are the important clinical manifestations and complications of mammalian bites?

Clinical Considerations

Several factors weigh into the clinical manifestations of mammalian bites and their potential complications. Bite location affects management strategies and infection risk. Preschool-aged children are more likely to be bitten by a dog on the head and face since these structures are typically at the level of a dog's mouth; as children get older, they are more likely to be bitten on their extremities, similar to adults.[1] The source of the bite (human or animal, type of animal) and the timing of the injury both impact the clinical presentation. Treatment is often delayed for feline bites that appear superficial or insignificant until signs of infection are clinically evident. Infection from feline bites is often due to *Pasteurella multocida*, which causes rapid-onset cellulitis with intense localized pain, swelling, and erythema within 12 to 18 hours of the bite.[1,9,10] Canine bites can cause significant tissue destruction, sometimes requiring subspeciality consultation.

When examining bite wounds, physicians must remember that there may be other, less significant wounds that need attention as well. Physical examination should include an overall assessment of the patient's clinical status, including vital signs. Depending on the time elapsed between bite and presentation, abnormal vital signs such as hypotension, respiratory rate abnormalities, and tachycardia can also be signs of sepsis or shock. Physicians should examine the location of the bites and note characteristics of length, width, and depth; puncture versus laceration; drainage; presence of retained foreign body; and extension of any surrounding edema and erythema. Assess for areas of tenderness in the surrounding structures (bones, muscles, joints), as well as lymphadenopathy, especially if there has been a delay in seeking care. A thorough neurovascular examination of the affected area should also be performed. Other components of the physical examination can be conducted as clinically indicated. For example, if the bite is located in the head or neck region, an examination of the scalp and skull should be conducted to assess for signs of fracture. A neurologic examination should also be considered.

Routine imaging of bite wounds is not indicated, but imaging should be considered if there is concern for a retained foreign body or injury complication like an abscess that is not clinically apparent. The prevalence of positive imaging findings in victims of bite wounds is not well reported.[11] However, plain x-rays or ultrasonography may be useful in discovering any retained radiopaque foreign bodies.[11] Ultrasonography is an excellent imaging modality for the detection of an abscess. Advanced imaging such as CT and MRI may be indicated if there is concern for additional traumatic injury (eg, a skull fracture) or an infectious complication (eg, osteomyelitis or a septic joint).[2,11] If the physical examination of an acute bite is consistent with superficial damage and there are no other clinical concerns, imaging is unnecessary.

Potential Complications

Complications from animal bites can occur days to weeks after the initial bite. These include osteomyelitis, tenosynovitis, tendonitis, orbital cellulitis, meningitis, and brain abscess, among others depending on the site of the injury.[1] In these cases, the history and physical examination are especially critical.

Osteomyelitis, for example, often presents with continued swelling and erythema of the involved area, with prolonged fever, or with persistent pain. Tenosynovitis or tendonitis will present similarly but with pain overlying a tendon, significant pain with tendon stretching, or with a mass overlying a tendon sheath.[1]

Patients with closed-fist human bites have a high risk of bone, joint, and tendon infections that can lead to permanent range-of-motion limitations. Violation of the joint capsule can also occur in these injuries, predisposing patients to significant infection. Most commonly, the third digit metacarpophalangeal joint of the dominant hand is affected. After impact with the mouth and teeth, bacterial inoculation occurs. As the person relaxes their hand from the closed to the open position, bacteria can translocate proximally, increasing susceptibility to tendon or deeper infections.[1] Patients with deep hand infections will typically present with significant pain and swelling, and with restricted movement of the digits.[1]

Patients who have suffered bites on the face near the eye or upper cheek can present with ongoing periorbital edema and erythema, pain with extraocular movements, proptosis, visual changes, or other ocular symptoms that suggest an orbital or periorbital infection. Although quite rare, in patients who present with a headache, fever, neck stiffness, or altered mental status, meningitis or intracerebral abscess should be considered.[12]

CRITICAL DECISION

What is the appropriate course of action for wound management in the emergency department?

Initial management begins prior to arrival in the emergency department. This includes cleaning and irrigating the wound with soap and water, pain control with over-the-counter medications, stopping any bleeding, and dressing the wound for transportation to a physician for evaluation. Copious irrigation of the wound is beneficial and should be performed. Tap water has been found to be as effective as sterile saline for this purpose.[4,13] In some cases, these actions will have been performed by EMS personnel or by the victim's family or bystanders.

If possible, information regarding an animal's vaccination status and whereabouts should be obtained by on-scene personnel or the victim's family, and the animal (domestic or wild) should be captured by animal control officers. In the emergency department, it is critical to obtain a thorough history during the evaluation of a bite victim. The circumstances of the bite — what caused the injury, where the victim was when the injury occurred, and when the injury occurred — and what initial aid, if any, was rendered to the victim, as well as other relevant information, such as law enforcement or animal control involvement, should be elicited. Additionally, the patient's pertinent medical history should be obtained, including any underlying medical conditions that can impact management and their immunization status, including their last tetanus vaccination.

Adequate pain control should be initiated. In the pediatric population, intranasal fentanyl at a dose of 2 μg/kg (with a maximum of 100 μg per dose) with or without intranasal midazolam at a dose of 0.2 mg/kg (with a maximum of 10 mg per dose) is an effective, safe, and rapid method for pain control.[14] Mammalian bites should be considered contaminated; therefore, cleaning and copious irrigation with water or saline are indicated. If there is concern that the animal may be rabid, then consider irrigating the wound with diluted povidone-iodine solution.[4] Proper irrigation has the added benefit of assisting the physician with assessing the depth and extension of the bite wound. Any devitalized tissue should be debrided, and the wound should be carefully explored. The physician should consider which wounds are appropriate for primary closure in the emergency department. These can include bites with no underlying injury, bites in immunocompetent patients, bites on the face or scalp, and simple wounds requiring simple single-layer closure.[4,5,8] Facial bites should be thoroughly irrigated, debrided as necessary, and treated with prophylactic antibiotics.[8] These wounds pose a cosmetic risk and are distressing for patients as well as families. Additional scenarios that warrant antibiotic prophylaxis include cat bites; deep puncture wounds; bites to the hand, genital area or in close proximity to a joint; moderate to severe wounds; crush injuries; and bites in immunocompromised patients (*Table 2*).[8] Physicians should also take into account the nature of the wound (location, mechanism, timing) and their comfort level with suturing such a wound.

Bite wounds that are at higher risk of infection and, therefore, not to be closed include heavily contaminated bites; bites to the extremities older than 8 to 12 hours; facial wounds older than 24 hours; bites from cats, humans, monkeys, or livestock; or bites in high-risk patients, such as those with immunocompromising conditions.[4,5,8] In these circumstances, good wound care should be practiced, antibiotics should be provided if clinically indicated, closure should be delayed, and the appropriate subspecialty consultation should be obtained by the physician.

Indications for Antibiotic Therapy
Moderate or severe bite wounds with edema or crush injury
Puncture wounds, especially if penetration of bone, tendon sheath, or joint has occurred
Deep or surgically closed facial wounds
Hand and foot bite wounds
Genital area bite wounds
Wounds in immunocompromised and asplenic people
Wounds with signs of infection
Cat bite wounds

TABLE 2. Indications for antibiotic therapy

Bite wounds should never be sealed with a tissue adhesive, no matter their age, appearance, or location. When suturing bite wounds, remember to provide appropriate local anesthesia. Although injectable anesthetics are generally well tolerated in adult patients, this may not be the case for pediatric patients. Consider the use of a topical anesthetic, such as lidocaine-epinephrine-tetracaine (LET), which is quite effective. Additionally, the use of intranasal medications for pain control may be of benefit.[14] For pediatric patients who are difficult to suture despite appropriate local anesthetic and intranasal medications, consider the use of moderate sedation with an agent such as ketamine.

Antibiotic Therapy

The preferred initial antibiotics for most bite wounds are amoxicillin-clavulanic acid or, if intravenous therapy is used, ampicillin-sulbactam. These cover common aerobic and anaerobic flora in most mammals.[1,5,8] If patients have a penicillin allergy, oral or parenteral treatment with trimethoprim-sulfamethoxazole plus clindamycin is an acceptable alternative.[1,5,8] Coverage for methicillin-resistant *Staphylococcus aureus* (MRSA) should be considered for severe bite wounds or any bite wound in patients with a history of a MRSA infection, especially if a post-bite infection develops. Patients who present with post-bite infections should have any exudate cultured and should be started on antimicrobials appropriate to the clinical situation. Antibiotics should be narrowed once culture results are available.

The duration of antibiotic therapy depends on its purpose. For prophylaxis, a 3- to 5-day course is sufficient, with close monitoring within 24 to 48 hours of initial evaluation for signs and symptoms of infection. If there is evidence of soft tissue infection, 7 to 14 days of therapy is indicated, depending on the severity and whether an abscess is present. If the bone or joint is involved, a 4- to 6-week course of antibiotics will likely be required.[1,5,15]

CRITICAL DECISION

When is it appropriate to provide prophylaxis for rabies and tetanus?

Rabies Postexposure Prophylaxis: General Principles

Rabies is caused by RNA viruses of the rhabdoviridae family and is transmitted in saliva or infected tissues (brain and nervous system), usually after a bite. Urine, feces, and blood are not considered infective. The virus causes devastating effects on the CNS, producing a progressive

Rabies Prophylaxis Recommendations	
Action	**Management**
Wound cleaning	All wounds should be thoroughly cleaned and irrigated with soap and water.
Human rabies immune globulin (HRIG)	If possible, the full dose (20 IU/kg) should be infiltrated around any wounds; any remaining volume should be administered IM at an anatomic site distant from vaccine administration.
Rabies vaccine	HDCV or PCECV 1 mL, IM (deltoid area or, for pediatric patients, the anterolateral thigh), one each on days 0, 3, 7, and 14. For immunocompromised individuals, a fifth dose may be given on day 28.

TABLE 3. Rabies prophylaxis recommendations (no prior vaccine)

Rabies Prophylaxis Recommendations	
Action	**Management**
Wound cleaning	All wounds should be thoroughly cleaned and irrigated with soap and water.
Human rabies immunoglobulin (HRIG)	Not indicated
Rabies vaccine	HDCV or PCECV 1 mL, IM (deltoid area or, for pediatric patients, the anterolateral thigh), one each on days 0 and 3.

TABLE 4. Rabies prophylaxis recommendations (previously vaccinated)

encephalomyelitis. Once a patient is symptomatic, rabies is almost always fatal. The incubation period can last from a few days to several months. During the prodromal phase, patients can present with nonspecific respiratory and GI symptoms. This is typically followed by an acute neurologic phase that is marked by nuchal rigidity, convulsions, marked agitation, hallucinations, and other bizarre behaviors such as hydrophobia or aerophobia.[16]

In the Unites States, rabies is usually confined to wild animals (more than 90% of cases), and there are robust rabies surveillance and control programs.[17,18] Almost every state in the United States has statutes mandating rabies vaccination for domestic animals. Among domestic animals, cats account for most reported rabies cases. Rodents and lagomorphs (eg, rabbits and pikas) can theoretically carry rabies; however, rabies infection among these animals is exceedingly rare, and there has been no known case of human transmission after a bite from animals in these groups. A recent report highlighted a mild increase in wild animal cases during the reporting period, particularly among bats, racoons, foxes, and skunks. Texas, Virginia, Pennsylvania, North Carolina, Colorado, and New York accounted for almost half of all rabid animal cases reported in 2018.[18] The US Department of Agriculture has been using fixed-wing aircraft since the mid-1990s to spread oral rabies vaccine to wildlife and has been successful in reducing cases (especially for coyotes, foxes, and racoons), with efforts that continue to this day.[18] Cases of rabies in humans are rare, with 1 to 3 cases reported annually, but up to 55,000 patients in the United States each year are treated with the rabies postexposure prophylaxis regimen.[17,18]

In all patients, postexposure management begins with thorough cleaning and copious irrigation of the wound. Postexposure prophylaxis should be given to any patient with potential or confirmed exposure to rabies. The regimen given depends on whether patients previously had the rabies prophylaxis series or not. It consists of the rabies vaccine (either human diploid cell vaccine [HDCV] or purified chick embryo cell vaccine [PCEC]) and human rabies immune globulin (HRIG) given on days 0, 3, 7, and 14. HRIG is dosed at 20 IU/kg, irrespective of the age of the patient. As much immune globulin as possible is infiltrated directly around the wound, and any remaining volume is administered intramuscularly in a location distant from the vaccination site. If the patient previously had postexposure prophylaxis, no immune globulin is indicated, and the rabies vaccine is administered only on days 0 and 3. (*Tables 3* and *4*).

Bats, skunks, racoons, coyotes, foxes, and wild mammals in general should be considered rabid, and prophylaxis should be given for all bites from these species unless it is known that there is no rabies in the area or the animal can be captured and tested.[15] Postexposure prophylaxis is not indicated if the bite came from a vaccinated domestic dog or cat, or in cases of unknown vaccination status, the dog or cat is well appearing and can be captured and observed for 10 days. If the animal develops signs of rabies infection, then prophylaxis should be immediately given. Wild animals should be assumed to be rabid and prophylaxis should be initiated while laboratory confirmation of rabies is pending if the animal is captured. If the bite involves a rodent or lagomorph or other domesticated animal, prophylaxis is generally not indicated, although if there is any question, physicians can consult their local or state health departments. In general, if there is any concern about rabies exposure, prophylaxis should be offered to the patient. Rabies is a reportable disease and emergency department physicians should work with their local health authorities regarding testing when appropriate.

✔ Pearls

- A thorough history and physical examination should be conducted on all patients who sustain mammalian bite wounds. Particular attention should be given to ensure the wound does not involve deep structures that may require subspecialty consultation. Practice good wound care in the emergency department by cleaning with soap and water and copious irrigation.

- Not all bite wounds require antibiotic prophylaxis, but patients with bites from dogs or cats should be prescribed appropriate coverage.

- Update tetanus immunizations for patients seeking care for mammalian bite wounds in the emergency department.

- Provide patients and families with information about animal bite prevention as part of their discharge instructions.

	Clean, Minor Wounds		All Other Wounds	
Number of previous tetanus doses	DTaP, Tdap	TIG	DTaP, Tdap	TIG
< 3 or unknown	Yes	No	Yes	Yes
> 3	No (if < 10 yrs since last dose)	No	No (if < 5 yrs since last dose)	No
	Yes (if > 10 yrs since last dose)	No	Yes (if > 5 years since last dose)	No

In children < 7 years, DTaP is preferred.
In adults and children > 7 years, Tdap is preferred.
Adapted from: The American Academy of Pediatrics' Red Book 2021-2024.
Report of the Committee on Infectious Disease. 32nd edition.

TABLE 5. Tetanus prophylaxis recommendations

Rabies Postexposure Prophylaxis: Specific Populations

The CDC recommends pre-exposure prophylaxis in high-risk populations, including veterinarians, veterinarian technicians, some international travelers, and some laboratory workers, among other groups.[17] These groups are given three doses of the vaccine on days 0, 7, and 21 or 28. If the individual has a potential exposure in the future, HRIG will not be indicated, and the abbreviated postexposure vaccination schedule will be followed.

Rabies vaccine is quite well tolerated, especially in pediatric patients. In adults, common side effects include mild localized reactions at the injection site, such as pain, erythema, and swelling; mild systemic reactions such as headache and myalgia have also been observed.

Tetanus Prophylaxis

Tetanus is caused by a neurotoxin produced by *Clostridium tetani* and can manifest in several clinical forms, including generalized and local tetanus. The organism is found throughout the world, inhabiting soil as well as animal intestinal tracts. With the advent of very effective immunization, particularly in countries with robust immunization programs, tetanus infection is not commonly seen. Animal bites do increase the risk of tetanus exposure, and ensuring adequate protection is an essential component of appropriate patient care. There are four forms of the disease: neonatal, localized, cephalic, and generalized, with generalized disease accounting for more than 80% of cases.[19] Generalized tetanus presents between 3 and 21 days after infection with cephalocaudal spread of muscle spasms that ultimately result in lockjaw and opisthotonos; death can occur quickly from diaphragmatic spasm or laryngospasm.[19] Management of tetanus involves supportive care and the administration of a single dose of tetanus immune globulin (TIG). This is effective in halting disease progression but not in reversing the effects of the toxin. Notably, tetanus is entirely preventable due to an effective immunization.

There are recommended tetanus immunization schedules for pediatric patients in the United States, as well as routine booster schedules.[15] Patients of any age who present to the emergency department with an animal wound should be asked about their tetanus vaccination status. If their vaccination status is not up to date, the tetanus immunization should be offered. The regimen given depends on the number of immunizations previously received and whether the wound is clean and minor (*Table 5*). Like the rabies vaccine, the tetanus vaccine is generally well tolerated, with common side effects including local reactions such as pain and swelling at the injection site.

Other Postexposure Prophylaxis Considerations

Patients bitten by other humans should have their hepatitis B immunization status checked. A nonimmunized patient who has been bitten by a person who is known to have hepatitis B or whose hepatitis status is unknown should be vaccinated against hepatitis B and be given hepatitis B immune globulin.[19]

CRITICAL DECISION

What factors determine appropriate patient disposition?

Predicting which mammalian bite patients will do well and which will not can be difficult. Most cases of mammalian bites that show no evidence of deep tissue infection or deep structure involvement at initial presentation can be discharged from the emergency department with appropriate management, including return precautions and follow-up. Subspecialty consultation should be considered in cases of lacerations that involve deep structures of the face or extremities, vascular injury, associated fractures, or complex facial lacerations. In some instances, hospital admission may be indicated. Patients with signs of moderate to severe infection, including systemic symptoms, will benefit from intravenous antibiotic therapy in addition to local wound care. Other patients who are candidates for admission include those who require operative intervention, such as cases of complex tenosynovitis or deep tissue infection, and those with underlying medical conditions (eg, immunocompromised states or diabetes). Special consideration for admission should be given to patients with cat bites to the hand or digits. These wounds are notorious for rapid deterioration from infection and can lead to significant morbidity, especially when presentation is delayed.[10] If there are concerns for medication compliance, lack of follow-up, or other extenuating circumstances, brief admission to initiate antibiotic therapy and arrange proper follow-up is reasonable.

Summary

Mammalian bites are a common reason to seek care in the emergency department. A thorough history and physical examination assist with appropriate management decisions. Radiographic studies are usually not indicated but may be ordered for select cases. Providing good wound care while in the emergency department and administering timely antibiotic treatment and rabies prophylaxis, when appropriate, will help ensure good patient outcomes.

CASE RESOLUTIONS

■ CASE ONE

There were no signs of a fracture or retained foreign body. The wounds did not require repair, but were thoroughly cleaned and irrigated. The parents were instructed in proper wound management and were provided strict return precautions. A 7-day course of amoxicillin-clavulanic acid was prescribed, and the parents were instructed to have the patient follow-up with his primary care physician within 48 hours. Tetanus vaccination was not indicated. The social worker assisted with reporting the incident to animal control. The child's parents confirmed with the dog's owners that the dog's immunizations were up to date and the animal was at home. Arrangements were made to have the dog observed for the next 10 days for any signs that may indicate rabies infection.

The child completed his antibiotic course and did well. The dog exhibited no signs of rabies during the observation period.

■ CASE TWO

The physician recognized that a bat exposure associated witih face scratches potentially indicated a radbies exposure. Rabies prophylaxis was recommended, including HRIG. The child was given the standard rabies vaccine dose (1 mL in the anterolateral aspect of the thigh) and HRIG (20 IU/kg), and arrangements were made for the family to return on days 3, 7, and 14 for the remaining vaccine doses. The child was up to date with her tetanus immunizations and did not require additional vaccine or TIG.

The family returned as instructed and completed the rabies vaccine course. The child did well, but the bat was never found.

■ CASE THREE

Although the physician was experienced with laceration repair, the injury was complex and at high risk for poor cosmetic and infectious outcomes. The patient was given pain medication and intravenous antibiotics (ampicillin-sulbactam), while plastic surgery was consulted. The surgeon agreed to take the patient to the operating suite for a thorough washout and repair of the wound. Before leaving the emergency department, the patient was given a dose of tetanus vaccine because his last dose was 11 years ago, and discussion was had about rabies prophylaxis for an unprovoked dog bite. The patient ultimately refused the rabies series.

After surgical repair, he was discharged with wound care instructions and 7 days of prophylactic amoxicillin-clavulanic acid and ultimately did well.

REFERENCES

1. Bula-Rudas FJ, Olcott JL. Human and animal bites. *Pediatr Rev.* 2018 ct;39(10):490-500.

2. Ellis R, Ellis C. Dog and cat bites. *Am Fam Physician.* 2014;90(4):239-243.

3. Cook JA, Sasor SE, Soleimani T, et al. An epidemiological analysis of pediatric dog bite injuries over a decade. *J Surg Res.* 2020 Feb;246:231-235.

4. Edens MA, Michel JA, Jones N. Mammalian bites in the emergency department: recommendations for wounds closure, antibiotics, and postexposure prophylaxis. *Emerg Med Pract.* 2016;18(4):1-20.

5. Hurt JB, Maday KR. Management and treatment of animal bites. *JAAPA.* 2018 Apr;31(4):27-31.

6. Harrison M. A 4-year review of human bite injuries presenting to emergency medicine and proposed evidence-based guidelines. *Injury.* 2009;40(8):826-830.

7. Smith KM, Smith KF, D'Auria JP. Exotic pets: health and safety issues for children and parents. *J Pediatr Health Care.* 2012;26(2):e2-e6.

8. Rasmussen D, Landon A, Powell J, Brown GR. Evaluating and treating mammalian bites. *JAAPA.* 2017 Mar;30(3):32-36.

9. Abrahamian FM, Goldstein EJC. Microbiology of animal bite wound infections. *Clinical Microbiology Reviews.* 2011;24(2):231-246.

10. Kheiran A, Palial V, Rollett R, et al. Cat bite: an injury not to underestimate. *J Plast Surg Hand Surg.* 2019 Dec;53(6):341-346.

11. Young PM, Bancroft LW, Peterson JJ, et al. Imaging spectrum of bites, stings, and their complications: pictorial review. *AJR Am J Roentgenol.* 2009 Sep;193(3 suppl):S31-41.

12. Zajkowska J, Król M, Falkowski D, et al. Capnocytophaga canimorsus – an underestimated danger after dog or cat bite – review of literature. *Przegl Epidemiol.* 2016;70(2):289-295.

13. Moscati RM, Mayrose J, Reardon RF, et al. A multicenter comparison of tap water versus sterile saline for wound irrigation. *Acad Emerg Med.* 2007 May;14(5):404-409.

14. Ryan PM, Kienstra AJ, Cosgrove P, Vezzetti R, Wilkinson M. Safety and effectiveness of intranasal midazolam and fentanyl used in combination in the pediatric emergency department. *Am J Emerg Med.* 2019 Feb;37(2):237-240.

15. Committee on Infectious Diseases, American Academy of Pediatrics; Bite wounds. In: Kimberlin DW, Barnett ED, Lynfield R, Sawyer M, eds. *Red Book: 2021-2024 Report of the Committee on Infectious Diseases.* 32nd edition. American Academy of Pediatrics; 2021;169-175.

16. Chitra S. Mani, Dennis L. Murray. Rabies. *Pediatrics in Review.* 2006 Apr;27(4) 129-136.

17. Rabies status: assessment by country. Centers for Disease Control and Prevention. https://www.cdc.gov/rabies/resources/countries-risk.html

18. Ma X, Monroe BP, Cleaton JM, et al. Rabies surveillance in the United States during 2018. *JAMA.* 2020 Jan;256(2):195-208.

19. Rhinesmith E, Fu L. Tetanus disease, treatment, management. *Pediatrics in Review* 2018 Aug;39(8): 430-432.

✖ Pitfalls

- Failing to recognize that bite wounds from bats, racoons, foxes, skunks, or coyotes are at risk for rabies transmission.

- Administering rabies prophylaxis for all dog and cat bites. If the animal that bit the patient can be observed for 10 days, prophylaxis is not indicated unless the animal exhibits signs of or is confirmed to have rabies.

- Suturing wounds from animal bites without thoroughly cleaning and irrigating the wound prior to closure.

- Failing to thoroughly inspect wounds or to consider radiographic imaging when there is a possibility of associated fracture or a retained foreign body.

Atrial Bigeminy

By Amal Mattu, MD, FACEP
Dr. Mattu is a professor, vice chair, and director of the
Emergency Cardiology Fellowship in the Department
of Emergency Medicine at the University of Maryland
School of Medicine in Baltimore.

Objective

On completion of this article, you should be able to:
■ Recognize atrial bigeminy on an ECG.

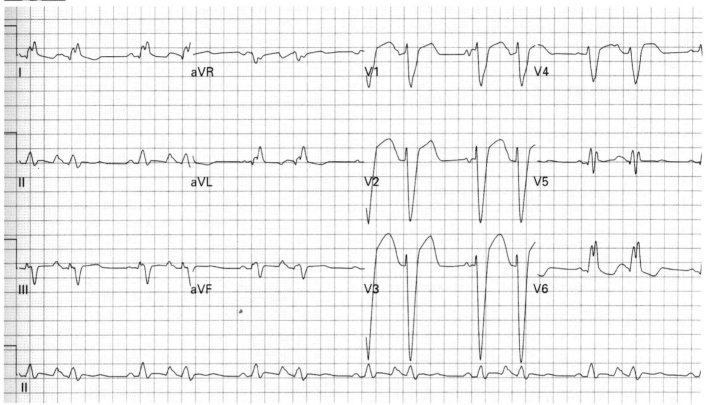

FIGURE 1. A 65-year-old man with palpitations

The ECG depicts a sinus rhythm with premature atrial contractions (PACs) in a pattern of atrial bigeminy, rate 75, nonspecific intraventricular conduction delay. The QRS complexes appear in groups of two and are separated by brief pauses that create a regularly irregular rhythm. The presence of grouped beats, or regular irregularity, is usually the result of either PACs or second-degree atrioventricular block (Mobitz I or II). In this case, the second QRS in each group is preceded by a P wave that differs in morphology from its predecessor. This second P-QRS complex is also followed by a short pause, which is characteristic of a PAC. In fact, the most common overall cause of a pause in the cardiac rhythm is a preceding PAC. When every second QRS complex is the result of a PAC, atrial bigeminy is diagnosed. The QRS complexes are markedly wide. The differential diagnosis of wide QRS complexes includes hypothermia, hyperkalemia, Wolff-Parkinson-White syndrome, aberrant ventricular conduction (eg, bundle branch block), ventricular ectopy, paced beats, and certain medications. In the absence of diagnostic criteria for any of the above, the term "nonspecific intraventricular conduction delay" is used. Although the QRS complexes resemble a left bundle branch

block (LBBB), the presence of Q waves, even small ones, in the lateral leads excludes the diagnosis of LBBB (*Figure 2*).

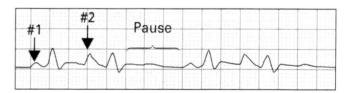

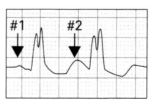

FIGURE 2. Premature atrial contractions in a bigeminy pattern. Note the presence of two different P-wave morphologies (#1 and #2) as well as the compensatory pause. P wave #1 likely results from a sinus node–originated beat, while P wave #2 results from an ectopic atrial focus.

From **Mattu A, Brady W.** *ECGs for the Emergency Physician 2.* BMJ Publishing. Reprinted with permission.

Twisting Intestines: Bilious Emesis

By Heather Jones, DO; Zachary Burroughs, MD; and Ann Dietrich, MD

Prisma Health-Upstate, Greenville, South Carolina

Reviewed by Sharon Mace, MD, FACEP

Objective

On completion of this article, you should be able to:

- Recall the differential diagnosis for bilious emesis in the pediatric population.

CASE PRESENTATION

A 5-day-old boy (full term, no significant medical history) presents with vomiting. His parent reports that the patient had been vomiting for the past few days and got progressively worse. By the time of presentation, his oral intake has decreased to only 1 ounce instead of his usual 2 to 3 ounces. At his pediatrician's office on the same day that he presented to the emergency department, the infant's weight was down 10% from his birth weight.

His vital signs include P 177, R 52, and T 36.9°C (98.4°F); his SpO$_2$ is 98% on room air. On examination, he has a slightly sunken anterior fontanelle, a global decrease in tone, and a distended abdomen, which makes him fussy when palpated. There are no masses or hepatosplenomegaly, and he has a normal capillary refill time. The infant's bib at bedside reveals bilious emesis (*Figure 1*).

Discussion

Infants can present with vomiting for a variety of reasons. Color and context of the vomitus are important factors for narrowing down causes. Vomitus often has a slight yellow tinge, but any green or bright yellow vomitus contains a large amount of bile and is considered bilious.[1] Bilious emesis in a child younger than 1 year should prompt evaluation for obstructive lesions including duodenal atresia, Hirschsprung disease, meconium ileus, and malrotation with volvulus. Any neonate with vomiting warrants a careful history that focuses on onset and duration of vomiting, nature of the vomitus, associated GI symptoms, and involvement of other organ systems.[2]

Duodenal atresia classically presents with bilious emesis and without abdominal distention. Maternal history may reveal polyhydramnios that was caused by the distal intestine's inability to absorb amniotic fluid. Diagnosis can be made with plain x-rays that show a double bubble sign. Distal small bowel atresia, jejunal or ileal, typically presents with bilious vomiting and abdominal distention 12 to 24 hours after feeding is initiated. Eighty percent of infants with distal atretic segments fail to pass meconium in the first 24 hours of life. The differential diagnosis for failure to pass meconium within the first 48 hours of life includes intestinal atresia, meconium ileus, and Hirschsprung disease. Meconium ileus typically presents in infants with cystic fibrosis. Meconium becomes impacted in the terminal ileum and leads to a partial obstruction due to its increased viscosity from a lack of chloride transporters. Both intestinal atresia and meconium ileus must be differentiated from long-segment Hirschsprung.[3] Hirschsprung disease results from the failure of ganglion cells to migrate into the bowel wall.[4] Plain x-rays of intestinal atresia and long-segment Hirschsprung classically show multiple air-fluid levels that are proximal to the obstruction in the upright or lateral decubitus position. In the setting of meconium ileus, air-fluid levels are less likely to be seen due to the high viscosity of the meconium, but haziness or a ground-glass appearance may be seen in the right lower quadrant. Contrast studies are often required to reach a definitive diagnosis because the small and large bowel of neonates are difficult to distinguish. Water soluble enemas are useful in differentiating atresia from meconium ileus and Hirschsprung disease. A small colon suggests an obstruction that is proximal to the ileocecal valve. Abdominal ultrasound can distinguish meconium ileus from ileal atresia and can identify concomitant intestinal malrotation.[3] Rectal biopsy remains the gold standard in the diagnosis of Hirschsprung disease.[4]

Midgut volvulus is defined as a segment of intestine that twists on itself, which leads to an obstruction and

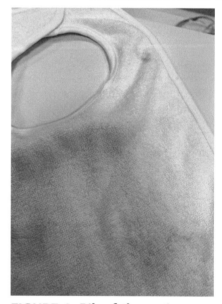

FIGURE 1. Bib of the patient upon presentation to the emergency department

reduced blood flow to the involved segment. Midgut malrotation is a defect in the normal embryonic rotation of the gut. Volvulus can occur independently of malrotation, but malrotation increases the risk of volvulus in infants and children. Volvulus secondary to malrotation typically presents in the first few weeks of life, with approximately 60% of cases occurring prior to 1 year old.[5]

The presentation of malrotation depends on the age and acuity of the case. Acute cases present with emesis that is classically bilious, but it can be nonbilious. Abdominal distention is a late finding in acute cases. Hemodynamic instability and hematochezia can occur over the first few hours of presentation. In older children and adults, presentation can be more variable. A small portion of patients with malrotation may present with chronic, intermittent obstructive symptoms, including abdominal pain and bilious vomiting. Infants with malrotation can present with failure to thrive and reflux symptoms.[5]

Pathophysiology

During embryonic development, the intestines develop in three portions: the foregut, midgut, and hindgut. At 4 to 6 weeks' gestation, the midgut develops rapidly, herniates into the umbilical cord, and returns to the abdominal cavity around the 8th to 10th week after undergoing a 270° counterclockwise rotation around the blood supply. Genetic mutations in the BCL6 gene affect the signaling pathway of normal gut rotation and can lead to a variety of midgut malrotation types including nonrotation, incomplete rotation, reverse rotation, and anomalous fixation of the mesentery. The most common type is nonrotation. Midgut malrotation is estimated to occur in around 1 in 6000 live births.[5] The ligament of Treitz is absent in malrotation, which causes an absence of the duodenal C loop and the presence of the duodenum to the right of the spine with the jejunum coiled in the right upper quadrant. The cecum is also not fixed and usually resides in the right upper quadrant.[2]

Complications

If diagnosis or surgical intervention is delayed, mesenteric ischemia can lead to gangrene of the small bowel. Once necrosis of the bowel occurs, resection is required. If necrosis and subsequent resection are extensive enough, short bowel syndrome can occur, which puts patients at risk of a variety of nutritional deficiencies. With early surgical correction, patients may experience slow return of bowel function, which may delay initiation of enteral nutrition. Some patients may require prolonged courses of total parenteral nutrition (TPN).[5]

Management

Diagnosis and management of intestinal volvulus are dictated by clinical presentation. For cases of intestinal perforation, physical examination findings of abdominal distention, rebound, or guarding may be present and indicate peritonitis. Rapid resuscitation and emergent operative exploration are indicated when peritonitis or sustained hemodynamic instability is present. If patients are hemodynamically stable, the diagnosis of intestinal obstruction with volvulus can be confirmed with radiological evaluation such as abdominal plain x-rays or an upper GI and small bowel follow-through. Nasogastric decompression can be initiated, and electrolyte disturbances should be corrected prior to surgery. Broad-spectrum antibiotics should also be administered prophylactically.[4]

The Ladd procedure is performed to reduce the volvulus. This procedure involves rotating the bowel counterclockwise, dividing the mesenteric (Ladd) bands, placing the small bowel on the right side and the large bowel on the left side of the abdomen, and performing an appendectomy. The procedure does not correct malrotation but widens the mesenteric pedicle to reduce the future risk of volvulus. Bowel viability is assessed, and resection is performed as indicated.[6]

FIGURE 2. Upper GI showing proximal duodenum is mildly dilated with tapering of the duodenum resulting in beaklike configuration of the proximal transverse duodenum. There is evidence of high-grade obstruction at this point, but a small amount contrast passed more distally making a caudal and rightward turn before refluxing back into the proximal duodenum. Configuration consistent with malrotation with midgut volvulus.

CASE RESOLUTION

An intravenous line was established, and a normal saline bolus was given. Initial laboratory tests and imaging were obtained, with laboratory values significant for a markedly elevated procalcitonin of 20 ng/mL and C-reactive protein level of 270 mg/L. A two-view abdominal series showed air-fluid levels that were concerning for obstruction. An upper GI series was obtained and showed high-grade duodenal obstruction with configuration consistent with malrotation with midgut volvulus. Given concern for midgut volvulus, surgery was consulted, and the patient was emergently taken to the operating room for an exploratory laparotomy. The patient was found to have a 720° volvulus, and 35 cm of necrotic small bowel was resected. An ostomy and mucous fistula were created. He was transferred to the pediatric ICU postoperatively for continued ventilatory support and prophylactic antibiotics. He was extubated on the second postoperative day and was started on enteral feeds the next day after bowel function returned. His hospital course was complicated by high ostomy output, for which he required TPN. The patient was able to undergo ostomy reversal 6 weeks after his initial operation and was discharged home a week later on full oral feeds.

REFERENCES

1. Lorenzo CD. Approach to the infant or child with nausea and vomiting . UpToDate. https://www.uptodate.com/contents/approach-to-the-infant-or-child-with-nausea-and-vomiting
2. Rus MC, Doughty CB. Vomiting. In: Shaw KN, Bachur RG, Chamberlain J, Lavelle J, Nagler J, Shook JE, eds. *Fleisher & Ludwig's Textbook of Pediatric Emergency Medicine.* 8th edition. Wolters Kluwer; 2020:548-555.
3. Kliegman R, Stanton BWS, Schor NF, Behrman RE, Nelson WE. Intestinal atresia, stenosis, and malrotation. In: Kliegman R, ed. *Nelson Textbook of Pediatrics.* 21st edition. Elsevier; 2020:1950-1953.
4. Kliegman R, Stanton BWS, Schor NF, Behrman RE, Nelson WE. Motility disorders and Hirschsprung disease. In: Kliegman R., ed. *Nelson Textbook of Pediatrics.* 21st edition. Elsevier; 2020:1955-1965.
5. Coste AH, Anand S, Nada H, Ahmad H. Midgut volvulus. StatPearls. Updated September 12, 2022. https://www.ncbi.nlm.nih.gov/books/NBK441962/
6. Alani M, Rentea RM. Midgut malrotation. StatPearls. Updated August 1, 2022. https://www.ncbi.nlm.nih.gov/books/NBK560888/

Established Status Epilepticus Treatment Trial (ESETT)

By Mallori Wilson, MD, LT, MC, USN; and Daphne P. Morrison Ponce, MD, CDR, MC, USN
Naval Medical Center, Portsmouth, Virginia

Reviewed by Andrew Eyre, MD, MS-HPEd

Objective

On completion of this article, you should be able to:

■ Discuss the use of anticonvulsant medications for status epilepticus.

Kapur J, Elm J, Chamberlain JM, et al. Randomized trial of three anticonvulsant medications for status epilepticus. *NEJM.* 2019 Nov; 381(22):2103-2113.

KEY POINTS

■ Morbidity and mortality associated with status epilepticus are reduced with early seizure cessation.

■ Fosphenytoin, levetiracetam, and valproate resulted in seizure termination within 60 minutes of drug infusion completion in approximately 50% of patients.

■ One-third of patients do not respond to appropriately dosed benzodiazepines for convulsive seizures.

The morbidity and mortality associated with status epilepticus are reduced with early seizure cessation. Up to one-third of seizures are benzodiazepine refractory, and only fosphenytoin is FDA-approved for benzodiazepine-refractory status epilepticus in adults; no such drug is FDA-approved for the pediatric population. Potential treatments are not well studied, so Kapur et al aimed to compare the efficacy and safety of three of the most common antiepileptics in adults and children in the emergency department.

The authors conducted a multicenter, prospective, randomized, double-blinded, superiority-inferiority clinical trial to compare the effectiveness and safety of fosphenytoin, levetiracetam, and valproate. Patients older than 2 years were enrolled in emergency departments across 57 hospitals in the United States once they had generalized convulsive seizures that lasted longer than 5 minutes or recurred within 30 minutes after appropriate benzodiazepine treatment. Patients were excluded for trauma, hypoglycemia, hyperglycemia, cardiac arrest, pregnancy, incarceration, having already received a nonbenzodiazepine antiepileptic, or an allergy or contraindication to the trial medications.

Following appropriate benzodiazepine dosing, study participants received one of the trial drugs from a "use next" medication box that was age stratified. The trial drugs of fosphenytoin (20 mgPE/kg, max 1,500 mgPE), levetiracetam (60 mg/kg, max 4,500 mg), or valproate (40 mg/kg, max 3,000 mg) were administered as infusions via pumps programmed over 10 minutes with a predetermined rate. Rescue therapy was administered, if clinically indicated, 20 minutes after trial treatment was completed.

The primary efficacy outcome was termination of clinical seizures with improved responsiveness 60 minutes after the trial treatment was completed without the need for additional antiepileptic therapy. The primary safety outcome was a composite of life-threatening hypotension and arrhythmia. The secondary efficacy outcomes

included time to seizure cessation (when audio recording was available), ICU admission, ICU length of stay, and hospital length of stay. The secondary safety outcomes included death, intubation within 1 hour after starting the trial drug, recurrent seizure 1 hour after starting the trial drug, and anaphylaxis.

Randomization was conducted via response-adaptive comparative effectiveness design. The first planned interim analysis was at 400 enrollments, with the potential for early trial cessation if criteria for success or futility were met. The primary analysis was based on the intention-to-treat population (unique patients for efficacy and all enrollments for safety).

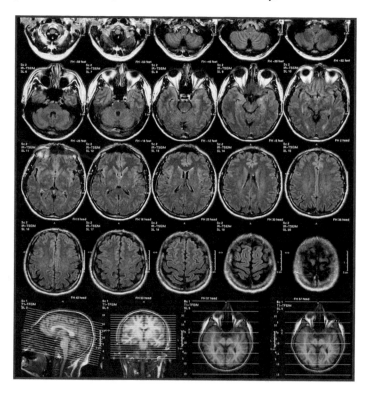

The fosphenytoin (n = 118), levetiracetam (n = 145), and valproate (n = 121) groups had similar baseline characteristics. Eligibility criteria deviation was 27% and included the following factors: timing of trial drug to benzodiazepine administration (50 patients), inadequate cumulative benzodiazepine dose (26 patients), enrollment of patients without status epilepticus (33 patients). The majority of enrollments (87%) had a final diagnosis of status epilepticus; 10% had a final diagnosis of nonepileptic seizure.

The primary efficacy outcome was achieved in 45% of the fosphenytoin, 47% of the levetiracetam, and 46% of the valproate group. The primary safety outcome was not statistically significant, with life-threatening hypotension or arrhythmia in 3.2% of the fosphenytoin, 1.3% of the levetiracetam, and 1.6% of the valproate group. Only 39 patients met the primary efficacy outcome and had audio recordings, which was used to determine seizure duration. The median time from drug start to seizure cessation was 11.7 minutes for fosphenytoin, 10.5 minutes for levetiracetam, and 7.0 minutes for valproate. Similarly, seizure recurrence and other safety outcomes did not differ significantly.

There was no significant difference in seizure termination among the three treatment groups, with approximately half of patients meeting the primary outcome in each group. There was also no significant difference in safety, although intubation and hypotension were more common with fosphenytoin and death was more frequent with levetiracetam. Prior observational studies showed varying efficacies among these three drugs. The limitations of this study include unblinding (although it mostly occurred after the primary outcome was determined); the relatively large enrollment of nonepileptic seizure diagnoses (10%); determining seizure cessation clinically instead of based on EEG findings; determining dosing from published experience, with the most-efficacious dosing unknown; more restrictive maximum-rate infusion of fosphenytoin, limiting the maximum dose for patients over 75 kg; not recording nonserious adverse events more than 24 hours after enrollment; and large eligibility deviations (primarily due to benzodiazepine's timing or dosing).

Disclosure

We are military service members. This work was prepared as part of our official duties. Title 17 U.S.C. § 105 provides that "Copyright protection under this title is not available for any work of the United States Government." Title 17 U.S.C. § 101 defines a United States Government work as a work prepared by a military service member or employee of the United States Government as part of that person's official duties.

The views expressed in this review article are those of the authors and do not necessarily reflect the official policy or position of the Department of the Navy, Department of Defense, or the United States Government.

Critical Decisions in Emergency Medicine's series of LLSA reviews features articles from ABEM's 2021 Lifelong Learning and Self-Assessment Reading List. Available online at acep.org/moc/llsa and on the ABEM website.

Closed Thoracic Lavage Rewarming

By Steven Warrington, MD, MEd
MercyOne Siouxland, Sioux City, Iowa

Objective

On completion of this article, you should be able to:

- Disscuss closed thoracic lavage for hypothermia.

Introduction

There are many active and passive methods of rewarming the hypothermic patient, with active rewarming generally used for symptomatic or arresting individuals. In patients with cardiac arrest, active extracorporeal blood warming with cardiopulmonary bypass may be the best option but may not be readily available at all locations. In those situations, other methods of active, or invasive, rewarming, such as thoracic lavage, may be considered.

Contraindications

- Mild or moderate hypothermia that may respond to less invasive measures without a poor outcome
- Significant coagulopathy
- Infection overlying sites of insertion
- Known pleurodesis or other known significant adhesion of the lung pleura to the thoracic pleura

Benefits and Risks

Thoracic lavage is beneficial because it rewarms faster than less invasive techniques due to the large, vascularized body surface area involved. Additionally, compared to extracorporeal blood warming, it can be performed without significant equipment or personnel aside from what is readily available in the emergency department.

Risks include those attributed to the procedure of tube thoracostomy. It is difficult to determine whether complications come from this procedure or from concomitant physiologic changes and damage from hypothermia and associated comorbidties. Some suggest that chest tubes on the left side can increase the risk of dysrhythmias or decrease the impact of closed chest compressions on arrested patients' circulation. Acute respiratory distress syndrome, pneumonia, and renal failure have all been documented in patients with arrest and thoracic lavage.

Alternatives

The technique described is a two-chest-tube system; however, there are also single-chest-tube techniques of closed thoracic lavage, as well as open thoracic lavage for rewarming. Single-tube techniques rely on infusion and suction, with time to allow for energy transfer. Open thoracic lavage is similar to performing a thoracotomy (without entering the pericardium)and uses warmed fluids over the heart and in the hemithorax, adding suction to allow for repeated boluses of warmed fluids.

Peritoneal lavage is another invasive alternative that involves a large body surface area to aid in rapid rewarming. Extracorporeal blood warming is an alternative that can be done with a bypass or dialysis system if available. There are also passive rewarming techniques such as warm air convection systems, inhalational air, and gastric or bladder lavages.

Reducing Side Effects

Sterile technique and saline are recommended for use, although some literature suggest that tap water may not significantly increase infection rates when used for lavage.

Special Considerations

Thoracic lavage requires large amounts of warmed saline, which ideally would be readily available with commercial warming equipment. In reality, most departments will not readily have the volume of warmed saline required for the intervention, but 1-liter bags of saline warmed in a standard microwave have reportedly been used. Warm a bag of saline in the microwave for 60 seconds, agitate (shake) it to distribute heat evenly, heat for another 60 seconds, and agitate once more. The saline should be at least 38°C (reported as 38.3°C in a 650-W microwave). Some literature recommend infusing solutions up to 42°C for rewarming.

Invasive techniques like thoracic lavage are generally reserved for patients with severe (ie, <30°C) hypothermia. Those without severe hypothermia but with significant dysrhythmias from hypothermia may also benefit from thoracic lavage. Other measures can be started simultaneously, such as warmed intravenous fluids, air convection systems, inhaled warmed air, or lavage of other spaces (eg, bladder, stomach, peritoneal cavity). Additionally, in some cases, open thoracic lavage may

TECHNIQUES

1. **Determine** if the patient requires invasive rewarming and if closed thoracic lavage will be performed.
2. **Consider** instituting passive rewarming while preparing for closed thoracic lavage.
3. **Place** the first chest tube anterior and superior, around the second to fourth intercostal space in the midclavicular line.
4. **Place** a second chest tube inferior and posterior, around the fifth to sixth intercostal space in the midposterior axillary line.
5. **Infuse** warmed fluids through the anterior superior chest tube while allowing it to drain from the posterior inferior tube.
6. **Monitor** "in" and "out" fluid amounts.
7. **Consider** if thoracic lavage of the contralateral side may provide benefit and, if so, repeat the above steps.
8. **Remove** the anterior superior tube when finished and close the site. Leave the posterior inferior tube to allow drainage. Dress the site as appropriate.

be indicated over closed lavage, such as in patients with a penetrating thoracic injury as well.

Another consideration is whether to perform a closed-system lavage on one side or both. The literature suggests that there are possible risks of performing a lavage on the left side of the chest, such as a decreased impact of closed-chest compressions. However, increased warming of the myocardium may occur when entering the left side of the chest. The ideal route (ie, unilateral, specific side, or bilateral) is unclear from the current literature.

Inferior Shoulder Dislocation

By William Chan, MD; and Victor Huang, MD
New York-Presbyterian Queens Hospital, Flushing

Reviewed by John Kiel, DO, MPH

Objective

CASE PRESENTATION

A 70-year-old woman presents with right shoulder pain, deformity, and decreased range of motion after she tripped and fell on the sidewalk. She is unable to adduct her arm.

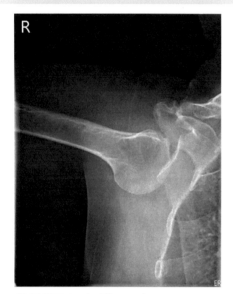

FIGURE 1. Axillary view, pre reduction

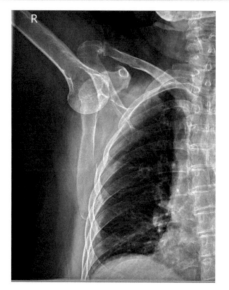

FIGURE 2. Anterior posterior view, pre reduction

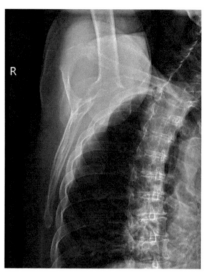

FIGURE 3. Lateral scapula view, pre reduction

Shoulder dislocation is one of the most common dislocations seen in the emergency department and represents 50% of all major joint dislocations.[1] In 2017, there were approximately 400,000 visits for dislocations in the United States.[2] Although anterior dislocations are frequently seen in the emergency department, inferior dislocations (ie, luxatio erecta) represent only 0.5% of all shoulder dislocations.[3]

The two main mechanisms of injury typically require high-energy trauma. First is axial loading through a fully abducted arm, which drives the humeral head through the weaker inferior glenohumeral ligaments.[4] The second is a hyperabduction force to the arm, which levers the proximal humerus on the acromion and results in injury to the inferior and middle glenohumeral ligaments.[4]

Physical Examination

Given the unique clinical presentation of this dislocation, diagnosis can often be made from a physical examination alone. The arm is typically in a fixed abducted position above the patient's head, with the humeral head palpable in the axilla (termed luxatio erecta, meaning "erect dislocation").[4] Classically, the elbow is flexed and the forearm is pronated.[4] The brachial plexus and axillary artery course in the axilla, inferior to the glenohumeral joint.[5] Physicians should have a high index of suspicion of possible neurovascular injury because the humeral head disrupts this space in an inferior dislocation.

Imaging

Plain x-rays are used to confirm the diagnosis and look for associated fractures. The humeral head is displaced inferiorly from the glenoid fossa. A distinct radiologic feature of inferior dislocations is that the humeral head is typically parallel to the spine of the scapula, whereas in anterior dislocations, the arm is adducted and the shaft of the humerus is parallel with the chest wall.[4] Further imaging can be performed, including CT to evaluate for associated fracture and MRI to look for rotator cuff tears, labral tears, and joint capsule injury.[6] When indicated, CT angiography should be considered for vascular injuries.

Management

Closed reduction should be performed in the emergency department. Two methods have been described for this reduction. The first method is traction-countertraction, in which axial traction is applied in the direction of the abducted humerus and countertraction is provided by a rolled sheet across the top of the shoulder.[4,6] However, this reduction can be difficult and typically requires procedural sedation.[6]

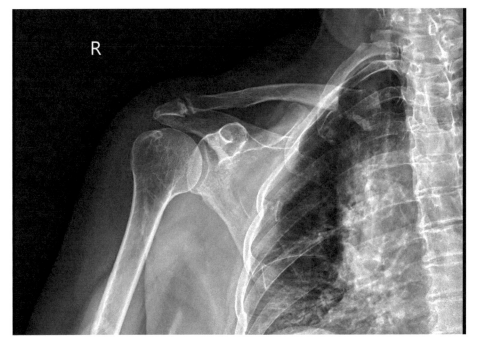

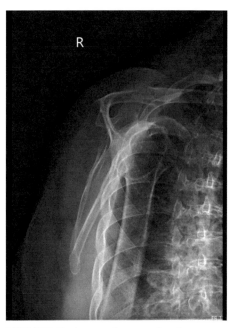

FIGURE 4. Anterior posterior view, post reduction

FIGURE 5. Lateral scapula view, post reduction

The second method involves rotating the head of the humerus from an inferior position to an anterior position relative to the glenoid.[4,6,7] The patient should be supine and the physician should stand on the affected side next to the head of the patient. One hand should be placed on the lateral aspect of the mid shaft of the humerus, and the humeral head should be pushed to the anterior position.[6,7] Meanwhile, the other hand should be positioned over the medial epicondyle, while gentle, superior-directed force is provided.[6,7] The resulting action converts the inferior dislocation to an anterior dislocation.[4,6,7]

From this position a variety of anterior dislocation reduction maneuvers can be performed.

In most cases, nonoperative treatment with sling immobilization for 2 to 3 weeks followed by physical therapy is appropriate.[4] Operative management may be needed for neurovascular injury, fracture-dislocation, capsular reconstruction, rotator cuff injury, and irreducible dislocations when the humeral head "buttonholes" through the inferior capsule.[3,4,7] One review of 199 patients from 101 articles found that 15 patients (8%) required operative management.[4]

CASE RESOLUTION

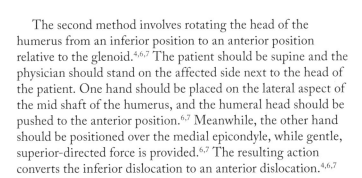

The patient was given 50 μg of fentanyl IV, and an intra-articular block was performed with 10 mL of 1% lidocaine without epinephrine. The two-step closed reduction maneuver was performed to convert the inferior dislocation into an anterior dislocation. The Park method was then performed for reducing the anterior dislocation.

REFERENCES

1. Alkaduhimi H, van der Linde JA, Flipsen M, van Deurzen DF, van den Bekerom MP. A systematic and technical guide on how to reduce a shoulder dislocation. Turk *J Emerg Med.* 2016 Nov 18;16(4):155-168.

2. Rui P, Kang K. National Hospital Ambulatory Medical Care Survey: 2017 emergency department summary tables. National Center for Health Statistics. https://www.cdc.gov/nchs/data/nhamcs/web_tables/2017_ed_web_tables-508.pdf

3. Groh GI, Wirth MA, Rockwood CA Jr. Results of treatment of luxatio erecta (inferior shoulder dislocation). *J Shoulder Elbow Surg.* 2010 Apr;19(3): 423-426.

4. Nambiar M, Owen D, Moore P, Carr A, Thomas M. Traumatic inferior shoulder dislocation: a review of management and outcome. *Eur J Trauma Emerg Surg.* 2018 Feb;44(1):45-51.

5. Orebaugh SL, Williams BA. Brachial plexus anatomy: normal and variant. *Sci World J.* 2009 Apr 28;9:300-312.

6. Yao F, Zhang L, Jing J. Luxatio erecta humeri with humeral greater tuberosity fracture and axillary nerve injury. *Am J Emerg Med.* 2018 Oct;36(10): 1926.e3-1926.e5.

7. Nho SJ, Dodson CC, Bardzik KF, Brophy RH, Domb BG, MacGillivray JD. The two-step maneuver for closed reduction of inferior glenohumeral dislocation (luxatio erecta to anterior dislocation to reduction). *J Orthop Trauma.* 2006 May;20(5):354-7.

Headache and Blurred Vision

By Joshua S. Broder, MD, FACEP
Dr. Broder is a professor and the residency program director in the Department of Emergency Medicine at Duke University Medical Center in Durham, North Carolina.

Objective

On completion of this article, you should be able to:

■ Discuss the usefulness of imaging in evaluating for idiopathic intracranial hypertension.

CASE PRESENTATION

A 25-year-old man presents with 2 weeks of worsening right-sided headache. He is nauseated and has vomited once. He notes blurring of his vision and slightly decreased peripheral vision on the right side. He denies any trauma, fever, or other neurologic deficits. Vital signs are BP 147/83, P 74, R 15, and T 36.9°C (98.4°F); SpO_2 is 99% on room air. His body mass index is 22.

The patient is awake and alert and has a normal general physical examination. His neurologic examination is notable for a right-sided visual field deficit. His visual acuity is 20/40 OD and 20/20 OS. The emergency physician is unable to visualize the fundus with a nondilated examination. The patient's noncontrast head CT scan is normal. The emergency physician obtains MRI and MR venography (MRV), considering a differential diagnosis of stroke, multiple sclerosis, and optic neuritis.

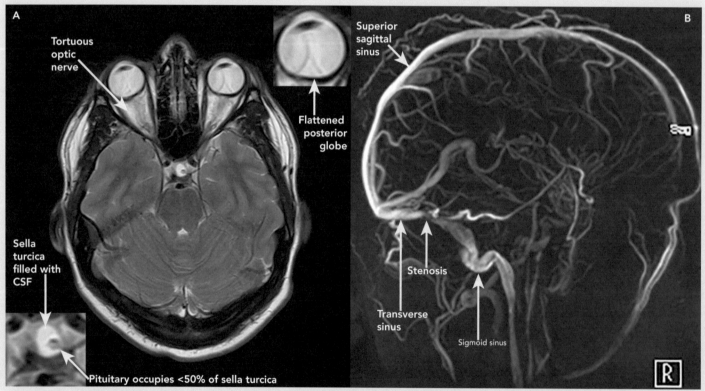

FIGURE 1. MRI and MRV. *A.* MRI with contrast, T2-weighted sequence. MRI shows an empty sella (defined as the pituitary occupying less than 50% of the fossa), flattening of the posterior globes, and tortuosity of optic nerves. *B.* MRV shows severe stenosis of the transverse sinus. Together, these findings suggest intracranial hypertension.

Discussion

Idiopathic intracranial hypertension (IIH) cannot be excluded by any current imaging study, but CT and MRI are often performed to evaluate for other causes of headache or neurologic signs and symptoms, such as stroke, optic neuritis, and multiple sclerosis. MRV and CT venography can demonstrate abnormalities of the cerebral venous sinuses such as thrombosis or stenosis. A variety of MRI findings have been described, but none have a high enough sensitivity to rule out IIH. Some findings are highly specific and strongly suggest the diagnosis (*Table 1*). Physicians should, therefore, not rely on imaging to eliminate IIH from the differential diagnosis. Confirmation or rejection should be by CSF pressure measurement after lumbar puncture.

MRI Finding	Sensitivity (95% CI)	Specificity (95% CI)
Empty sella sign	62.2 (48.0-74.7)	90.7 (84.8-94.4)
Posterior globe flattening	56.3 (46.5-65.6)	95.3 (85.7-98.6)
Optic nerve tortuosity	36.9 (26.8-48.2)	88.4 (82.1-92.7)
Transverse sinus stenosis	84.4 (65.9-93.9)	94.9 (91.7-96.9)

TABLE 1. MRI sensitivity and specificity

REFERENCES

1. Kwee RM, Kwee TC. Systematic review and meta-analysis of MRI signs for diagnosis of idiopathic intracranial hypertension. *Eur J Radiol* 2019;116:106-115.

CASE RESOLUTION

Lumbar puncture was performed. The opening pressure was greater than 55 cm of water (normal ≤20-25 cm of water). After 27 mL of CSF was removed, the closing pressure was 28 cm of water. The patient reported improvement in his headache following the procedure. He was prescribed acetazolamide and referred to neurology for consideration of venous sinus stenting.

Feature Editor: Joshua S. Broder, MD, FACEP. See also *Diagnostic Imaging for the Emergency Physician* (Winner of the 2011 Prose Award in Clinical Medicine, the American Publishers Award for Professional and Scholarly Excellence) and *Critical Images in Emergency Medicine* by Dr. Broder.

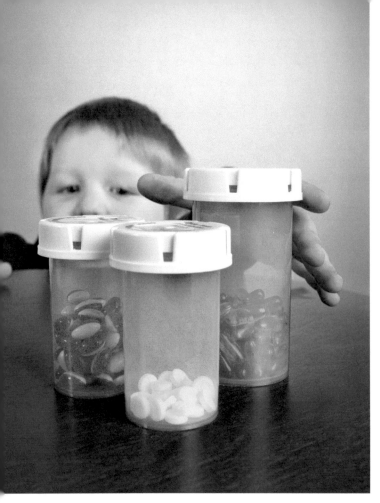

Seek and You Shall Find

Pediatric Toxic Ingestions

LESSON 4

By Vandana Thapar, MD; Cynthia Orantes, MD, FAAP; and Latonia Miller, MD, MS

Dr. Thapar is an associate professor, Dr. Orantes is a fellow, and Dr. Miller is a resident at the University of Texas Houston Health Center in Texas

Reviewed by Ann Dietrich, MD, FAAP, FACEP

Objectives

On completion of this lesson, you should be able to:

1. List the elements of the primary assessment and approach when presented with an unknown acute toxin ingestion.

2. State which medications activated charcoal is effective against and when to use multidose activated charcoal.

3. Explain which diagnostic tests and procedures aid in identifying toxins and their treatments.

4. Describe how to identify, distinguish, and manage common toxidromes.

5. Name drugs on the "one pill can kill" list.

6. State which antidotes are effective against different toxins.

From the EM Model

1.0 Signs, Symptoms, and Presentations
    1.3 General
        1.3.55 Toxidromes
17.0 Toxicologic Disorders
    17.1 Drug and Chemical Classes

■ CRITICAL DECISIONS ■

- How should a suspected acute toxin ingestion be approached?

- What details should be obtained when gathering the history of patients with acute toxin ingestions?

- What should be assessed during the physical examination of patients with acute toxic ingestions?

- What specific tests should be performed when the ingested toxin is unknown?

- When should activated charcoal be used to treat acute toxin ingestions?

- What are the symptoms of anticholinergic toxidromes, and how are they managed?

- How are other clinical toxidromes identified and managed?

- How are calcium channel blocker and β-blocker toxidromes differentiated from one another?

- When should poison control be contacted?

With the wide range of toxins that children ingest, identifying the specific toxidrome takes a bit of detective work on the part of emergency physicians. The toxic ingestions encountered in the emergency department, including sedative-hypnotics, anticholinergics, and sympathomimetics, can have overlapping presentations, and unfortunately, their incidence is rising. Emergency physicians must know the symptoms and diagnostic tests to differentiate and appropriately treat toxidromes in the vulnerable pediatric population.

■ CASE ONE

A 15-year-old girl with a history of major depressive disorder was found unresponsive at home by family with an empty bottle of her headache medication next to her. On arrival, she is obtunded, has a dry flush, and has dilated pupils. Her vital signs include BP 82/45, R 22, and T 39.5°C(103.1°F); her SpO$_2$ is 99% on room air. A pulse oximetry saturation of 99% in room air. Her point-of-care glucose level is 92 mg/dL.

■ CASE TWO

A 15-year-old boy accompanied by his mother presents via EMS. His mother called EMS because the patient complained of dizziness, shortness of breath, and chest discomfort after he came home from a party early in the morning. He has not urinated for a while. The patient reports he went to a "pill party," where kids bring pills from their families' medicine cabinets. He does not know what he has taken. The patient is lying down with the head of his bed at 30° and is holding his head as if he has a headache or is dizzy. His vital signs include BP 96/60, P 40, R 16, and T 36.5°C (97.7°F). He is able to answer questions but seems slightly anxious. He is immediately placed on monitors, and an ECG is completed and shows sinus bradycardia. An intravenous line is placed, and 20 mL/kg of normal saline is administered.

Introduction

In 1974, the term toxidrome was coined to describe the constellation of signs and symptoms after exposure to a specific toxin group. From 2008 to 2011, emergency departments across the United States saw more than 1.1 million patients per year for drug poisoning; the pediatric population, specifically, averaged 28.8 visits per 10,000 over 4 years. As science and society continue to evolve, so too does the medicine cabinet, and the rate of pediatric toxic ingestion continues to increase. Psychosocial barriers, socioeconomic barriers, mental disability, and limited social interaction in a modernized society also contribute to this increased rate. Acute poisonings have evolved from the era of tricyclic antidepressant, rat poisoning, and iron tablet ingestions to diphenhydramine, button battery, and synthetic and illicit substance ingestions. Toxic ingestions present in a bimodal distribution: in those younger than 5 years and in adolescents. Studies report unintentional ingestion is more common in children younger than 5 years because of their tendency to put things in their mouths. Adolescents, by contrast, tend to experience acute toxidromes secondary to chronic use of substances, intentional self-harm, peer pressure, or chasing euphoric effects.

CRITICAL DECISION

How should a suspected acute toxin ingestion be approached?

When emergency physicians evaluate altered pediatric patients, they should suspect acute toxic ingestion, especially in those younger than 5 years or those with a history of toxic ingestion. On presentation, these children should immediately be placed on cardiac monitoring and supplemental oxygen if in respiratory distress. Intravenous access should be obtained, and blood and urine specimens should be collected for analysis. Their airway, breathing, circulation, and need for decontamination (ABCDs) should be rapidly assessed along with their vital signs. Hemodynamically unstable patients with signs of respiratory distress and reduced airway protection may require intubation. Symptoms of tachycardia and hypotension may require fluid administration and vasopressors. When patients present from an unknown location, rather than from home, after exposure to aerosolized toxins or topical contaminants, they should be decontaminated, and health care personnel should use personal protective equipment. Patients' clothing may also need to be removed so contaminated body parts can be irrigated. Alternatively, if patients are hemodynamically stable, cardiovascularly intact, able to protect their airway, and breathing without effort, laboratory tests should be ordered. Additional information can also be obtained from family to aid in diagnosis and management.

CRITICAL DECISION

What details should be obtained when gathering the history of patients with acute toxin ingestions?

Emergency physicians can gain more details of the history from patients' family, friends, bystanders, and EMS. The history should include information on whether the substance was ingested, inhaled, or touched; the dosage or strength of the substance; the number of pills or liquid volume consumed or the number of pills remaining in the bottle; the time of ingestion; any coingestions; and symptoms or complaints just prior to presentation. Time of ingestion is especially important because some toxins can be managed more aggressively with activated charcoal, cathartics, and antidotes within the first few hours of presentation.

CRITICAL DECISION

What should be assessed during the physical examination of patients with acute toxic ingestions?

For an acute toxin ingestion or exposure, a thorough physical examination can help distinguish between the nuanced effects of

✔ Pearls

- Early identification of toxidromes and early treatment can dramatically change patient outcomes.

- ß-blocker overdose is associated with hypoglycemia, while calcium channel blocker overdose is associated with hyperglycemia.

- Early phone calls to poison control are an essential part of managing toxic ingestions.

some drugs or medications. The severity of the toxicity can also be seen in the patients' vital signs, volume status, and mentation. Acute toxin ingestions can lead to variable body temperature, heart rate, blood pressure, and respiratory rate. When assessing patients' neurologic status and mentation, their family or guardians or EMS, possibly, can provide their baseline status. Patients' pupillary size and response to light should be assessed, and they should be monitored for hallucinations, agitation, and seizures. Other areas to evaluate include the mucous membranes, capillary refill time, skin moisture (dry versus moist), and urine output (to assess for urinary retention.) Many toxidromes have overlapping symptomatology, and presentations can be complicated when more than one substance was ingested at a time.

CRITICAL DECISION

What specific tests should be performed when the ingested toxin is unknown?

Diagnostic and laboratory testing are crucial for identifying end-organ failure secondary to toxic ingestions. Specific tests to include in the workup include the following: a point-of-care glucose test; complete metabolic panel; blood gas analysis; acetaminophen, salicylate, and ethanol levels; urine drug screen; urinalysis (pH is important when managing salicylate ingestion); urine or serum pregnancy test, serum osmolality (for ingestion of toxic alcohols); antiepileptic medication levels; creatine kinase and myoglobin levels; and an ECG (for suspected dysrhythmia or conduction delay). A point-of-care glucose reading on arrival of an acutely altered patient can help determine whether the altered mental status is from hypo- or hyperglycemia. The collection of various drug levels such as acetaminophen and salicylate can help diagnose common coingestions.

CRITICAL DECISION

When should activated charcoal be used to treat acute toxin ingestions?

Activated charcoal works by adsorbing the potential toxin. Activated charcoal's small pores increase its surface area so that it can adhere to more of the toxin, thereby decreasing the amount of toxin available for the body to absorb. Poison control recommends that activated charcoal be administered for toxins it is effective against in patients who present within 2 hours of drug ingestion and have a stable mental status and airway (including those who are intubated). If aspirated, activated charcoal can cause a pneumonitis, which can increase morbidity and mortality. Activated charcoal works well on large substances, organic substances, and those with poor water solubility. It binds poorly to alcohols, iron, lithium, acids, alkaline electrolytes, arsenic, and heavy metals. Multidose activated charcoal works well against drugs that undergo enterhepatic reabsorption like carbamazepine, theophylline, phenobarbital, dapsone, and quinine. Multidose activated charcoal is thought to decrease these toxins' reabsorption, thereby decreasing their overall effects on the body.

CRITICAL DECISION

What are the symptoms of anticholinergic toxidromes, and how are they managed?

Not all anticholinergics are one and the same; cyclic antidepressants can cause a variety of symptoms. Patients with acute cyclic antidepressant toxicity may initially appear stable but have the potential to rapidly decompensate, usually within the first 2 hours following ingestion. The sudden change in presentation can be attributed to the many effects of cyclic antidepressants in the body: Cyclic antidepressants function as sodium channel blockers, histamine receptor blockers, anticholinergics, norepinephrine and serotonin reuptake inhibitors, and α-1 receptor blockers. As a sodium channel blocker, cyclic antidepressants slow the depolarization of cardiac myocytes, leading to a widened QRS complex, prolonged QTc interval, and hypotension. By preventing the reuptake of norepinephrine, cyclic antidepressant toxidromes can cause tachycardia and hypertension followed by hypotension (after norepinephrine depletion). Their common histamine-receptor-blocker effects include sedation and even coma. Effects from α-1 receptor blockade can also cause sedation as well as orthostatic hypotension and miosis. These symptoms help distinguish cyclic antidepressant toxicity from other anticholinergic toxidromes.

In children, acute anticholinergic toxicity can occur with ingestions greater than 5 mg/kg and can lead to cardiovascular toxicity with refractory hypotension, acidosis, and dysrhythmias. An ECG should be immediately obtained, with close attention paid to signs of toxicity including tachycardia and intraventricular conduction delays as seen in a widened QRS complex (QRS >120 ms), right axis deviation of QRS complexes (tall terminal R wave in aVR >3 mm, R/S ratio >0.7), prolonged QTc (>440-460 ms, if symptomatic), and in some cases, right bundle branch blocks.

The treatment for acute cyclic antidepressant toxicity is sodium bicarbonate in 1 to 2 mEq/kg IV boluses, particularly if cardiovascular toxicity is suspected to alkalinize the serum pH to between 7.50 and 7.55. Sodium bicarbonate should be continued if the QRS complex continues to widen on ECG. Potential therapies for intractable cardiovascular toxicity include lidocaine 1.5 mg/kg/dose coadministered with sodium bicarbonate. Other potential therapies are intralipid therapy and extracorporeal membrane oxygenation (ECMO).

Hypotension secondary to acute cyclic antidepressant toxicity is managed with volume resuscitation using intravenous crystalloid fluids followed by vasopressor support with norepinephrine, if needed.

Neurologic findings found in cyclic antidepressant toxicity include altered mental status, agitation, a lower-than-normal

✖ Pitfalls

- Disregarding the importance of obtaining a thorough history that includes events leading up to the presentation and any potential exposures.

- Failing to prepare for hemodynamic and airway complications in pediatric patients with altered mental status.

- Failing to identify reversible causes of toxin ingestions, toxins with known antidotes, and ingestions that cause significant disease, such as drugs on the "one pill kills" list and acetaminophen toxidromes.

Common Toxidrome Class	Associated Symptomatology		Treatment or Antidote
Cholinergic: organophosphates, carbamates, pilocarpine	Diarrhea Diaphoresis Urination Miosis Bradycardia Bronchorrhea/broncho secretions	Emesis Lacrimation Lethargic DUMBBELS or SLUDGE	Carbamates: atropine IV 0.05 mg/kg/dose Organophosphates: initial dose of atropine IV 0.05 mg/kg. If not responding, double dose every 3-5 min until bronchorrhea is reduced. Maximum dose 0.5-1 mg IV. Pralidoxime 25-50 mg/kg/dose IV over 30-60 min, followed by 20 mg/kg/hr. Continue therapy for 24-72 hr.
Anticholinergic: antihistamines, cyclic antidepressants, doxylamine, atropine, benztropine, phenothiazines, scopolamine, cyclopentolate, jimson weed, and deadly nightshade.	Tachycardia Hyperthermia Flushed, dry skin "Red as a beet" "Dry as a bone" "Hot as a hare" "Blind as a bat" "Mad as a hatter" "Full as a flask"	Urinary urgency/retention Dilated pupils Delirium/hallucinations	Most anticholinergics: physostigmine 0.02 mg/kg (max of 0.5 mg) IV slowly over 5 minutes. Can repeat after 10-15 min. Cyclic antidepressants: sodium bicarbonate in 1-2 mEq/kg IV boluses. Titrate to pH 7.5 with additional boluses or continuous infusion.
Sympathomimetic: cocaine, amphetamines, ephedrine, phencyclidine, pseudoephedrine, methamphetamine, MDMA (ecstasy).	Mydriasis Sweating Dilated pupils Tachycardia	Hypertension Hyperthermia Seizures	Benzodiazepines 0.1 mg/kg/dose, first line for agitation, hypertension, and seizures
Hallucinogen: LSD, mescaline, PCP, psilocybin, dimethyltryptamine (DMT), ketamine, salvia	Mydriasis Hallucinations/delusions Tachycardia	Hypertension Synesthesia Agitation Seizure	Supportive care
Narcotics: morphine, heroin, fentanyl, oxycodone, hydrocodone, meperidine	Miosis Drowsiness	Euphoria Bradypnea	Naltrexone, naloxone, methadone, buprenorphine
Sedative: benzodiazepines, barbiturates, eszopiclone, zaleplon, zolpidem	Miosis Drowsiness Slurred speech Bradypnea Hypotension Hyperpnea Tachypnea	Metabolic acidosis Hyperthermia Tinnitus Confused Agitated Seizure "DKA like"	Supportive care Benzodiazepines: flumazenil Barbiturate: supportive care, sodium bicarbonate drip to alkalize urine, hemodialysis
Serotonin agonists: SSRIs, MAOIs	Autonomic instability Hypertonicity Hyperreflexive Tremor Agitated Altered mental status Diaphoretic	Hyperthermic Rhabdomyolysis Metabolic acidosis Renal failure DIC Shock	Supportive care Forced diuresis for rhabdomyolysis Serial ECG, if QTc interval is >560 ms then start magnesium
Neuroleptic malignant syndrome: haloperidol, clozapine, risperidone, olanzapine, metoclopramide, chlorpromazine	Autonomic instability Hypertonicity Altered mental status Hyperthermia Metabolic acidosis Rhabdomyolysis		Supportive Benzodiazepines Dantrolene Bromocriptine

TABLE 1. Common toxidromes

seizure threshold, hallucinations, lethargy, and coma. Seizures are commonly associated with widened QRS complexes greater than 100 ms on ECG. Benzodiazepines can be used to manage seizures and agitation. Antipsychotic medications should be used cautiously because they can further exacerbate cardiac conduction, resulting in a wider QRS complex and prolonged QTc interval.

Other common cholinergic toxidromes are organophosphate and carbamate toxicities from exposure to insecticides or pesticides. Both agents work by inhibiting the function of acetylcholinesterase, which leads to more acetylcholine in the synaptic cleft of the neuromuscular junction and strong muscarinic and nicotinic responses. Presenting symptoms can include defecation, urination, miosis, bronchorrhea, bronchospasms, bradycardia, emesis, lacrimation, and salivation (*Table 1*). Thus, the diagnosis of cholinergic toxicity is often made clinically; however, a comprehensive history (eg, exposures and the time since symptoms started) and physical examination are also important for a correct and timely diagnosis. If cholinergic toxicity is suspected on presentation, then special attention must be paid to airway, breathing, and circulation, as well as decontamination — clothing can be hazardous and can even prolong patients' exposure period. Staff should wear the proper personal protective equipment because exposure can occur through skin contact or inhalation as well. Severe toxicity can present with altered mentation and respiratory failure that requires intubation. Death from cholinergic toxicity can be attributed to heightened nicotinic receptor activity that causes bronchospasm, bradycardia, and bronchorrhea. An atropine trial should be considered early to confirm suspicions of a cholinergic toxidrome; results are considered positive if symptoms cease after administration of atropine. Cholinergic toxicity should also be treated with pralidoxime, which inhibits both muscarinic and nicotinic effects. Seizures that accompany cholinergic toxicity should be treated with benzodiazepines. Rarely, patients may also develop neurotoxicity symptoms 1 to 3 weeks post exposure.

CRITICAL DECISION

How are other clinical toxidromes identified and managed?

Sympathomimetic toxidrome presentations often get confused with the anticholinergic toxidrome because both can present with acute agitation, tachycardia, and hyperthermia (see *Table 1*). However, unlike anticholinergic toxicity, patients with sympathomimetic toxicity will also present with diaphoresis and hyperactive bowel sounds but will not have urinary retention. Unlike cyclic antidepressant toxicities, sympathomimetic toxicities do not commonly present with cardiac conduction delays on ECG; however, if the ECG detects a widened QRS complex dysrhythmia 1 to 2 mEq/kg of sodium bicarbonate is the recommended treatment. Sympathomimetics function by blocking fast sodium channels in the CNS, cardiovascular, respiratory, GI, and integumentary systems. Patients with mild toxicity may need only brief observation for 4 to 6 hours. For patients with severe toxicity, usually indicated by agitation and seizures, the primary treatment is benzodiazepines or phenobarbital. The first-line treatment for hypertension secondary to sympathomimetic toxicity is benzodiazepines. If blood pressures remain elevated or a hypertensive emergency is anticipated, sodium nitroprusside or phentolamine can be considered. For cocaine ingestions specifically, β-blockers should be avoided because they can worsen hypertension through unopposed α-adrenergic receptor stimulation. Urinalysis may reveal myoglobinuria (positive blood but no RBCs noted on microscopy), and serum electrolytes may reveal hyperkalemia and an elevated creatine kinase — rhabdomyolysis is a common complication of sympathomimetic toxicity. Volume resuscitation with isotonic crystalloid fluids is the recommended treatment. In cases of hypertensive emergency, neurologic findings, or acute headaches, a noncontrast head CT is indicated given the increased risk of cocaine-induced cerebrovascular accidents.

CRITICAL DECISION

How are calcium channel blocker and β-blocker toxidromes differentiated from one another?

Calcium channel blockers have a higher incidence of mortality compared to β-blockers in an overdose ingestion.

β-blocker medications at therapeutic doses are mostly β1 selective; at toxic doses, they can stimulate both β1- and β2-adrenergic receptors. Symptoms of toxicity from overdose occur because of effects on the cardiovascular system. β1-receptor blockade decreases heart rate, heart contractility, and blood pressure through inhibition of fast sodium channels. β2-blockade can also cause bronchoconstriction, which combined with β1-blockade effects can lead to respiratory failure in cases of toxicity. β2 effects can also cause hypoglycemia due to the stimulation of gluconeogenesis and inhibition of glycogenolysis. In patients with β-blocker toxicity who are alert and interactive and present in under 2 hours from ingestion, activated charcoal may help but should be used with caution because these patients can decline rapidly. Glucagon helps in β-blocker toxicity by bypassing β-adrenergic receptor stimulation and activating cyclic adenosine monophosphate (cAMP) to treat hypoglycemia, hypotension, and bradycardia. If glucagon is ineffective, then epinephrine and dopamine may be helpful for patients with both bradycardia and hypotension, while atropine may be helpful for patients with bradycardia. ECMO may be needed if pharmacologic interventions are ineffective; hemodialysis is not useful in β-blocker toxicity.

There are three different classes of calcium channel blockade; in smaller doses, they each have a specific effect, but in overdose, they all affect cardiac contractility, interfere with the atrioventricular (AV) node, and cause peripheral dilation. Patients may present awake and alert, but their mental status can decline rapidly secondary to cardiovascular collapse. Unlike β-blocker overdose, calcium channel overdose presents with hyperglycemia, which is secondary to a calcium-mediated decrease in insulin release. Like patients with a β-blocker overdose, patients with a calcium channel blocker overdose whose mental status is normal should receive activated charcoal if they have presented within 2 hours of ingestion. Atropine, calcium, and intravenous fluids should be given for patients with bradycardia; if ineffective, then vasopressors and external pacemakers may be required. If hyperglycemia occurs, high-dose insulin in a 1-unit/kg bolus and a 0.5-units/kg/hr drip can be used to lower the glucose level. If pharmacologic and external pacing interventions are ineffective, then ECMO may be needed for calcium channel blocker overdoses as well.

CRITICAL DECISION

When should poison control be contacted?

Poison control should be contacted for all suspected toxin ingestions after patients are stablized. Contacting Poison Control early can help direct patient management, including whether they should be observed, admitted, or transferred for specialized care. Poison Control can be contacted at 1-800-222-1222.

Summary

Pediatric toxic ingestion has become a more common presentation in emergency departments across the United States, and early identification is paramount. Managing the ABCDs and gathering a thorough history, including input from patients' family or friends, can glean useful information to identify the toxin, the time frame of ingestion, the quantity ingested, and any possible coingestions. Patients should be assessed for hemodynamic instability, and laboratory and other diagnostic

CASE RESOLUTIONS

■ CASE ONE

The emergency physician suspected a cyclic antidepressant overdose because this medication is often prescribed for migraine prophylaxis. Following a primary assessment, the patient was placed on cardiac and respiratory monitoring, and laboratory and ECG testing were obtained. After the ECG revealed a widened QRS complex and prolonged QTc interval, the physician promptly initiated intravenous sodium bicarbonate for cardiotoxicity.

■ CASE TWO

Laboratory tests were sent, and the bedside glucose level was 280 mg/dL. The patient's blood pressure suddenly dropped to 60/40 mm Hg, so another fluid bolus and atropine were administered, and the patient was intubated. The emergency physician suspected a calcium channel blocker overdose, but the patient was outside of the 2-hour presentation window for treatment with activated charcoal.

A cardiology consultation was requested. An internal jugular line was placed in case transvenous pacing became necessary. A calcium chloride bolus was given, and the drip was started at 0.3 mL/kg/hr, with monitoring every 30 minutes. The patient was safely transported to the pediatric ICU, where he became unstable and required ECMO.

tests like ECGs should be ordered based on presentation. Most toxins can be treated with supportive measures, but some may require more therapeutic interventions with medications like bicarbonate, benzodiazepines, or atropine. Poison Control can be a useful resource for guiding the diagnosis and management of toxidromes.

REFERENCES

1. In: Tenenbein M, Macias CG, Sharieff GQ, Yamamoto LG, Schafermeyer R, eds. *Strange and Schafermeyer's Pediatric Emergency Medicine*. 5th ed. McGraw Hill; 2019.

2. Mangus CW, Canares TL. Toxic ingestions: initial management. *Pediat Rev*. 2018 Apr 1;39(4):219-221.

3. Fine JS. Poisoning. In: McInerny TK, Adam HM, Campbell DE, DeWitt TG, Foy JM, Kamat DM, eds. *American Academy of Pediatrics Textbook of Pediatric Care*. 2nd ed. American Academy of Pediatrics; 2016.

4. Velez LI, Shepherd JG, Goto CS. Approach to the child with occult toxic exposure. UpToDate. Updated April 19, 2022. www.uptodate.com/contents/approach-to-the-child-with-occult-toxic-exposure

5. Bird S. Organophosphate and carbamate poisoning. UpToDate. Updated March 27, 2023. https://www.uptodate.com/contents/organophosphate-and-carbamate-poisoning

6. Su MK, Goldman M. Anticholinergic poisoning. UpToDate. Updated February 8, 2023. www.uptodate.com/contents/anticholinergic-poisoning

7. O'Connor AD, Padilla-Jones A, Gherkin RD, Levine M. Prevalence of rhabdomyolysis in sympathomimetic toxicity: a comparison of stimulants. *J Med Toxicol*. 2015 Jun;11(2)195-200.

8. Get help online or by phone. Poison Control National Capital Poison Center. https://www.poison.org/

9. Meehan TJ, Erikson TB. Chapter 112: general approach to the poisoned patient. In: Schafermeyer R, Tenebein M, Macias CG, Sharieff GQ, Yamamoto LG, eds. *Strange and Schafermeyer's Pediatric Emergency Medicine*. 4th edition. McGraw Hill; 2014.

CME Questions

Reviewed by Michael S. Beeson, MD, MBA, FACEP

Qualified, paid subscribers to *Critical Decisions in Emergency Medicine* may receive CME certificates for up to 5 ACEP Category I credits, 5 *AMA PRA Category 1 Credits*™, and 5 AOA Category 2-B credits for completing this activity in its entirety. Submit your answers online at acep.org/cdem; a score of 75% or better is required. You may receive credit for completing the CME activity any time within 3 years of its publication date. Answers to this month's questions will be published in next month's issue.

1 What is true about canine bites?

A. Canine bites are low force injuries
B. The extremities are most often involved in pediatric patients
C. The majority of bites are reported as provoked
D. The majority of bites involve animals that are known to the victim

2 What is true about feline bites?

A. Most feline bites are reported by victims as provoked
B. Most feline bites involve the face
C. Signs of infection post injury typically develop very slowly
D. The full extent of damage is always apparent on clinical examination

3 What is recommended to prevent animal bites?

A. Not approaching unfamiliar dogs
B. Not leaving young children alone with animals
C. Pet socialization
D. All of the above

4 Which statement is true regarding examining mammalian bites?

A. All mammalian bites require imaging to rule out a foreign body
B. Clinicians should examine the location and characteristics of the bite; the presence of drainage or erythema, and any evidence of a retained foreign body
C. Feline bites are often associated with a fracture
D. Punctures from feline bites are typically superficial in nature

5 Imaging is most likely indicated in which circumstance?

A. A superficial, linear cheek wound without crepitus, deformrity, or signs of foreign body
B. A suspected abscess
C. A suspected bat bite that cannot be readily discovered on physical examination
D. All bite wounds

6 Which bite wound is most appropriate for primary wound closure in the emergency department?

A. A cat bite to the face
B A deep stellate facial woundfrom a large dog bite sustained 6 hours ago
C. A laceration to the left metacarpophalangeal joint that occurred after a punch during an altercation
D. A superficial dog bite to the calf of the left leg that is 4 cm long, 3 cm wide, and more than 18 hours old

7 In which circumstance is rabies prophylaxis (vaccine and immune globulin) most likely indicated?

A. A bat lands on the head of someone sitting on their porch in the daytime
B. A pet rabbit bites its owner on the nose
C. A dog bites a neighbor
D. A squirrel bites a person, runs away, and cannot be located

8 Which rabies prophylaxis is recommended for patients receiving it for the first time after an at-risk animal exposure?

A. Human diploid cell vaccine (HDCV) or purified chick embryo cell vaccine (PCECV) on days 0 and 3
B. Human diploid cell vaccine (HDCV) or purified chick embryo cell vaccine (PCECV) on days 0 and 3 plus human rabies immune globulin (HRIG) on day 0
C. Human diploid cell vaccine (HDCV) or purified chick embryo cell vaccine (PCECV) on days 0, 3, 7, and 21
D. Human diploid cell vaccine (HDCV) or purified chick embryo cell vaccine (PCECV) on days 0, 3, 7, and 21 plus human rabies immune globulin (HRIG) on day 0

9 Which patient should be given tetanus prophylaxis?

A. A 20-year-old person with a long, superficial dog scratch to the torso whose last tetanus immunization was 7 years ago
B. A 30-year-old person whose last tetanus immunization was 8 years ago who presents with a large, contaminated dog bite to the leg
C. A fully immunized 5-year-old child with a cat bite to the hand
D. A fully immunized 12-month-old baby who was bitten by a dog

10 Which action demonstrates appropriate patient management following a mammalian bite?

A. Rabies prophylaxis for all bite wounds
B. Subspeciality consultation for all bite wounds
C. Tetanus prophylaxis for all bite wounds
D. Timely follow up with the patient's primary care physician or subspecialist

11 Which ingested material is activated charcoal ineffective against?

A. Carbamazepine
B. Iron
C. Phenobarbital
D. Theophylline

12 **What is the recommended time frame for administering activated charcoal in toxic ingestions it is effective against?**

   A.   within 2 hours of ingestion
   B.   within 4 hours of ingestion
   C.   within 12 hours of ingestion
   D.   within 24 hours of ingestion

13 **Which ingestion-antidote pairing is incorrect?**

   A.   β-blocker and physostigmine
   B.   Calcium channel blocker and atropine
   C.   Cocaine and benzodiazepines
   D.   Morphine and naloxone

14 **Which toxidrome is treated only with supportive care?**

   A.   Anticholinergic
   B.   Hallucinogenic
   C.   Narcotic
   D.   Sedative

15 **Which toxidrome contaminates patients' clothing and warrants decontamination and use of personal protective equipment by medical staff?**

   A.   Anticholinergic
   B.   Cholinergic
   C.   Hallucinogenic
   D.   Narcotic

16 **What is the first-line antidote for β-blocker toxicity?**

   A.   Dopamine
   B.   Epinephrine
   C.   Glucagon
   D.   Hemodialysis

17 **What is a common complication of sympathomimetic toxicity?**

   A.   Bradycardia
   B.   Bronchorrhea
   C.   Respiratory distress
   D.   Rhabdomyolysis

18 **Which symptom is seen in anticholinergic but not sympathomimetic toxidromes?**

   A.   Agitation
   B.   Hyperthermia
   C.   Tachycardia
   D.   Urinary retention

19 **A 3 year old was found with her mother's hair-straightening lye product on her face. It created a burn on her cheek and neck, but no lesions are seen in the patient's mouth, lips, or nares. She is not having any difficulty breathing or drooling, and she was able to eat crackers with milk on her way to the emergency department. What is the most appropriate treatment?**

   A.   Chest x-ray in 6 hours and if negative, discharge home
   B.   Emergent GI consult for endoscopy
   C.   Intubation in case of difficulty breathing
   D.   Observation and discharge with return precautions for any GI upset

20 **Which medication worsens hypertension in cases of cocaine ingestion?**

   A.   ACE inhibitors
   B.   β-blockers
   C.   Calcium channel blockers
   D.   Central agonists

ANSWER KEY FOR JANUARY 2022, VOLUME 36, NUMBER 1

1	2	3	4	5	6	7	8	9	10	11	12	13	14	15	16	17	18	19	20
A	B	C	D	D	D	D	D	A	A	B	A	A	D	D	C	B	D	C	B

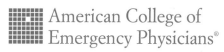

American College of
Emergency Physicians®

ADVANCING EMERGENCY CARE

Post Office Box 619911
Dallas, Texas 75261-9911

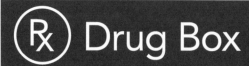 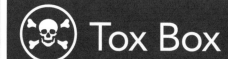

Fluvoxamine in Outpatient COVID-19

By Frank LoVecchio, DO, MPH, FACEP
Valleywise Health and ASU Phoenix, Arizona

Objective
On reading this column you should be able to
■ Recall the determiniation of the use of fluvoxamine in outpatient COVID-19.

Fluvoxamine binds to the sigma-1 receptor on immune cells, resulting in reduced production of inflammatory cytokines in mice. In vitro, fluvoxamine reduces inflammatory gene expression in human endothelial cells and macrophages. Randomized trials have studied the use of fluvoxamine for the treatment of nonhospitalized patients with COVID-19, with equivocal results. IDSA has not endorsed routine use, as a meta-analysis did not show a mortality benefit. The NIH COVID-19 Treatment Guidelines Panel has taken a neutral position.

Adverse Effects, Monitoring, and Drug-Drug Interactions
When fluvoxamine is used to treat psychiatric conditions, the most common adverse effects are nausea, diarrhea, indigestion, neurologic effects (eg, asthenia, insomnia, somnolence, anxiety, headache), and rarely suicidal ideation. Fluvoxamine is a cytochrome P450 (CYP) 2D6 substrate and a potent inhibitor of CYP1A2 and CYP2C19, and a moderate inhibitor of CYP2C9, CYP2D6, and CYP3A4. Fluvoxamine can enhance the serotonergic effects of other SSRIs or monoamine oxidase inhibitors (MAOIs), resulting in serotonin syndrome; therefore, it should not be used within 2 weeks of receipt of other SSRIs or MAOIs. Fluvoxamine may enhance the effects of antiplatelets and anticoagulants.

Considerations in Pregnancy
The association of SSRI use in the late third trimester with a small, increased risk of primary persistent pulmonary hypertension in newborns has not been excluded, although the absolute risk is likely low. The risk of fluvoxamine use in pregnancy for the treatment of COVID-19 should be balanced with the potential benefit.

Adverse effects due to SSRI use in children are similar to those in adults, although children and adolescents appear to have higher rates of behavioral activation and vomiting than adults. There are no data on the use of fluvoxamine for the prevention or treatment of COVID-19 in children.

In summary, there is insufficient evidence to recommend either for or against the use of fluvoxamine for the treatment of outpatient COVID-19. Clinicians should be aware of the toxicity and drug interactions. Fluvoxamine 100 mg PO twice daily for 10 days is commonly prescribed.

REFERENCE
Reis G, Dos Santos Moreira-Silva EA, Silva DCM, et al. Effect of early treatment with fluvoxamine on risk of emergency care and hospitalisation among patients with COVID-19: the TOGETHER randomised, platform clinical trial. *Lancet Glob Health.* 2022 Jan;10(1):e42-e51 https://www.covid19treatmentguidelines.nih.gov/therapies/ immunomodulators/fluvoxamine/

Precautions
Nirmatrelvir/ritonavir is not recommended in patients with severe renal impairment (eGFR <30 mL/min) or severe hepatic impairment until more data are available.

Nirmatrelvir/ritonavir is contraindicated if allergic and with drugs that are highly dependent on CYP3A for clearance, and for which elevated concentrations are associated with serious and/or life-threatening reactions. It is contraindicated with drugs that are potent CYP3A inducers where significantly reduced nirmatrelvir or ritonavir plasma concentrations may be associated with the potential for loss of virologic response and possible resistance.

Pediatric Cannabis (THC) Ingestions

By Christian A. Tomaszewski, MD, MS, MBA, FACEP
University of California, San Diego Health

Objective
On reading this column you should be able to
■ Describe the effects of pediatric cannabis ingestions.

Delta-9-tetrahydrocannibinol (THC) is the primary psychoactive agent in cannabis. With legalization, attractive edible formulations, often infused with excess THC (eg, 500 mg in one package) are increasingly ingested inadvertently by children. Symptomatic ingestions can lead to involved workups (if history is unobtainable) along with rare ICU admission or intubation.

Mechanism
■ THC agonist at CB1 (& CB2)– main psychoactive.
■ CBD antagonist or weak binding at CB1/2 – anticonvulsant, anxiolytic.

Pharmacokinetics
■ Doses.
  ● ≥ 25 mg in adults to alter cognitive/psychomotor performance.
  ● As little as 5 mg causes pediatric intoxication.
■ Timing.
  ● Effects start 30-60 min post-ingestion.
  ● Peak blood levels ~4 h (range 1-8 h).
  ● Duration of effect 6-24 h.

Clinical Manifestations
■ *CNS:* lethargy, sedation, hypotonia, ataxia, seizures.
■ *Cardiac:* tachycardia, hypertension, hypotension.
■ *Eyes:* horizontal nystagmus, conjunctival injection, mydriasis (rare).
■ *GI:* nausea, vomiting.
■ *Resp:* depression.
■ *Metabolic:* rare increased lactate.

Diagnostics
■ Screening glucose level.
■ Urine drug screen may be positive for THC-COOH.
■ Workup for AMS if hx unclear (±CT/LP/EEG).

Treatment
■ May try naloxone or flumazenil to reverse out non-THC AMS.
■ Benzodiazepines for seizures.
■ Dexmedetomidine or benzos for agitation.
■ Airway protection – rare cases have required intubation.

Critical decisions
in emergency medicine

Volume 36 Number 3: **March 2022**

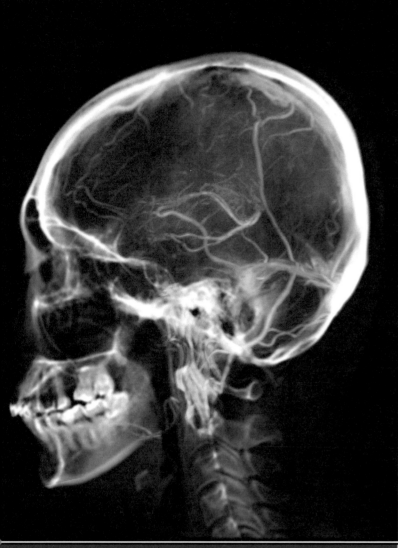

All in Vein

Cerebral venous thrombosis (CVT) is an uncommon cause of cerebrovascular disease, accounting for up to 1% of all strokes in adults. CVT is a challenging diagnosis to make due to a wide range of clinical presentations; hence, a high degree of clinical suspicion is required to make the diagnosis.

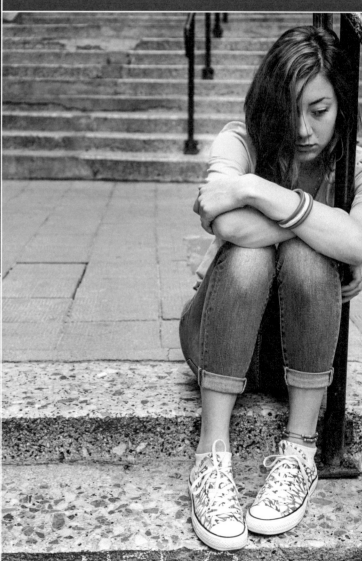

Out of It

Altered mental status encompasses a broad differential spanning almost all physiologic systems, from metabolic encephalopathy to infection or traumatic brain injury. The ability to quickly and accurately determine the etiology of a patient's altered behavior is a key skill for emergency physicians.

THE OFFICIAL CME PUBLICATION OF THE AMERICAN COLLEGE OF EMERGENCY PHYSICIANS

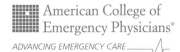
American College of Emergency Physicians®
ADVANCING EMERGENCY CARE

Critical decisions
in emergency medicine

Critical Decisions in Emergency Medicine is the official CME publication of the American College of Emergency Physicians. Additional volumes are available.

EDITOR-IN-CHIEF

Michael S. Beeson, MD, MBA, FACEP
Northeastern Ohio Universities, Rootstown, OH

SECTION EDITORS

Joshua S. Broder, MD, FACEP
Duke University, Durham, NC

Andrew J. Eyre, MD, MHPEd
Brigham & Women's Hospital/
Harvard Medical School, Boston, MA

John Kiel, DO, MPH
University of Florida College of Medicine,
Jacksonville, FL

Frank LoVecchio, DO, MPH, FACEP
Maricopa Medical Center/Banner Phoenix Poison
and Drug Information Center, Phoenix, AZ

Amal Mattu, MD, FACEP
University of Maryland, Baltimore, MD

Christian A. Tomaszewski, MD, MS, MBA, FACEP
University of California Health Sciences,
San Diego, CA

Steven J. Warrington, MD, MEd
MercyOne Siouxland, Sioux City, IA

ASSOCIATE EDITORS

Tareq Al-Salamah, MBBS, MPH, FACEP
King Saud University, Riyadh, Saudi Arabia/
University of Maryland, Baltimore, MD

Wan-Tsu W. Chang, MD
University of Maryland, Baltimore, MD

Ann M. Dietrich, MD, FAAP, FACEP
University of South Carolina College of Medicine,
Greenville, SC

Kelsey Drake, MD, MPH, FACEP
St. Anthony Hospital, Lakewood, CO

Walter L. Green, MD, FACEP
UT Southwestern Medical Center, Dallas, TX

John C. Greenwood, MD
University of Pennsylvania, Philadelphia, PA

Danya Khoujah, MBBS
University of Maryland, Baltimore, MD

Sharon E. Mace, MD, FACEP
Cleveland Clinic Lerner College of Medicine/
Case Western Reserve University, Cleveland, OH

Nathaniel Mann, MD
Greenville Health System, Greenville, SC

George Sternbach, MD, FACEP
Stanford University Medical Center, Stanford, CA

Joseph F. Waeckerle, MD, FACEP
University of Missouri-Kansas City School of Medicine,
Kansas City, MO

EDITORIAL STAFF

Mark Paglia, Senior Manager
cdem@acep.org

Melissa Mills, Associate Editor

ISSN2325-0186 (Print)   ISSN2325-8365 (Online)

Contents

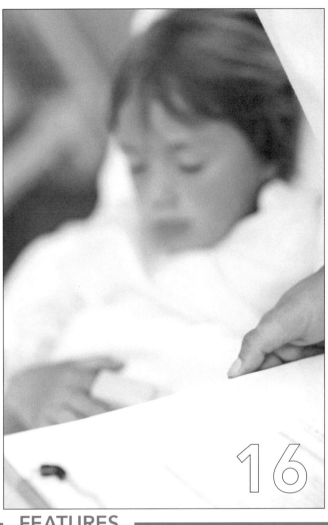

Lesson 5 4

All in Vein
Cerebral Venous Thrombosis
By Reem Alfalasi, MBChB; and Saef Izzy, MD, MBChB
Reviewed by Tareq Al-Salamah, MBBS, MPH, FACEP

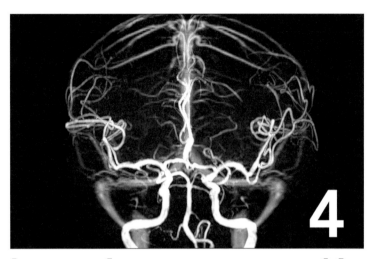

Lesson 6 16

Out of It
Approach to the Pediatric Patient With Altered Mental Status
By Jonathan M. Newsome, MD; Megan K. Long, MD, FAAP; and
Nipa V. Sanghani, MD, FAAP
Reviewed by Ann Dietrich, MD, FAAP, FACEP

FEATURES

The Critical ECG — Cerebral T-Wave Patterns..8
 By Amal Mattu, MD, FACEP

The LLSA Literature Review — Breastfeeding Patients 9
 By Courtney Sakas, MD; and Laura Welsh, MD
 Reviewed by Andrew J. Eyre, MD, MS-HPEd

Clinical Pediatrics — Ileocolic Intussusception...10
 By Katherine Guess, MD; and Aderonke Ojo, MBBS, MHA
 Reviewed by Sharon E. Mace, MD, FACEP

Critical Cases in Orthopedics and Trauma — Monteggia Fracture 12
 By Richard Courtney, DO; and Drew Clare, MD
 Reviewed by John Kiel, DO, MPH

The Critical Procedure — Partial Drainage of Subcutaneous Hematoma.....................14
 By Steven J. Warrington, MD, MEd, MS

The Critical Image — Injury after a fall...26
 By Joshua S. Broder, MD, FACEP

CME Questions 28
 Reviewed by Kelsey Drake, MD; Nathaniel Mann, MD; and Ann Dietrich, MD, FAAP, FACEP

Drug Box — Acetazolamide 30
 By Frank LoVecchio, DO, MPH, FACEP

Tox Box — Flecainide Overdose...30
 By Christian A. Tomaszewski, MD, MS, MBA, FACEP

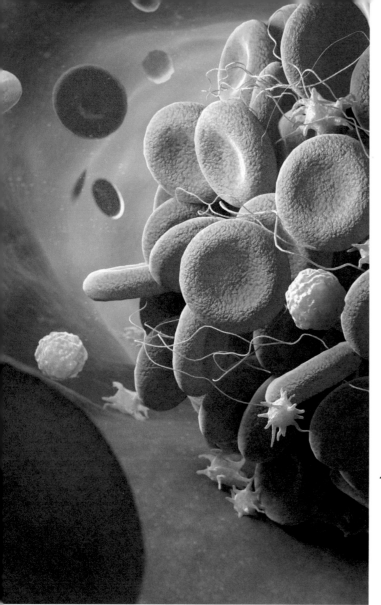

All in Vein

Cerebral Venous Thrombosis

LESSON **5**

By Reem Alfalasi, MBChB; and Saef Izzy, MD, MBChB
Dr. Alfalasi is a critical care fellow in the Department of
Anesthesiology at Columbia University Irving Medical Center in
New York, New York, and Dr. Izzy is a neurocritical care faculty
member in the Department of Neurology at Brigham and
Women's Hospital in Boston, Massachusetts.

Reviewed by Tareq Al-Salamah, MBBS, MPH, FACEP

Objectives

On completion of this lesson, you should be able to:

1. Identify signs and symptoms of CVT.
2. List risk factors associated with the development of CVT.
3. Describe the pathophysiology that contributes to the development of CVT.
4. Recognize the appropriate diagnostic workup of patients with concerns for CVT.
5. Identify the appropriate treatment and disposition of patients with CVT.

From the EM Model

12.0 Nervous System Disorders
    12.8 Other Conditions of the Brain
        12.8.4 Cerebral Venous Sinus Thrombosis

■ CRITICAL DECISIONS ■

- When should cerebral venous thrombosis be suspected?

- Which risk factors contribute to the development of CVT?

- What is the appropriate diagnostic workup for CVT?

- What are common diagnostic pitfalls in the workup of CVT?

- What is the appropriate management of CVT?

Cerebral venous thrombosis (CVT) is an uncommon cause of cerebrovascular disease, accounting for up to 1% of all strokes in adults. CVT is a challenging diagnosis to make due to a wide range of clinical presentations; hence, a high degree of clinical suspicion is required to make the diagnosis. Although most cases are associated with favorable outcomes, delays in diagnosis are associated with higher rates of complications, disability, and even death.

■ CASE ONE

A 78-year-old man presents via EMS for altered mental status. The patient's daughter states that he was recently diagnosed with metastatic colon cancer and has complained of a headache over the past 2 days. He appeared lethargic last night and was unresponsive this morning. His vital signs are blood pressure 210/118, heart rate 48, respiratory rate 12, temperature 36.6°C (97.9°F), and SpO2 98% on room air. On observation, the patient appears somnolent and altered. On examination, the patient has a GCS score of 7, asymmetric pupils, and left upper and lower extremity weakness. He is emergently intubated and started on hypertonic saline. The head of the bed is elevated to 30 degrees.

■ CASE TWO

A 22-year-old woman presents with a 2-week history of a headache. She states that the headache has been progressively worsening, describes it as diffuse and dull, and says it is associated with numbness in her right hand. Her past medical history is significant for obesity and taking oral contraceptive pills. The patient's neurological exam is suggestive of right upper extremity numbness and weakness but is otherwise unremarkable.

■ CASE THREE

A 32-year-old woman G2P1001 presents via EMS with a seizure. The patient's seizure terminated with 4 mg of IV lorazepam. Her vitals are blood pressure 110/67, heart rate 79, respiratory rate 16, temperature 37.2°C (99°F), and SpO2 98% on room air. The patient is 28 weeks pregnant, and her pregnancy is complicated with gestational diabetes. Her finger stick glucose is 178 mg/dL. On reassessment at 45 minutes after presentation, the patient is alert and oriented and back to her baseline. She states that she has been experiencing blurring vision and a worsening frontal headache over the past week.

Introduction

A thrombus in the cerebral venous system develops because of imbalances between prothrombotic and thrombolytic factors. Risk factors leading to CVT are similar to those that lead to venous thromboembolism and can be described by Virchow's triad (blood stasis, hypercoagulability, and endothelial injury). Once a clot is formed, pressure builds up within the cerebral venous system, and the integrity of the blood-brain barrier is disrupted, leading to vasogenic edema and cerebral hemorrhage. Increased pressures can also lead to decreased cerebral perfusion pressures, resulting in ischemia and cytotoxic edema. Increased cerebral venous pressures contribute to hydrocephalus development, which can lead to increased intracranial pressures and, in some cases, to cerebral herniation and devastating neurological outcomes.

CRITICAL DECISION

When should cerebral venous thrombosis be suspected?

CVT can present on a broad spectrum, ranging from no symptoms to subtle presentations or critical life-threatening conditions such as intracranial hemorrhage, elevated intracranial pressure (ICP), and rarely, cerebral herniation. Hence, a high degree of suspicion is required for diagnosis. CVT should be suspected in young patients with a stroke, a stroke that crosses typical arterial distributions, multiple cortical or subcortical hemorrhagic infarctions, or a stroke that presents with atypical features such as altered mental status, seizures, or a headache. CVT should also be suspected in pregnant women with a headache with neurologic deficits, seizures, or a history of taking oral contraceptive pills.

CRITICAL DECISION

Which risk factors contribute to the development of CVT?

More than 85% of CVT cases have one or more identifiable risk factors. When an imbalance between a prothrombotic and thrombolytic state occurs, a clot can form within the cerebral venous system. Many of these risk factors can be described by Virchow's triad (blood stasis, hypercoagulability, and endothelial injury). Risk factors include lupus; hematological conditions such as thrombophilia, thrombotic thrombocytopenic purpura, and heparin-induced thrombocytopenia; systemic or parameningeal infections and infections of the face or sinuses; malignancies; pregnancy and puerperium; and medications such as oral contraceptive pills (*Table 1*).

CRITICAL DECISION

What is the appropriate diagnostic workup for CVT?

Angiography is the gold standard in the diagnosis of CVT. However, due to advances in imaging techniques, it has been largely replaced by CT venography (CTV) and magnetic resonance venography (MRV). Angiography is rarely performed outside of cases that require endovascular therapies. A noncontrast CT can diagnose less than one-third of CVT cases by detecting a hyperattenuation of the affected venous sinus. Hence, a negative noncontrast CT cannot rule out CVT. Indirect signs of CVT on noncontrast CT include hydrocephalus, intracranial hemorrhage, venous infarct, or edema. In cases with a high degree of suspicion, imaging with venography can detect a thrombus by identifying a

✔ Pearls

- Edema or hemorrhage near a major venous sinus is suspicious for CVT.

- The highest rate of CVT recurrence is within the first year, affecting up to 15% of patients. The annual rate of recurrence after that is 6.5%.

- Cavernous sinus thrombosis is a subset of CVT that does not represent the majority of clinical presentations. Hence, symptoms such as chemosis, ophthalmoplegia, proptosis, and orbital pain are not the most common presentations of CVT.

filling defect. MRV is superior to CTV in detecting parenchymal lesions, is associated with a lower risk of contrast-related adverse reactions, and does not expose the patient to ionizing radiation. However, in contrast to CTV, MRV is more expensive, is not readily available, cannot be performed on patients with ferromagnetic devices, and has a higher probability of developing motion artifacts.

No single laboratory test is useful in diagnosing CVT, as it is often a radiographic diagnosis. However, laboratory results can help identify underlying conditions contributing to the development of CVT. The patient's initial workup should include a complete blood count, a chemistry panel, prothrombin time, activated partial thromboplastin time, and an erythrocyte sedimentation rate. Once the diagnosis of CVT is confirmed, a workup to identify precipitating factors is warranted. More than 30% of patients with CVT have an underlying thrombophilia. Thus, blood work should be drawn before the administration of anticoagulation (unless doing so will delay anticoagulant therapy), or 2 to 4 weeks after discontinuation of anticoagulants, as treatment can interfere with laboratory values and the diagnosis of thrombophilias. The hematology department should be consulted for further testing and management. A D-dimer test does not typically help diagnose or rule out CVT. Additionally, look for other precipitating factors such as systemic or parameningeal infections.

CRITICAL DECISION

What are common diagnostic pitfalls in the workup of CVT?

Due to the broad spectrum of possible clinical presentations, CVT can mimic other conditions and can be easily misdiagnosed; hence, a high degree of suspicion is required for diagnosis. It is estimated that up to 40% of CVT patients have a concomitant intracranial hemorrhage because of increased venous pressure. CVT bleed can present as a lobar hemorrhage with bilateral parenchymal lesions or a cerebral infarct that crosses multiple arterial territories. Altered mental status is a common presentation of CVT in the elderly population who are, in general, less likely to present with a headache compared to the younger population.

✖ Pitfalls

- Failing to recognize that a negative noncontrast CT of the head does not rule out CVT, as less than one-third of scans demonstrate a thrombus by detecting hyperattenuation of the affected sinus.

- Admitting a patient to a floor bed in the setting of clinical stability on presentation, which is not recommended due to the high risk of rapid clinical deterioration early in the course of CVT. Patients should be admitted to a stroke unit or a unit with a higher level of care, such as the ICU.

- Failing to recognize that altered mental status or unusual behavior in this patient population could signify underlying seizure activity, requiring antiepileptic therapy and an EEG.

Name	Description
Thrombophilias	Protein C and S deficiency, factor V Leiden mutation, G20210A mutation, hyperhomocysteinemia, antiphospholipid syndrome, antithrombin deficiency
Infections	CNS, parameningeal, systemic infections
Hematologic	Heparin-induced thrombocytopenia, essential thrombocytosis, paroxysmal nocturnal hemoglobinuria, thrombotic thrombocytopenic purpura
Medications	Asparaginase, tamoxifen, oral contraceptive pills, steroids, methotrexate
Others	Pregnancy and puerperium, vasculitides, dehydration, head trauma, arteriovenous malformations, hyperthyroidism

TABLE 1. Cerebral Venous Thrombosis Risk Factors

CRITICAL DECISION

What is the appropriate management of CVT?

Anticoagulation is the cornerstone therapy for the management of CVT. Anticoagulation facilitates recanalization, prevents clot propagation, and is considered safe in CVT management, even in CVT cases with a concurrent intracranial hemorrhage. It is still important to consult colleagues in neurology, hematology, and related departments in cases of CVT. There is limited literature suggesting that treating CVT with low-molecular-weight heparin (LMWH) or unfractionated heparin (UFH) is associated with a lower dependency rate or death. UFH is still the preferred agent in clinically unstable patients or patients who undergo an invasive procedure such as a decompressive hemicraniectomy. This is due to the availability of reversal agents, a short half-life, and the ability to closely monitor patients. Patients are initially managed with heparin during the acute phase of the illness and then transitioned to an oral anticoagulant. Monotherapy with aspirin is inadequate for the management of CVT. Endovascular therapy is indicated in patients who continue to decompensate despite maximal medical therapy. These include catheter-directed thrombolysis or mechanical thrombectomy. However, these complex decisions are often made in conjunction with hematologists, neurologists, neurointensivists, and interventional radiologists. Patients with rapid deterioration and concerns for cerebral herniation should undergo ICP-reducing measures such as hyperventilation, elevation of the head of the bed, administration of hypertonic intravenous solutions such as mannitol or hypertonic saline, and in severe cases, decompressive craniectomy.

Summary

CVT is uncommonly encountered in the emergency department. It can present vaguely, mimicking other more common presentations, such that a high degree of suspicion is required to diagnose this condition. Although patients with neurological signs and symptoms are often worked up with a noncontrast CT scan of the head, these scans are usually unremarkable in patients with CVT and, if abnormal, often present with indirect signs that can deter the clinician from making the diagnosis. Patients diagnosed with CVT should be started on anticoagulation, even in the presence of an intracranial bleed due to CVT. Admission to a neurointensive care unit is recommended due to the high risk of decompensation during the acute phase.

CASE RESOLUTIONS

CASE ONE

The patient's presentation raised concern for a space-occupying lesion with increased intracranial pressures and possible cerebral herniation. His workup included a noncontrast CT scan of his brain that revealed significant right temporoparietal intracerebral hemorrhage with cerebral edema with signs of uncal herniation and an area of hyperattenuation in the cerebral venous system that was concerning for CVT. CTV was obtained and showed a thrombus in the right transverse sinus. Therefore, a heparin drip was initiated, and the patient was admitted to the neurointensive care unit for further management. His condition continued to deteriorate despite maximal medical therapy, which warranted a decompressive craniectomy.

CASE TWO

The patient's workup included a lumbar puncture that showed normal opening pressures. Her noncontrast CT scan of the head revealed a delta sign, suggesting CVT. A CTV was diagnostic for superior sagittal sinus thrombosis. She was started on a heparin drip and admitted to the neurointensive care unit for further management. During her workup, she was diagnosed with factor V Leiden thrombophilia and was advised to consider nonhormonal birth control options. She remained clinically stable during her hospital course and was discharged on aspirin and warfarin. Her outpatient MRV in 3 months revealed a complete recanalization of her cerebral venous system.

CASE THREE

The patient's acute onset blurry vision was concerning for a stroke. Her workup included a noncontrast CT head scan, which showed a left parieto-occipital intracranial hemorrhage (ICH) with a 2-mm midline shift. CT angiography was unremarkable. During her first day of hospitalization, she experienced multiple seizures and worsening of her mental status, which required intubation. Given her risk factors and the clinical course of the ICH, CVT was suspected. Therefore, CTV was obtained and showed thrombosis in the proximal left transverse sinus. The patient was started on a heparin drip, and neurosurgery was consulted for an evaluation. Repeat CT and CTV showed expansion of the ICH size with worsening midline shift; there was also a significant increase in venous clot burden despite starting heparin. The patient underwent catheter-directed thrombolysis and was started on maximal intracranial hypertension treatment, including mannitol, external ventricular drain, and sedation.

REFERENCES

1. Centers for Disease Control and Prevention. Traumatic brain injury and concussion. https://www.cdc.gov/traumaticbraininjury/index.html
2. Dmytriw AA, Song JSA, Yu E, Poon CS. Cerebral venous thrombosis: state of the art diagnosis and management. *Neuroradiology.* 2018;60(7):669-685.
3. Gulati D, Strbian D, Sundararajan S. Cerebral venous thrombosis: diagnosis and management. *Stroke.* 2014;45(2):e16-e18.
4. Piazza G. Clinician update cerebral venous thrombosis. *Circulation.* 2012;1704-1709.
5. Saposnik G, Barinagarrementeria F, Brown RD Jr, et al. Diagnosis and management of cerebral venous thrombosis: a statement for healthcare professionals from the American Heart Association/American Stroke Association. *Stroke.* 2011;42(4):1158-1192.
6. Coutinho JM. Cerebral venous thrombosis. *J Thromb Haemost.* 2015;13 suppl 1:S238-S244.
7. Devasaqayam S, Wyatt B, Leyden J, Kleinig T. Cerebral venous sinus thrombosis incidence is higher than previously thought: a retrospective population-based study. *Stroke.* 2016;47(9):2180-2182.
8. Coutinho JM, Zuurbier SM, Aramideh M, Stam J. The incidence of cerebral venous thrombosis: a cross-sectional study. *Stroke.* 2012;43(12):3375-3377.
9. Zuurbier SM, Hiltunen S, Lindgren E, et al. Cerebral venous thrombosis in older patients. *Stroke.* 2018;49(1):197-200.
10. Long B, Koyfman A, Runyon MS. Cerebral venous thrombosis: a challenging neurologic diagnosis. *Emerg Med Clin North Am.* 2017;35(4):869-878.
11. Patel SI, Obeid H, Matti L, Ramakrishna H, Shamoun FE. Cerebral venous thrombosis: current and newer anticoagulant treatment options. *Neurologist.* 2015;20(5):80-88.
12. Bushnell C, Saposnik G. Evaluation and management of cerebral venous thrombosis. *Continuum (Minneap Minn).* 2014;20(2 Cerebrovascular Disease):335-351.
13. Silvis SM, Aguiar de Sousa D, Ferro JM, Coutinho JM. Cerebral venous thrombosis. *Nature Rev Neurol.* 2017;13:555-565.
14. Bousser MG, Ferro JM. Cerebral venous thrombosis: an update. *Lancet Neurol.* 2007;6(2):162-170.
15. Seneviratna A, Pallemulle R. Cerebral venous thrombosis in a post-partum patient. *Sri Lankan J Anaesthesiol.* 2019;27(1):97-99.
16. Lu A, Shen PY, Dahlin BC, Nidecker AE, Nundkumar A, Lee PS. Cerebral venous thrombosis and infarct: review of imaging manifestations. *Applied Radiol.* 2016;45(3):9-17.
17. Zuurbier SM, Coutinho JM. Cerebral venous thrombosis. In: Islam M, eds. *Thrombosis and Embolism: From Research to Clinical Practice. Advances in Experimental Medicine and Biology.* Vol 906. 2016.
18. Sharma C, Yadav A, Singh SS, Mehrotra M, Prakash A. Obstetric cerebral venous thrombosis: a clinical dilemma. *J Clin Diagn Res.* 2019;13(8).
19. Behrouzi R, Punter M. Diagnosis and management of cerebral venous thrombosis. *Clin Med (Lond).* 2018;18(1):75-79.
20. Ageno W, Beyer-Westendorf J, Garcia DA, Lazo-Langner A, McBane RD, Paciaroni M. Guidance for the management of venous thrombosis in unusual sites. *J Thromb Thrombolysis.* 2016;41(1):129-143.
21. Hartel M, Kluczewska E, Gancarczyk-Urlik E, Pierzchała K, Bien K, Zastawnik A. Cerebral venous sinus thrombosis. *Phlebology.* 2015;30(1):3-10.
22. Khealani BA, Wasay M, Saadah M, et al. Cerebral venous thrombosis: a descriptive multicenter study of patients in Pakistan and Middle East. *Stroke.* 2008;39(10):2707-2711.
23. Ferro JM, Canhão P, Bousser MG, Stam J, Barinagarrementeria F; ISCVT Investigators. Cerebral vein and dural sinus thrombosis in elderly patients. *Stroke.* 2005;36(9):1927-1932.
24. Martinelli I, Sacchi E, Landi G, Taioli E, Duca F, Mannucci PM. High risk of cerebral-vein thrombosis in carriers of a prothrombin-gene mutation and in users of oral contraceptives. *N Engl J Med.* 1998;338(25):1793-1797.
25. Guimarães J, Azevedo E. Phytoestrogens as a risk factor for cerebral sinus thrombosis. *Cerebrovasc Dis.* 2005;20(2):137-138.
26. Davie CA, O'Brien P. Stroke and pregnancy. *J Neurol Neurosurg Psychiatry.* 2008;79(3):240-245.
27. Wasay M, Bakshi R, Bobustuc G, et al. Cerebral venous thrombosis: analysis of a multicenter cohort from the United States. *J Stroke Cerebrovasc Dis.* 2008;17(2):49-54.
28. Gosk-Bierska I, Wysokinski W, Brown RD Jr, et al. Cerebral venous sinus thrombosis: Incidence of venous thrombosis recurrence and survival. *Neurology.* 2006;67(5):814-819.
29. Ogata T, Kamouchi M, Kitazono T, et al. Cerebral venous thrombosis associated with iron deficiency anemia. *J Stroke Cerebrovasc Dis.* 2008;17(6):426-428.
30. Alper G, Berrak SG, Ekinci G, Canpolat C, Erzen C. Sagittal sinus thrombosis associated with thrombocytopenia: a report of two patients. Pediatr Neurol. 1999;21(2):573-575.
31. Otite FO, Patel S, Sharma R, et al. Trends in incidence and epidemiologic characteristics of cerebral venous thrombosis in the United States. *Neurology.* 2020;95(16):e2200-e2213.

The Critical ECG
Cerebral T-Wave Patterns

By Amal Mattu, MD, FACEP
Dr. Mattu is a professor, vice chair, and director of the
Emergency Cardiology Fellowship in the Department
of Emergency Medicine at the University of Maryland
School of Medicine in Baltimore.

Objective

On completion of this article, you should be able to:
- Discuss how cerebral disorders affect T waves.

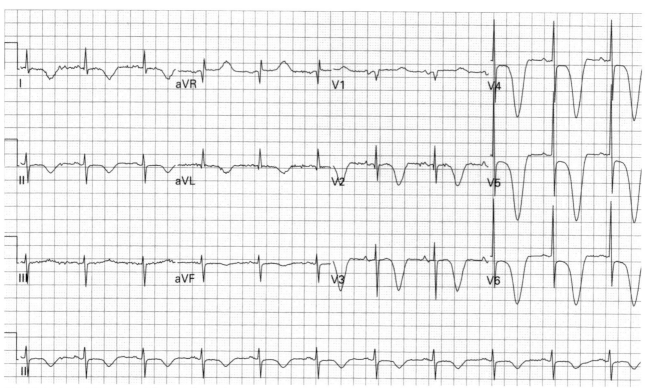

FIGURE 1. A 77-year-old man found unconscious at home.

Sinus rhythm, rate 64, left anterior fascicular block, left ventricular hypertrophy, prolonged QT interval, T-wave abnormality suggestive of diffuse cardiac ischemia versus intracranial hemorrhage (*Figure 1*). The most prominent abnormality is the presence of giant T-wave inversions in the precordial leads. T-wave inversions of this magnitude in patients with a depressed level of consciousness are highly suggestive of a large intracranial hemorrhage and, in fact, are often referred to as "cerebral T-wave patterns." These T-wave abnormalities may be present in nonhemorrhagic cerebral disorders as well (eg, cerebral edema, ischemic stroke), but less commonly. They may be present in the limb leads, although they tend to be most prominent in the precordial leads, where their magnitude may be 20 mm or more. A prolonged QT interval typically is associated with these cerebral T waves. Rarely, T-wave inversions of this magnitude occur in cardiac ischemia, but those patients are likely to have a normal mental status. The exact reason why cerebral disorders can cause these unusual T waves is uncertain. This patient did, in fact, have a large intracranial hemorrhage and died within 2 days (*Figure 2*).

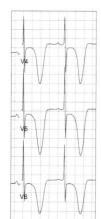

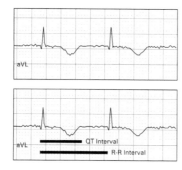

For this rate, the QT interval > one-half the R-R interval — the QT interval is prolonged for this rate.

FIGURE 2. CNS disasters can produce a range of ECG abnormalities. In this instance, the patient demonstrates deeply inverted T waves. The QT interval is also prolonged, another manifestation of a significant CNS event. Determination of the QT interval can be performed via several different methods, including Bazett's formula or a comparison of the QT interval relative to the R-R interval. In this simple bedside determination, the QT interval is compared to the R-R interval; in sinus rhythm with rates between 60 and 100 per minute, a normal QT interval should be less than one-half the related R-R interval for that rate.

*From **Mattu A, Brady W**. ECGs for the Emergency Physician 2. London: BMJ Publishing. Reprinted with permission.*

The Literature Review
Breastfeeding Patients

By Courtney Sakas, MD; and Laura Welsh, MD
Department of Emergency Medicine, Boston
University, Boston, Massachusetts

Objective

On completion of this article, you should be able to:

- Discuss best practices for treating breastfeeding patients.

Black AD. Managing the breastfeeding patient in the emergency department. *Ann Emerg Med.* 2020 Jan;75(1):105-110.

KEY POINTS

- Indiscriminate "pump and dump" advice can be harmful and cause early weaning.
- There are free and low-cost resources that can be easily accessed on shift to help guide medication use in breastfeeding patients.
- The breastfeeding patient differs from the pregnant patient; breastfeeding patients have more safe options for pain control and imaging studies.
- Few illnesses are absolute contraindications to breastfeeding, and it is generally safe for patients to continue to breastfeed while ill.

The lack of education surrounding breastfeeding patients in the emergency department can lead to well-intentioned but confusing advice for patients. Often, to protect themselves and the infant, the breastfeeding patient is advised to "pump and dump" if they are exposed to certain medications, contrast agents, or infectious illnesses. However, this advice can be misguided and harmful. Even a brief interruption in breastfeeding can lead to disruptions in milk production and result in early weaning. Even if a breastfeeding patient is not exposed to potentially harmful substances, a prolonged emergency department wait time without the ability to pump at regular intervals can interrupt milk supply and increase the risk of complications such as mastitis.

Medications that are contraindicated in pregnancy are not necessarily contraindicated in the breastfeeding patient. For instance, NSAIDs and opioids with shorter half-lives (eg, fentanyl and morphine) are safe options for analgesia. If an oral opioid is needed, hydrocodone is the oral agent preferred by the Academy of Breastfeeding Medicine, with a recommended dose of 30 mg or less daily. Hydromorphone has a long half-life, and oxycodone concentrates in the breast milk — both should therefore be avoided. If procedural sedation is performed, midazolam, fentanyl, propofol, and etomidate are safe, but there are insufficient data on ketamine to support its use in breastfeeding patients. When determining the safety of other classes of medications, physicians should consider the concentration of the substance in the breast milk relative to the patient's blood; if the drug can be absorbed orally by the infant; and if the drug could interfere with breast milk supply or affect the taste of breast milk, thereby reducing the infant's desire to feed.

Contrast and radiation exposure recommendations also change in breastfeeding patients compared to pregnant patients. X-rays confer no risk to the breastfed infant, and CT scans with contrast are also safe. There are no reports of direct harm to a breastfed infant from iodinated contrast in the breast milk. MRI imaging with gadolinium is safe according to the American College of Radiology, as the infant dose is negligible compared to the patient dose. Nuclear medicine study safety depends on the specific isotope used and the half-life of that agent. For instance, a hepatobiliary iminodiacetic acid (HIDA) scan requires no interruption in breastfeeding, but a V/Q scan requires a 13-hour interruption in breastfeeding due to its radioactive half-life. For all nuclear studies, there is no need to "pump and dump," as the breast milk can be saved until the radioactivity has dissipated.

Infectious disease is another area that can be confusing in regard to breastfeeding recommendations. In general, ordinary infections frequently encountered in the emergency department are not a reason to discontinue breastfeeding. The few absolute contraindications to breastfeeding are Ebola, HIV, Marburg, Lassa, smallpox, African trypanosomiasis, rabies, HTLV-1, and brucellosis. If a breastfeeding patient has an airborne illness like varicella or tuberculosis, direct breastfeeding should be avoided, but pumping is safe. Zoster infection is only a contraindication if the breastfeeding patient has lesions across their breast. Mastitis is not a contraindication unless there is an associated abscess, in which case it is recommended to discard breast milk for the first 24 hours of antibiotics.

Emergency physicians do not often receive formal education on human lactation, and these knowledge gaps can harm the nursing infant or breastfeeding relationship. If a physician has questions regarding the safety of medications, many online resources exist, including LactMed (an online database) and InfantRisk (a website and an app). Additionally, as most newborns nurse about every 2 to 3 hours, providing a patient with a breast pump while in the emergency department can help preserve supply and prevent painful complications like clogged ducts or mastitis.

Critical Decisions in Emergency Medicine's series of LLSA reviews features articles from ABEM's 2022 Lifelong Learning and Self-Assessment Reading List. Available online at acep.org/moc/llsa and on the ABEM website.

Ileocolic Intussusception

By Katherine Guess, MD; and Aderonke Ojo, MBBS, MHA
Baylor College of Medicine, Houston, Texas

Reviewed by Sharon E. Mace, MD, FACEP

Objective

On completion of this article, you should be able to:

■ Discuss the presentation and management of ileocolic intussusception.

CASE PRESENTATION

A previously healthy and fully vaccinated 7-month-old girl presents with a 1-day history of nonbloody and nonbilious emesis. Prior to presentation, she vomited six times. The emesis consisted of undigested food. She is now unable to tolerate any PO without vomiting. Her last urine output was 12 hours ago, and her last bowel movement occurred the previous day and was nonbloody. Her parents note that the child appears uncomfortable and is less active than usual. She does not have a fever and has had no sick contacts.

This patient's vital signs were BP 90/56, P 148, R 36, and T 38°C (100.4°F); SpO2 was 99% on room air. She was lethargic and had dry mucous membranes. She had clear breath sounds bilaterally, and her abdomen was soft and nontender, with no organomegaly. A point-of-care glucose was 40 mg/dL. She received a D10 bolus and a 40 cc/kg normal saline bolus. Ultrasound of the abdomen revealed an ileocolic intussusception.

Clinical Presentation

While the presentations of intussusception may vary, the typical picture is a healthy infant, 6 months to toddler age, who presents with acute onset of intermittent episodes of abdominal pain interspersed with asymptomatic periods. Children often pull their knees toward their chest in order to find relief from the pain. While this is a common finding with this presentation, it is not specific for the diagnosis. Additional nonspecific findings include nausea, vomiting, and diarrhea. Children are often misdiagnosed with gastroenteritis because of the overlapping symptomatology. Later findings of intussusception include bloody or "red currant jelly" stools, a palpable "sausage-like" mass in the abdomen, lethargy, and altered mental status. The classic triad of intermittent abdominal pain, bloody stools, and a palpable abdominal mass is frequently taught as the most common presentation for children with intussusception, but multiple studies confirm that less than 40% of cases present with these symptoms simultaneously. To complicate the diagnosis even further, patients may be completely asymptomatic at the time of presentation.

Differential Diagnosis

The differential diagnosis is broad and includes gastroenteritis, constipation, bowel obstruction, malrotation, volvulus, infectious diarrheas, appendicitis, sepsis, meningitis, head injury, or toxic ingestions in children who present with an altered mental state.

Pathophysiology

Intussusception involves telescoping of the bowel within itself and is the most common abdominal emergency in children less than 2 years old. Intussusceptions may be ileoileal, ileocolic, jejunojejunal, jejunoileal, or colocolic, but the majority of intussusceptions involve the terminal ileum and adjacent colon. Ileocolic intussusceptions comprise 90% of this type of bowel pathology.

The underlying pathogenesis leading to intussusception is poorly understood, and as many as 90% of cases are idiopathic. A very small percentage of these children may have a lead point. Lead points are typically discovered in surgery following a failed attempt to reduce the intussusception radiologically. Investigators suggest that lymphoid hyperplasia caused by viral or bacterial infections serve as lead points, areas that disturb peristalsis and contribute to the development of the intussusception.

Management

A majority of intussusceptions are successfully reduced with an air enema by a pediatric radiologist. Many institutions continue to use barium enemas for reduction, but air enemas have a higher success rate at 84%. A patient with intussusception who is fluid depleted should be fluid resuscitated prior to reduction, and a surgery consultation should be obtained prior to radiology reduction in case the intussusception is nonreducible or if the rare complication of perforation occurs from the reduction. Most patients can be safely discharged home after a period of observation in the emergency department, or in the observation unit if they are able to tolerate PO with return precautions.

Complications

If intussusception is misdiagnosed or the diagnosis is delayed, the obstruction caused by the bowel telescoping may lead to vascular compromise or obstruction and subsequent bowel necrosis and perforation. Patients with prolonged intussusception may present with altered mental status, syncope, peritonitis, and hypovolemic or septic shock. Recurrent intussusception occurs in about 10% to 20% of patients, and 50% of these children recur within the first week after the initial reduction. This is one reason why a period of observation postreduction is recommended. Parents should be given clear instructions for when to return.

Association With Infections and Vaccines

Infectious etiologies, including viral gastroenteritis or bacterial enteritis, have been associated with intussusception in infants and children. Adenovirus and human herpes virus 6 (HHV-6) infections have been associated with subsequent development of intussusception, and concurrent infections of these two viruses increase the risk of intussusception even further.

A previously distributed rotavirus vaccine was associated with a more than 30-fold increase in the development of intussusception and was removed from the market in 1999. It has been replaced with two oral vaccines. While intussusception remains a rare adverse effect following administration of the rotavirus vaccines, physicians agree that the protection from viral gastroenteritis caused by rotavirus outweighs the risk of intussusception. Children with a history of intussusception should not receive either rotavirus vaccine.

Bowel abnormalities such as Meckel diverticula, polyps, mesenteric nodes, lymphoma, duplication, and hemangiomas

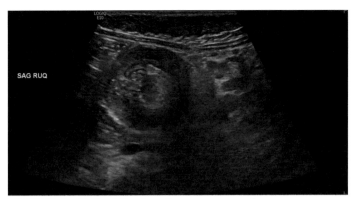

FIGURE 1. Coiled-Spring Appearance of Intussusception Seen on Ultrasound of Right Upper Quadrant

may also serve as lead points. Diagnoses including Henoch-Schönlein purpura, cystic fibrosis, nephrotic syndrome, and Peutz-Jeghers syndrome predispose children to intussusception as well.

CASE RESOLUTION

Treatment included a 5 mL/kg D10 bolus and a 20 mL/kg normal saline bolus. The child's glucose level improved to 140 mg/dL. Pediatric radiology and pediatric surgery consultations were obtained. The child underwent a successful, uncomplicated reduction of the intussusception with an air enema and was discharged home after a brief period of observation.

REFERENCES

1. Waseem M. Intussusception. *Ped Emerg Care.* 2008; 24(11):793-800.
2. Mandeville K, Chien M, Willyerd FA, et al. Intussusception: clinical presentations and imaging characteristics. *Ped Emerg Care.* 2012;28(9):842-844.
3. Weihmiller SN, Buonomo C, and Bachur R. Risk stratification of children being evaluated for intussusception. *Pediatrics.* 2011;127(2):e296-e303.
4. Applegate KE. Intussusception in children: evidence-based diagnosis and treatment. *Ped Radiol.* 2009;39 suppl 2:S140-S143.
5. Cade M, Nylund M, Denson LA, and Noel JM. Bacterial enteritis as a risk factor for childhood intussusception: a retrospective cohort study. *J Pediatrics.* 2010;156(5): 761-765.
6. Burnett E, Parashar UD, and Tate JE. Associations of intussusception with adenovirus, rotavirus, and other pathogens: a review of the literature. *Pediatr Infec Dis J.* 2020;13:13.
7. Burnett E, Kabir F, Trang NV, et al. Infectious etiologies of intussusception among children <2 years old in 4 Asian countries. *J Infect Dis.* 2020;221(9):1499-1505.
8. Lappalainen S, Ylitalo S, Arola A, et al. Simultaneous presence of human herpesvirus 6 and adenovirus infections in intestinal intussusception of young children. *Acta Paediatr.* 2012;101(6):663-670.
9. Shui IM, Patel M, Parashar UD, et al. Risk of intussusception following administration of pentavalent rotavirus vaccine in US infants. *JAMA.* 2012;307(6):590-604.
10. Buttery JP, Standish J, and Bines JE. Intussusception and rotavirus vaccines: consensus on benefits outweighing recognized risk. *Pediatr Infect Dis J.* 2014; 33(7):772-773.
11. Centers for Disease Control and Prevention (CDC). Addition of history of intussusception as a contraindication for rotavirus vaccination. *MMWR Morb Mortal Wkly Rep.* 2011 Oct 21;60(41):1427.
12. Kee HM, Park JY, Yi DY, Lim IS. A case of intussusception with acute appendicitis. *Pediatr Gastroenterol Hepatol Nutr.* 2015 Jun;18(2):134-137.

Critical Cases in Orthopedics and Trauma

Monteggia Fracture

By Richard Courtney, DO; and Drew Clare, MD
University of Florida College of Medicine, Jacksonville, Florida

Reviewed by John Kiel, DO, MPH

Objective

On completion on this article, you should be able to:

- Recognize a Monteggia fracture.

CASE PRESENTATION

A 51-year-old right-handed man with no significant medical history presents after being assaulted with a large blunt object. He was struck all over without loss of consciousness. He has left proximal forearm pain. On examination, the patient has a 2-cm wound to the left proximal forearm along the dorsal/ulnar aspect that is hemostatic. The left arm is neurovascularly intact.

X-rays of the left arm revealed an open proximal ulnar fracture with an anteriorly displaced radial head consistent with an open Monteggia fracture (*Figure 1*). The patient received cefazolin 2 g IV and a tetanus booster in the trauma center. He was temporarily placed in a posterior long arm splint until he could be taken to the operating room by the orthopedic surgery team for debridement and washout as well as open reduction and internal fixation.

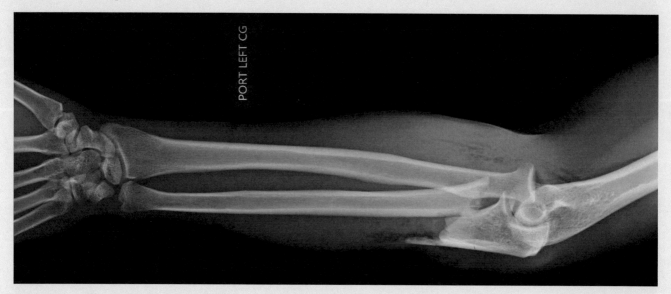

FIGURE 1. Elbow X-Ray Lateral View

Discussion

A Monteggia fracture is defined as a fracture of the proximal third of the ulna with associated radial head dislocation. José Luis Bado created the most commonly used classification system in which the fracture/dislocation pattern is divided into four categories:

- Type 1: Fracture of the proximal or middle third of the ulna with anterior dislocation of the radial head.
- Type 2: Fracture of the proximal or middle third of the ulna with posterior dislocation of the radial head.
- Type 3: Fracture of the ulnar metaphysis (distal to the coronoid process) with lateral dislocation of the radial head.
- Type 4: Fracture of the proximal or middle third of the ulna and anterior dislocation of the radial head.[1, 2]

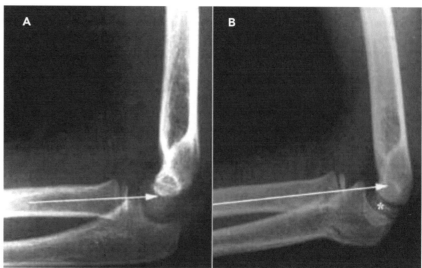

FIGURE 2. Radiocapitellar Line A is normal; B is abnormal, indicating dislocation.[5]

Type 1 fractures tend to be more common in the pediatric population, while type 2 fractures are the most common among adult patients. The mechanism of injury varies between the different types, with direct trauma to the ulna and axial loading injuries being the most common.[3]

Radial head dislocation can be subtle and is sometimes missed, leading to a delay in the diagnosis and treatment.[4] Diagnosis of radial head dislocation can be made by drawing the radiocapitellar line to evaluate if the line runs through the capitellum (*Figure 2*). If the line does not cross through the capitellum, this is suggestive of a radial head dislocation.

If radial head dislocation is missed, this can lead to a chronic unreducible dislocated radial head, resulting in pain and limited supination/pronation.[4] Additionally, dislocation of the radial head can lead to posterior interosseous nerve palsy, resulting in the loss of thumb and metacarpophalangeal joint extension, with preserved wrist extension.[5]

Management in the emergency department involves reduction of the ulnar fracture and dislocated radial head in consultation with orthopedic surgery. The majority of these injuries in adults require operative intervention with open reduction and internal fixation. Additionally, all open fractures require emergent orthopedic consultation for extensive washout.[6]

CASE RESOLUTION

The patient was taken to the operating room by the orthopedic surgery team for debridement and washout as well as open reduction and internal fixation (*Figure 3*). He had an uncomplicated postoperative course and was subsequently lost to follow-up.

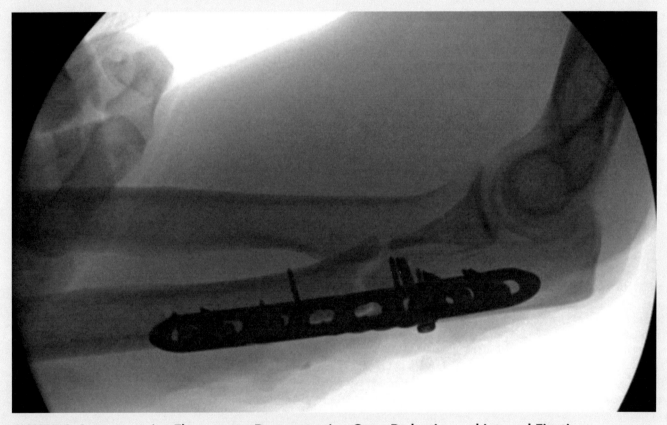

FIGURE 3. Intraoperative Fluoroscopy Demonstrating Open Reduction and Internal Fixation

REFERENCES

1. Bado JL. The Monteggia lesion. *Clin Orthop Relat Res*. 1967;50:71-86.
2. Beutel BG. Monteggia fractures in pediatric and adult populations. *Orthopedics*. 2012;35:138-144.
3. Eathiraju S, Mudgal CS, Jupiter JB. Monteggia fracture-dislocations. *Hand Clin*. 2007 May;23(2):165-177.
4. Perron AD, Hersh RE, Brady WJ, Keats TE. Orthopedic pitfalls in the ED: Galeazzi and Monteggia fracture-dislocation. *Am J Emerg Med*. 2001 May;19(3):225-228.
5. Yoshida N, Tsuchida Y. Posterior interosseous nerve palsy due to Bado type-III Monteggia fracture. *Case Reports*. 2018.
6. Delpont M, Louahem D, Cottalorda J. Monteggia injuries. *Orthop Traumatol Surg Res*. 2018;104(1S):S113-S120.

The Critical Procedure

Partial Drainage of Subcutaneous Hematoma

By Steven Warrington, MD, MEd
MercyOne Siouxland, Sioux City, Iowa

Objective

On completion of this article, you should be able to:

■ Demonstrate a partial drainage of subcutaneous hemtaoma.

Introduction

Subcutaneous hematomas are not uncommon and are generally left alone in the emergency department. However, certain situations may warrant partial drainage, such as if the skin is under significant tension and the clinician has concern for skin necrosis. Another consideration is if the patient has significant discomfort due to the size and pressure of the hematoma, which may warrant consideration for drainage or partial drainage.

Contraindications

■ Overlying infection

Benefits and Risks

The primary benefit of performing a partial drainage of a subcutaneous hematoma is to alleviate symptoms and decrease the risk of overlying skin necrosis. Partial drainage with this specific technique may also leave less of a scar than one of the alternative methods. There is a potential cosmetic benefit of not attempting partial drainage, depending on the site and size of the hematoma.

The primary risks associated with the procedure are introducing infection to the hematoma, creating a new hematoma or rebleeding, and having a poor cosmetic outcome. While failure of a procedure is often a risk, failure of this procedure as a whole is less likely, as it is only intended for partial drainage.

Alternatives

There are multiple potential approaches when faced with a subcutaneous hematoma. First, the clinician may just reassure the patient and not attempt any drainage. While it is an option, as these may resolve on their own, there are publications noting various risks such as necrosis, decreased mobilization in the elderly, and infections, with eventual operative management. Second, the physician may opt to attempt full drainage of the hematoma. This may be done in multiple fashions, such as with traditional scalpel and deloculation or other methods described in the literature, such as with a Yankauer suction tip. Finally, a consultant may be involved for possible operative drainage or evacuation.

Reducing Side Effects

Due to the high risk of infection, it has been recommended that sterile technique and saline be used, but there is some literature to suggest tap water may not cause a significant increase in the rate of infections when used for lavage. Additional side effects to consider are rebleeding or worsening the hematoma. The available literature suggests using compression after the procedure, but there are no specific data to determine if the approach provides any short- or long-term benefit.

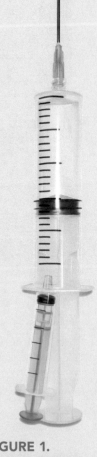

━━ TECHNIQUE ━━

1. **Consider** preprocedure ultrasound to define the area affected and use point-of-care ultrasound during the procedure to monitor the location of the needle tip.
2. **Obtain** the patient's consent and then obtain the materials and equipment for the procedure.
3. **Sterilize** and prep the area.
4. **Attach** a 16G needle/catheter to a 50-mL or larger syringe, with a 10-mL syringe available.
5. **Insert** the 16G needle through the skin that has been prepped toward the hematoma.
6. **Aspirate** on the syringe to create suction and place the smaller syringe into the space between the barrel flange and plunger flange to ensure constant negative pressure is created (*Figure 1*).
7. **Advance** the needle tip into the hematoma and pass through the hematoma repeatedly and in different tracts.
8. **Empty** the syringe and repeat as necessary.
9. **Dress** the site. Consider compression dressing.
10. **Instruct** the patient on signs of infection and follow-up care. Consider a short course of antibiotic therapy.

FIGURE 1.
Syringe Setup.
A small syringe is inserted between the base and plunger of the 50-mL syringe.

Special Considerations

The first thing to consider is the risk of infection for an undrained hematoma versus a drained hematoma. Although the risk of a sterile hematoma turning into an infected hematoma is often discussed in the literature, no original studies were found discussing rates of traumatic hematomas (noniatrogenic) converting to infected hematomas. Additionally, there was no original literature found on the risk of converting a sterile hematoma to an infected hematoma due to attempted drainage. It is important to note that the authors that originally described the technique recommended a short course (3 days) of antibiotics following the procedure.

The second point to consider is the difficulty of determining a hematoma versus other causes of swelling. Point-of-care ultrasound may be helpful to ensure fluid collection and to define the rough location of edges of the fluid collection. Furthermore, doing the procedure under ultrasound can help to ensure that the needle stays within the fluid collection and does not unnecessarily pass into healthy tissue, causing more pain and potential further bleeding.

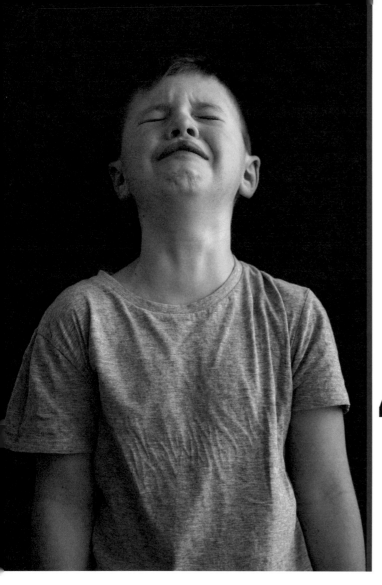

Out of It

Approach to the Pediatric Patient With Altered Mental Status

LESSON 6

By Jonathan M. Newsome, MD; Megan K. Long, MD, FAAP; and Nipa V. Sanghani, MD, FAAP

Dr. Newsome is a resident in the Department of Emergency Medicine, Dr. Long is an assistant professor of Pediatric Emergency Medicine, and Dr. Sanghani is an assistant professor in the Department of Emergency Medicine and assistant medical director of Pediatric Emergency Medicine at UTHealth Houston in Texas.

Reviewed by Ann Dietrich, MD, FAAP, FACEP

Objectives

On completion of this lesson, you should be able to:

1. Describe the different etiologies of altered mental status in a pediatric patient.
2. Explain when to order neuroimaging on a child and what type of neuroimaging to order based on the differential diagnosis.
3. Describe the optimal treatments for altered mental status depending on the cause.
4. Explain when it is reasonable to send a pediatric patient that presented with altered mental status home.
5. Discuss when a pediatric patient with altered mental status should be transferred to a tertiary care center for further evaluation and treatment.

From the EM Model

1.0 Signs, Symptoms, and Presentations
    1.3 General
        1.3.1. Altered Mental Status

■ CRITICAL DECISIONS ■

- How important are airway, breathing, and circulation in patients with altered mental status?
- How should the GCS be used in patients presenting after trauma?
- What presentations may have elevated intracranial pressures, and how can they be treated?
- When should neuroimaging be ordered in children with altered mental status?
- What signs are consistent with drug overdose, and what treatment is appropriate?

Altered mental status encompasses a broad differential diagnosis, spanning almost all physiologic systems; from metabolic encephalopathy to infection or traumatic brain injury (TBI). The ability to quickly and accurately determine the etiology of a patient's altered behavior is a keen skill emergency physicians must possess, and managing these patients may be a particularly daunting challenge.

CASE ONE

A 3-month-old boy presents via EMS after being found unresponsive during a nap. His mother says that she initiated CPR while EMS was en route. When EMS reached the patient, he was unresponsive, with P 160 and SpO2 100%. The patient's mother says that he has been in his usual state of health lately and does not have any other symptoms. On arrival, his vital signs are BP 120/60, P 100, R 35, and T 36.9°C (98.4°F); SpO_2 is 98% on room air.

At the hospital, the baby has a 10-minute seizure that resolves after a dose of lorazepam. On examination, the patient is postictal and unresponsive. A small bruise is noted on his ear. The baby appears to have some irregular respirations intermittently but is maintaining his airway. The cardiac and abdominal examinations are unremarkable. The patient is withdrawing to pain. While examining the patient, he has a second seizure that lasts 20 minutes. Another dose of lorazepam is given, and the patient is loaded with levetiracetam.

CASE TWO

A 6-year-old boy is brought in for unresponsiveness that started while he was riding in the car with his mother. The patient was in a booster seat and was wearing a seatbelt when he suddenly shot his head up, screamed, and slumped over. Prior to this, he had been in his normal state of health without other symptoms; his mother denies possible ingestion.

The patient has a history of a repaired left hypoplastic heart with a Fontan procedure, and he had a pacemaker placed at age 3 years. He is currently on aspirin but missed a few doses. His immunizations are up to date. His vital signs are BP 100/65, P 125, R 30, and T 37.1°C (98.8°F); SpO_2 is 100% on room air.

On examination, the patient is initially unresponsive. Within a few minutes, he starts to slowly arouse. He is agitated, crying, and uncooperative. He seems to have facial droop while crying. The patient has a holosystolic murmur that is 3/6, but he has a normal lung and abdominal examination. The patient is flailing his arms and legs, but his left arm and leg do not seem to be moving as much as the right side.

CASE THREE

A 14-year-old boy presents via ambulance. His mother states that he has appeared very sleepy today and is difficult to arouse. He has no history of recent illness, and he appeared to be in his usual state of health yesterday. He has a history of depression but is not taking any medications. His mother denies any further medical history.

On evaluation, the patient is sleeping but rouses to voice. His speech is intelligible but is short when answering questions, and he falls quickly back to sleep. His respirations appear to be deep and fast; he is protecting his airway and has a pulse oximetry of 100%. His vital signs include P 120 and T 36.6°C (99.7°F) but are otherwise normal. Further examination reveals warm skin without the presence of a rash, 5-mm pupils that are reactive bilaterally, and normal cardiac and pulmonary examinations. Aside from somnolence, he appears to be oriented without further neurologic deficits.

Introduction

Altered mental status (AMS) is a continuum that includes confusion, delirium, lethargy (stupor or obtundation), and coma. In the younger pediatric population, confusion and delirium may be hard to recognize, so physicians need to be vigilant. Children may be unable to express themselves, and children who have AMS may present as a child "acting out" or "throwing a tantrum." Moreover, infants may present with inconsolable crying or poor feeding and somnolence.

AMS can be seen with a wide array of metabolic, neurologic, traumatic, and infectious diseases as well as toxic ingestions. Airway, breathing, and circulation (ABCs) must always be assessed first. Once the ABCs are evaluated and determined to be stable or stabilized, a thorough history and physical examination are key in tailoring the appropriate workup of the pediatric patient. When obtaining a history, it is important to decipher the timing of the AMS to determine if the onset was acute or chronic and to discover any events that preceded the onset, such as trauma, seizure, fevers, and ingestions. It is crucial to ascertain any medical or surgical history that may predispose children to seemingly adult causes of AMS, such as stroke, sickle cell disease, congenital cardiac conditions, or surgery. When performing a physical examination, a thorough neurological examination may be the key to deciding which laboratory studies or imaging to order. A global neurologic deficit suggests a differential of toxic exposure or ingestion; metabolic encephalopathy; or infectious causes, such as encephalitis, meningitis, or sepsis. On the other hand, a focal neurologic deficit should lead a clinician to consider a workup for stroke, intracranial hemorrhage (trauma, aneurysm), or tumor.

Based on the direction that a detailed history and physical steers the physician, a wide array of laboratories and imaging can be ordered. For serum studies, a complete blood count (CBC), electrolytes, hepatic function panel, blood gas, glucose level, acetaminophen level, alcohol level, and aspirin level can be ordered. Urine pregnancy, urine drug screen, and urinalysis can also be sent to help determine the cause of the AMS. Other more invasive testing may be required, such as a lumbar puncture (LP). Diagnostic imaging such as CT or MRI may also be needed to fully evaluate and diagnose the child.

CRITICAL DECISION

How important are airway, breathing, and circulation in patients with altered mental status?

Traumatic injuries account for the highest rate of death and disability in the pediatric population, with TBI contributing the most to this statistic. Altered sensorium in pediatric patients presenting after traumatic injury may have a diversity of causes, including blunt head trauma, hemorrhagic shock, or severe pain. The pediatric population has a disproportionately large head compared to body size and weaker cervical musculature, which predisposes children to sustain more head injuries than adults following trauma. Rapid assessment of the patient's ABCs, in addition to disability and complete exposure (ABCDE) to assess for injuries, are time-critical actions.

CRITICAL DECISION

How should the GCS be used in patients presenting after trauma?

The Glasgow Coma Scale (GCS) is a quick assessment tool that quantifies a patient's mental status. The scale has been modified for patients 2 years old and younger to account for development. In addition to a patient's airway and breathing status, the GCS can be helpful when considering intubation; however, patients may present in respiratory failure without a depressed GCS score. A GCS score of 8 or less in the setting of traumatic injury should prompt early intubation, with careful consideration of the anatomic differences of the pediatric airway. TBI can be graded with the GCS; a GCS score of 3 to 8 indicates severe TBI, 8 to 12 indicates moderate TBI, and 13 to 15 indicates mild TBI.[1] The table below summarizes the Pediatric GCS (*Table 1*).[2,3] In addition, a pediatric GCS can be done using MDCalc: https://www.mdcalc.com/pediatric-glasgow-coma-scale-pgcs.

Decision tools such as the PECARN Pediatric Head Injury/Trauma Algorithm can help guide emergency physicians when deciding to order advanced imaging on pediatric patients.[4,5] Factors such as a depressed GCS score, severity of injury mechanism, findings of scalp occipital or parietal hematomas (in children younger than 2 years), evidence of skull fracture, loss of consciousness, or persistent vomiting should increase suspicion for TBI, necessitating CT examination versus observation and reassessment. A clinical calculator for PECARN for pediatric head injury can be found on MDCalc: https://www.mdcalc.com/pecarn-pediatric-head-injury-trauma-algorithm.

CRITICAL DECISION

What presentations may have elevated intracranial pressures, and how can they be treated?

In a child who presents with severe head trauma, hypovolemia and hypoxia drastically worsen patient outcomes and should be promptly addressed.[6] A full neurologic examination should be performed in a comatose patient after initial resuscitative efforts are complete. The neurologic examination includes pupillary examination, brain stem testing (oculocephalic reflex, corneal reflex, and cough reflex), and motor response to stimulation. Worsening mental status, anisocoria, and abnormal posturing should prompt concern for increased intracranial pressure and brain herniation. Changes in vital signs, including hypertension, bradycardia, and irregular respirations (Cushing's triad), are associated with brain herniation. These patients should be intubated and hyperventilated (only used with herniating patients) to prevent hypercarbia; management with either 3% saline 5 mL/kg IV or mannitol 0.25 to 1 g/kg IV is also appropriate, although newer guidelines suggest the superiority of hypertonic saline to mannitol.[7] Pediatric neurosurgery should be consulted immediately for patient evaluation and surgical decompression and evacuation of a hemorrhage, when appropriate.

Pediatric patients with mild to moderate head trauma who have evidence of a depressed skull fracture or intracranial hemorrhage on CT imaging should be transferred to a facility with pediatric neurosurgery for evaluation and surgical intervention, if needed. Patients less than 2 years old with a questionable history or injuries inconsistent with the reported

	Infant (<2 years old)	Child/Adult	Score (Max15)
Eye Opening	Opens eyes spontaneously	Opens eyes spontaneously	4
	Opens to voice	Opens to voice	3
	Opens to pain	Opens to pain	2
	Eyes do not open	Eyes do not open	1
Verbal Response	Coos and babbles	Oriented	5
	Irritable, cries	Confused	4
	Cries to pain	Inappropriate words	3
	Moans to pain	Incomprehensible sounds	2
	No response	No response	1
Motor Response	Moves purposefully	Obeys commands	6
	Withdraws to touch	Localizes to pain	5
	Withdraws to pain	Withdraws to pain	4
	Abnormal flexion posturing	Abnormal flexion posturing	3
	Abnormal extension posturing	Abnormal extension posturing	2
	No response	No response	1

TABLE 1.   Pediatric and Adult GCS

mechanism should raise suspicion for nonaccidental trauma, and further testing should include a skeletal survey x-ray series, evaluation of liver function tests, and an ophthalmologic examination to assess for retinal hemorrhages.

Children with mild head injury, including concussions and a single nondisplaced skull fracture (without intracranial bleeding), can be safely discharged home with follow-up with their primary care physician, provided there is no concern for nonaccidental trauma and they have returned to their neurologic baseline in the emergency department. If there is concern for nonaccidental trauma, social work and child protective services should be consulted to determine a safe discharge.

Vascular

The most common cause of spontaneous, nontraumatic, intracranial hemorrhages are arteriovenous malformations (AVMs). AVMs are more likely to cause repetitive episodes of bleeding, with worsening morbidity and mortality with each subsequent bleed.[8] Aneurysms are less likely but may result in a sentinel bleed. These lesions are both arterial in nature and can result in a subarachnoid hemorrhage. Patients with these lesions usually have an acute onset of symptoms such as headache (sometimes described as the worst headache of their lives), vomiting, focal neurological symptoms (depending on where the hemorrhage is located), and AMS.

Cerebral vascular accidents (strokes) are rare in the pediatric population, with an incidence of 1.2 to 13 cases per 100,000 for ischemic and hemorrhagic strokes combined.[9] Pediatric patients with sickle cell disease (6%-9%), congenital heart defect (most common cause), and cancer have a higher incidence of stroke than the general pediatric population. A central venous thrombosis can also be seen in children as a sequela of ear and sinus infections. Children have a highly variable presentation influenced by age and the vasculature affected. Patients usually present with a focal neurologic deficit (hemiparesis with facial weakness). Older children may present with headaches, whereas children younger than 4 years may present with seizures.

A cavernous hemangioma is a low-flow venous lesion that can cause a patient to have an intracranial hemorrhage.[8] This usually results in the subacute onset of symptoms. The patient would again start off with a headache and vomiting that may worsen over time as blood starts to accumulate within the cranium. The patient may develop a focal neurologic deficit and AMS as it expands.

Patients may need a CT head with a CT angiogram to look for vascular abnormalities, stroke, and hemorrhage emergently. If the patient is stable, an MRI brain with a magnetic resonance angiography and magnetic resonance venography for more in-depth imaging can be done.

Initial management is focused on stabilization and supportive care. Pediatric patients with sickle cell disease need an acute blood transfusion to reduce the amount of hemoglobin (Hgb) S to less than 30%.[8] Children with intracranial hemorrhage may need pediatric neurosurgical intervention to evacuate a hematoma in a ruptured aneurysm or to cauterize an AVM. Thrombolytics are experimental in pediatrics and are rarely used. If the patient has a large stroke, a thrombectomy may be considered. In the event that the patient has an ischemic stroke and needs thrombolytics or a thrombectomy, the patient should be transferred to a pediatric stroke center, and the therapies should be given in consultation with a pediatric neurologist. More than 75% of children have long-term morbidity, including learning difficulties, seizures, and hemiparesis.[8]

Infection

Infections account for 28% of pediatric emergency department visits per year.[10] AMS secondary to infection can range from somnolence to coma, and patients can quickly deteriorate if appropriate therapy is not administered.

Sepsis and Septic Shock

Septic shock is defined as severe infection resulting in hypotension with signs of end-organ dysfunction. AMS, vital sign derangements (eg, fever or hypothermia), poor capillary refill, or hypotension should raise suspicion for septic shock. Appropriate history and physical examination may provide evidence of a specific infectious etiology. Infectious workup typically includes point-of-care glucose, CBC with differential, complete metabolic panel, blood cultures, urinalysis with urine culture, lactic acid, and procalcitonin. LP should be performed when central nervous system (CNS) infection is suspected, once the patient is stabilized. A chest x-ray is only warranted in an altered patient that has signs of respiratory disease. Elevated white blood cells, procalcitonin, lactic acid, and metabolic acidosis help establish a diagnosis of septic shock.

Once shock has been identified, the patient must be quickly resuscitated with intravenous antibiotics and fluids.[11] Appropriate volume administration usually ranges from 20 to 60 mL/kg until stabilization of the patient's hemodynamic status is achieved. Vasopressor support should be added if the patient remains hemodynamically unstable after fluid administration; usually, norepinephrine is used in septic shock. Sources of septic infection include pneumonia, urinary tract infection, intra-abdominal infection, or CNS infection. If a rash is present, suspicion for meningococcemia (petechia and purpura) and toxic shock syndrome (sunburn-like rash followed by desquamation) should increase, and the patient should be evaluated and treated as necessary.

Empiric antibiotic therapy should be given within 1 hour of suspecting a patient has sepsis. Regimens are subdivided into age groups based on prevalence of causative pathogens. In neonates between 0 and 28 days old, ampicillin and gentamicin (or cefotaxime) are preferred, plus or minus acyclovir. Common pathogens associated with infection in this age group include Group B Streptococcus, Escherichia coli, Listeria, Enterococcus, and herpes simplex virus (HSV). Older infants and children can be treated with vancomycin and ceftriaxone as empiric therapy.

In infants with a history of prematurity, a physician should also consider the diagnosis of necrotizing enterocolitis (NEC) in conjunction with sepsis. This would necessitate clindamycin or metronidazole as empiric antibiotic therapy.[12] Infants with NEC may present with a change in feeding habits, hematochezia, vomiting, or other signs that are suggestive of bacteremia. These infants may also show findings of pneumatosis intestinalis on abdominal x-ray. Ultimately, these patients need management at a facility with pediatric surgeon availability.

Meningitis and Encephalitis

Infections of the CNS associated with AMS include encephalitis and meningitis. Encephalitis is an infection of the brain parenchyma, while meningitis is an infection of the meninges. Viruses are the most common cause of encephalitis and meningitis, but bacterial and fungal CNS infections typically have a more severe course. Encephalitis may also be secondary to noninfectious causes, such as autoimmune processes. Signs of CNS infections include fever, hypothermia, vomiting, diarrhea, poor feeding, bulging fontanelle (in infants), irritability, lethargy, seizures, neurologic deficit, and neck stiffness or nuchal rigidity.[13]

In patients less than 3 months old, the most common bacterial meningitic infections are caused by Group B Streptococcus and E. coli. In infants and children, Streptococcus pneumoniae and Neisseria meningitidis are the most common pathogens. Haemophilus influenzae should also be considered in unvaccinated children. Enteroviruses contribute to the majority of viral meningitis cases, but HSV should be considered in neonates presenting with vesicular lesions of the skin, eye, or mouth, or if the mother has a history of genital herpes infection. Recent studies suggest the highest risk for HSV infection is less than 14 days of age.[14]

Treatment of suspected meningitis should be given as quickly as possible. Ideally, blood cultures and cerebral spinal fluid (CSF) studies are obtained prior to antibiotic administration, but if the patient is too unstable or has signs of herniation,

---

✔ Pearls

- A child throwing a tantrum may be exhibiting signs of AMS.
- A thorough history and physical examination are vital to deciphering the cause of AMS in a pediatric patient.
- If a patient with a history of sickle cell disease or a congenital heart defect presents with a focal neurological defect, have a high suspicion for a stroke.

antibiotics should be administered without CSF. Unfortunately, meningitis has a high morbidity and mortality even with appropriate management. Newborns and neonates should receive ampicillin and cefotaxime or ampicillin and an aminoglycoside.[15] Infants and children older than 1 month should receive vancomycin and ceftriaxone. Antibiotic therapy should not be withheld in lieu of CT imaging of the brain, which is indicated when the patient is immunocompromised, shows signs of focal neurologic deficit, has papilledema, or has known CNS disease.[15] In addition, recent evidence supports the use of empiric acyclovir in neonates less than 21 days old.[16]

Abscesses and Empyema

Physicians who encounter patients with a combination of AMS and focal findings should always be suspicious of a cerebral or epidural abscess or subdural empyema. Cerebral abscesses can also result from an untreated congenital heart disease, endocarditis, or a dental infection. The peak incidence is between the ages of 4 and 7 years. Subdural empyema may be a consequence of bacterial meningitis, sinusitis, or otitis media. Epidural abscesses, although rare, can result from osteomyelitis of the skull and orbital cellulitis or sinusitis or otitis.

CRITICAL DECISION

When should neuroimaging be ordered in children with altered mental status?

A thorough history from the family about recent bacterial infections can assist with making the correct diagnosis. A head CT is crucial in diagnosing patients with focal infections. In addition to starting these patients on empiric antibiotics (usually vancomycin and ceftriaxone), pediatric neurosurgery needs to be consulted immediately for possible drainage of the abscess or empyema.

Neuroimaging

In children who require neuroimaging before LP, blood cultures should be obtained and empiric antibiotics administered before imaging. LP should be performed as soon as possible after neuroimaging is completed, provided that the imaging has not revealed any contraindications.

Indications for neuroimaging before LP include severely depressed mental status (coma), papilledema, focal neurologic deficit, history of hydrocephalus, presence of a CSF shunt, or recent history of CNS trauma or neurosurgery.

Seizure

Seizures are a common reason pediatric patients have AMS. The most common type of seizures seen in the pediatric population include febrile seizures and epileptic generalized tonic-clonic seizures.

Febrile seizures are seizures that occur when a patient (6 months to 5 years of age) has a rapid elevation in temperature. The majority of the fevers are secondary to viral infections. Simple febrile seizures are generalized tonic-clonic seizures that last less than 15 minutes, with the majority of them lasting less than 5 minutes. These children usually return to baseline quickly and are not toxic appearing. The American Academy of Pediatrics guidelines recommend evaluating for the source of the fever and discharging home with the child's guardians, with good return precautions. Pediatric patients with a complex febrile seizure (ie, a febrile seizure that lasts longer than 15 minutes or a focal seizure) require a more thorough evaluation to identify any underlying conditions.

Most epileptic generalized tonic-clonic seizures last less than 5 minutes, but if they last longer, the recommendation is to give a benzodiazepine (eg, midazolam or lorezepam [0.1 mg/kg IV]) or diazepam (0.1-0.2 mg/kg IV). The airway should be monitored, and the patient should receive respiratory support as needed. If the seizure is sustained, levetiracetam (20 mg/kg IV loading dose), levetiracetam (60 mg/kg), or fosphenytoin (20 mg/kg IV loading dose) are second-line medications. If all the medications fail and the patient remains in status epilepticus, then the patient should either receive a repeat dose of second-line medication or be placed under anesthetic doses of thiopental, midazolam, pentobarbital, or propofol in consultation with a tertiary care center pediatric intensivist. The patient may exhibit bradypnea or respiratory failure secondary to the medications even if the seizures have stopped. In this case, the patient may also require respiratory support and admission to the pediatric ICU (PICU).

Whether a patient presents with a febrile seizure, first-time seizure, or breakthrough seizures, patients may have a postictal period lasting anywhere from a few minutes to 24 hours. Over time, their mental status slowly returns to baseline on its own. If their mentation does not return to normal, then a workup of what caused the seizure needs to be done. Differentials such as trauma, CNS infections, electrolyte abnormalities, and inborn errors of metabolism (IEM) need to be considered.

Metabolic Derangement

The main metabolic causes of AMS in children include diabetic ketoacidosis (DKA), diabetes insipidus, hyponatremia, hypoglycemia, hypocalcemia, thyroid abnormalities, IEM, and congenital adrenal hyperplasia (CAH).

DKA

Patients with DKA can present with AMS or irritability, and a small percentage can present with full coma or stupor. Consider DKA when a patient is altered with irregular breathing (Kussmaul breathing) or has a history of polyuria, polydipsia, diabetes, or autoimmune disease. Protecting the airway when indicated and performing a physical examination to assess for any preceding focus of infection is important in the initial diagnosis; serum laboratory studies, including venous blood gas, serum ketones, and chemistry, should also be performed. Patients may have reactive leukocytosis on CBC without an infectious etiology.

Life-threatening complications of DKA include cerebral edema, hyperkalemia, hypokalemia, hypophosphatemia, and hemodynamic instability leading to cardiovascular collapse. Risk factors for cerebral edema include age less than 3 years,

---

✖ Pitfalls

- Ordering a head CT on every pediatric patient with a head injury.
- Giving insulin to a child in DKA in the first hour of resuscitation.
- Missing nonaccidental trauma in a nonverbal child.

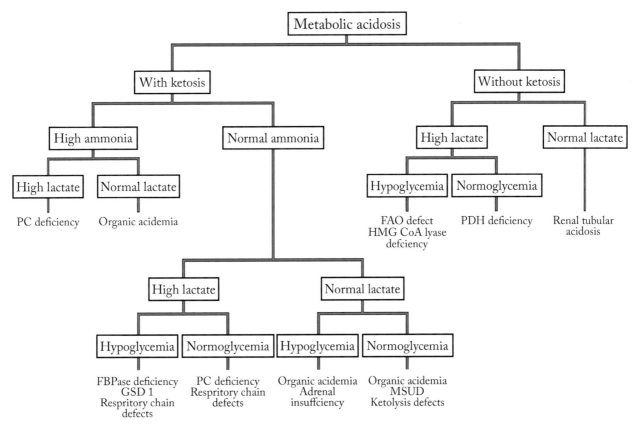

FIGURE 1. Metabolic Acidosis With and Without Ketosis

giving insulin in the first hour of treatment, new-onset diabetes, elevated blood urea nitrogen, low PCO_2, failure of serum sodium to rise with hyperglycemia correction, and use of bicarbonate in the treatment regimen.[8] Patients with evidence of fluid deficit should be treated with isotonic crystalloid fluids 10 to 20 mL/kg in the first hours of management until peripheral perfusion has improved and urine output has returned. Insulin should be given at 0.05 to 0.1 unit/kg/hr, and glucose can be added to intravenous fluids when serum glucose is less than 300 mg/dL.[8] Potassium replacement in the form of potassium acetate and potassium phosphate should be started at the same time as the insulin infusion is initiated, typically beginning with 40 mEq/L total. Patients should have serum glucose checks every hour to titrate insulin drip as well as frequent repeat electrolyte and pH measures every 2 to 4 hours initially.[8] Patients with severe DKA with a pH less than 7.0, AMS, or necessary ventilation or pressure support should be managed in the PICU.

IEM

Similar to the diagnosis of new-onset DKA, the diagnosis of IEM requires a high index of clinical suspicion. Suspect IEM in infants and toddlers, especially if they are vomiting, not tolerating feeds, irritable, lethargic, seizing, tachypneic, or hypothermic. They may have had a history of failure to thrive, developmental delay, or regression of developmental milestones. Patients with IEM may present after having a prolonged fasting period, and infants may present with a brief resolved unexplained event (BRUE) or sudden infant death syndrome (SIDS). Initial laboratory workup should include CBC, chemistry, blood gas, glucose, ammonia level, uric acid level, liver function tests, and urinalysis.[8] Consultation with an IEM specialist early is recommended, even prior to transfer to a tertiary care facility.

It is helpful to learn broad categories of IEM to help with initial diagnosis and management in the emergency department. For example, IEM can be divided into aminoacidopathies, fatty acid oxidation disorders, urea cycle disorders, fatty acid oxidation defects, mitochondrial disorders, disorders of carbohydrate metabolism, lysosomal storage disorders, and peroxisomal disorders. Typical laboratory abnormalities include some derangement of acid-base, hyperammonemia, and hypoglycemia. Patients may also have infection as a preceding factor to metabolic crisis.

Metabolic acidosis due to buildup of abnormal metabolites causing an anion gap occurs most commonly in organic acidemias, but it can also be seen in amino acid disorders, mitochondrial disorders, and disorders of carbohydrate metabolism (*Figure 1*).[17] Urine pH can be helpful in differentiating between renal tubular acidosis (RTA) and IEM as the cause of a metabolic acidosis. A urine pH of less than 5 would be an appropriate renal compensation to an IEM--driven metabolic acidosis, as the kidneys would excrete uric acid. However, for RTA, urinary pH would be greater than 5. In a patient with an unexplained acid-base disorder, suspect IEM, and order additional laboratory studies, including serum pyruvate, lactate, and quantitative amino acid analysis as well as urine organic acids.

Hyperammonemia should be concerning for an IEM when the ammonia level is greater than 100 μmol/L. The specimen should be drawn without a tourniquet when possible and be placed on ice to send to the laboratory. Urea cycle disorders typically have hyperammonemia to greater than 300 μmol/L. These patients also present with respiratory alkalosis due to hyperpnea as a result of elevated ammonia level. Hyperammonemia is neurotoxic and must be acutely managed with hemodialysis and, for patients with urea cycle disorders, the medication sodium phenylacetate-sodium benzoate.[18]

Management of airway and circulation are primary for IEM. Respiratory support, including intubation, may be needed since metabolites can cause respiratory and CNS depression. Fluid resuscitation with normal saline is preferred to improve circulation and treat dehydration, which could be a precipitating factor for presentation to the emergency department. Lactated Ringer solution should be avoided because it can worsen lactic acidosis. Patients should be kept without oral or intravenous intake of amino acids or carbohydrates until the diagnosis is confirmed, as these can increase toxic metabolites.[19] However, hypoglycemia should be treated as soon as it is recognized to prevent catabolism and improve mental status. For IEM, hypoglycemia should be treated with dextrose 8 to 10 mg/kg/min in the form of D10W via peripheral IV in order to suppress catabolism. The goal for the serum glucose range is 100 to 120 mg/dL, so in some cases, insulin at a rate of 0.05 unit/kg/min must be started and titrated to maintain normoglycemia.[8]

Hypoglycemia

Any child with AMS should have a rapid serum glucose test. Hypoglycemia is defined as serum glucose less than 50 mg/dL with or without symptoms. In the absence of ketones, hypoglycemia should trigger consideration of hyperinsulinism or fatty acid oxidation defect. Hypoglycemia can have various causes not related to IEM and may present with irritability, poor feeding, or seizure. Other causes of hypoglycemia include but are not limited to large tumors (Wilms), decreased intake or decreased absorption (fasting or acute diarrhea), hypopituitarism, hypothyroidism, toxic ingestion (beta-blocker or alcohol, salicylates), and sepsis. Outside the scope of IEM, the recommended management for hypoglycemia in an altered pediatric patient is to give intravenous dextrose 3 to 5 mL/kg of 10% dextrose solution (D10W). This can be given easily in a peripheral IV. Higher concentrations pose logistical issues with administration. Serum glucose should be monitored frequently until levels are consistently greater than 70 mg/dL. Mental status may gradually improve, depending on the initial degree of lethargy. Hypoglycemic seizures should be managed with anticonvulsants if they are not improving with glucose management.

Other rare causes of hypoglycemia, in addition to IEMs, include hyperinsulinism and hypopituitarism. Hypoglycemia associated with hypopituitarism is rare and may be congenital (perinatal injury or genetic or developmental CNS defects, such as anencephaly) or acquired (infiltrative disorders, trauma, CNS surgery, or tumors). Hypopituitarism may present with dramatic symptoms, including hypoglycemia or hypotension in vulnerable patients with recent CNS trauma or surgery, short stature, or hypogonadism who undergo a stressful event or illness. Diagnostic evaluation should include an evaluation for any concerns about underlying conditions (such as sepsis) and ideally laboratory studies serum cortisol, plasma ACTH, and chemistries, drawn with the hypoglycemic episode if possible. The results of these studies are not necessary prior to emergent treatment with IV hydrocortisone 50 mg/m². Other treatments, such as antibiotics and fluid resuscitation, should be initiated if sepsis is suspected. Patients should be treated based on clinical presentation. If surface area is unavailable for dosing of hydrocortisone, 1 to 2 mg/kg hydrocortisone IV can be given; it is often easiest to think "small, medium, and large" (ie, 25 mg, 50 mg, and 100 mg, respectively) for infants, school-aged children,

and teens, respectively. Neonates may need smaller doses, such as 12.5 mg. The most important aspect is to give steroids early to help improve cortisol levels and manage adrenal crisis.[20]

Patients with CAH and adrenal insufficiency may present with addisonian crisis or salt-wasting crisis. Laboratory studies may show hyponatremia, hyperkalemia, and hypoglycemia in CAH. They may have ambiguous genitalia (females are usually diagnosed at birth with ambiguous genitalia, whereas males may present in crisis at a few weeks of age because they do not have ambiguous genitalia) or precocious puberty. Salt-wasting crisis presents first at 2 to 3 weeks of age (typically males) when a newborn screen for 21-hydroxylase deficiency, the most common form of CAH, may not yet have resulted. For this reason, all altered neonates should have a bedside glucose measurement and a physical examination, including external genital examination, early in the course of the assessment. Salt-wasting crisis must be managed emergently with stress-dose hydrocortisone, prompt fluid resuscitation, and frequent electrolyte monitoring.

Hyponatremia

Hyponatremia is defined by a serum sodium less than 135 mEq/L, although clinical signs and symptoms usually do not begin until the sodium level is less than 125 mEq/L. AMS can result from hyponatremia due to syndrome of inappropriate antidiuretic hormone production (SIADH). SIADH is associated with infectious conditions such as bacterial pneumonia, bacterial meningitis, and very commonly in Rocky Mountain spotted fever. Patients who are altered to the level of severe lethargy or seizures should receive 3% saline 3 mL/kg IV every 10 to 20 minutes as needed, and the initial etiology should be treated as well (antibiotics in the case of bacterial infection).

Thyroid Abnormalities

Consider thyroid abnormalities in patients who present with AMS and hemodynamic instability. Patients with thyroid storm (very uncommon in infants, increases in frequency as the child enters adolescence) may present with delirium or stupor but will also have symptoms typical of hyperthyroidism (ie, goiter, exophthalmos, tachycardia, and congestive heart failure). The presence of high fever is what differentiates thyroid storm from typical hyperthyroidism. Temperature may be greater than 41°C (105.8°F). The most threatening complications of thyroid storm are heart failure, hypotension, and pulmonary edema. Thyroid studies, including free T4, TSH, and T3, should be drawn. Patients are managed with propranolol 10 μg/kg IV over 15 minutes, iodine, and methimazole 20 to 30 mg every 6 to 12 hours.[8]

Consider neonatal thyrotoxicosis in irritable and tachycardic neonates with a maternal history of hyperthyroidism. It is a rare but life-threatening disease that occurs in just 1% to 5% of infants born to mothers with hyperthyroidism. Infants are treated with propranolol 1 mg/kg three times daily as well as iodine drops.[21]

Hypocalcemia (Hypoparathyroidism)

Hypocalcemia can present with apathy, lethargy, or seizures as signs of AMS. Patients may have a history of muscle cramps, spasms, or paresthesias. On examination, patients may have Chvostek sign (tapping over the facial nerve elicits cheek muscle twitching) or Trousseau sign (carpopedal spasm following ischemia from an inflated blood pressure cuff).[22,23] Emergent treatment for hypocalcemia is with 10% calcium gluconate 1 mL/kg IV over 15 minutes.

CRITICAL DECISION

What signs are consistent with drug overdose, and what treatment is appropriate?

Toxic Ingestion/Exposure

Pediatric intentional or unintentional ingestions have been increasing over recent years, including during the COVID-19 pandemic, when pediatric volumes initially decreased.[24,25] As is the typical theme for approaching patients with AMS, primary evaluation of those presenting after ingestion begins with the ABCDEs and is supplemented by establishing IV access and placing the patient on monitors, including cardiac, pulse oximetry, and capnography, if available. Identifying the correct agent and total ingested amount is often difficult because younger children are often unable to say what they ingested, while older children or teenagers presenting after intentional ingestion may not provide a reliable history. If possible, ascertain the type and amount of the substance ingested, if there are any coingested substances, the timing of ingestion, whether the ingestion was intentional, and what symptoms are present. These answers, along with toxicologic screening tests, will be important in narrowing the broad differential of poisoning agents. The following subsections highlight five important pediatric toxidromes.

Anticholinergic Ingestion

Medications with anticholinergic properties include antihistamines, tricyclic antidepressants, scopolamine, and doxylamine. Concern should be raised for anticholinergic toxicity in patients presenting with anticholinergic symptoms (eg, mydriasis, dry mucous membranes, tachycardia, and urinary retention); more serious CNS affects, such as confusion, anxiety, delirium, hallucinations, and seizures, are associated with severe poisoning. A mnemonic for symptoms of anticholinergic toxicity is "red as a beet, dry as a bone, blind as a bat, mad as a hatter, hot as a hare, and full as a flask."

Several recent viral internet challenges have been associated with adolescent injury, including the Tide Pod® challenge and the boiling water challenge. Diphenhydramine has become a popular drug of abuse among teenagers due to its wide availability and the TikTok craze of ingesting large amounts of it for its hallucinogenic potential.[26] These challenges underscore the importance of being up to date with current social media trends, as this may prove beneficial in determining the correct etiology of a toxidrome.

Treatment is mostly symptomatic treatment and supportive care. An ECG should be performed to monitor for widened QRS intervals or prolonged QTc. If the ingestion is within the hour and the patient has a normal mental status, activated charcoal can be used to bind the drug. If a patient presents with seizure, lorazepam (0.1 mg/kg IV) or diazepam (0.1-0.2 mg/kg IV) can be used. If a patient with a clear pure anticholinergic poisoning is severely agitated and has both peripheral and central signs of toxicity, physostigmine (0.02 mg/kg IV slowly over 3 minutes) can be used to improve sensorium. This dose can be repeated every 10 to 15 minutes to a maximum dose of 2 mg. It should be noted that physostigmine can precipitate a seizure if it is given too quickly or at too high of a dose. Atropine should be available to counter severe cholinergic effects that may occur. It may also be dangerous to give physostigmine if the patient has ingested multiple substances. Because physostigmine can potentially have severe risks, physicians may favor benzodiazepines to treat anticholinergic delirium.[8]

Cannabinoid Intoxication

New political landscapes have given rise to increased availability of cannabinoid-containing products in the United States. Subsequently, there has been a rise in the number of pediatric patients presenting with cannabinoid overdose.[28] Cannabis-containing food products (commonly referred to as "edibles"), including cookies, brownies, or candies, may be easily mistaken as normal treats by children. Pediatric ingestions of small amounts of these products can lead to intoxication because they typically contain high concentrations of tetrahydrocannabinol (THC), the primary psychoactive compound in cannabis. Smoking or vaping are other popular forms of cannabis consumption among adolescents.

The most common presenting sign of cannabinoid overdose is lethargy and ataxia.[27] Patients may also present agitated, delirious, or in severe cases, comatose. Other physical examination findings include hypotonia, tachycardia, and hypoventilation.[28] A toxicologic workup is appropriate; however, cannabinoid intoxication is a clinical diagnosis and should not be reliant on a urine drug screen, as THC metabolites can be detected in urine for 3 days after a single use, to more than 30 days in chronic users.[29] Furthermore, synthetic cannabinoid metabolites may not be detected by a urine drug screen. Treatment of cannabinoid toxicity is supportive and should address abnormal vital signs and respiratory derangements. Agitation or anxiety can be treated with benzodiazepines. At this time, there are no strong data to support the use of activated charcoal in the management of ingested cannabis.

Carbon Monoxide Poisoning

Carbon monoxide (CO) is a clear and odorless gas that can be produced from a variety of sources such as automobiles, gas-burning ovens and heaters, and house fires. CO is a molecule that competes with oxygen for binding on the Hgb molecule, decreasing the amount of oxygen delivered to tissues. There are approximately 5,000 annual visits to pediatric emergency departments as a result of CO poisoning.[30] Symptoms of CO poisoning include nausea, vomiting, headache, and lethargy. Infants, who are typically unable to describe traditional symptoms, may present with increased fussiness, obtundation, or feeding intolerance. In addition, infants may be more prone to the effects of CO secondary to the presence of fetal Hgb and an increased respiratory rate. Because symptoms of CO poisoning are often nonspecific, a thorough history may provide important contextual clues leading to an appropriate diagnosis. Patients presenting from the scene of a fire should have their airway evaluated, and other coexposures such as cyanide toxicity should also be considered.

In patients who present with suspected CO exposure, a carboxyhemoglobin level is warranted, and 100% oxygen should be administered via nonrebreather mask. Hyperbaric oxygen therapy should be administered if the CO level is greater than 25% (20% in pregnant patients), if there is loss of consciousness or a depressed GCS score, severe metabolic acidosis (pH less than 7.1), or if organ dysfunction is present.[31] Considerations for pediatric patients requiring hyperbaric oxygen include myringotomy if the child is too young to equalize pressure in their middle ear. Children and infants should be kept warm during their therapy.

Opioid Intoxication

Opiates and opiate-derivatives are commonly abused by adolescents, leading to frequent overdose cases seen in the emergency department.[32] Younger children may also present after accidental ingestion of prescription opioids found within their household. Prescription medications such as fentanyl patches, buprenorphine, and methadone may cause life-threatening intoxication in children with a single dose. Symptoms of opiate intoxication include respiratory depression, AMS, miosis, and decreased bowel sounds. Hypothermia, hypotension, and muscle rigidity may also be present.

The mainstay treatment of opiate intoxication is rapid reversal with naloxone while providing respiratory support with 100% O2 via nonrebreather mask, or bag-valve-mask ventilation if the patient is apneic. Children less than 20 kg should receive naloxone 0.1 mg/kg IV or IO (maximum 2 mg per dose); children greater than 20 kg should receive 2 mg IV or IO. This dose may be repeated (maximum 10 mg total) until the patient's respiratory and mental status improve.[33] Intubation should be considered if initial doses of naloxone are ineffective. Intoxication with long-acting opiates such as methadone and buprenorphine may require a naloxone infusion. The hourly infusion rate should be set at two-thirds of the naloxone dose required to restore consciousness and an appropriate respiratory rate.[34]

In addition to the typical laboratory workup for patients presenting with AMS, patients with opiate toxicity should also have an ECG, acetaminophen level, and creatine kinase (CK) level. An ECG can assess for prolonged QT interval, which can occur with methadone overdose. An acetaminophen level may be elevated and require further management, as many prescription opiates also contain acetaminophen. Finally, a CK level is helpful in further management because patients with opiate toxicity are at risk of rhabdomyolysis secondary to rigidity.

Admission is warranted with infants and young children receiving naloxone or adolescents who have taken a long-acting opiate. Older children who respond appropriately to initial naloxone administration can be observed in the emergency department and discharged after 2 hours of monitoring if no further dosing of naloxone is required and if there is no concern that the patient ingested a long-acting opiate. Depending on the age of the child and circumstances of the ingestion, psychiatric services and social services may be necessary prior to disposition.

Salicylate Overdose

Salicylate-containing products, including acetylsalicylic acid, accounted for more than 16,000 poisonings in 2019.[35] Acute ingestion of salicylates can lead to several clinical manifestations; severe toxicity is associated with noncardiogenic pulmonary edema and AMS, including coma. Initial symptoms of overdose may include tinnitus, nausea, vomiting, and diarrhea. Clinically, tachypnea, hyperpyrexia, and tachycardia may be evident.

Salicylates affect the medullary respiratory center, causing increased respiratory rate, leading to a respiratory alkalosis. Salicylates also inhibit oxidative phosphorylation in mitochondria, which contributes to an elevated anion gap metabolic acidosis. Because acidosis enhances conversion of salicylates into their protonated form, tachypnea is an important compensatory mechanism in maintaining acid-base homeostasis by respiratory excretion of carbon dioxide. Intubation should be avoided unless the patient demonstrates respiratory failure (ie., hypoxia or bradypnea), as it is typically difficult to achieve minute volumes necessary to maintain the protective alkalosis.

Treatment options for salicylate overdose include activated charcoal, volume resuscitation, urine alkalinization with sodium bicarbonate, and hemodialysis for severe poisonings. Laboratory salicylate levels can help determine appropriate treatment pathways. Symptoms of salicylate toxicity may appear at a level greater than 30 mg/dL. Activated charcoal given at 1 g/kg (max 50 g) can be given to nonaltered patients with acute salicylate ingestions. Volume resuscitation should commence as patients usually have very high insensible losses from tachypnea. Alkalinization of urine enhances excretion of salicylates from blood and can be done with administration of sodium bicarbonate (1 mmol/kg initial bolus followed by 5% dextrose in water containing sodium bicarbonate and potassium). The goal for urinary output should be 1 to 1.5 mL/kg/hr,and urine pH should be maintained at greater than 7.5. Hemodialysis is indicated when levels exceed 90 mg/dL for acute ingestions and should be considered early in patients presenting with AMS secondary to salicylate overdose.[36]

Summary

Managing the altered pediatric patient is a formidable task that requires broad knowledge of several potential etiologies. The first priority is management of the patient's ABCs. The child should be placed on appropriate monitoring devices, and intravenous access and appropriate laboratory studies should be obtained. During and following stabilization, the child should be evaluated with a thorough history and physical examination to determine the underlying etiology of the child's altered sensorium; the differential diagnosis should include traumatic injury, infection, metabolic or neurologic abnormalities, or a toxidrome. The astute emergency physician will corroborate abnormal vital signs and physical examination findings with important answers to history questions that should provide the clues needed to tailor further workup and treatment.

REFERENCES

1. Traumatic Brain Injury. Centers for Disease Control and Prevention, National Center for Injury Prevention and Control. https://www.cdc.gov/traumaticbraininjury/index.html

2. Holmes JF, Palchak MJ, MacFarlane T, Kuppermann N. Performance of the pediatric Glasgow coma scale in children with blunt head trauma. *Acad Emerg Med.* 2005;12:814.

3. Teasdale G, Jennett B. Assessment of coma and impaired consciousness. A practical scale. *Lancet.* 1974;2:81.

4. Kuppermann N, Holmes JF, Dayan PS, et al; Pediatric Emergency Care Applied Research Network (PECARN). Identification of children at very low risk of clinically-important brain injuries after head trauma: a prospective cohort study. *Lancet.* 2009 Oct 3;374(9696):1160-1170.

5. Cho S, Hwang S, Jung JY, et al. Validation of Pediatric Emergency Care Applied Research Network (PECARN) rule in children with minor head trauma. *PLoS One.* 2022 Jan 18;17(1):e0262102.

6. American College of Surgeons. Committee on Trauma. *Advanced Trauma Life Support: Student Course Manual.* 10th ed. American College of Surgeons; 2018.

CASE RESOLUTIONS

■ CASE ONE

Imaging and laboratory studies were ordered for the unresponsive 3-month-old boy who had two prolonged seizures requiring anticonvulsants in the emergency department. A chest x-ray showed multiple rib fractures in different stages of healing, and a bone survey showed bilateral femur corner fractures. The liver function test and lipase levels were elevated. A head CT showed a large subdural bleed with a midline shift. Neurosurgery was consulted, and the patient was taken to the operating room for evacuation of the hematoma. Afterwards, he was admitted to the ICU. In the ICU, the patient was found to have retinal hemorrhages. This was a case of nonaccidental trauma.

■ CASE TWO

The unresponsive 6-year-old boy was thought to have been postictal from a seizure. This patient's aura, along with the facial droop and decreased movement of his left upper and lower extremity, were unusual. A CT head was ordered for concern of a ruptured aneurysm, which revealed a massive ischemic stroke. A code stroke was called, and the neurology team arrived. A CT angiography found a large basilar artery stroke. The patient was intubated in the emergency department. Tissue plaminogen activator was administered, and he was taken to the catheterization laboratory for a thrombectomy. Within days, the patient returned to baseline and was discharged home with no deficits.

■ CASE THREE

The 14-year-old boy's somnolence, abnormal breathing rate, and tachycardia were concerning. Given his vital sign derangements and history of depression, a toxicologic panel was ordered, and a salicylate level was noted to be elevated to 60 mg/dL. The patient received a bolus dose of sodium bicarbonate and was started on a bicarbonate drip. A Foley catheter was placed to monitor urine output and pH, and the patient was admitted to the PICU.

7. Fenn NE 3rd, Sierra CM. Hyperosmolar therapy for severe traumatic brain injury in pediatrics: a review of the literature. *J Pediatr Pharmacol Ther.* 2019;24(6):465-472.

8. Shaw KN, Bachur EG, Chamberlain J, Lavelle J, Nagler J, Shook JE, eds. *Fleisher & Ludwig's Textbook of Pediatric Emergency Medicine.* 8th ed. Wolters Kluwer; 2021.

9. Tsze DS, Valente JH. Pediatric stroke: a review. *Emerg Med Int.* 2011;2011:734506.

10. Hasegawa K, Tsugawa Y, Cohen A, Camargo CA Jr. Infectious disease-related emergency department visits among children in the US. *Pediatr Infect Dis J.* 2015;34(7):681-685.

11. Weiss SL, Peters MJ, Alhazzani W, et al. Surviving sepsis campaign international guidelines for the management of septic shock and sepsis-associated organ dysfunction in children. *Pediatr Crit Care Med.* 2020;21:e52.

12. Smith MJ, Boutzoukas A, Autmizguine J, et al. Antibiotic safety and effectiveness in premature infants with complicated intraabdominal infections. *Pediatr Infect Dis J.* 2021;40:550.

13. Kostenniemi UJ, Norman D, Borgström M, Silfverdal SA. The clinical presentation of acute bacterial meningitis varies with age, sex and duration of illness. *Acta Paediatr.* 2015;104:1117.

14. Cruz AT, Freedman SB, Kulik DM, et al. HSV study group of the Pediatric Emergency Medicine Collaborative Research Committee. Herpes simplex virus infection in infants undergoing meningitis evaluation. *Pediatrics.* 2018 Feb;141(2):e20171688.

15. Tunkel AR, Hartman BJ, Kaplan SL, et al. Practice guidelines for the management of bacterial meningitis. *Clin Infect Dis.* 2004;39:1267.

16. Long SS, Pool TE, Vodzak J, Daskalaki I, Gould JM. Herpes simplex virus infection in young infants during 2 decades of empiric acyclovir therapy. *Pediatr Infect Dis J.* 2011 Jul;30(7):556-561.

17. Gibson K, Halliday JL, Kirby DM, et al. Mitochondrial oxidative phosphorylation disorders presenting in neonates: clinical manifestations and enzymatic and molecular diagnoses. *Pediatrics.* 2008;122:1003.

18. Summar ML, Mew NA. Inborn errors of metabolism with hyperammonemia: Urea cycle defects and related disorders. *Pediatr Clin North Am.* 2018 Apr;65(2):231-246.

19. Ellaway CJ, Wilcken B, Christodoulou J. Clinical approach to inborn errors of metabolism presenting in the newborn period. *J Paediatr Child Health.* 2002 Oct;38(5):511-517.

20. Miller BS, Spencer SP, Geffner ME, et al. Emergency management of adrenal insufficiency in children: advocating for treatment options in outpatient and field settings. *J Investig Med.* 2019 Feb 28.

21. Kliegman RM, St. Geme J, eds. *Nelson Textbook of Pediatrics.* 21st ed. Elsevier; 2020.

22. Mohebbi MR, Rosenkrans KA, Jung MJ. Chvostek's and Trousseau's signs in a case of hypoparathyroidism. *J Clin Diagn Res.* 2013 May;7(5):970.

23. Ahmed MA, Martinez A, Mariam S, Whitehouse W. Chvostek's sign and hypocalcaemia in children with seizures. *Seizure.* 2004 Jun;13(4):217-222.

24. Mazer-Amirshahi M, Sun C, Mullins P, et al. Trends in emergency department resource utilization for poisoning-related visits, 2003-2011. *J Med Toxicol.* 2016 Sep;12(3):248-254.

25. Chaiyachati BH, Agawu A, Zorc JJ, Balamuth F. Trends in pediatric emergency department utilization after institution of coronavirus disease-19 mandatory social distancing. *J Pediatr.* 2020;226:274-277.e1.

26. Minhaj FS, Leonard J. Dangers of the TikTok Benadryl challenge. Contemporary PEDS J. 2021 Jan;38:1. https://www.contemporarypediatrics.com/view/dangers-of-the-tiktok-benadryl-challenge

27. Richards JR, Smith NE, Moulin AK. Unintentional cannabis ingestion in children: A systematic review. *J Pediatr.* 2017 Nov;190:142-152.

28. Wong KU, Baum CR. Acute cannabis toxicity. *Pediatr Emerg Care.* 2019 Nov;35(11):799-804.

29. Moeller KE, Kissack JC, Atayee RS, Lee KC. Clinical interpretation of urine drug tests: what clinicians need to know about urine drug screens. *Mayo Clin Proc.* 2017 May;92(5):774-796.

30. Macnow TE, Waltzman ML. Carbon monoxide poisoning in children: Diagnosis and management in the emergency department. *Pediatr Emerg Med Pract.* 2016 Sep;13(9):1-24.

31. Hampson NB, Dunford RG, Kramer CC, Norkool DM. Selection criteria utilized for hyperbaric oxygen treatment of carbon monoxide poisoning. *J Emerg Med.* 1995 Mar-Apr;13(2):227-231.

32. McCabe SE, West BT, Veliz P, McCabe VV, Stoddard SA, Boyd CJ. Trends in medical and nonmedical use of prescription opioids among US adolescents: 1976-2015. *Pediatrics.* 2017 Apr;139(4):e20162387.

33. American Academy of Pediatrics Committee on Drugs. Naloxone dosage and route of administration for infants and children: addendum to emergency drug doses for infants and children. *Pediatrics.* 1990 Sep;86(3):484-485.

34. Perry HE, Shannon MW. Diagnosis and management of opioid- and benzodiazepine-induced comatose overdose in children. *Curr Opin Pediatr.* 1996;8(3):243-247.

35. Gummin DD, Mowry JB, Beuhler MC, et al. 2019 annual report of the American Association of Poison Control Centers' National Poison Data System (NPDS): 37th annual report. *Clin Toxicol (Phila).* 2020 Dec;58(12):1360-1541.

36. Palmer BF, Clegg DJ. Salicylate toxicity. *N Engl J Med.* 2020 Jun 25;382(26):2544-2555.

Injury after a fall

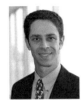

By Joshua S. Broder, MD, FACEP
Dr. Broder is a professor and the residency program director in the Department of Emergency Medicine at Duke University Medical Center in Durham, North Carolina.

Objectives

On completion of this article, you should be able to:

■ Discuss which imaging tests are needed when central cord syndrome is suspected.

CASE PRESENTATION

A 55-year-old woman presents after a fall from standing after drinking five glasses of wine. The patient struck her chin and upper lip, avulsing a maxillary incisor. She did not lose consciousness and was able to stand after the fall, but she complains of bilateral upper extremity pain and difficulty moving her arms. Vital signs are BP 160/92, P 105, E 11, and T 36.7°C (98.0°F); SpO$_2$ is 100% on room air.

The patient is awake and alert, although intoxicated. Her primary survey is intact. She has swelling of her upper lip, and her left central maxillary incisor is loose. A cervical collar is in place, and the patient denies midline posterior neck tenderness. There is no evident swelling or deformity of her upper extremities, but she complains of severe pins and needles pain with light touch to either arm below the elbow. Her upper extremity extension and flexion and grip appear weak, 2/5, although it is unclear how much her exam is limited by pain. Her lower extremity neurologic examination is normal. Noncontrast head CT is normal (*Figure 1*). Cervical spine CT shows no fractures or but demonstrates extensive degenerative disease and spinal canal narrowing at the C4 to C6 levels. The emergency physician obtains an MRI of the cervical spine (*Figure 2*).

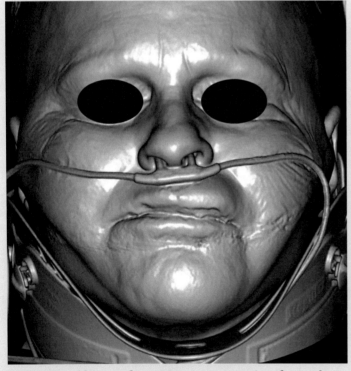

FIGURE 1. Skin surface 3D reconstruction from the patient's facial CT. The reconstruction emphasizes the mechanism of injury, spinal hyperextension. The patient also has swelling of the upper lip from falling forward.

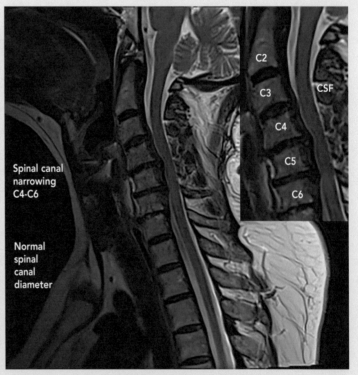

FIGURE 2. Cervical MRI without contrast, T2-weighted sequence. Above and below the level of spinal stenosis, cerebrospinal fluid is seen surrounding the spinal cord. At the level of severe stenosis, the spinal cord is tightly bounded within the canal.

Central cord syndrome is an incomplete spinal cord injury occurring from a cervical spine hyperextension mechanism, leading to spinal cord compression, particularly in patients older than 50 years with existing spinal stenosis. The clinical syndrome includes upper extremity weakness and hyperesthesia, often with sparing of the lower extremities. Particularly in patients with altered mental status, subtle weakness may be overlooked and upper extremity pain may be erroneously attributed to arm injuries. CT may be negative for acute injuries such as fracture or subluxation while commonly demonstrating chronic degenerative changes and canal stenosis.[1] MRI without contrast should be pursued when the condition is suspected based on history and examination findings, even when CT does not demonstrate traumatic injuries.[2]

While some spontaneous improvement is common, long-term disability from arm weakness can occur. Rapid decompression (<24 hours after injury) is associated with better neurologic outcomes.[3] One study found that early surgery is associated with increased mortality, but a systematic review did not find such a relationship.[3,4]

CASE RESOLUTION

The patient underwent C5 corpectomy and C4 to C6 anterior cervical discectomy and fusion. After surgery, her hyperesthesia resolved, and her strength improved, with 4+/5 strength in triceps extension and 5/5 strength in other muscle groups.

REFERENCES

1. Kunam VK, Velayudhan V, Chaudhry ZA, Bobinski M, Smoker WRK, Reede DL. Incomplete cord syndromes: clinical and imaging review. Radiographics. 2018;38:1201-1222.
2. Expert Panel on Neurological I, Musculoskeletal I, Beckmann NM, et al. ACR Appropriateness Criteria® Suspected Spine Trauma. J Am Coll Radiol. 2019;16:S264-S285.
3. Anderson KK, Tetreault L, Shamji MF, et al. Optimal timing of surgical decompression for acute traumatic central cord syndrome: a systematic review of the literature. Neurosurgery. 2015;77 suppl 4:S15-S32.
4. Samuel AM, Grant RA, Bohl DD, et al. Delayed surgery after acute traumatic central cord syndrome is associated with reduced mortality. Spine (Phila Pa 1976). 2015;40:349-356.

CME Questions

Reviewed by Michael S. Beeson, MD, MBA, FACEP

Qualified, paid subscribers to *Critical Decisions in Emergency Medicine* may receive CME certificates for up to 5 ACEP Category I credits, 5 *AMA PRA Category 1 Credits*™, and 5 AOA Category 2-B credits for completing this activity in its entirety. Submit your answers online at acep.org/cdem; a score of 75% or better is required. You may receive credit for completing the CME activity any time within 3 years of its publication date. Answers to this month's questions will be published in next month's issue.

1   What is the rate of recurrence of CVT in the first year after occurrence?

   A.   6.5%
   B.   15%
   C.   18%
   D.   23%

2   Which cerebral venous sinus is most commonly affected in CVT?

   A.   Cavernous
   B.   Inferior petrosal
   C.   Inferior sagittal
   D.   Superior sagittal

3   What is the most common cause of CVT in developing countries?

   A.   Infection
   B.   Malignancy
   C.   Pregnancy
   D.   A and C

4   What is the recommended imaging modality to diagnose CVT?

   A.   Angiography
   B.   Noncontrast CT of the head
   C.   Noncontrast MRI of the brain
   D.   CTV or MRV

5   Which drugs increase the risk of developing CVT?

   A.   Asparaginase, methotrexate, and tamoxifen
   B.   Steroids, danazol, and lithium
   C.   Vitamin A, ecstasy, and IV immune globulin
   D.   All of these

6   What is the leading cause of death in the acute phase of CVT?

   A.   Hydrocephalus
   B.   Pulmonary embolism
   C.   Seizure
   D.   Transtentorial herniation

7   What is the prevalence of intracranial hemorrhage in patients with CVT?

   A.   10%-20%
   B.   30%-40%
   C.   45%
   D.   50%-60%

8   What is the anticoagulant of choice during the acute phase of CVT?

   A.   Low-molecular-weight heparin
   B.   Unfractionated heparin
   C.   Warfarin
   D.   A and B

9   Which factors are associated with poor outcomes in CVT?

   A.   Male sex, altered mental status, and age greater than 37
   B.   Posterior fossa lesions, GCS score less than 9, and seizures
   C.   Underlying malignancy, large parenchymal lesions, and hypertension
   D.   All of these

10   What is the prevalence of seizures in patients diagnosed with CVT?

   A.   5%
   B.   10%
   C.   30%
   D.   45%

11   A 14-year-old girl presents after ingesting several pills of aspirin 12 hours prior to arrival. She is somnolent but rouses to voice. She has an increased respiratory rate. What is the most likely acid-base disturbance?

   A.   Respiratory acidosis with metabolic acidosis
   B.   Respiratory acidosis with metabolic alkalosis
   C.   Respiratory alkalosis with metabolic acidosis
   D.   Respiratory alkalosis with metabolic alkalosis

12   A 12-year-old boy presents after being ejected during a motor vehicle crash. The patient moans, but his speech is otherwise incomprehensible. He withdraws his extremities and opens his eyes to pain. What is this patient's GCS score?

   A.   7
   B.   8
   C.   9
   D.   10

13   An unresponsive 18-kg 4-year-old boy presents via EMS after being found down by his parent. He was started on 100% oxygen via nonrebreather mask en route due to slow respirations; the child had normal pulse oximetry and other vital signs. On examination, the child has pinpoint pupils and depressed respirations, and he rouses only to noxious stimulus. After placing him on monitors and establishing intravenous access, what is the next step in management?

   A.   Administer naloxone 0.1 mg/kg IV
   B.   Consult toxicology
   C.   Order a urine drug screen to evaluate for opiate ingestion
   D.   Perform emergent endotracheal intubation

14 What symptoms are most suggestive of anticholinergic toxicity?

A. Ataxia and lethargy
B. Dry mucous membranes, mydriasis, tachycardia, and urinary retention
C. Miosis and respiratory depression
D. Tinnitus, vomiting, and increased respiratory rate with deep respirations

15 How quickly should empiric antibiotic therapy be administered to patients with signs of sepsis?

A. 1 hour
B. 2 hours
C. 6 hours
D. 8 hours

16 A 1-year-old girl presents after a witnessed 3-ft fall off a bed onto a hardwood floor. She started crying immediately, and the parents believe that the patient hit her head. She has not had any episodes of vomiting and is currently awake. There are no external signs of skull fracture or hematoma, and the child is acting normally according to the parents. According to the PECARN trial, can this child be dispositioned without head imaging?

A. No, the child's GCS score warrants a CT scan after a period of observation
B. No, the child's mechanism warrants an immediate CT scan
C. Yes, the child can be discharged after 24 hours of observation in the inpatient unit if no further symptoms develop
D. Yes, the child can be observed in the ED or discharged and observed at home by the parents for 4 to 6 hours

17 A 15-year-old boy presents after being ejected from his dirt bike. The patient was not wearing a helmet at the time of injury, and witnesses report that he lost consciousness. On arrival, the patient is moaning with unintelligible speech, and he only opens his eyes to pain. He withdraws his extremities to pain without localizing. Based on his GCS score, what would this patient's brain injury be described as?

A. Concussion
B. Mild traumatic brain injury
C. Moderate traumatic brain injury
D. Severe traumatic brain injury

18 What are the best first steps in management for pediatric patients who present with any degree of altered mental status?

A. Assess the patient for signs of external trauma
B. Assess the patient's airway, breathing, and circulation for respiratory or hemodynamic compromise
C. Perform a comprehensive history and physical examination to determine the most likely cause of the altered mental status
D. Place an IV and send appropriate laboratory workup

19 What finding is not an indication to obtain intracranial imaging prior to performing a lumbar puncture?

A. High fever
B. History of hydrocephalus
C. Papilledema
D. Presence of a CSF shunt

20 A 9-year-old girl presents with agitation and uncontrollable crying following a referral from a pediatrician. The patient was discharged from another hospital yesterday after spending 1 night there. The blood work, urinalysis, chest x-ray, and abdominal ultrasound obtained there were normal. Today, her parents state that she is not "walking properly," despite the fact that she walked into the room by herself with both parents on either side of her. The parents deny any trauma and say that the patient had a cough and congestion last week. Her vital signs and examination are unremarkable. CN II-XII are intact. The child follows commands when asked, but does not speak. When asked what her name is or who her parents are, she offers only a blank stare. What is the most likely diagnosis?

A. Cerebrovascular accident
B. Diabetic ketoacidosis
C. Encephalitis
D. Inborn error of metabolism

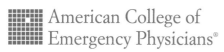

American College of
Emergency Physicians®

ADVANCING EMERGENCY CARE ___/_

Post Office Box 619911
Dallas, Texas 75261-9911

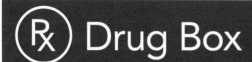 Drug Box

Acetazolamide

By Frank LoVecchio, DO, MPH, FACEP
Valleywise Health and ASU, Phoenix, Arizona

Objective
On completion of this column, you should be able to:
- Summarize how to prescribe acetazolamide.

Introduction
Acetazolamide is used to treat glaucoma, epilepsy, and altitude sickness. It may be used long term for the treatment of open-angle glaucoma and short term for acute angle-closure glaucoma until surgery. Acetazolamide is a diuretic and carbonic anhydrase inhibitor, and its main mechanism of action is decreasing the amount of hydrogen ions and bicarbonate in the body.
 Historically, acetazolamide has been used to treat periodic paralysis, heart failure, menstrual-related epilepsy, and symptoms associated with dural ectasia in individuals with Marfan syndrome. It has also been used to prevent methotrexate-induced kidney damage by alkalinizing one's urine; however, this is no longer recommended. Off-label uses are numerous, with a notable potential use for the emergency physician as a respiratory stimulant in stable hypercapnic COPD.

Dosage
Altitude illness: 500 to 1,000 mg/day in divided oral doses every 8 to 12 hours (immediate release tablets) or divided every 12 to 24 hours (extended release capsules). To reduce side effects, a recommended alternative dose is 125 mg twice daily, beginning either the day before (preferred) or on the day of ascent. In situations of rapid ascent (such as rescue or military operations), 1,000 mg/day is recommended, with the addition of dexamethasone.
Secondary or acute (closed-angle) glaucoma: Initial dose of 250 to 500 mg, with a maintenance dose of 125 to 250 mg every 4 hours. Giving 250 mg every 12 hours has been effective in the short-term treatment of some patients.

Side Effects
Common adverse effects of acetazolamide include paresthesia, fatigue, drowsiness, depression, decreased libido, bitter or metallic taste, nausea, vomiting, abdominal cramps, diarrhea, black feces, polyuria, kidney stones, metabolic acidosis, and electrolyte changes (eg, hypokalemia and hyponatremia). Less common adverse effects include Stevens-Johnson syndrome, anaphylaxis, and blood dyscrasias.

Contraindications
Contraindications include hypersensitivity to acetazolamide, sulfonamides, or any component of the formulation; hepatic disease or insufficiency; decreased sodium or potassium levels; adrenocortical insufficiency; cirrhosis; hyperchloremic acidosis, severe renal disease or dysfunction; and long-term use in noncongestive angle-closure glaucoma.
 Although the FDA-approved product labeling states this medication is contraindicated with other sulfonamide-containing drug classes, the scientific basis of this statement is very weak.
 Acetazolamide is not recommended in pregnancy.

Significant Drug Interactions
Acetazolamide may alter levels of some common antiepileptic drugs and should be avoided with salicylate use.

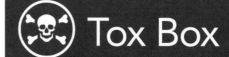 Tox Box

Flecainide Overdose

By Christian A. Tomaszewski, MD, MS, MBA, FACEP
University of California San Diego Health

Objective
On completion of this column, you should be able to:
- Discuss how to identify an overdose of flecainide.

Introduction
Flecainide is a class Ic antidysrhythmic drug that blocks cardiac sodium channels, leading to hypotension and ventricular dysrhythmias in overdose. With its narrow therapeutic window, life-threatening toxicity can occur after chronic dosing errors, especially in renal dysfunction, or within hours of an acute overdose ≥1 g.

Toxicokinetics
- Absorption
  - High oral bioavailability, 90%
  - Peak level 3 hours postingestion
  - High volume of distribution, 8 to 9 L/kg (not dialyzable)
- Metabolism (half-life 12-24 hours)
  - Primarily hepatic
  - 30% excreted by kidney unchanged

Mechanism
- Blocks cardiac fast sodium channels
- Slows cardiac conduction
- Decreased cardiac contractility

Clinical Manifestations
- *CNS:* dizziness, visual disturbance, headache, and seizure
- *GI:* nausea and vomiting
- *Cardiac:* hypotension, bradycardia, and ventricular tachydysrhythmias

Diagnostics
- Screening glucose and acetaminophen levels
- Electrolytes, calcium, and magnesium
- ECG: QRS widening, prolonged PR, and elevated terminal 0 ms in aVR
- Flecainide levels are generally uavailable.

Treatment
- May give activated charcoal orally if <1 hour postingestion and can protect airway
- Hypertonic sodium bicarbonate for wide QRS (target 7.45-7.55)
- Hypotension
  - IV fluid bolus for hypotension
  - Norepinephrine for fluid unresponsive hypotension
- Correct electrolyte abnormalities (eg, hypokalemia and hypomagnesemia)
- Lidocaine or amiodarone may help with ventricular tachycardia.
- Refractory hypotension
  - IV lipid emulsion 20% 100 ml bolus (1.5 ml/kg; may repeat)
  - Consider ECMO for refractory shock.

Disposition
- If asymptomatic, monitor for up to ~6 hours after oral overdose.
- If symptomatic or ECG changes, monitor until resolution.

Critical decisions
in emergency medicine

Volume 36 Number 4: **April 2023**

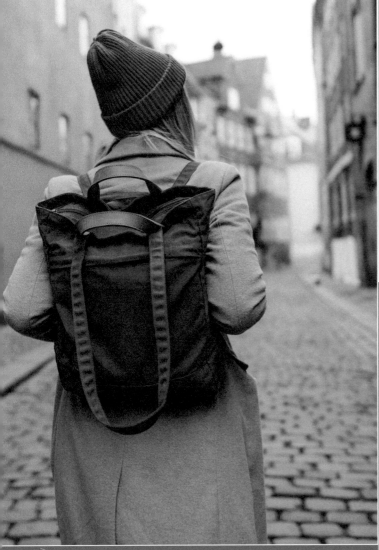

Travel Bug

Modern travel's ease and speed expose travelers to conditions rarely encountered at home, where they typically seek treatment. With international travel on the rise after the COVID-19 pandemic brought it to a temporary halt, emergency physicians must be prepared to evaluate and manage patients whose recent travel may inform their diagnosis.

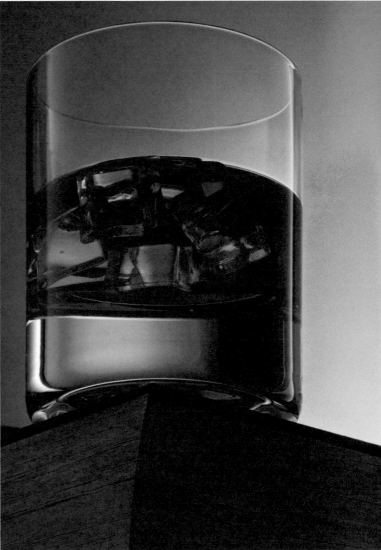

Tipsy-Turvy

Alcohol intoxication is a common presentation for adults, but lately, patients are presenting at younger ages. Whether alcohol ingestion is intentional or accidental, children face different adverse reactions than their adult counterparts. Emergency physicians must recognize these complications and be able to manage various alcohol poisonings.

THE OFFICIAL CME PUBLICATION OF THE AMERICAN COLLEGE OF EMERGENCY PHYSICIANS

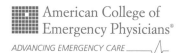
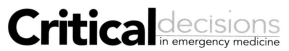

Criticaldecisions
in emergency medicine

Critical Decisions in Emergency Medicine is the official CME publication of the American College of Emergency Physicians. Additional volumes are available.

EDITOR-IN-CHIEF

Michael S. Beeson, MD, MBA, FACEP
Northeastern Ohio Universities, Rootstown, OH

SECTION EDITORS

Joshua S. Broder, MD, FACEP
Duke University, Durham, NC

Andrew J. Eyre, MD, MHPEd
Brigham & Women's Hospital/
Harvard Medical School, Boston, MA

John Kiel, DO, MPH
University of Florida College of Medicine,
Jacksonville, FL

Frank LoVecchio, DO, MPH, FACEP
Maricopa Medical Center/Banner Phoenix Poison
and Drug Information Center, Phoenix, AZ

Amal Mattu, MD, FACEP
University of Maryland, Baltimore, MD

Christian A. Tomaszewski, MD, MS, MBA, FACEP
University of California Health Sciences,
San Diego, CA

Steven J. Warrington, MD, MEd
MercyOne Siouxland, Sioux City, IA

ASSOCIATE EDITORS

Tareq Al-Salamah, MBBS, MPH, FACEP
King Saud University, Riyadh, Saudi Arabia/
University of Maryland, Baltimore, MD

Wan-Tsu W. Chang, MD
University of Maryland, Baltimore, MD

Ann M. Dietrich, MD, FAAP, FACEP
University of South Carolina College of Medicine,
Greenville, SC

Kelsey Drake, MD, MPH, FACEP
St. Anthony Hospital, Lakewood, CO

Walter L. Green, MD, FACEP
UT Southwestern Medical Center, Dallas, TX

John C. Greenwood, MD
University of Pennsylvania, Philadelphia, PA

Danya Khoujah, MBBS
University of Maryland, Baltimore, MD

Sharon E. Mace, MD, FACEP
Cleveland Clinic Lerner College of Medicine/
Case Western Reserve University, Cleveland, OH

Nathaniel Mann, MD
Greenville Health System, Greenville, SC

George Sternbach, MD, FACEP
Stanford University Medical Center, Stanford, CA

Joseph F. Waeckerle, MD, FACEP
University of Missouri-Kansas City School of Medicine,
Kansas City, MO

EDITORIAL STAFF

Suzannah Alexander, Editorial Director
salexander@acep.org

Sydney King
Managing Editor

Joy Carrico
Assistant Editor

Kyle Powell, Graphic Artist

ISSN2325-0186 (Print)   ISSN2325-8365 (Online)

Contents

Lesson 7 4

Travel Bug
Fever Following Travel
By Meghan Nodurft-Froman, MPH; and Elizabeth DeVos, MD, MPH
Reviewed by Kelsey Drake, MD, MPH, FACEP

Lesson 8 26

Tipsy-Turvy
Pediatric Alcohol Poisoning
By Mauro Rodriguez, DO; and Jyothi Lagisetty, MD, EMT-P, FACEP
Reviewed by Ann M. Dietrich, MD, FAAP, FACEP

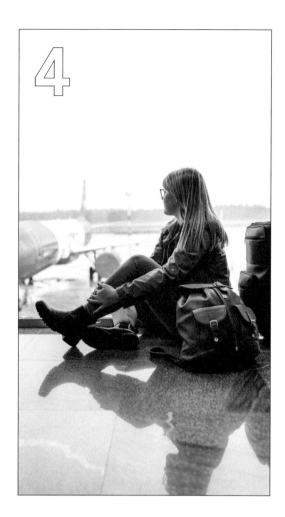

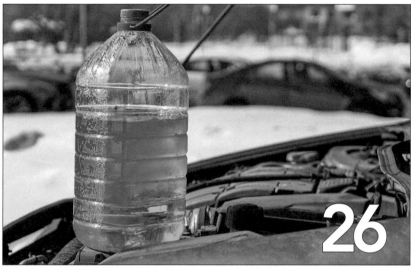

26

FEATURES

Clinical Pediatrics — Pediatric THC Toxicity 16
   By E. Mason Jackson, MD; and Erik S. Fisher, MD
   Reviewed by Sharon E. Mace, MD, FACEP

The LLSA Literature Review — Procedural Sedation 18
   By Johnothan Smileye, MD; and Michael E. Abboud, MD, MSEd
   Reviewed by Andrew J. Eyre, MD, MHPEd

The Critical ECG — Mobitz I Atrioventricular Conduction 20
   By Amal Mattu, MD, FACEP

Critical Cases in Orthopedics and Trauma — Subtalar Dislocation 22
   By Jonathan Jong, DO; and Victor Huang, MD, CAQ-SM
   Reviewed by John Kiel, DO, MPH

The Critical Procedure — Dental Splint With Skin-Closure Strips and
      Cyanoacrylate Tissue Adhesive 25
   By Steven J. Warrington, MD, MEd

The Critical Image —Abnormal Density in Chest X-Ray 32
   By Joshua S. Broder, MD, FACEP

CME Questions 34

Drug Box — Gabapentin 36
   By Frank LoVecchio, DO, MPH, FACEP

Tox Box — Aconite Poisoning 36
   By Christian Tomaszewski, MD, MS, MBA, FACEP

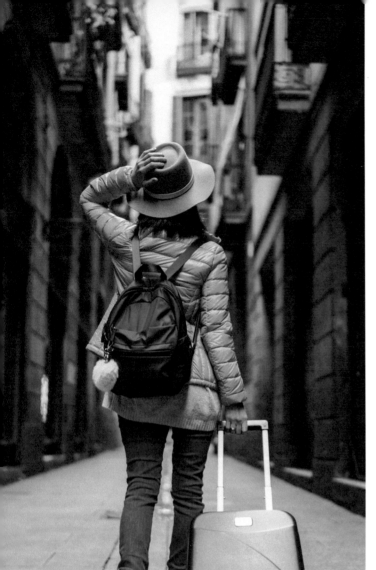

Travel Bug
Fever Following Travel

LESSON 7

By Meghan Nodurft-Froman, MPH; and Elizabeth DeVos, MD, MPH

Ms. Nodurft-Froman ran COVID-19 testing and vaccine operations through UF Health in Gainesville, Florida. Dr. DeVos is an associate professor of emergency medicine and the medical director of International Emergency Medicine Education at the University of Florida, Jacksonville.

Reviewed by Kelsey Drake, MD, MPH, FACEP

Objectives

On completion of this lesson, you should be able to:

1. List the elements of a complete travel history.
2. Identify and manage cases of suspected malaria.
3. Identify and manage cases of suspected viral hemorrhagic fever.
4. Synthesize an assessment based on the involved organ systems and travel history to identify high-risk conditions in febrile returned travelers.
5. Recognize reportable causes of fever in returned travelers.

From the EM Model
1.0 Signs, Symptoms, and Presentations
    1.1 Abnormal Vital Signs
        1.1.2 Fever

CRITICAL DECISIONS

- What specific details should be obtained when inquiring about a patient's travel history?

- How should suspected malaria be approached, and what other diseases should be considered?

- What are the potential causes of hemorrhagic fever, and how should they be managed?

- What diseases should be considered in a febrile returned traveler with respiratory complaints, abdominal pain, or neurologic symptoms?

- Which diseases should be reported to the CDC?

Modern travel's ease and speed expose travelers to conditions rarely encountered at home, where they typically seek treatment. With international travel on the rise after the COVID-19 pandemic brought it to a temporary halt, emergency physicians must be prepared to evaluate and manage patients whose recent travel may inform their diagnosis.

■ CASE ONE

A 35-year-old woman presents with generalized malaise, fever, chills, headache, and abdominal pain over the past week. Initial laboratory results show mild anemia and thrombocytopenia with a normal WBC count. Additional history details about recent travel are gathered. The patient reveals that she returned from Uganda in East Africa 14 days ago, where she was visiting her grandparents. She did not take any prophylactic medications during her trip.

■ CASE TWO

A 40-year-old man presents with a 2-day history of sudden-onset fever, fatigue, and myalgia, followed by a 1-day history of vomiting, diarrhea, and abdominal pain. Today, he has bloody stools. The patient explains that he returned from Guinea in West Africa 10 days ago, where he was volunteering in a rural hospital. He initially felt okay when he returned home.

■ CASE THREE

A 53-year-old diabetic woman with a body mass index of 35 presents with a cough, shortness of breath, and an associated fever. Her temperature is 39°C (102.2°F), and she is tachycardic and tachypneic with increased work of breathing. She reports returning from a work conference in Southern Brazil 10 days ago.

Before the COVID-19 pandemic, it was estimated that as many as 64% of travelers became ill abroad.[1] In light of the pandemic, it is difficult to say how that statistic holds up. However, as the situation stabilizes, we will again be able to determine the degree of risk a traveler assumes when venturing out.

Most travel-related illnesses are mild and self-limiting, generally presenting with upper respiratory or gastrointestinal (GI) symptoms.[2] However, more serious conditions, including COVID-19, malaria, dengue fever, rickettsial infections, and typhoid fever, are diagnosed with varying frequencies in returned travelers with systemic febrile illness. Factors that can complicate diagnostic accuracy include difficulties in establishing timelines and identifying exposures, geographic variation in risk, differing incubation periods, and significant overlap in clinical presentations.

Travel-related diseases can pose significant challenges to physicians who do not encounter these conditions regularly, and COVID-19 has completely overwhelmed the issue for the past 2 years. However, preparation and an organized clinical approach allow physicians to reduce the risks associated with these common disorders, as people increasingly return to international travel.

CRITICAL DECISION

What specific details should be obtained when inquiring about a patient's travel history?

In addition to the usual components of a patient's history of past and present illness, emergency physicians should gather a careful travel history, which can indicate risk for various travel-related diseases. Physicians should identify, at minimum, the geographic region of travel, the reason for travel, the timeline of travel, possible exposures, pre-travel immunizations, and chemoprophylaxis.

Travel Destination

Disease risk varies significantly by region. For example, a febrile patient who returns from Sub-Saharan Africa may be more likely to have malaria than someone who returns from another region where dengue fever or other diseases are more prominent.[3] Similarly, rickettsial infections, yellow fever, enteric fever, and many other diseases are endemic to certain areas, so a patient's exposure varies greatly based on the region of travel (*Table 1*).

Timeline

It is essential to establish a travel and exposure timeline, including details about the duration of the trip, timing of exposure, and timing of illness in relation to travel. Some studies suggest that longer trips are correlated with an increased risk and incidence of illness.[1] Furthermore, due to the variation of incubation periods, the timing of illness related to travel can help measure a patient's risk for certain conditions.

Pre-travel History and Chemoprophylaxis

Emergency physicians should also evaluate a patient's pre-travel preparation. Travelers who visit a clinic before departure are less likely to present with fever, acquire malaria, or experience severe disease than those who depart without a pre-trip assessment. For example, if a patient is suspected of having malaria, the physician should inquire as to whether the patient received chemoprophylaxis at a travel clinic and, if so, should assess compliance with the prescribed regimen. In one case series of United States civilians, 6% of patients with malaria reported adherence to appropriate chemoprophylaxis.[4]

Although the incidence is less likely, a traveler who has taken chemoprophylactic medications can still acquire malaria.

Other Historical Details

To further narrow the differential diagnosis and risk stratify the case, emergency physicians should seek to identify possible exposures, such as a history of freshwater swimming, known ingestions of contaminated food or water, interactions with farm animals, or reported insect bites.[5]

Details about a traveler's accommodations and activities can provide critical information as well. Business travelers can experience different exposures than adventure travelers or front-line humanitarian workers. Possible risk factors should be investigated: Did the patient have bed nets or screens? Was the patient in a rural or urban environment? Was the patient staying in a hotel, camping, or visiting farms? These factors can suggest differing susceptibilities to various infections.

Region	Incubation Period of <10 Days	Incubation Period of <21 Days	Incubation Period of >21 Days	Incubation Period of Months
Caribbean	• Chikungunya • Dengue • Zika	•Leptospirosis		
Central America	• Dengue • Zika	• Enteric fever • Leptospirosis	• Leishmaniasis	• Chagas disease • Leishmaniasis
South America	• Dengue • Yellow fever • Zika	• Enteric fever • Leptospirosis	• Leishmaniasis	• Chagas disease • Leishmaniasis
South Central Asia	• Chikungunya • Dengue • SARS	• Enteric fever		
Southeast Asia	• Chikungunya • Dengue • SARS	• Japanese encephalitis • Enteric fever • Leptospirosis	• Leishmaniasis	• Leishmaniasis
Sub-Saharan Africa	• Hemorrhagic fevers • Yellow fever	• Hemorrhagic fevers • Enteric fever	• Filariasis • Leishmaniasis • Schistosomiasis	• Filariasis • Leishmaniasis
Widespread	• Malaria • COVID-19	• HIV • Malaria	• Hepatitis A, E • HIV • Malaria	• Malaria • Tuberculosis

TABLE 1. Selected infectious diseases by region and typical incubation period

Travelers who were visiting friends or family are at increased risk for certain illnesses due to increased exposure to local populations.

In addition, physicians should ask whether the patient sought medical care overseas. Whether the patient went to a clinic or local hospital or purchased medications from a local pharmacy can be valuable information. In many countries, antibiotics and other medications can be purchased without a prescription. This information can help explain a delayed or atypical clinical presentation.

COVID-19 has elevated travelers' awareness of travel restrictions and quarantines — typical public health measures aimed at reducing the spread of serious emerging infectious diseases. Although recommendations change frequently, identifying precautions and the traveler's adherence to them should be a routine part of travel and vaccination histories. The mode of travel may further provide insight into the risk of acquiring infectious diseases. Although air filtration and rapid turnover in air travel typically reduce risk, multiple respiratory viruses, including COVID-19, have been linked to transmission during flight.[6,7,8]

CRITICAL DECISION

How should suspected malaria be approached, and what other diseases should be considered?

Several epidemiological studies of fever in returned travelers indicate that when a specific etiological diagnosis is made, malaria is the most frequently identified illness.[3,9,10] However, differentiating malaria from other travel-related systemic febrile illnesses can be challenging due to the nonspecific findings that are associated with this condition.

Malaria is caused by *Plasmodium* parasites spread via an *Anopheles* mosquito vector (*Figure 1*). Five *Plasmodium* species

cause malaria in humans: *P. falciparum*, *P. vivax*, *P. ovale*, *P. malariae*, and *P. knowlesi*. Other confounding causes of acute febrile illness in the returned traveler are also vector-borne; for example, dengue, Zika, yellow fever, and chikungunya are all arboviruses whose primary vector is the *Aedes aegypti* mosquito.

Malaria, particularly in uncomplicated infections, is characterized by symptoms shared by other minor viral illnesses.[11] Early symptoms of uncomplicated malaria include fever, malaise, myalgia, headache, and chills. The classic paroxysms of chills and fever, followed by diaphoresis, are infrequently observed with falciparum malaria infections.[2] The nonspecific early findings of malaria overlap significantly with other causes of acute febrile illness in returned travelers, such as dengue, chikungunya, and Zika (*Figure 2*). Although myalgia is common with malarial infections, it is usually less severe than with dengue, and muscle tenderness is less prominent with malaria than with leptospirosis or typhus.[11]

Malaria is also less likely to present with a rash than dengue, chikungunya, Zika, typhus, enteric fever, or meningococcal septicemia.[11] Petechiae are often associated with viral hemorrhagic fevers (VHFs) but are rarely seen with malaria. Petechiae are only found in severe falciparum malaria infections associated with complications such as disseminated intravascular coagulation.[11] High fevers, splenomegaly, thrombocytopenia, mild jaundice, and abdominal tenderness are commonly found in patients infected with malaria.

Knowing the geographic area of travel, as well as the travel timeline, can aid physicians. Although significant overlap exists in endemic areas of malaria, dengue, chikungunya, Zika, African trypanosomiasis, and leptospirosis, a travel timeline can help differentiate them. Chikungunya, dengue, and Zika have incubation periods of less than 2 weeks, while the incubation period for malaria varies by species. The incubation period for *P. falciparum* is around 12 to 14 days, with a range from 7 to 30 days. The overwhelming majority of cases of *P. falciparum* malaria occur within 1 month of return, but *P. vivax* and *P. ovale* infections can present months or even years after the initial infection.[12]

Complications of malaria can develop rapidly and include encephalopathy, hypoglycemia, acidosis, acute renal failure, pulmonary edema, hepatic dysfunction, intravascular hemolysis, disseminated intravascular coagulation, and shock. Because of the rapid onset of complications, patients with signs of severe malaria or a parasite load of greater than 5% should be treated immediately with intravenous antimalarials. Pregnant patients and children are more susceptible to morbidity and mortality related to malarial infection, so physicians should be vigilant about detecting severe disease in these populations, even in mild-appearing cases.

Malaria is diagnosed based on demonstration of the parasite, which is accomplished via thick and thin blood smears or by more advanced methods, including rapid antigen tests and polymerase chain reaction (PCR) techniques.[11] A febrile traveler who has returned from an endemic area should promptly have thick and thin blood smears examined for the parasite, after notifying the lab personnel about the concern for the infrequently seen disease. When suspicion is high and the parasite cannot be visualized, the patient should undergo repeat blood smears every 12 to 24 hours for 2 days.[11] In cases of altered mental status and fever after traveling to endemic areas, CSF should be evaluated to rule out other causes of encephalopathies. CSF in patients with malaria is usually normal or demonstrates nonspecific, mildly elevated protein and mild pleocytosis.[13]

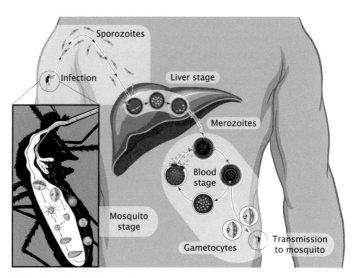

FIGURE 1. **Life cycle of the malaria parasite**

Treatment varies based on the severity of the illness, drug susceptibility, and species of the parasite. Due to increasing drug resistance in endemic areas, the WHO recommends artemisinin-based compounds as the first-line therapy for falciparum malaria infections.[1,14] In addition to initial therapy to treat erythrocytic forms, patients with *P. vivax* or *P. ovale* infections require primaquine to eradicate the dormant liver hypnozoites and to prevent relapse.[11] The CDC maintains a malaria hotline, where physicians can receive diagnostic and treatment advice from a Division of Parasitic Diseases and Malaria (DPDM) expert. The CDC Malaria Hotline can be reached Monday through Friday from 9 am to 5 pm Eastern time at 855-856-4713; for after-hours assistance with diagnosis or management of suspected malaria cases, clinicians can call the CDC Emergency

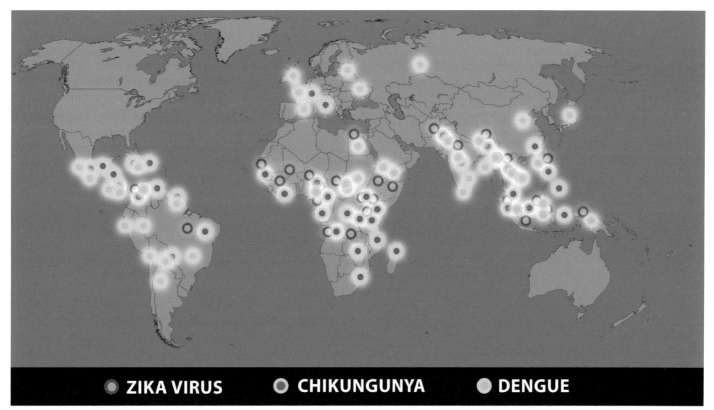

ZIKA VIRUS **CHIKUNGUNYA** **DENGUE**

FIGURE 2. **Global distribution of arboviruses**

Operations Center at 770-488-7100 and ask to speak to the DPDM expert on call.[15]

Although no emergency treatment is required, the clinical presentation of Zika can overlap greatly with malaria and is another important consideration in the febrile returned traveler, particularly for women of childbearing age. In cases of suspected Zika, emergency physicians should follow state guidelines for testing and can find information related to regions with active Zika outbreaks on the CDC "Zika Travel Information" website.[16]

Dengue, chikungunya, and Zika have been specifically mentioned, but it is worth noting that other diseases can present similarly. Therefore, emergency physicians should consider a broad differential for returned travelers who present with acute febrile illness, including acute HIV, enteric fever, leptospirosis, African trypanosomiasis, yellow fever, visceral leishmaniasis, hepatitis, influenza, tick-borne rickettsioses, and many other illnesses.

CRITICAL DECISION

What are the potential causes of hemorrhagic fever, and how should they be managed?

The WHO defines acute hemorrhagic fever syndrome as an acute onset of fever of less than 3 weeks' duration in a severely ill patient, plus any two of the following:
- Hemorrhagic or purpuric rash
- Epistaxis
- Hematemesis
- Hemoptysis
- Blood in stools
- Other hemorrhagic symptoms and no known predisposing host factors for hemorrhagic manifestations.[17]

Hemorrhagic fevers can be caused by viral, bacterial, or rickettsial diseases. Viral causes can be classified into the following families: filoviruses (Ebola and Marburg), arenaviruses (Lassa fever, Junin, Machupo, Lujo, Sabia, and Chapare), flaviviruses (yellow fever, dengue, Omsk hemorrhagic fever, and Kyasanur Forest disease), and bunyaviruses (Crimean-Congo hemorrhagic fever, Rift Valley fever, and Hantaan hemorrhagic fever). Each virus is associated with a specific host species, and human infection is incidental. These host-virus associations generally limit the distribution of each disease to specific geographic areas, although travelers can carry disease to nonendemic areas. Human-to-human spread can cause significant outbreaks, as exemplified by recent Ebola outbreaks in West and Central Africa.[18]

Ebola Virus Disease

Ebola virus disease sets itself apart from other causes of hemorrhagic fever by its virulence and mortality. Mortality rates have reached as high as 70% to 90% in prior epidemics.[19,20] Ebola viruses are found in several African countries. The West African Ebola epidemic of 2014 to 2016 turned the virus into a household name.[18]

The Ebola and Marburg viruses, of the filovirus family, are among the most virulent diseases in humans.[20] Unlike other causes of VHF, the primary reservoir for Ebola is uncertain, although many believe that fruit bats serve this role.[21] Humans can contract the virus through contact with infected bats, primates, or other humans. Once humans are infected, the disease can spread rapidly. Human-to-human transmission occurs through direct contact with bodily fluids from an infected person, by contact with objects that have been contaminated with such bodily fluids, and even through contact with the semen of men who previously recovered from the disease.[22,23]

The combination of virulence and mortality of both Ebola and other causes of VHF makes transmission prevention a critically important focus. Early symptoms of VHF can be similar to, and therefore difficult to distinguish from, other febrile illnesses. During an outbreak, screening of febrile patients for travel to endemic areas and symptoms concerning for VHF should be routine at the entry point to the health care system. Physicians must maintain a high degree of suspicion in any patient who has recently traveled from an endemic area or has had contact with someone with VHF and who presents with fever, muscle aches, severe headache, diarrhea, vomiting, abdominal pain, or any unexplained hemorrhage.

If VHF is suspected, extreme caution must be taken to prevent transmission within the health care facility. The patient should immediately be placed in an isolation room with a designated bathroom or bedside commode. Health care workers should act in designated roles to minimize the number of workers who contact the patient. All personnel who interact with the patient should wear appropriate personal protective equipment and should be recorded in a log. For a comprehensive review of appropriate personal protective equipment, see the CDC guidelines. The facility's infection control program and the local health department should be notified, and the patient's workup should continue using only dedicated equipment in compliance with local protocols. For further details on the approach to triage, see the algorithm published by the CDC.[24]

If clinical suspicion is high after initial evaluation, testing should proceed in conjunction with the local health department. Various forms of testing are available, including PCR, enzyme-linked immunosorbent assay, virus isolation, and immune globulin M and immune globulin G for patients later in the disease course. For most causes of VHF, no specific treatment exists. Management should therefore be supportive (ie, intravenous fluids, electrolyte replacement, supplemental oxygen, vasopressors, and mechanical ventilation) and combined with the treatment of other infections, as needed.

Dengue Virus Infection

Dengue virus infection is the most common mosquito-borne illness worldwide.[25,26] Transmission is ubiquitous throughout the subtropics and tropics, with more than half the world's population at risk of infection.[27] Manifestations of dengue virus infection can range from acute febrile illness, commonly referred to as dengue fever, to dengue hemorrhagic fever and dengue shock syndrome.

The primary vector for dengue virus transmission is the Aedes aegypti mosquito. The incubation period ranges from 3 to 14 days, but symptoms usually begin 4 to 7 days after being bitten by an infected mosquito. Dengue fever can present as an

acute febrile illness; it is colloquially referred to as "breakbone fever" due to the associated arthralgia. The WHO recommends considering dengue fever when fever is accompanied by two or more of the following symptoms:
- Severe headache
- Retro-orbital pain
- Joint pain
- Myalgia
- Nausea
- Vomiting
- Swollen glands
- Rash[28]

Hemorrhagic manifestations, such as epistaxis and scattered petechiae, are seen in cases of uncomplicated dengue infection; however, they can also indicate more severe disease. Patients with dengue fever can also present with abdominal pain, lethargy, restlessness, or elevated liver transaminase levels, but these symptoms should alert physicians to possible severe dengue infection.

Symptoms of severe disease usually manifest 2 to 5 days after the onset of typical dengue fever.[29] In addition to fever, patients with dengue hemorrhagic fever exhibit the following triad of features:
- Evidence of increased vascular permeability;
- Marked thrombocytopenia (100,000 cells/mm3 or less); and
- Spontaneous bleeding or signs of hemorrhagic tendency.[30]

The term dengue shock syndrome is used when dengue is accompanied by signs of circulatory failure, such as hypotension, narrow pulse pressure, or weak pulses, in addition to features of dengue hemorrhagic fever. Historically, the virus has been classified into dengue fever, dengue hemorrhagic fever, and dengue shock syndrome. Although these terms are still frequently used in clinical practice, nomenclature has more recently been simplified to dengue with or without warning signs and severe dengue.[30] In the updated classification system, severe dengue fever is defined by severe plasma leakage, severe hemorrhage, or severe organ impairment. Understanding both systems can help physicians recognize signs of more serious illness and communicate effectively with consulting services.

Signs of increased vascular permeability include pleural effusion, ascites, or hemoconcentration, which can be diagnosed with bedside ultrasound, chest x-ray, or a CT scan of the chest and abdomen. These complications usually begin 3 to 7 days after the onset of typical dengue fever, usually coinciding with the time of defervescence. The sequelae of profound vascular leakage can include respiratory distress and overt shock.[30]

Hemorrhagic manifestations of dengue virus infection include spontaneous bleeding, generally petechiae or ecchymoses, or evidence of hemorrhagic tendency. Hemorrhagic tendency is demonstrated by a positive tourniquet test (*Figure 3*). The test is performed by taking the patient's blood pressure and then inflating the blood pressure cuff on the arm to midway between the systolic and diastolic blood pressures, keeping it inflated for 5 minutes. The pressure is then released for 2 minutes. The skin beneath the cuff is examined for petechiae, and the number of petechiae is recorded. The test is considered positive if there are 10 or more petechiae per 1 square inch of skin. A positive test indicates microvascular fragility and a hemorrhagic tendency.

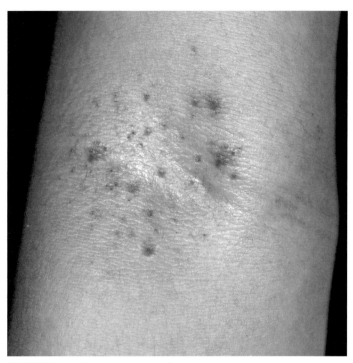

FIGURE 3. **Positive tourniquet test**

Although dengue is generally a clinical diagnosis, more advanced confirmatory testing exists. Management is supportive, consisting primarily of volume resuscitation and analgesia. Pain management should be achieved with agents other than nonsteroidal anti-inflammatory agents, as these are contraindicated in cases of dengue fever.[2]

CRITICAL DECISION

What diseases should be considered in a febrile returned traveler with respiratory complaints, abdominal pain, or neurologic symptoms?

As with other travel-related illnesses, it is essential to elicit a detailed travel history to identify potentially important exposures. For undifferentiated fevers in returned travelers, the involved organ systems can provide additional clues for the diagnosis. The approach to fever in the returned traveler with respiratory symptoms, abdominal pain, or neurologic symptoms should begin with the consideration of non–travel-related causes, then expand to a differential diagnosis that includes travel-related etiologies.

Respiratory Complaints and Fever

On March 11, 2020, the WHO declared COVID-19 a global pandemic, and in just 24 months, it has led to the highest number of global deaths in the past 20 years, with over 500 million confirmed cases and more than 6 million deaths worldwide.[31] As borders reopen, travel restrictions are lifted, and COVID-19 becomes endemic, emergency physicians must consider it in the differential diagnosis for febrile patients returning from travel. It is important to understand the various classifications of symptomatic COVID-19 infection, available laboratory testing, and pertinent imaging findings in COVID-19 disease.[32,33]

Symptomatic cases of COVID-19 are classified as nonsevere, severe, and critical. Approximately 80% of symptomatic cases present as nonsevere with fever, changes in taste or smell, myalgias, and respiratory tract symptoms.33 Most cases that present to the emergency department are classified as either severe or critical because the CDC guides patients to seek emergency care for symptoms including shortness of breath, chest pain, new confusion, somnolence, and cyanosis.[34] A severe presentation is defined by an SpO_2 level less than 90%, which is an indication for hospital admission.[33] Critical COVID-19 includes acute respiratory distress, sepsis, septic shock, or any other condition requiring life-sustaining assistance.[33] Research shows that the most common reason for COVID-19 ICU admission is hypoxemic respiratory failure, while bacterial and fungal coinfections are a major cause of morbidity and mortality among COVID-19 cases.[33]

Laboratory testing complements clinical findings in determining a COVID-19 diagnosis. After a reverse transcription PCR (RT-PCR) positive SARS-CoV-2 result, a complete blood count (CBC) may reveal lymphopenia, which can be profound in severe disease. Chemistry and liver-function testing can evaluate for organ injury along with other COVID-19 complications.[33] Associated severe illnesses may include diabetic ketoacidosis or thrombotic events; appropriate laboratory testing should be considered if these are suspected. Chest x-ray is usually the first step in the evaluation of respiratory symptoms in COVID-19, but CT to evaluate for pulmonary embolism or other concurrent lung pathology should be considered in patients with severe respiratory symptoms (*Figures 4 and 5*).[33]

Research shows that SARS-CoV-2 variants, especially the variants of concern, are mutating at an accelerated rate in comparison to similar coronaviruses. To indicate the level of transmissibility and disease severity, variants are classified as variants of interest, variants of concern, or variants of high consequence (*Table 2*).[35] Emergency physicians should note the circulating variants and their frequently changing clinical implications.

Before the COVID-19 pandemic, respiratory complaints associated with fever occurred in about one in seven cases in the returned traveler.[3] Although the vast majority of cases are attributable to common bacterial and viral pathogens, it is important to note that travelers in close contact with the local population, such as those visiting family or staying in relatives'

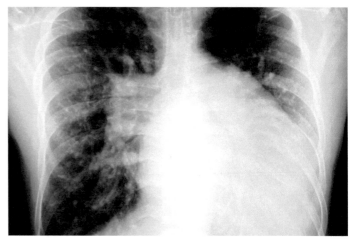

FIGURE 4. **Chest x-ray showing ground-glass opacities in a COVID-19 patient**

homes, are at an increased risk for pneumonia and influenza as compared to tourists and business travelers.[3] Some other considerations include legionellosis, acute schistosomiasis, Q fever, leptospirosis, severe acute respiratory syndrome (SARS), and Middle East respiratory syndrome (MERS).

Historical factors can cause physicians to investigate more uncommon causes of travel-related respiratory illness. Patients with a history of travel that includes farm work, particularly with cattle, goats, and sheep, should be evaluated for acute Q fever caused by Coxiella burnetii, which is typically transmitted in aerosolized animal excrement or contaminated soil (*Figure 6*). Unpasteurized milk is another source of the pathogen. Incubation is approximately 3 weeks, and patients can present with pulmonary symptoms, headaches, and other nonspecific symptoms. Emergency physicians should also be aware that Q fever can progress to endocarditis or vascular infections.[36]

Adventure travelers who participate in boating and swimming activities in Sub-Saharan Africa or Southeast Asia are at risk for Katayama fever due to acute schistosomiasis. In these patients, an immunologic response to the schistosoma worms can cause fever, nonproductive cough, bronchospasm, urticaria, fatigue, and organomegaly. Pulmonary infiltrates on x-ray and eosinophilia typically present 4 to 6 weeks after travel. The diagnosis is primarily clinical.[37,38]

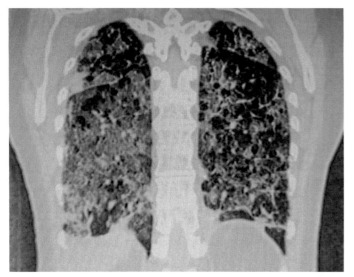 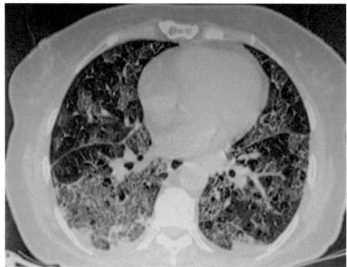

FIGURE 5. **CT of the chest showing bilateral ground-glass opacities in a COVID-19 patient**

In recent years, outbreaks of progressive viral respiratory syndromes have occurred. Maintaining awareness of ongoing public health syndromic surveillance, appropriate personal protection, and patient isolation can aid in timely diagnosis and prevent further disease spread. For the SARS outbreak of 2002 to 2003, infection risk was highest in health care workers, those caring for or slaughtering wildlife for human consumption, male sex, advanced age, and air travelers. The SARS coronavirus, transmitted by aerosolized droplets, has an incubation period of approximately 4 to 6 days and typically presents with a fever greater than 38°C (100.4°F) as well as evidence of pneumonia or acute respiratory distress syndrome (ARDS) on chest x-ray.[39,40]

Similarly, the CDC currently recommends that patients with fever and pneumonia be assessed for MERS if they have returned from travel from the Arabian peninsula within the last 14 days, if they have had close contact with such a traveler, if they are febrile with respiratory complaints after spending time in a health care facility (as a visitor, employee, or patient) in a territory where health care–associated cases of MERS have recently been identified, or if they have had close contact with a MERS patient. Emergency physicians should follow established guidelines for testing and reporting in such cases.[41]

Abdominal Pain and Fever

Concerning features such as jaundice, organomegaly, or hematochezia should encourage physicians to pursue an expanded workup and to search for potential exposures. Laboratory studies and imaging (stool microscopy, stool culture and sensitivity, stool ova and parasites, stool serology, hemoccult testing, blood cultures, or other advanced diagnostic tools) should be ordered as clinically indicated. Empiric treatment should be based on the suspected diagnoses.

Aspects of patients' presentations can guide emergency physicians to narrow the differential for fever and abdominal pain in the returned traveler. For example, a chief complaint of watery diarrhea can suggest enterotoxigenic Escherichia coli, cryptosporidiosis, giardiasis, cholera, or a rotavirus.

A history of bloody diarrhea can suggest an invasive or inflammatory etiology, including both bacterial and parasitic causes, such as enterohemorrhagic *E. coli*, enteroinvasive *E. coli*, *Salmonella*, shigellosis, *Campylobacter enteritis*, *Yersinia enterocolitica*, or *Entamoeba histolytica*, although these often present with watery diarrhea as well.

Jaundice can imply hepatitis, severe malaria, leptospirosis, yellow fever, dengue, or other VHFs as the etiology of patients' abdominal pain. Organomegaly can suggest malaria, leishmaniasis, amoebic liver abscess, enteric fever, brucellosis, schistosomiasis, or hepatitis. Petechiae can be due to leptospirosis, yellow fever, dengue, or other VHFs. Abdominal pain and fever accompanied by a rash should alert emergency physicians to VHFs, brucellosis, or enteric fever, among other illnesses. Shigellosis should be considered in patients with diarrhea, febrile seizures, and a history of travel. In patients with fever, abdominal pain, and eosinophilia associated with pulmonary symptoms, physicians should consider helminthic sources, such as hookworms or roundworms.

Traveler's Diarrhea

Diarrhea and gastroenteritis are among the most common travel-related complaints. Although it is important to consider more concerning etiologies, most patients with fever, abdominal pain, and diarrhea are suffering from traveler's diarrhea, a mild and self-limited disorder that generally resolves within 3 to 7 days.[42] Primary treatment is targeted at fluid resuscitation, as needed. Antibiotic and antimotility agents can be used to limit the severity and duration of symptoms. When there is suspicion for enterohemorrhagic *E. coli* (eg, a history of bloody stools), caution should be used, as antibiotic treatment is associated with an increased risk of hemolytic uremic syndrome.

Bacterial and viral pathogens associated with traveler's diarrhea generally have an incubation period of 6 to 72 hours; the incubation period for protozoal pathogens is considerably longer, around 1 to 2 weeks.[42] Markedly elevated fever and blood or pus in the stool are uncommon and should raise suspicion for another etiology.

Enteric Fever

Enteric fever, caused by *Salmonella* Typhi or *Salmonella* Paratyphi, can produce fever and abdominal pain, particularly an undifferentiated prolonged fever. The presentation of the disease is somewhat nonspecific. When suspicion exists, malaria should be ruled out, and other diagnoses should be considered, including hepatitis, VHFs, bacterial enteritis, dengue, brucellosis, rickettsial infections, leptospirosis, amoebic liver abscesses, acute HIV, cholera, amoebic dysentery, and parasitic etiologies, such as *Giardia* and *Cryptosporidium*.

The incidence of enteric fever is highest in South and Southeast Asia, but it should also be considered for travelers returning from Africa, East Asia, West Asia, Central America, and South America.[43,44] The incubation period for enteric fever ranges from 5 to 21 days.[45] Humans are the only hosts of *Salmonella* Typhi and *Salmonella* Paratyphi, and both ill and asymptomatic chronic carriers can shed bacteria in their stool. Most cases are transmitted via contaminated food or water. However, transmission has been described in health care workers

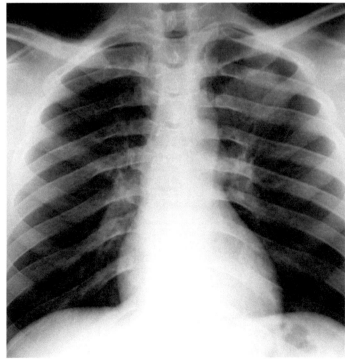

FIGURE 6. Lung x-ray of a patient with Q fever

(exposed via both patient and specimen contact) and between male sexual partners.[45]

Risk factors for transmission include consumption of contaminated water or ice, food washed in contaminated water, raw fruits and vegetables grown in fields fertilized with sewage, food and drinks from street vendors, flooding, and suboptimal hand washing practices.[46] Patients should be asked about their immunization history because many travelers who acquire typhoid fever have not been appropriately immunized and the vaccine can be less than 75% effective.[46]

The initial presentation of enteric fever is variable, but fever is generally present in the early stages. Vital signs can show relative bradycardia compared to what is expected for the degree of fever, sometimes referred to as pulse-temperature dissociation or the Faget sign. The classically described "rose spots" of typhoid fever are groups of faint, salmon-colored, blanching maculopapules primarily found on the trunk; when present, they are usually evident during the latter part of the first week or during the second week of infection.[45] Abdominal pain, nausea, vomiting, anorexia, hepatosplenomegaly, myalgia, and headache can also be present. Patients with severe infection can present with GI bleeding, intestinal perforation with resulting peritonitis, septic shock, or altered mental status.[45]

A definitive diagnosis of *Salmonella* Typhi or *Salmonella* Paratyphi is made by isolation of the organism. Physicians should consider ordering stool and blood cultures during the initial evaluation. Stool cultures are often negative during the first week of the disease course, while blood cultures are commonly positive.

An important treatment consideration is the increasing rate of multidrug-resistant strains of *Salmonella* Typhi and strains with decreased ciprofloxacin susceptibility.[45] For severe or complicated disease courses, ceftriaxone is considered the first-line empiric therapy. Antibiotic therapy for uncomplicated disease courses depends on the risk of antibiotic resistance; azithromycin is typically recommended for empiric treatment of enteric fever acquired in areas with high fluoroquinolone resistance.

COVID-19

GI symptoms are the first presenting complaint in up to one-third of COVID-19 patients. As many as half have diarrhea, and two-thirds have nausea and vomiting. While respiratory symptoms may be more profound, it is important to consider COVID-19 risk factors and exposures when patients present with GI complaints.[47]

Neurological Complaints and Fever

Altered Mental Status

Altered mental status in febrile travelers returning from malaria-endemic regions requires emergent evaluation for cerebral malaria, bacterial meningitis, and encephalitis. Venezuelan equine encephalitis, Japanese encephalitis, and tick-borne encephalitis should also be considered, depending on the area of travel. Tick-borne encephalopathies are most common in Eastern European outdoor adventurers. Neisseria meningitidis should be considered for those patients who have visited Sub-Saharan Africa's meningitis belt, which encompasses 26 countries from Senegal to Ethiopia, although outbreaks are sometimes seen in other parts of the world as well. Although a vaccine is now required for Muslim pilgrims who travel to Mecca after a 1987 outbreak, the vaccination does not cover all strains, so physicians should remain alert for meningococcal meningitis. Cryptococcal meningitis and tuberculous meningitis are further considerations for immunocompromised patients with prolonged travel and those who have lived among local populations in Sub-Saharan Africa.

Seizure

The two most common causes of seizures worldwide, neurocysticercosis and schistosomiasis, can present with fever, but they are uncommon in casual travelers.[48] Seizures with a febrile diarrheal illness should raise concern for shigellosis. Patients who present with febrile seizures after travel to endemic areas should also be evaluated for Japanese encephalitis, dengue hemorrhagic fever, and cerebral malaria.[48] Japanese encephalitis is a mosquito-borne flavivirus that is vaccine preventable. Travelers to rural and peri-urban areas in Southeast Asia and the Western Pacific are at the highest risk of exposure. Although only 1 in 250 infections presents with serious clinical disease, those that do can present with fever, headaches, seizures, parkinsonian features, and even coma. In severe disease courses, the case fatality rate reaches 30%, and up to another 30% can experience permanent neuropsychological problems.[48,49]

The specific diagnosis should be based on serologic and CSF confirmatory studies, and treatment is typically symptomatic. Refer to the previous discussions on dengue shock syndrome and malaria for further information. Remember that pregnant women, children, nonimmune populations, and those taking inadequate chemoprophylaxis are at increased risk for cerebral malaria.

✔ Pearls

- Review assessments for international travel screening or other CDC and WHO information to help identify high-risk patients.

- Remember infections with seasonal variation can present at atypical times due to varying times of transmission in other geographic areas.

- Repeat blood smears within 12 to 24 hours of presentation for patients with suspected malaria if initial testing is negative because sensitivity improves with repeated tests.

- Consider enteric fever for causes of prolonged fever when malaria has been excluded.

- Conduct additional laboratory testing and imaging to rule out lethal COVID-19 complications when a patient has severe COVID-19 (defined as hypoxia with >50% lung involvement).

CRITICAL DECISION

Which diseases should be reported to the CDC?

In the interest of public health, the CDC must be informed of the diagnosis of several infectious diseases. It is the responsibility of the physician, not the patient, to notify the CDC. Such diseases are designated as either reportable or notifiable. It is mandatory to report cases of any disease with a reportable designation; reporting a notifiable disease is voluntary. Each state determines what diseases fall under each category, so reportable diseases are unique to each state. Physicians, hospitals, and laboratories should report cases to the local health department, which then shares the information with the CDC. Some laboratories automatically report positive results, but physicians should be familiar with the procedures in their individual practice settings.

Reporting cases of certain infectious diseases serves many purposes — the most important of which is to help to slow the spread of communicable diseases. Reporting cases also facilitates surveillance, which can help to identify sources of outbreaks; allows public health organizations to plan preventive measures and control strategies; and expedites the initiation of appropriate treatment options. Specific diseases receive reportable designations based on virulence, communicability, and the potential for morbidity and mortality. Notifiable infectious diseases are compiled by the CDC, including those that are unique to the returned traveler, and are maintained in an annual table at the National Notifiable Diseases Surveillance System website.[50]

Summary

Although travel-related diseases are uncommonly seen in emergency departments in the United States, prompt recognition and appropriate management are essential for the safety of patients as well as for the individuals with whom they come into contact. Emergency physicians must be adept at taking a complete travel history, including prophylaxis and immunizations, and should be comfortable forming an appropriate differential diagnosis based on history and physical examination.

Travel history, incubation period, and organ-system involvement should lead physicians toward specific diagnoses. Physicians should maintain an increased index of suspicion for people with higher-risk exposures, such as adventure travelers, humanitarian workers, those visiting friends and relatives, and those with fevers lasting longer than 1 week. In addition, physicians must ensure that patients are appropriately isolated, personal protection protocols are followed, and diseases of concern are reported.

REFERENCES

1. Hill DR. Health problems in a large cohort of Americans traveling to developing countries. *J Travel Med.* 2000;7(5):259-266.
2. D'Andrea S, De Wulf A. Global travelers. In: Tintinalli JE, Ma OJ, Yealy DM, et al, eds. *Tintinalli's Emergency Medicine: A Comprehensive Study Guide.* 9th ed. McGraw-Hill Education; 2020:1079-1091.
3. Wilson ME, Weld LH, Boggild A, et al. Fever in returned travelers: results from the GeoSentinel surveillance network. *Clin Infect Dis.* 2007;44(12):1560-1568.
4. Cullen KA, Arguin PM; Centers for Disease Control and Prevention. Malaria surveillance — United States, 2011. *MMWR.* 2013 Nov 1;62(ss05):1-17.
5. Fairley JK. Posttravel evaluation: general approach to the returned traveler. In: Centers for Disease Control and Prevention. *CDC Yellow Book 2020: Health Information for International Travel.* Oxford University Press; 2020. https://wwwnc.cdc.gov/travel/yellowbook/2020/posttravel-evaluation/general-approach-to-the-returned-traveler
6. Bielecki M, Patel D, Hinkelbein J, et al. Air travel and COVID-19 prevention in the pandemic and peri-pandemic period: a narrative review. *Travel Med Infect Dis.* 2021;39:101915.
7. Khatib AN, Carvalho AM, Primavesi R, To K, Poirier V. Navigating the risks of flying during COVID-19: a review for safe air travel. *J Travel Med.* 2020;27(8):taaa212.
8. Khatib AN, McGuinness S, Wilder-Smith A. COVID-19 transmission and the safety of air travel during the pandemic: a scoping review. *Curr Opin Infect Dis.* 2021;34(5):415-422.
9. Schlagenhauf P, Weld L, Goorhuis A, et al. Travel-associated infection presenting in Europe (2008-12): an analysis of EuroTravNet longitudinal, surveillance data, and evaluation of the effect of the pre-travel consultation. *Lancet Infect Dis.* 2015;15(1):55-64.
10. Freedman DO, Weld LH, Kozarsky PE, et al. Spectrum of disease and relation to place of exposure among ill returned travelers. *N Engl J Med.* 2006;354(2):119-130.
11. White NJ, Ashley EA. Malaria. In: Jameson J, Fauci AS, Kasper DL, Hauser SL, Longo DL, Loscalzo J, eds. *Harrison's Principles of Internal Medicine.* 20th ed. McGraw-Hill Education; 2018.
12. Wilson ME. Posttravel evaluation: fever. In: Centers for Disease Control and Prevention. *CDC Yellow Book 2020: Health Information for International Travel.* Oxford University Press; 2020. https://wwwnc.cdc.gov/travel/yellowbook/2020/posttravel-evaluation/fever
13. Misra UK, Kalita J, Prabhakar S, Chakravarty A, Kochar D, Nair PP. Cerebral malaria and bacterial meningitis. *Ann Indian Acad Neurol.* 2011;14(suppl 1):S35-S39.
14. World Health Organization. *Guidelines for the Treatment of Malaria.* 3rd ed. World Health Organization; 2015. https://www.who.int/publications/i/item/guidelines-for-malaria 441/1/9789241549127_eng.pdf
15. Steele S. CDC malaria hotline—when the caller is ill abroad. Centers for Disease Control and Prevention. Published August 12, 2013. https://blogs.cdc.gov/global/2013/08/12/cdc-malaria-hotline-when-the-caller-is-ill-abroad/
16. Zika travel information. Centers for Disease Control and Prevention. Updated December 10, 2021. https://wwwnc.cdc.gov/travel/page/zika-travel-information

✗ Pitfalls

- Neglecting to ask about recent travel or to collect a thorough travel history when indicated.

- Ignoring personal safety precautions and appropriate isolation procedures.

- Forgetting appropriate reporting protocols.

- Overlooking patients at increased risk for more severe disease, including children, pregnant women, elderly patients, and immunocompromised individuals.

- Disregarding alternate sources of chest pain and shortness of breath in patients with COVID-19, such as pulmonary embolism, especially in returned travelers with the additional risk factor of immobilization on long flights.

CASE RESOLUTIONS

■ CASE ONE

The emergency physician suspected malaria for the 35-year-old woman who presented with generalized malaise, fever, chills, headache, and abdominal pain. Thick and thin smears were ordered, which revealed falciparum malaria with a parasite density of 3%. At the time of diagnosis, she exhibited no manifestations of severe malaria. She was treated with artemether-lumefantrine twice a day for 3 days and made a complete recovery.

■ CASE TWO

The 40-year-old man with bloody stools was isolated, and mandatory transmission-based precautions were undertaken. Laboratory tests revealed elevated blood urea nitrogen and creatinine levels, elevated liver enzymes, leukopenia, and thrombocytopenia. PCR confirmed the diagnosis of Ebola virus disease. The patient was treated supportively with intravenous fluids, electrolyte replacement, blood product transfusions, and eventually mechanical ventilation. Despite these efforts, he died 7 days later.

■ CASE THREE

The 53-year-old woman's respiratory status worsened; she required intubation for mechanical ventilation. Her CT scan showed ground-glass opacities. Urine antigens for Legionella pneumophila and Streptococcus pneumoniae were both negative; viral panels for influenza, respiratory syncytial virus, parainfluenza virus, and adenovirus were all negative; and sputum cultures for acid-fast bacilli showed no growth. The emergency physician sent a nasopharyngeal specimen for RT-PCR testing for SARS-CoV-2, which returned positive. The patient received aggressive supportive care in the ICU and, after a 30-day hospitalization, was stabilized enough for extubation.

17. World Health Organization. WHO Recommended Surveillance Standards. https://apps.who.int/iris/bitstream/handle/10665/65517/WHO_CDS_CSR_ISR_99.2.pdf

18. Ebola (Ebola virus disease). Centers for Disease Control and Prevention. https://www.cdc.gov/vhf/ebola/history/chronology.html

19. Bray M, Murphy FA. Filovirus research: knowledge expands to meet a growing threat. J Infect Dis. 2007;196(suppl 2):S438-S443.

20. Feldmann H, Geisbert TW. Ebola haemorrhagic fever. Lancet. 2011;377(9768):849-862.

21. Hayman DTS, Yu M, Crameri G, et al. Ebola virus antibodies in fruit bats, Ghana, West Africa. Emerg Infect Dis. 2012;18(7):1207-1209.

22. Crozier I. Ebola virus RNA in the semen of male survivors of Ebola virus disease: the uncertain gravitas of a privileged persistence. J Infect Dis. 2016;214(10):1467-1469.

23. Uyeki TM, Erickson BR, Brown S, et al. Ebola virus persistence in semen of male survivors. Clin Infect Dis. 2016;62(12):1552-1555.

24. US Department of Health and Human Services; Centers for Disease Control and Prevention. Identify, Isolate, Inform: Emergency Department Evaluation and Management of Patients Under Investigation for Ebola Virus Disease. https://www.cdc.gov/vhf/ebola/pdf/ed-algorithm-management-patients-possible-ebola.pdf

25. Barlam TF, Kasper DL. Approach to the acutely ill infected febrile patient. In: Jameson J, Fauci AS, Kasper DL, Hauser SL, Longo DL, Loscalzo J, eds. Harrison's Principles of Internal Medicine. 20th ed. McGraw-Hill Education; 2018.

26. Bhatt S, Gething PW, Brady OJ, et al. The global distribution and burden of dengue. Nature. 2013;496(7446):504-507.

27. Brady OJ, Gething PW, Bhatt S, et al. Refining the global spatial limits of dengue virus transmission by evidence-based consensus. PLoS Negl Trop Dis. 2012;6(8):e1760.

28. Dengue and severe dengue. World Health Organization. https://www.who.int/news-room/fact-sheets/detail/dengue-and-severe-dengue

29. Kuhn JH, Charrel RN. Arthropod-borne and rodent-borne virus infections. In: Jameson J, Fauci AS, Kasper DL, Hauser SL, Longo DL, Loscalzo J, eds. Harrison's Principles of Internal Medicine. 20th ed. McGraw-Hill Education; 2018.

30. World Health Organization. Dengue: Guidelines for Diagnosis, Treatment, Prevention and Control. New Edition 2009. https://apps.who.int/iris/bitstream/handle/10665/44188/9789241547871_eng.pdf?sequence=1&isAllowed=y

31. Wilder-Smith, A. COVID-19 in comparison with other emerging viral diseases: risk of geographic spread via travel. Trop Dis Travel Med Vaccines. 2021;7(1):3.

32. WHO coronavirus (COVID-19) dashboard. World Health Organization. https://covid19.who.int

33. Long B, Carius BM, Chavez S, et al. Clinical update on COVID-19 for the emergency clinician: presentation and evaluation. Am J Emerg Med. 2022;54:46-57.

34. COVID-19. Centers for Disease Control and Prevention. https://www.cdc.gov/coronavirus/2019-ncov/if-you-are-sick/steps-when-sick.html

35. Tay JH, Porter AF, Wirth W, Duchene S. The emergence of SARS-CoV-2 variants of concern is driven by acceleration of the substitution rate. Mol Biol Evol. 2022;39(2):msac013.

36. Delord M, Socolovschi C, Parola P. Rickettsioses and Q fever in travelers (2004-2013). Travel Med Infect Dis. 2014;12(5):443-458.

37. Puylaert CAJ, van Thiel PP. Images in clinical medicine. Katayama fever. N Engl J Med. 2016 Feb 4;374(5):469.

38. Doherty JF, Moody AH, Wright SG. Katayama fever: an acute manifestation of schistosomiasis. BMJ. 1996;313(7064):1071-1072.

39. World Health Organization, Department of Communicable Disease Surveillance and Response. Consensus Document on the Epidemiology of Severe Acute Respiratory Syndrome (SARS). World Health Organization; 2003. https://apps.who.int/iris/bitstream/handle/10665/70863/WHO_CDS_CSR_GAR_2003.11_eng.pdf?sequence=1&isAllowed=y

40. Case definitions for surveillance of severe acute respiratory syndrome (SARS). World Health Organization. Updated May 1, 2003. https://www.who.int/publications/m/item/case-definitions-for-surveillance-of-severe-acute-respiratory-syndrome-(sars)

41. People who may be at increased risk for MERS. Centers for Disease Control and Prevention. https://www.cdc.gov/coronavirus/mers/risk.html

42. Connor BA. Preparing international travelers: travelers' diarrhea. In: Centers for Disease Control and Prevention. CDC Yellow Book 2020: Health Information for International Travel. Oxford University Press; 2020. https://wwwnc.cdc.gov/travel/yellowbook/2020/preparing-international-travelers/travelers-diarrhea

43. Crump JA, Luby SP, Mintz ED. The global burden of typhoid fever. Bull World Health Organ. 2004;82(5):346-353.

44. Mogasale V, Maskery B, Ochiai RL, et al. Burden of typhoid fever in low-income and middle-income countries: a systematic, literature-based update with risk-factor adjustment. *Lancet Glob Health.* 2014;2(10):e570-e580.

45. Pegues DA, Miller SI. Salmonellosis. In: Jameson J, Fauci AS, Kasper DL, Hauser SL, Longo DL, Loscalzo J, eds. *Harrison's Principles of Internal Medicine.* 20th ed. McGraw-Hill Education; 2018.

46. Jackson BR, Iqbal S, Mahon B; Centers for Disease Control and Prevention. Updated recommendations for the use of typhoid vaccine — Advisory Committee on Immunization Practices, United States, 2015. *MMWR.* 2015;64(11):305-308. https://www.cdc.gov/mmwr/preview/mmwrhtml/mm6411a4.htm

47. Han MH, Zunt JR. Neurologic aspects of infections in international travelers. *Neurologist.* 2005;11(1):30-44.

48. Japanese encephalitis. World Health Organization. Published December 31, 2015. http://www.who.int/mediacentre/factsheets/fs386/en/

49. Thakur KT, Zunt JR. Approach to the international traveler with neurological symptoms. *Future Neurology.* 2015;10(2):101-113.

50. Nationally notifiable infectious diseases and conditions, United States, annual data for 2019. Centers for Disease Control and Prevention. https://wonder.cdc.gov/nndss/nndss_annual_tables_menu.asp

Pediatric THC Toxicity

By E. Mason Jackson, MD; and Erik S. Fisher, MD

Prisma Health Upstate, University of South Carolina School of Medicine, Greenville, South Carolina

Reviewed by Sharon E. Mace, MD, FACEP

Objective

On completion of this article, you should be able to:

■ Determine how to manage THC toxicity in pediatric patients.

CASE PRESENTATION

A 17-year-old boy presents via EMS to a level-2 pediatric trauma center as a critical arrival due to altered mental status, headache, and possible seizure activity. His blood glucose level is 168 mg/dL en route, and he receives 5 mg of midazolam for possible seizure-like activity. EMS also administers 2 mg of naloxone without any effect. On arrival, the patient is obtunded with a Glasgow Coma Scale score of 9 (E2 V2 M5), tachycardic with a systolic blood pressure around 100 mm Hg, and hypoxic, requiring oxygen administration via nasal cannula. The patient's pupils are 5 mm and fixed bilaterally, and he is reported to have had a severe headache prior to his alteration of consciousness. A cardiopulmonary examination is unremarkable, and there are no focal neurologic deficits.

The patient is taken to radiology for emergent CT imaging of his brain, which does not reveal any acute trauma, fracture, or hemorrhage to explain his abrupt alteration in mentation. A broad workup is initiated, including a complete blood count and comprehensive metabolic panel, and the results are overwhelmingly normal. There are no acute findings on chest x-ray, and urinalysis and electrocardiogram are also normal. Toxicologic workup reveals negative acetaminophen and salicylate levels. However, urine drug screen is positive for cannabinoids. The patient can ventilate, oxygenate, and maintain a patent airway despite his sedation; thus, intubation is deferred. Once the patient's family arrives at the bedside, they present the clinical team with a bottle of sublingual δ-8 tetrahydrocannabinol (δ-8 THC) oil that the patient uses recreationally at home.

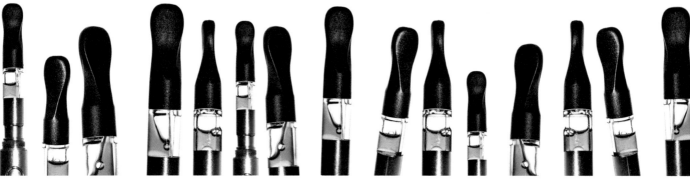

Discussion

For the past 4,000 years, cannabis and chemical derivatives have been used for medicinal purposes as well as drugs of abuse. Δ-9 tetrahydrocannabinol (δ-9 THC), the first cannabinoid isolated from *Cannabis sativa* and *C. indica*, is well understood as the primary psychoactive component of marijuana (*Figure 1*). Cannabinoids exert numerous biological effects through their interaction at specific G-protein receptors, namely cannabinoid receptors 1 and 2 (CB_1 and CB_2, respectively).

CB_1 receptors are densely present throughout the brain and are responsible for complex effects on learning, cognition, and mood, with the exact mechanism still unknown. However, there are relatively few CB_1 receptors in the brainstem, which likely explains the lack of coma, altered level of consciousness, and respiratory depression seen with other drugs of abuse. Meanwhile CB_2 receptors are theorized to have complex anti-inflammatory properties, which are not well understood. Stimulation of these receptors, whether by exogenous cannabinoids or endocannabinoids, leads to presynaptic cell hyperpolarization and decreased neurotransmitter release.

Despite the legalization of marijuana and cannabinoids, structurally related compounds that are not derived from *Cannabis* spp. are also growing in consumption, and they hold similar potent effects. A hemp-derived legal alternative to δ-9 THC, δ-8 THC, has been growing in consumption (*Figure 2*). As cannabinoid drugs gain popularity and prevalence, it is imperative that emergency physicians recognize these drugs in overdose, which disproportionally affects the pediatric population.

Δ-8 THC comes in a variety of formulations and strengths, making it difficult to quantify the total amount of drug ingested. Preparations of δ-8 THC include gummies, oil tinctures, and vape liquid. Doses range from 30 to 40 mg/mL (1-1.5 mg/gtt) of oil to 10 to 25 mg per gummy. When this variability is mixed with the lack of FDA regulation regarding purity and its relatively new presence on the market, δ-8 THC toxicity becomes hard to assess and manage. With the pediatric population, flavored

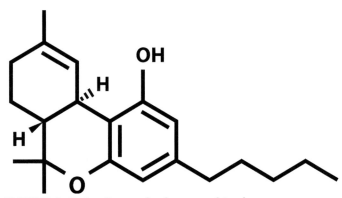

FIGURE 1. Delta-9 tetrahydrocannabinol

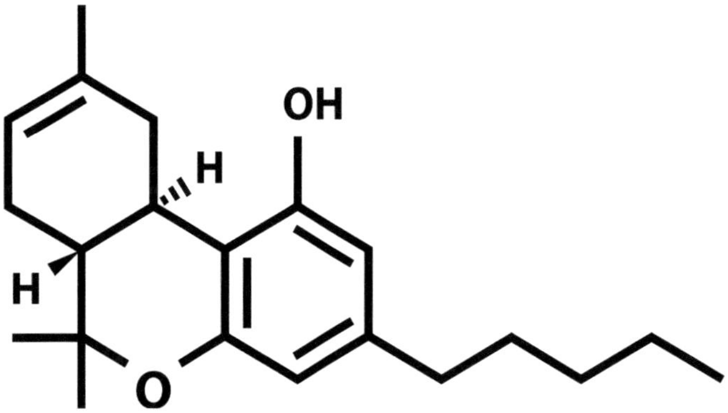

FIGURE 2. Delta-8 tetrahydrocannabinol

gummies and colorful bottles of THC oil pose a significant ingestion risk.

Clinical Features

Since the literature surrounding synthetic or atypical cannabinoids, such as δ-8 THC, is sparse, δ-9 THC is often used as a reference. *Goldfrank's Toxicologic Emergencies* specifically references hashish, the pressed resin of the *C. sativa* plant, as causing obtundation in pediatric patients within 30 to 75 minutes at a dose of 250 to 1,000 mg. The spectrum of THC toxicity in pediatric patients ranges from mild psychomotor slowing to lethargy, seizure, vital sign derangements, and apnea. Clearly, a child, who is more focused on the flavored gummy or liquid, can quickly ingest a large enough amount of the drug to cause life-threatening symptoms.

Treatment

With both δ-8 and δ-9 THC, there is no specific antidotal therapy. Supportive care is the mainstay of therapy and revolves around airway protection, ruling out coingestant and concomitant pathology, seizure treatment, and vital sign management.

CASE RESOLUTION

The patient's mental status improved throughout his stay in the emergency department. He was able to answer brief questions but was significantly somnolent. No focal or generalized seizure activity was observed. He was admitted to the pediatric hospitalist service for further observation and later said that he took "20 drops" of δ-8 THC oil, which he increased from his "daily 8 drops" because he no longer thought it was working. This roughly translates to an ingested dose of 20 mg to 800 mg, depending on whether these were actual drops or milliliters. The patient returned to his baseline mental status and was discharged from the hospital the following day without any residual deficits.

REFERENCES

1. Iwanicki JL. Hallucinogens. In: Walls RM, Hockberger RS, Gausche-Hill M, et al, eds. *Rosen's Emergency Medicine: Concepts and Clinical Practice.* Vol 2. 9th ed. Elsevier; 2018:1907-1909.
2. Lapoint JM. Cannabinoids. In: Nelson LS, Howland MA, Lewin NA, Smith SW, Goldfrank LR, Hoffman RS, eds. *Goldfrank's Toxicologic Emergencies.* 11th ed. McGraw-Hill Education; 2019:1111-1123.
3. Babalonis S, Raup-Konsavage WM, Akpunonu PD, Balla A, Vrana KE. Δ8-THC: legal status, widespread availability, and safety concerns. *Cannabis Cannabinoid Res.* 2021;6(5):362-365.
4. US Food and Drug Administration. 5 things to know about delta-8 tetrahydrocannabinol. Updated September 14, 2021. https://www.fda.gov/consumers/consumer-updates/5-things-know-about-delta-8-tetrahydrocannabinol-delta-8-thc

Procedural Sedation

By Johnothan Smileye, MD; and Michael E. Abboud, MD, MSEd
Department of Emergency Medicine, University of Pennsylvania

Reviewed by Andrew J. Eyre, MD, MHPEd

Objective

On completion of this article, you should be able to:
- Identify the proper usage and dosage of propofol for deep procedural sedation in both adults and children in the emergency department.

Miller KA, Andolfatto G, Miner JR, Burton JH, Krauss BS. Clinical practice guideline for emergency department procedural sedation with propofol: 2018 update. *Ann Emerg Med.* 2019 May 1;73(5):470-480.

KEY POINTS

- Propofol provides short-acting anesthesia that has been well documented in the literature for use in the emergency department for procedural sedation in both adults and children.

- Relative contraindications for propofol include propofol allergy, elderly patients, infants younger than 6 months, and ASA Class III or higher.

- Propofol should be administered by a clinician qualified to administer deep sedation and ideally with at least two individuals present: one dedicated to sedation and continuous patient monitoring and another performing the procedure.

- Propofol can be administered as a bolus or infusion, with higher doses in children, and can be coadministered with analgesics, including ketamine and fentanyl.

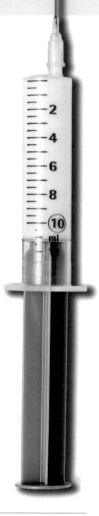

Propofol is an ultra-short-acting agent that provides both anesthesia and amnesia to patients. Its use has been well documented in the emergency department for procedural sedation. Despite its safety, the use of propofol in children is much lower than in adults. This article provides updated evidence-based guidelines for the use of propofol in the emergency department for deep procedural sedation.

Patients undergoing procedural sedation with propofol require continuous monitoring both via monitoring equipment and direct visualization, including continuous cardiac monitoring, capnography, and pulse oximetry as well as careful monitoring of the patient's respiratory rate and blood pressure (cycled at least every 5 minutes) throughout the procedure and recovery. Supplemental oxygen should also be administered throughout the procedure, as this provides longer periods of normal oxygenation if the patient becomes hypopneic or apneic. Young children are especially at risk, given their smaller pulmonary reserve.

Emergency department procedural sedation requires a clinician who is trained and qualified to administer deep sedation. The team should be composed of at least two personnel: one dedicated to the procedure and a second dedicated to sedation, patient monitoring, and any potential resuscitative interventions. If only one clinician performs both the procedure and sedation, then they must immediately stop the procedure to perform resuscitation, if needed.

Propofol can be given as a bolus or infusion. Propofol infusions are becoming more popular, as they minimize the risk of respiratory depression, hypotension, and suboptimal sedation seen at propofol's peak and trough. Bolus dosing in adults is an initial bolus of 0.5 to 1.0 mg/kg, with additional boluses of 0.25 to 0.5 mg/kg every 1 to 3 minutes as needed. Infusion dosing should be titrated between 100 and 150 µg/kg/min (6-9 mg/kg/hr). Consider starting on the lower end of the dosage range for elderly patients as well as obese patients, as propofol dosing should be based on lean body mass and not total body weight. Children require higher doses to achieve a desired level of sedation. Use an initial bolus dose of 2 mg/kg in patients 3 years or younger and 1.5 mg/kg in older children and teenagers, with additional boluses of 0.5 to 1 mg/kg every 1 to 3 minutes as needed. For infusions in children, use 100 to 250 µg/kg/min (6-15 mg/kg/hr).

Propofol does not have analgesic properties, so patients undergoing painful procedures may benefit from propofol coadministration with an analgesic agent. Ketamine is often coadministered with propofol (ketofol) in a 1:1 mixture in a single syringe at the same mL/kg volume as single-agent propofol, which provides a faster onset of deep sedation and analgesia. Fentanyl is also commonly administered with propofol for analgesia.

Critical Decisions in Emergency Medicine's series of LLSA reviews features articles from ABEM's 2022 Lifelong Learning and Self-Assessment Reading List. Available online at acep.org/moc/llsa and on the ABEM website.

Patients should receive fentanyl prior to receiving propofol to decrease the risk of respiratory depression that can occur with coadministration.

The most common adverse effect of propofol is transient hypotension, which is seen in both adults and children. As such, special consideration should be given to administering propofol to critically ill or hypotensive patients. Respiratory depression, including hypoxia or apnea, can be seen in any patient but is more common in adults than in children. The use of airway adjuncts (eg, bag-valve-mask ventilation and intubation) are rarely needed. Rare side effects include injection site pain and nausea and vomiting. Propofol infusion syndrome has not been documented in the literature for emergency department procedural sedation.

One absolute contraindication for the use of propofol is a previous propofol allergy. Relative contraindications include children younger than 6 months old or under 5 kg, patients older than 75 years, and patients with an American Society of Anesthesiologists (ASA) Physical Status Classification System Class III and above. Previous soybean or egg allergy (both used in the manufacturing of propofol) is no longer considered a contraindication, as data does not support this concern.

Mobitz I Atrioventricular Conduction

By Amal Mattu, MD, FACEP

Dr. Mattu is a professor, vice chair, and director of the Emergency Cardiology Fellowship in the Department of Emergency Medicine at the University of Maryland School of Medicine in Baltimore.

Objective

On completion of this article, you should be able to:

- Identify nonconducted P waves, an AV block, and a left bundle branch block on ECG.

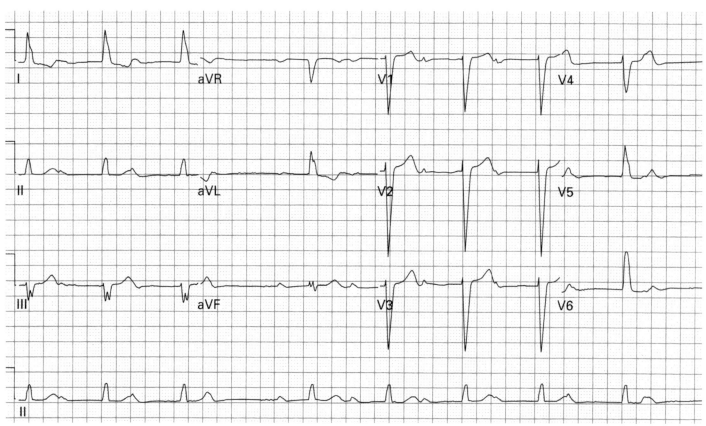

FIGURE 1. A 93-year-old woman presenting after a syncopal episode

Sinus rhythm with second-degree atrioventricular (AV) block type 1 (Wenckebach, Mobitz I), rate 50, left bundle branch block (LBBB). The atrial rate is approximately 60, although the approximate ventricular rate is 50 (*Figure 1*). Nonconducted P waves are present, and a constant P-P interval persists, indicating the presence of an AV block. For those P waves that are conducted, the PR interval appears to gradually increase preceding the nonconducted P waves.

The increasing PR interval defines Mobitz I AV conduction. The novice interpreter may miss the nonconducted P waves because both of the nonconducted P waves on the rhythm strip are "buried" within the T waves (*Figure 2*). LBBB is also present with expected ST-segment discordance — ST segments are normally deviated opposite to the terminal deflection of the QRS complex when LBBB is present (ie, when the terminal portion of the QRS complex points primarily upward, ST-segment depression is expected; when the terminal portion of the QRS complex points downward, ST-segment elevation is expected).

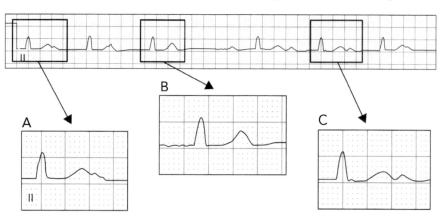

FIGURE 2. Nonconducted P waves. The P waves are partially obscured by the T wave in (A) and (C); the P wave is entirely obscured by the T wave in this beat (B).

From **Mattu A, Brady W.** *ECGs for the Emergency Physician 2.* BMJ Publishing; 2008:11,23. Reprinted with permission.

Subtalar Dislocation

By Jonathan Jong, DO; and Victor Huang, MD, CAQ-SM
NewYork-Presbyterian Queens

Reviewed by John Kiel, DO, MPH

Objective

On completion of this article, you should be able to:

■ Describe the typical presentation, management, and complications of subtalar dislocations.

■ **CASE PRESENTATION** ■

A 45-year-old man presents with left foot pain and deformity after he inverted his foot while running on uneven pavement. On examination, the foot is deformed, in fixed supination (*Figure 1*); it is neurovascularly intact; and there are no open skin breaks.

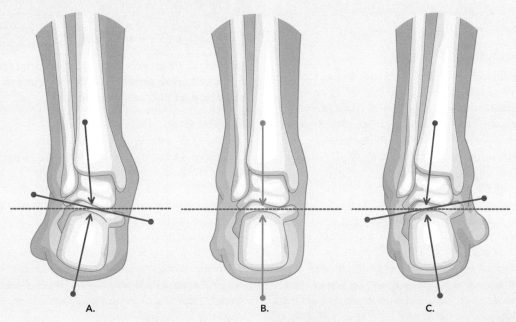

FIGURE 1. **Left foot showing pronation (A), normal positioning (B), and supination (C)**

Discussion

Subtalar dislocations are rare and involve the simultaneous disruption of the talocalcaneal and talonavicular joints (*Figure 2*). The joints are supported by strong ligaments and a tight joint capsule, such that dislocation often requires a high-energy mechanism.[1] As a result, they represent only 1% to 2% of all dislocations. Subtalar dislocations can be further classified into medial, lateral, anterior, and posterior dislocations based on the displacement of the midfoot.[2] Medial dislocations are the most common, representing about 65% of all subtalar dislocations, followed by lateral dislocations at about 35%.[2] Anterior and posterior dislocations are rare.

Mechanism of Injury

Subtalar dislocations are generally seen in younger men.[1] Commonly, the mechanism of injury is high energy, such as a motor vehicle crash or a fall from height. Medial subtalar dislocations can specifically result from athletic activities, such as basketball, due to forceful inversion with the foot in plantarflexion, while lateral dislocations occur with eversion in plantarflexion.[3]

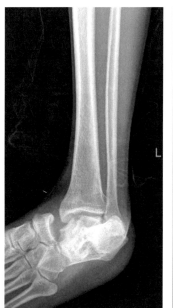
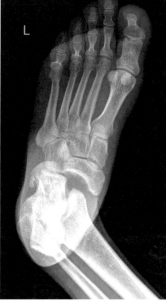

FIGURE 2. **Anterior-posterior (AP) and oblique x-rays of the left ankle demonstrating a medial subtalar dislocation**

Physical Examination

On examination, subtalar dislocations present with obvious displacement of the hindfoot. The foot is typically locked in supination for medial dislocations and in pronation for lateral dislocations.[3] The neurovascular examination is typically normal, but it is important to confirm pulses and perform a terse motor and sensory examination.

Imaging

Plain x-rays of the foot and ankle should be obtained pre- and postreduction. It is important to obtain a postreduction CT scan due to the prevalence of occult injuries (*Figure 3*).[4] In one case series of nine patients, all had occult injuries on CT; these additional findings changed the management of four patients. Associated injuries include fractures of the fifth metatarsal, talus, and malleolus as well as osteochondral fractures of the dislocated articular surfaces.[4,5]

Reduction Technique

These patients should undergo closed reduction as soon as possible. Procedural sedation is often required for successful reduction.[6] Patients should be positioned with their knee flexed to 90° to relax the gastrocnemius and soleus muscles. Reduction can then be performed with traction and countertraction, accentuating the deformity and then reversing the mechanism.

Definitive Management

Immobilization can be achieved with placement of a short-leg splint with stirrups and made non-weight bearing in crutches. The period of immobilization is controversial. In general, 4 weeks of immobilization is appropriate for most patients.[4] However, some evidence suggests a shorter immobilization period, with one prospective study advocating for 2 to 3 weeks followed by early range of motion exercises for better functional outcomes.[4,7]

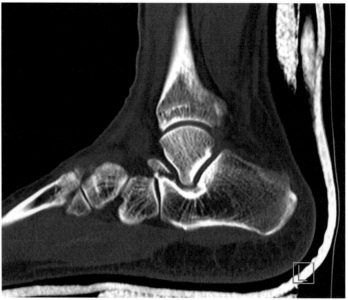

FIGURE 3. Postreduction CT demonstrating a fracture of the anterior process of the calcaneus and interval reduction of subtalar dislocation

Complications

Orthopedics or podiatry should be consulted for all subtalar dislocations. Open fractures, neurovascular compromise, and irreducible dislocations require emergent consultation. Occasionally, attempts at closed reduction are unsuccessful due to interposed soft tissue blocking the reduction.[3,4] These cases may require open reduction.

Long-term outcomes are influenced by various factors, including the dislocation type, associated bony and soft-tissue injuries, the high-energy mechanism, and length of immobilization.[4] Patients may suffer from post-traumatic arthritis, talus necrosis, and subtalar joint stiffness, although immediate closed reduction may help decrease the risk of developing these complications.[6]

CASE RESOLUTION

The patient was given fentanyl 100 µg IV and midazolam 2 mg IV. Closed reduction was performed with traction-countertraction, inversion followed by eversion. A postreduction CT scan showed a mildly displaced anterior process with a calcaneus fracture. The patient followed up with orthopedics and was managed nonoperatively in a short-leg cast for 4 weeks.

REFERENCES

1. DeLee JC, Curtis R. Subtalar dislocation of the foot. *J Bone Joint Surg Am.* 1982;64:433-437.

2. Bibbo C, Anderson RB, Davis WH. Injury characteristics and the clinical outcome of subtalar dislocations: a clinical and radiographic analysis of 25 cases. *Foot Ankle Int.* 2003;24(2):158-163.

3. Giannoulis D, Papadopoulos DV, Lykissas MG, Koulouvaris P, Gkiatas I, Mavrodontidis A. Subtalar dislocation without associated fractures: case report and review of literature. *World J Orthop.* 2015;6(3):374-379.

4. Perugia D, Basile A, Massoni C, Gumina S, Rossi F, Ferretti A. Conservative treatment of subtalar dislocations. *Int Orthop.* 2002;26(1):56-60.

5. Bibbo C, Lin SS, Abidi N, Berberian W, Grossman M, Gebauer G, Behrens FF. Missed and associated injuries after subtalar dislocation: the role of CT. *Foot Ankle Int.* 2001 Apr;22(4):324-328.

6. de Palma L, Santucci A, Marinelli M, Borgogno E, Catalani A. Clinical outcome of closed isolated subtalar dislocations. *Arch Orthop Trauma Surg.* 2008 Jun;128(6):593-598.

7. Lasanianos NG, Lyras DN, Mouzopoulos G, Tsutseos N, Garnavos C. Early mobilization after uncomplicated medial subtalar dislocation provides successful functional results. *J Orthop Traumatol.* 2011;12(1):37-43.

Dental Splint With Skin-Closure Strips and Cyanoacrylate Tissue Adhesive

By Steven J. Warrington, MD, MEd

MercyOne Siouxland, Sioux City, Iowa

Objective

On completion of this article, you should be able to:

■ Apply a dental splint, using skin-closure strips and cyanoacrylate tissue adhesive, to stabilize loose dentition.

While use of specialized or formal dental supplies is ideal for dental injuries and procedures, not all emergency departments are equipped with such materials. In instances without the materials to apply a more traditional dental splint, the use of readily available materials may be required. In these situations, skin-closure strips and cyanoacrylate tissue adhesive may be used to form a dental splint to stabilize loose dentition.

Contraindications

■ Allergy to a component of the adhesive or glue.

Benefits and Risks

Dental splints may help loose dentition remain stabilized, which may aid in healing and prevent complications. The goal of the dental splint is temporary stabilization and treatment to allow time for follow-up care with the appropriate consultant (eg, dentistry, oral maxillofacial surgery).

The primary risk for this procedure is an allergic reaction to a component of the adhesive or glue. Aside from that, there is also the risk of immediate failure of the procedure or failure prior to follow-up care. Furthermore, failure of a dental splint could lead to aspiration of a loose tooth.

Alternatives

Alternatives include not splinting the tooth or using more specialized materials. For example, temporary cement and a dental brace or metal bar may be used in place of the method discussed here. Additionally, a dental splint with only cyanoacrylate adhesive may be used (ie, without skin-closure strips) as an alternative.

Reducing Side Effects

There are minimal side effects from the procedure, aside from failure or applying the cyanoacrylate to unintended locations. Explaining to the patient the importance of remaining still in one position and applying the cyanoacrylate in a controlled manner may help reduce application of cyanoacrylate to unintended locations. Depending on the container the cyanoacrylate comes in, it may be beneficial to remove the applicator tip and apply from the tube itself.

Special Considerations

Drying of the dental surfaces prior to treatment and applying the cyanoacrylate drop by drop may yield better results. Another tip for an improved outcome is to consider having the patient bite on a tongue depressor to align the dentition and bite prior to the procedure.

TECHNIQUE

1. **Obtain** the patient's consent and obtain the materials and equipment for the procedure.

2. **Have** the patient bite along a tongue depressor to ensure the dentition to be splinted has the correct alignment and placement.

3. **Dry** the dentition to be splinted.

4. **Apply** the skin-closure strips (ie, wound-closure adhesive tape) to the involved dentition as well as the dentition to either side.

5. **Apply** the cyanoacrylate in a controlled fashion, drop by drop, along the skin-closure strips and where they meet individual teeth.

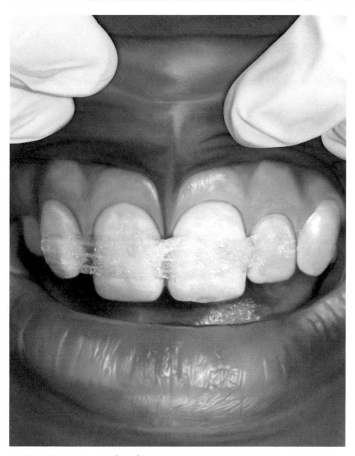

FIGURE 1. Dental splint setup.
Use n-butyl-2-cyanoacrylate tissue adhesive and skin-closure strips (wound-closure adhesive tape) to splint traumatized teeth.

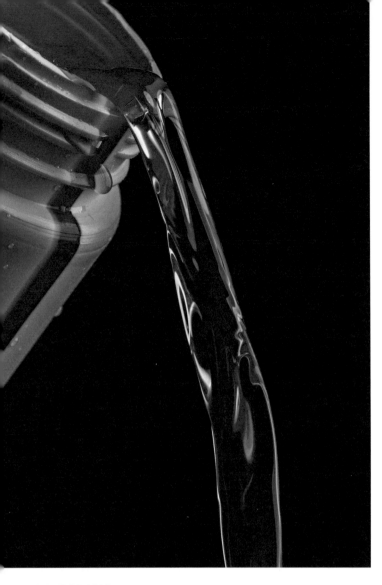

Tipsy-Turvy

Pediatric Alcohol Poisoning

LESSON 8

By **Mauro Rodriguez, DO** (not shown); and
Jyothi Lagisetty, MD, EMT-P, FACEP

Dr. Rodriguez is a categorical pediatrics resident and Dr. Lagisetty is a clinical assistant professor in the Department of Emergency Medicine and Pediatric Emergency Medicine at McGovern Medical School at the University of Texas Health Science Center in Houston.

Reviewed by **Ann M. Dietrich, MD, FAAP, FACEP**

OBJECTIVES

On completion of this lesson, you should be able to:

1. Discuss the clinical manifestations of alcohol poisoning in pediatric patients.

2. Differentiate the pathophysiology and clinical manifestations of ethanol, ethylene glycol, and methanol poisonings.

3. Explain the management of alcohol poisoning in the emergency department.

4. Describe the symptoms and predisposing factors associated with alcohol withdrawal.

5. List the treatment options for alcohol withdrawal.

FROM THE EM MODEL

14.0 Psychobehavioral Disorders
    14.1 Substance Use Disorders
        14.1.1 Alcohol Use Disorder

▬ CRITICAL DECISIONS ▬

■ What are the signs and symptoms of different types of alcohol poisoning?

■ How should suspected pediatric alcohol poisoning be assessed in the emergency department?

■ What is the antidote for ethanol poisoning?

■ How should alcohol withdrawal be managed?

■ What is the antidote for ethylene glycol and methanol poisoning?

Alcohol intoxication is a common presentation for adults, but lately, patients are presenting at younger ages. Whether pediatric alcohol ingestion is intentional or accidental, children face a multitude of different adverse reactions to alcohol when compared to their adult counterparts. Emergency physicians must recognize these complications and be able to manage various alcohol poisonings.

■ CASE ONE

A 16-year-old girl presents via EMS after being found unconscious in her room. She locked herself in her room for the past 24 hours after breaking up with her boyfriend following a significant argument. When EMS arrived, she was awake but drowsy. On arrival, she is bradycardic, appears confused, and only withdraws to pain. Her extremities are cool to the touch and appear clammy, and her clothing smells of alcohol.

■ CASE TWO

A 3-year-old boy presents via EMS after new-onset, witnessed, seizure-like activity. According to the patient's parents, the child was playing in the garage when he suddenly appeared dizzy and started walking wobbly. He had noticeably fast breathing before experiencing the seizure-like activity. On arrival, his respiratory rate is 50, but he does not have signs of increased work of breathing. His cardiac examination is unremarkable, and his capillary refill is 3 seconds. The neurologic examination is significant for a child who is lethargic, is unresponsive to voice but is responsive to pain, and has hypotonic extremities.

■ CASE THREE

A 17-year-old boy presents via EMS after having a syncopal episode during a flight from Switzerland to Houston, Texas. He got up during the flight to use the bathroom when he felt his heart pounding and his hands shaking before "blacking out." This is the second syncopal episode that he has experienced in the past month. He endorses drinking an estimated 500 mL of vodka a day plus occasional cigarette smoking. On examination, he is tachycardic and hypertensive. He has a nonintention tremor on neurologic examination, but his examination is otherwise normal.

Introduction

Initial alcohol abuse at a young age correlates with higher rates of developing alcohol dependence, with dependence rates decreasing in first-time users proportionally to alcohol introduction at an older age.[1] Although intentional alcohol use is commonly seen among teenagers and young adults, young children are more likely to present after accidental alcohol ingestion.[2] When inappropriately supervised, younger children are at an increased risk of accidental ingestion due to their innate curiosity. Poisoning can occur from a multitude of alcohols (including ethanol and parent alcohols, such as ethylene glycol and methanol) due to the fast rate of alcohol absorption and activity within the body. Emergency physicians must understand the presentation and management of pediatric patients with altered mental status due to alcohol ingestion because the timely initiation of appropriate treatment is critical to preventing permanent complications.

Terminology

Alcohol abuse is defined as a behavioral pattern of use that leads to significant impairment and interference with a patient's daily obligations, social life, personal safety, or judgment.[1] Alcohol dependence is a behavioral pattern of use leading to significant impairment and the development of tolerance, withdrawal, an inability to cut down, missed regular activities due to alcohol-seeking behaviors, and continued use despite acknowledgement of the abuse.[1] Alcohol intoxication is defined as an overdose in alcohol, typically used to refer to ethanol overuse but can be nonspecific to include other parent alcohols. Symptoms of alcohol intoxication vary depending on the type of alcohol consumed (Table 1). Ethanol is the most common type of alcohol intoxication seen in the emergency department, along with the occasional presentation of ethylene glycol, methanol, and isopropyl alcohol poisoning, among others. The toxic dose for ethanol in young children is 0.4 mL/kg of ethanol or a peak serum level of more than 50 mg/dL.[3]

Presentation	Ethanol	Ethylene Glycol	Methanol
Most common symptoms	The most common findings include bradycardia, hypothermia, behavioral changes, slurred speech, nystagmus, ataxia, respiratory depression, lethargy, and coma.	Abdominal pain, flank pain, decreased urine output, and hematuria can ensue due to the propensity to develop acute renal injury and calcium oxalate crystals.	Visual difficulties can ensue, from blurring to complete blindness.
Severity-dependent symptoms	Lower levels of serum ethanol concentration are associated with impaired judgment, abnormal behaviors, and short-term memory loss, whereas higher levels are associated with lethargy, disorientation, and even death.	Kussmaul respirations from metabolic acidosis, seizures, and hypotension can develop.	Kussmaul respirations from metabolic acidosis, seizures, and hypotension can develop.

TABLE 1. **Symptoms of different types of alcohol poisoning**

	Ethanol	Ethylene Glycol	Methanol
Products	• Aftershaves • Cosmetics • Cough syrups • Glass cleaners • Hand sanitizers • Kombucha • Mouthwash • Perfumes/colognes • Vanilla extract	• Antifreeze • Ballpoint pens • Cosmetics • Films • Brake fluids • Paints • Plastics • Stamp pad inks • Solvents	• Adhesives • Antifreeze • Paints • Shellacs • Tobacco smoke • Varnishes • Windshield washer fluid

TABLE 2. Consumer products with potentially toxic ingestants

Epidemiology

Ethanol consumption by children and adolescents is estimated to be around 11% of the total consumption in the United States.[2] Regardless of the type of alcohol, young children have a higher propensity for alcohol poisoning after consumption due to their smaller body surface area. Thousands of ethanol exposures are reported to Poison Control for children under 6 years of age, with nearly 90% of these exposures being secondary to a home product containing alcohol, such as hand sanitizer or mouthwash (*Table 2*).[2,4]

By contrast, adolescents primarily become symptomatic after binge drinking.[1] Alcohol abuse increases risk-taking behaviors among teenagers and young adults. Alcohol use is associated with fatal motor vehicle crashes, behavioral problems at school and work, delinquent behavior, use of other illicit substances, and riskier sexual behaviors (eg, having unprotected sex, multiple sex partners, or an unwanted pregnancy).[1,2] The American Academy of Pediatrics has recognized decreased rates of alcohol abuse among adolescents since strict laws on alcohol sales have been enacted.

CRITICAL DECISION

What are the signs and symptoms of different types of alcohol poisoning?

Ethanol Poisoning

Ethanol affects the central nervous system (CNS) by acting as a sedative due to GABA-mediated activation.[2,5] The degree of intoxication dictates the severity of the presentation. Lower levels of serum ethanol concentration are associated with impaired judgment, abnormal behaviors, and short-term memory loss, whereas higher levels are associated with lethargy, disorientation, and even death. The most common findings include bradycardia, hypothermia, behavioral changes, slurred speech, nystagmus, ataxia, respiratory depression, lethargy, and coma.[3,6] Hypotension and hypovolemia may also develop due to the propensity for increased urine output.[6] Although all ages are vulnerable to hypoglycemia, pediatric patients are most vulnerable to developing hypoglycemia that is severe enough to result in subsequent seizures, coma, and death.[3]

Ethanol Withdrawal

Withdrawal symptoms can be seen within 6 hours of cessation of alcohol consumption (*Table 3*). Because alcohol is a depressant, clinical features of withdrawal include anxiety, tachycardia, hypertension, fever, irritability, sweating, disorientation, gastrointestinal (GI) distress, tremors, seizures, and hallucinations occurring within hours of alcohol cessation.[6] The most concerning and uncommon symptom in pediatric patients is delirium tremens, which can be seen 2 to 3 days after cessation of alcohol. Delirium tremens exacerbates the above symptoms and can result in death if left untreated from circulatory collapse.[6] Clinical Institute Withdrawal Assessment for Alcohol-Revised (CIWA-Ar) scoring is an objective tool for scoring alcohol withdrawal to determine the severity.[5] Lastly, alcohol withdrawal can be associated with electrolyte abnormalities, such as hypokalemia and hypomagnesemia.[6]

Ethylene Glycol

Ethylene glycol poisoning shares many similarities with methanol intoxication. The three stages of ethylene glycol intoxication are defined by symptoms that vary based on the amount of time that has passed since ingestion (*Table 4*). Depending on the severity of intoxication, Kussmaul respirations from metabolic acidosis, seizures, and hypotension can develop. Specific to ethylene glycol poisoning, abdominal pain, flank pain, decreased urine output, and hematuria can

✔ Pearls

- Alcohol intoxication can cause hypoglycemia in all age groups but tends to be more prominent in toddlers and young children.

- Alcohol withdrawal can occur within 6 hours after alcohol cessation and may last up to 7 days; it is managed supportively.

- Ethylene glycol and methanol poisoning present similarly, with an increased osmolal gap and late anion gap metabolic acidosis; both are treated with fomepizole.

- Once absorbed by the body, ethanol must be metabolized to be cleared; there is no drug available to reverse the effects of ethanol poisoning.

ensue due to the propensity to develop acute renal injury and calcium oxalate crystals.[7,8]

Glyoxylate is the primary toxic metabolite formed by ethylene glycol poisoning. Alcohol dehydrogenase acts on ethylene glycol, converting it into glycolaldehyde. Aldehyde dehydrogenase subsequently makes glycolate. Due to oxidation, glycolate is further metabolized into glyoxylate, which can be identified in urine as calcium oxalate crystals.

Methanol

Methanol poisoning, from ingestion of products like windshield washer fluid, shares many similarities with ethylene glycol intoxication. Methanol intoxication is associated with abdominal pain, an osmolal gap, and late anion gap metabolic acidosis. Depending on the severity of intoxication, Kussmaul respirations from metabolic acidosis, seizures, and hypotension can develop. Specific to methanol poisoning, visual difficulties can ensue, from blurring to complete blindness.[5,7]

CRITICAL DECISION

How should suspected pediatric alcohol poisoning be assessed in the emergency department?

Laboratory Studies

Evaluation with laboratory studies is essential in patients with altered mental status due to suspected alcohol poisoning. A basic metabolic profile can help to evaluate for electrolyte abnormalities, hypoglycemia (most commonly in younger children), and an anion gap. Blood gas should be obtained to evaluate acid-base status. Drug-specific levels of ethanol, acetaminophen, and aspirin should be obtained, along with methanol, ethylene glycol, and isopropyl alcohol, if available. A urine drug screen can help screen for possible polysubstance abuse.[3,9] Special considerations should be taken for calcium derangement and urine oxalate crystals with ethylene glycol poisoning and an increased osmolal gap in alternative alcohol ingestion. In ethylene glycol and methanol intoxication, anion gap acidosis can take hours to develop, as metabolism with alcohol dehydrogenase and acetaldehyde dehydrogenase takes place.[8,10]

Imaging

No specific imaging is necessary for the diagnosis of alcohol poisoning, but imaging should be geared toward the working differential diagnosis. A chest x-ray may be particularly useful in children who present with concerning respiratory findings,

	Withdrawal symptoms can be seen within 6 hours of cessation of alcohol consumption, including:	
• Anxiety	• Hypertension	
• Delirium tremens	• Irritability	
• Disorientation	• Seizures	
• Fever	• Sweating	
• GI distress	• Tachycardia	
• Hallucinations	• Tremors	

TABLE 3. **Clinical features of alcohol withdrawal**

especially if there is concern for aspiration injury. If intubation is needed, a chest x-ray will be needed to evaluate appropriate endotracheal tube positioning. Depending on the presenting symptoms, a brain CT may be warranted if there is concern regarding trauma.[9]

CRITICAL DECISION

What is the antidote for ethanol poisoning?

There is no drug available to reverse the effects of ethanol poisoning. Once absorbed by the body, ethanol must be metabolized to be cleared. In adults, alcohol is metabolized at a rate of approximately 15 mg/dL/hr.[5] In children, ethanol is cleared by the liver at a rate of approximately 30 mg/dL/hr. The treatment is primarily supportive in terms of protecting the airway and nurturing the cardiovascular system. In severe overdoses, hemodialysis may be necessary to help eliminate alcohol from the blood.[3]

Patients with alcohol intoxication that require admission are at increased risk of developing Wernicke encephalopathy, which consists of a classic triad of ophthalmoplegia, ataxia, and confusion.[7] Although Wernicke encephalopathy is uncommon in pediatric patients, management with dextrose-containing fluids and daily thiamine supplementation should be considered for patients at risk of alcohol withdrawal, particularly in patients with neurologic manifestations. Thiamine supplementation must be started in patients who have chronic disease or have suspected nutritional determinants in addition to alcoholism.[11]

CRITICAL DECISION

How should alcohol withdrawal be managed?

Alcohol withdrawal should be managed supportively. Pediatric patients should be carefully considered for inpatient observation and management.[7] Although electrolyte disturbances (specifically hypokalemia and hypophosphatemia) are seen, they commonly correct without intervention. The use

	Stage 1	Stage 2*	Stage 3
Onset	<12 hours	12 to 36 hours	>48 hours
Symptoms	Neurologic abnormalities (eg, ataxia, slurred speech, nystagmus, headaches, lethargy, coma, and seizures)	Tachypnea, heart rate irregularities, cyanosis, pulmonary edema with subsequent respiratory distress, and circulatory shock	Decreased urine output, proteinuria or hematuria, and acute kidney injury

* Stage 2 is the period in which death is most common because the body is at the highest risk of going into shock.
TABLE 4. **Stages of ethylene glycol intoxication**

CASE ONE

The 16-year-old girl who was found unconscious was determined to have an improving neurologic status on presentation and, consequently, did not require intubation. She was worked up for toxic ingestion, and basic laboratory studies and an ECG were obtained. Given the patient's history of a recent breakup, self-isolation, and physical examination findings, there was clinical concern for alcohol poisoning with possible associated self-harm behaviors. Her initial serum ethanol level was 53 mg/dL, and her urine drug screen was positive for cannabinoids. Her management consisted of supportive care with isotonic intravenous fluids and close monitoring of her electrolytes. Once she was medically cleared, she was evaluated by child psychiatry. Her final disposition was inpatient psychiatry care due to uncovered suicidality.

CASE TWO

The 3-year-old boy with seizure-like activity was thought to have a toxic exposure, given the acuity of symptom onset. He was quickly intubated due to his neurologic status. Basic laboratory studies were obtained. His venous blood gas was concerning for metabolic acidosis with a pH of 7.15, PCO_2 of 20 mm Hg, and serum bicarbonate level of 13 mEq/L; his basic metabolic profile revealed an anion gap of 19. Urinalysis identified calcium oxalate crystals. Based on his history, anion gap metabolic acidosis, and positive urinalysis, there was high concern for ethylene glycol intoxication. Without obtaining confirmatory levels of ethylene glycol, treatment with fomepizole was initiated, and the patient was admitted to the pediatric ICU. He continued scheduled fomepizole administration until his blood pH normalized.

CASE THREE

The 17-year-old boy who presented after having a syncopal episode was recognized to have a high likelihood of alcohol dependence. This patient estimated consuming 500 mL of vodka daily. A direct flight from Switzerland to Houston takes about 11 hours, which would allow a sufficient time-lapse for symptoms of alcohol withdrawal to manifest. The initial workup included basic laboratory studies, drug levels, a urine drug screen, and a negative cardiac workup. His ethanol level was 98 mg/dL, and the urine drug screen was negative. His comprehensive metabolic profile showed hypokalemia at 2.0 and phosphorus at 1.9, which prompted admission. As an inpatient, he was started on daily thiamine with glucose-containing fluids to minimize the risk of developing Wernicke encephalopathy. Nutrition and adolescent medicine were consulted to address the electrolyte derangement, which was attributed to chronic alcohol abuse. Supportive care was continued, and the patient was safely discharged after his electrolyte balance was restored 7 days later.

of long-acting benzodiazepines that act on GABA receptors has been popularized, with chlordiazepoxide, diazepam, and lorazepam being the agents of choice. These drugs can be administered and tailored to prevent worsening withdrawal and control agitation, depending on CIWA-Ar scores.[7,12]

CRITICAL DECISION

What is the antidote for ethylene glycol and methanol poisoning?

Ethylene glycol and methanol intoxication should be treated in a timely manner when there is a high index of suspicion for intoxication with one of these agents. Thorough exposure and environmental histories are important in making an educated decision. The treatment is primarily supportive and should include close monitoring for respiratory and cardiovascular status. Pharmacologic treatment should not be delayed for blood concentration levels.

Fomepizole is the treatment of choice for these parent alcohols because it inhibits alcohol dehydrogenase and has relatively minimal side effects.[10,11] Alternatively, ethanol can be considered if fomepizole is unavailable because it has a higher affinity for alcohol dehydrogenase; however, the toxic effects of ethanol must also be considered. If significant acidosis is identified due to the metabolizing effects of alcohol dehydrogenase, sodium bicarbonate can prevent the end-organ damage effects that toxic acids have on the body.[11]

Summary

Alcohol poisoning can be a life-threatening medical condition that must be considered for patients presenting with altered mental status and other neurologic symptoms. Notably, children face a multitude of different adverse reactions to alcohol when compared to their adult counterparts, which must be taken into consideration when making management decisions. Although ethanol poisoning is primarily treated with supportive care, appropriate evaluation is needed to determine the necessary medical intervention, especially given its association with polysubstance abuse and mental health disorders. Timely recognition of alcohol withdrawal and intervention are crucial because severe presentations can be deadly. Alternative alcohol poisonings (eg, with ethylene glycol and methanol) present similarly but have different toxicities. Recognition of history, physical examination, and laboratory findings is vital in the initiation of treatment with fomepizole.

REFERENCES

1. Kokotailo PK; Committee on Substance Abuse. Alcohol use by youth and adolescents: a pediatric concern. *Pediatrics*. 2010 May;125(5):1078-1087.

2. Baum CR. Ethanol intoxication in children: epidemiology, estimation of toxicity, and toxic effects. UpToDate. Updated February 7, 2022. https://www.uptodate.com/contents/ethanol-intoxication-in-children-epidemiology-estimation-of-toxicity-and-toxic-effects

3. Baum CR. Ethanol intoxication in children: clinical features, evaluation, and management. UpToDate. Updated March 26, 2021. https://www.uptodate.com/contents/ethanol-intoxication-in-children-clinical-features-evaluation-and-management

4. Bronstein AC, Spyker DA, Cantilena LR Jr, Rumack BH, Dart RC. 2011 annual report of the American Association of Poison Control Centers' National Poison Data System (NPDS): 29th annual report. Clin Toxicol (Phila). 2012 Dec;50(10):911-1164.

5. Adinoff B, Bone GH, Linnoila M. Acute ethanol poisoning and the ethanol withdrawal syndrome. Med Toxicol Adverse Drug Exp. 1988 May-Jun;3(3):172-196.

6. Morgan MY. Acute alcohol toxicity and withdrawal in the emergency room and medical admissions unit. Clin Med (Lond). 2015 Oct;15(5):486-489.

7. Greenky D, Ball TT, Murray B. A neonate with metabolic acidosis: intentional ethylene glycol poisoning. Am J Emerg Med. 2021 Jun;44:e5-e478.

8. Sivilotti MLA. Methanol and ethylene glycol poisoning: pharmacology, clinical manifestations, and diagnosis. UpToDate. Updated January 7, 2020. https://www.uptodate.com/contents/methanol-and-ethylene-glycol-poisoning-pharmacology-clinical-manifestations-and-diagnosis

9. Velez LI, Shepherd JG, Goto CS. Approach to the child with occult toxic exposure. UpToDate. Updated May 13, 2020. https://www.uptodate.com/contents/approach-to-the-child-with-occult-toxic-exposure

10. Mégarbane B. Treatment of patients with ethylene glycol or methanol poisoning: focus on fomepizole. Open Access Emerg Med. 2010 Aug 24;2:67-75.

11. Sivilotti MLA. Methanol and ethylene glycol poisoning: management. UpToDate. Updated July 29, 2021. https://www.uptodate.com/contents/methanol-and-ethylene-glycol-poisoning-management

12. Ahwazi HH, Abdijadid S. Chlordiazepoxide. StatPearls [Internet]. 2022 Jan. https://www.ncbi.nlm.nih.gov/books/NBK547659

✖ Pitfalls

- Failing to consider polysubstance abuse in patients who present with alcohol poisoning, especially in the setting of altered mental status.

- Failing to consult Poison Control for additional resources and interventions for alcohol poisoning.

- Delaying treatment of suspected methanol or ethylene glycol poisoning due to a lack of serum concentration availability.

ADDITIONAL READING

1. Gaw CE, Osterhoudt KC. Ethanol intoxication of young children. Pediatr Emerg Care. 2019 Oct;35(10):722-730.

2. Estimated ethanol (and toxic alcohol) serum concentration based on ingestion. MDCalc. https://www.mdcalc.com/estimated-ethanol-toxic-alcohol-serum-concentration-based-ingestion

3. CIWA-Ar for Alcohol Withdrawal. MDCalc. https://www.mdcalc.com/ciwa-ar-alcohol-withdrawal

The Critical Image
Abnormal Density in Chest X-Ray

By Joshua S. Broder, MD, FACEP

Dr. Broder is a professor and the residency program director in the Department of Emergency Medicine at Duke University Medical Center in Durham, North Carolina.

Objective

On completion of this article, you should be able to:
- Interpret chest x-ray and CT findings in an acute respiratory illness.
- Identify the "spine sign" on lateral chest x-rays.

CASE PRESENTATION

A 35-year-old woman with granulomatosis with polyangiitis (formerly Wegener granulomatosis) and a left bronchial stent presents with a nonproductive cough, fever, dyspnea, and pleuritic left posterior thoracic pain for 1 week. She was seen 4 days earlier, had a normal chest x-ray (*Figure 1*), and was treated with amoxicillin without improvement. Her vital signs are blood pressure 110/70, heart rate 117, respiratory rate 18, temperature 39°C (102.2°F); SpO2 is 90% on room air.

The patient appears comfortable and in no distress. She is tachycardic but has no accessory heart sounds. Her breath sounds are decreased in the left lung base. She has no peripheral edema or leg tenderness. COVID testing is negative, and a chest x-ray is performed (*Figure 2*).

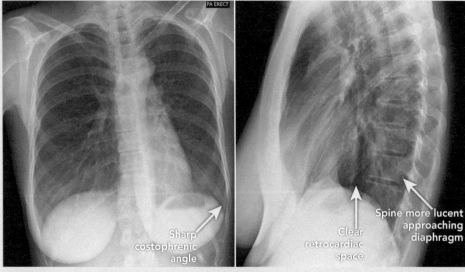

FIGURE 1. Initial PA chest x-ray showing clear lung fields and a normal (sharp) costophrenic angle; the lateral chest x-ray demonstrates normal findings, including a clear retrocardiac space and absent "spine sign"

On *frontal projection x-ray* (posterior-anterior [PA] or anterior-posterior [AP]), the heart may mask posterior chest pathology. Abnormal density in the region of the heart can offer a clue but may not be recognized. The *lateral chest x-ray* offers important additional diagnostic information and should be obtained if the patient's condition allows. On lateral view, the space behind the heart normally appears nearly black. The spine normally appears progressively darker nearer the diaphragm; more superior, the spine appears brighter as a consequence of attenuation of the x-ray beam by muscle and bone of the shoulder girdle. Increased

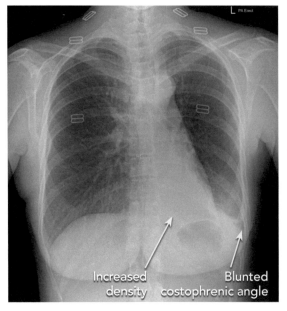
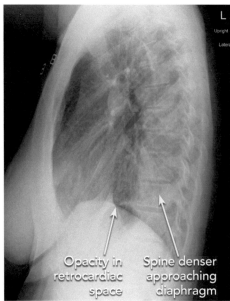

Figure 2. PA chest x-ray, 4 days later, showing a blunted costophrenic angle and increased cardiac density. The lateral view shows retrocardiac density and an abnormal "spine sign."

retrocardiac or spinal density is abnormal and may be caused by conditions such as infectious pneumonia, aspiration, a mass, or pleural fluid. Abnormal density overlying the spine is called an abnormal "spine sign."[1] Comparison with previous images is best practice and can assist in the recognition of subtle new abnormalities.

For complex patients (eg, immuno-compromised) or those with an equivocal or a negative chest x-ray, CT can provide supplemental information such as airway patency, as in this case (*Figure C*). If vascular abnormalities (eg, pulmonary embolism) are not suspected, intravenous contrast is often unnecessary.[2,3]

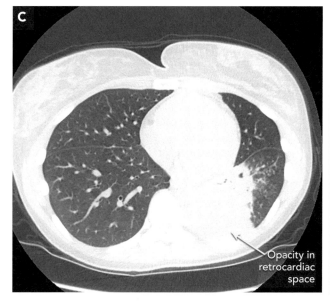
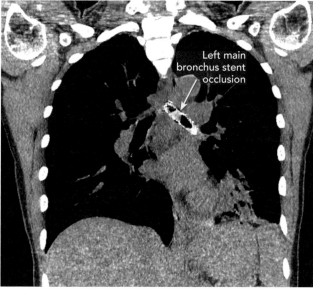

C. Axial CT image demonstrating a dense left lower lobe infiltrate posterior to the heart, which corresponds to the x-ray findings. Coronal reconstruction also demonstrates occlusion of the patient's left main bronchus stent. The patient has postobstructive pneumonia.

CASE RESOLUTION

The patient was treated with broad-spectrum intravenous antibiotics and admitted. Bronchoscopy was performed, the obstructed stent was cleared, and bronchoalveolar lavage was performed (*Figure D*).

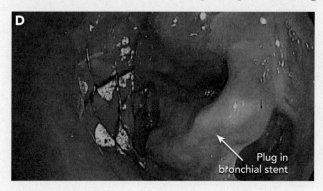
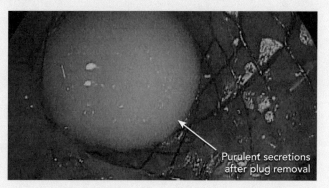

REFERENCES

1. Medjek M, Hackx M, Ghaye B, De Maertelaer V, Gevenois PA. Value of the "spine sign" on lateral chest views. *Br J Radiol.* 2015;88(1050):20140378.
2. Expert Panel on Thoracic Imaging; Lee C, Colletti PM, Chung JH, et al. ACR Appropriateness Criteria® Acute Respiratory Illness in Immunocompromised Patients. *J Am Coll Radiol.* 2019;16(11S):S331-S339.
3. Expert Panel on Thoracic Imaging; Jokerst C, Chung JH, Ackman JB, et al. ACR Appropriateness Criteria® Acute Respiratory Illness in Immunocompetent Patients. *J Am Coll Radiol.* 2018;15(11S):S240-S251.

Feature Editor: Joshua S. Broder, MD, FACEP. See also *Diagnostic Imaging for the Emergency Physician* (Winner of the 2011 Prose Award in Clinical Medicine, the American Publishers Award for Professional and Scholarly Excellence) and *Critical Images in Emergency Medicine* by Dr. Broder.

CME Questions

Reviewed by **Kelsey Drake, MD, MPH, FACEP**; and **Ann M. Dietrich, MD, FAAP, FACEP**

Qualified, paid subscribers to *Critical Decisions in Emergency Medicine* may receive CME certificates for up to 5 ACEP Category I credits, 5 *AMA PRA Category 1 Credits*™, and 5 AOA Category 2-B credits for completing this activity in its entirety. Submit your answers online at acep.org/cdem; a score of 75% or better is required. You may receive credit for completing the CME activity any time within 3 years of its publication date. Answers to this month's questions will be published in next month's issue.

1   Acute hemorrhagic fever syndrome includes a fever of what duration?

   A.   <1 week
   B.   <3 weeks
   C.   <1 month
   D.   >1 month

2   By what route is Ebola transmitted?

   A.   Contaminated food
   B.   Contaminated water
   C.   Direct contact with infected bodily fluids
   D.   Insect bite

3   A 45-year-old health care worker who returns from working in Sierra Leone in West Africa presents with a fever of 38.6°C (101.5°F), abdominal pain, and diarrhea. The physical examination is significant for a purpuric rash. What is the most appropriate next step?

   A.   Administer intravenous fluid bolus therapy
   B.   Contact the local health department
   C.   Place the patient in isolation
   D.   Place the patient on a cardiac monitor

4   A 35-year-old man who recently returned from a trip to Kenya in East Africa presents with fever and generalized malaise. Other than a temperature of 38.3°C (100.9°F), his vital signs are normal. His physical examination is unremarkable, CBC shows leukocytosis of 14,000 cells/mm3, a basic metabolic panel is unremarkable, and no Plasmodium is visualized on peripheral blood smears. What is the most appropriate next step?

   A.   Continue symptomatic care and repeat blood smears for 12 to 24 hours
   B.   Inform the patient that he does not have malaria and discharge home
   C.   Start intravenous treatment with an artemisinin-based compound therapy
   D.   Start outpatient chloroquine

5   Which condition is correctly paired with its usual incubation period?

   A.   Chikungunya — 3 weeks
   B.   Hepatitis E — 1 week
   C.   Malaria — <10 days to months
   D.   SARS — 2 weeks

6   Travelers from which geographic area are at the highest risk of acquiring enteric fever?

   A.   Caribbean
   B.   North America
   C.   South Asia
   D.   Western Europe

7   Which disease is correctly paired with its typical mode of transmission?

   A.   Chikungunya — deer tick
   B.   Ebola virus disease — undercooked food
   C.   Enteric fever — reduviid bug
   D.   Zika — Aedes aegypti mosquito

8   What is the most likely source of fever in a patient who presents for evaluation at 14 days after travel?

   A.   Chagas disease contracted in rural Latin America
   B.   Chikungunya contracted while hiking
   C.   Leishmaniasis contracted while volunteering in urban slums
   D.   Tuberculosis contracted while providing medical care

9   What is the most frequently identified cause of fever in the returned traveler when a specific etiological diagnosis can be made?

   A.   Dengue fever
   B.   Malaria
   C.   Neurocysticercosis
   D.   Yellow fever

10   What is the most common cause of new-onset seizure in adults worldwide?

   A.   Japanese encephalitis
   B.   Leshmaniasis
   C.   Neisseria meningitidis
   D.   Neurocysticercosis

11   Which symptom should raise concern for alcohol withdrawal rather than alcohol intoxication?

   A.   Anxiety
   B.   Dizziness
   C.   Lethargy
   D.   Vomiting

12 **What toxic metabolite is formed by ethylene glycol poisoning?**

A. Acetaldehyde
B. Beta-hydroxybutyrate
C. Formic acid
D. Glyoxylate

13 **A 3-year-old child is admitted with a peak serum ethanol level of 57 mg/dL. For which complication must the child be monitored?**

A. Hyperkalemia
B. Hypocalcemia
C. Hypoglycemia
D. Metabolic alkalosis

14 **A child presents with blurry vision after drinking a chemical from an unlabeled bottle. Given the patient's symptoms, which chemical ingestion is most likely?**

A. Brake fluid
B. Hand sanitizer
C. Mouthwash
D. Windshield washer fluid

15 **A 16-year-old boy presents with suspected alcohol poisoning about 2 hours ago. His ethanol levels are negative, his serum bicarbonate level is 15 mEq/L, his anion gap is normal, but he has an elevated osmolal gap. Which medication should be administered?**

A. Activated charcoal
B. Chlordiazepoxide
C. Fomepizole
D. Naloxone

16 **A 4-year-old girl presents with slurred speech and flank pain. Basic laboratory studies demonstrate a high anion gap metabolic acidosis. Which toxic ingestion is most likely?**

A. Ethanol
B. Ethylene glycol
C. Isopropyl alcohol
D. Methanol

17 **What symptoms or physical examination findings would be expected in a teenager with suspected ethanol poisoning?**

A. Hallucinations
B. Hypertension
C. Impaired judgment
D. Vision impairment

18 **At which point after ingestion is a child at the highest risk of death from ethylene glycol intoxication?**

A. <12 hours
B. 12 to 36 hours
C. 2 to 3 days
D. >1 week

19 **A 17-year-old girl presents via EMS after being found unconscious next to a spilled bottle of antifreeze. She is making incomprehensive sounds, does not open her eyes, and withdraws to painful stimuli. She is tachypneic and has labored breathing on room air. What is the best next step in management?**

A. Obtain a stat brain CT
B. Order toxic ingestion studies
C. Prepare to intubate the patient
D. Start treatment with fomepizole

20 **Which laboratory finding can be seen in the setting of ethylene glycol intoxication?**

A. Hypercalcemia
B. Hypoglycemia
C. Metabolic alkalosis
D. Oxalate crystals

ANSWER KEY FOR MARCH 2022, VOLUME 36, NUMBER 3

1	2	3	4	5	6	7	8	9	10	11	12	13	14	15	16	17	18	19	20
B	D	D	D	D	D	B	D	D	B	C	B	A	B	A	D	D	B	A	C

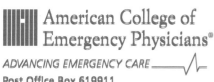
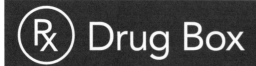

GABAPENTIN

By **Frank LoVecchio, DO, MPH, FACEP**
Valleywise Health and ASU, CHS, Phoenix, Arizona

OBJECTIVE

On completion of this column, you should be able to:
- Describe the use of gabapentin for acute and chronic pain.

Gabapentin is structurally similar to gamma-aminobutyric acid (GABA) but does not bind to $GABA_A$ or $GABA_B$ receptors. About two-thirds of patients who take gabapentin achieve good pain relief.

Mechanism of Action
Binds to presynaptic voltage-gated calcium channels with the alpha-2-delta-1 subunit. Thought to decrease excitatory neurotransmitters.

Indications
FDA approved for postherpetic neuralgia and partial seizures. Off-label use in neuropathic pain, fibromyalgia, restless leg syndrome, and diabetic complications. Viable option in alcohol dependence (as it is not hepatically metabolized) and as an adjunctive treatment for opioid dependence. Evidence for use in acute pain is sparse.
Recent review of evidence in acute and chronic pain: One study of acute postoperative pain (70 participants) showed no benefit of gabapentin compared to placebo. In chronic pain (15 studies; 1,468 participants), the NNT for improvement in combining trials was 4.3 (95% CI 3.5-5.7); 42% of patients improved on gabapentin versus 19% on placebo. The NNH for adverse events leading to withdrawal from a trial was insignificant. The NNT for effective pain relief in diabetic neuropathy was 2.9 (95% CI 2.2-4.3) and in postherpetic neuralgia was 3.9 (95% CI 3-5.7).

Dosing
General: 300 mg daily; then add 300 mg daily until desired effect
Postherpetic neuralgia: day 1: 300 mg once; day 2: 300 mg BID; day 3: 300 mg TID; titrated PRN for relief (no benefit in >1,800 mg/day)
Seizures: 300 mg TID; titrate based on response and tolerability; typical dosage 900 to 1,800 mg/day in three divided doses
Neuropathy: 300 to 3,600 mg/day
Restless leg syndrome: 300 mg daily 2 hours before bedtime
Alcohol dependence: 600 mg TID

Side Effects and Other Considerations
Most common side effects: dizziness, somnolence, ataxia
Less common: peripheral edema, diarrhea, nausea, vomiting
Contraindications: Hypersensitivity
Pregnancy/lactation: pregnancy category C; excreted through human breast milk
Precautions: CNS depressant; monitor for suicidality; do not discontinue suddenly

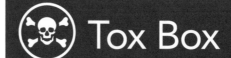

ACONITE POISONING

By **Christian Tomaszewski, MD, MS, MBA, FACEP**
University of California San Diego Health

OBJECTIVE

On completion of this column, you should be able to:
- Describe the management of aconite poisoning.

Aconitine and related alkaloids are natural plant toxins. Poisoning can occur from accidental or intentional ingestion of wild plants (monkshood, wolfsbane) or through improper use in some herbal medications. Two grams of root are potentially lethal.

Kinetics
- Absorbed rapidly after ingestion
- Half-life up to ~24 hours

Mechanism
- Binds to open state of voltage-sensitive sodium channels
- Contains aconitine, mesaconitine, and hypaconitine
- Potent cardiovascular and neurovascular toxin

Clinical Manifestations
- CNS — paresthesia, perioral or limb numbness, muscle weakness
- Cardiac — hypotension, variety of dysrhythmias with ventricular tachycardia as the most serious (eg, torsades de pointes, atrial fibrillation, bidirectional)
- GI — hypersalivation, nausea, vomiting, abdominal pain, diarrhea
- Pulmonary — respiratory paralysis

Diagnostics
- Screening glucose, electrolytes, calcium, magnesium, ECG
- Aconitine is detectable in urine or blood as send out.

Treatment
- Oral activated charcoal if <1 hr postingestion and can protect airway
- Atropine for symptomatic bradycardia
- IV fluid bolus for hypotension; norepinephrine for fluid unresponsive hypotension
- Correct electrolyte abnormalities (ie, hypokalemia, hypomagnesemia).
- Amiodarone or flecainide is the preferred antidysrhythmic for ventricular tachycardias; lidocaine and cardioversion have less success.
- Refractory hypotension may require cardiopulmonary bypass.

Disposition
- If asymptomatic, patient may be observed at home.
- If symptomatic (usually GI) or worse, monitor until resolution.

Critical decisions
in emergency medicine

Volume 36 Number 5: **May 2022**

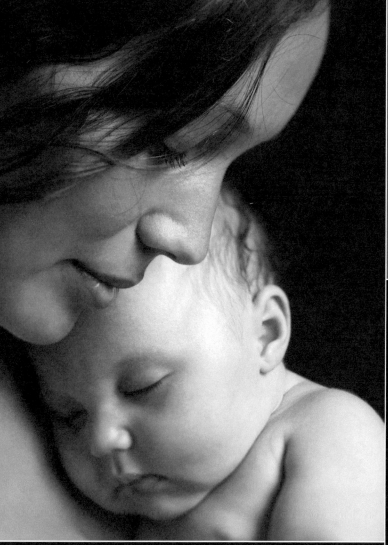

Born Yesterday

Postpartum emergencies can occur in the days, weeks, and even months following childbirth and are often seen in the emergency department. Because they vary in occurrence and severity, emergency physicians must think broadly to avoid missing or mistreating critical diagnoses and must be prepared to manage life-threatening cases.

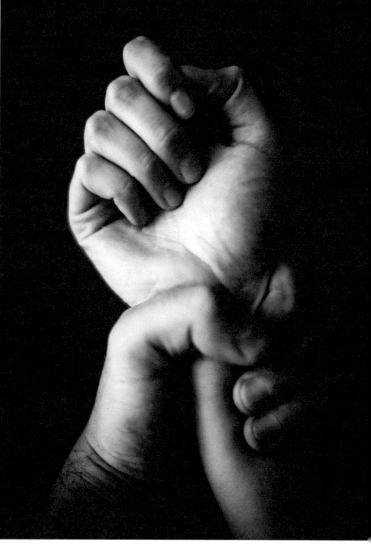

Warning Signs

Intimate partner violence affects millions of people each year, regardless of gender, age, race, and socioeconomic status. It can masquerade as a host of common complaints, including chronic pain, substance abuse, and depression. Consequently, this potentially lethal cycle can be particularly difficult for emergency physicians to identify and address.

THE OFFICIAL CME PUBLICATION OF THE AMERICAN COLLEGE OF EMERGENCY PHYSICIANS

Individuals in Control of Content

1. Nneka Azih, MD - Faculty
2. Jeffrey Bullard-Berent, MD - Faculty
3. Drew Clare, MD - Faculty
4. Neehar Kundurti, MD - Faculty
5. Hunter Lively, DO - Faculty
6. Amy Magdalany, PharmD - Faculty
7. Nicholas G. Maldonado, MD - Faculty
8. Shama Patel, MD - Faculty
9. Megan J. Rivera, MD - Faculty
10. Heather V. Rozzi, MD - Faculty
11. Ronya Silmi, MD - Faculty
12. Lisa E. Smale, DO - Faculty
13. Joshua S. Broder, MD - Faculty/Planner
14. Wan-Tsu W. Chang, MD - Faculty/Planner
15. Andrew J. Eyre, MD, MHPEd - Faculty/Planner
16. John Kiel, DO, MPH - Faculty/Planner
17. Frank LoVecchio, DO, MPH - Faculty/Planner
18. Sharon E. Mace, MD - Faculty/Planner
19. Amal Mattu, MD - Faculty/Planner
20. Christian A. Tomaszewski, MD, MS, MBA - Faculty/Planner
21. Steven J. Warrington, MD, MEd - Faculty/Planner
22. Tareq Al-Salamah, MBBS, MPH - Planner
23. Michael S. Beeson, MD, MBA - Planner
24. Ann M. Dietrich, MD - Planner
25. Kelsey Drake, MD, MPH - Planner
26. Walter L. Green, MD, FACEP - Planner
27. John C. Greenwood, MD - Planner
28. Danya Khoujah, MBBS - Planner
29. Nathaniel Mann, MD - Planner
30. George Sternbach, MD - Planner
31. Suzannah Alexander - Planner/Reviewer

Contributor Disclosures. In accordance with the ACCME Standards for Integrity and Independence in Accredited Continuing Education, all relevant financial relationships, and the absence of relevant financial relationships, must be disclosed to learners for all individuals in control of content before learners engage with the accredited education and in a format that can be verified at the time of accreditation. The following individuals have reported relationships with ineligible companies, as defined by the ACCME. These relationships, in the context of their involvement in the CME activity, could be perceived by some as a real or apparent conflict of interest. All relevant financial relationships have been mitigated to ensure that no commercial bias has been inserted into the educational content. Joshua S. Broder, MD, FACEP, is a founder and president of OmniSono Inc, an ultrasound technology company. Sharon E. Mace, MD, FACEP, performs contracted research funded by Biofire Corporation, Genetesis, Quidel, and IBSA Pharma. All remaining individuals with control over content have no relevant financial relationships to disclose.

This educational activity consists of two lessons, eight feature articles, a post-test, and evaluation questions; as designed, the activity should take approximately 5 hours to complete. The participant should, in order, review the learning objectives for the lesson or article, read the lesson or article as published in the print or online version until all have been reviewed, and then complete the online post-test (a minimum score of 75% is required) and evaluation questions. Release date May 1, 2022. Expiration date April 30, 2025.

Accreditation Statement. The American College of Emergency Physicians is accredited by the Accreditation Council for Continuing Medical Education to provide continuing medical education for physicians.

The American College of Emergency Physicians designates this enduring material for a maximum of 5 *AMA PRA Category 1 Credits™*. Physicians should claim only the credit commensurate with the extent of their participation in the activity.

Each issue of *Critical Decisions in Emergency Medicine* is approved by ACEP for 5 ACEP Category I credits. Approved by the AOA for 5 Category 2-B credits.

Commercial Support. There was no commercial support for this CME activity.

Target Audience. This educational activity has been developed for emergency physicians.

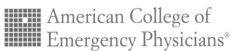

American College of Emergency Physicians®

ADVANCING EMERGENCY CARE

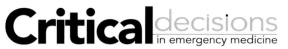

Critical Decisions in Emergency Medicine is the official CME publication of the American College of Emergency Physicians. Additional volumes are available.

EDITOR-IN-CHIEF

Michael S. Beeson, MD, MBA, FACEP
Northeastern Ohio Universities, Rootstown, OH

SECTION EDITORS

Joshua S. Broder, MD, FACEP
Duke University, Durham, NC

Andrew J. Eyre, MD, MHPEd
Brigham & Women's Hospital/ Harvard Medical School, Boston, MA

John Kiel, DO, MPH
University of Florida College of Medicine, Jacksonville, FL

Frank LoVecchio, DO, MPH, FACEP
Maricopa Medical Center/Banner Phoenix Poison and Drug Information Center, Phoenix, AZ

Amal Mattu, MD, FACEP
University of Maryland, Baltimore, MD

Christian A. Tomaszewski, MD, MS, MBA, FACEP
University of California Health Sciences, San Diego, CA

Steven J. Warrington, MD, MEd
MercyOne Siouxland, Sioux City, IA

ASSOCIATE EDITORS

Tareq Al-Salamah, MBBS, MPH, FACEP
King Saud University, Riyadh, Saudi Arabia/ University of Maryland, Baltimore, MD

Wan-Tsu W. Chang, MD
University of Maryland, Baltimore, MD

Ann M. Dietrich, MD, FAAP, FACEP
University of South Carolina College of Medicine, Greenville, SC

Kelsey Drake, MD, MPH, FACEP
St. Anthony Hospital, Lakewood, CO

Walter L. Green, MD, FACEP
UT Southwestern Medical Center, Dallas, TX

John C. Greenwood, MD
University of Pennsylvania, Philadelphia, PA

Danya Khoujah, MBBS
University of Maryland, Baltimore, MD

Sharon E. Mace, MD, FACEP
Cleveland Clinic Lerner College of Medicine/ Case Western Reserve University, Cleveland, OH

Nathaniel Mann, MD
Greenville Health System, Greenville, SC

George Sternbach, MD, FACEP
Stanford University Medical Center, Stanford, CA

EDITORIAL STAFF

Suzannah Alexander, Editorial Director
salexander@acep.org

Joy Carrico
Managing Editor

Sydney King
Managing Editor

Kyle Powell, Graphic Artist

ISSN2325-0186 (Print)   ISSN2325-8365 (Online)

Contents

Lesson 9 4
Born Yesterday
Postpartum Emergencies

By Hunter Lively, DO; and Drew Clare, MD
Reviewed by John Kiel, DO, MPH

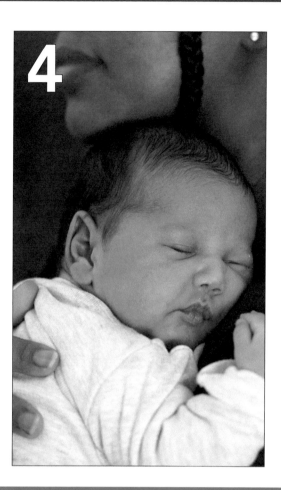

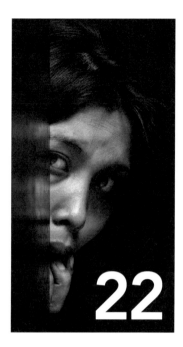

Lesson 10........22
Warning Signs
Identifying Intimate Partner Violence

By Heather V. Rozzi, MD, FACEP; and Lisa E. Smale, DO
Reviewed by Wan-Tsu W. Chang, MD

FEATURES

The Critical ECG — Ventricular Tachycardia..11
    By Amal Mattu, MD, FACEP

Clinical Pediatrics — Brain Abscess With Single Ventricle Anatomy Presenting as Stroke 12
    By Neehar Kundurti, MD, FAAP; and Jeffrey Bullard-Berent, MD, FAAP, FACEP
    Reviewed by Sharon E. Mace, MD, FACEP

The Critical Procedure — Dental Fracture Dressing 15
    By Steven J. Warrington, MD, MEd

The LLSA Literature Review — Cardioversion Strategies for Acute Uncomplicated
        Atrial Fibrillation...16
    By Megan J. Rivera, MD; and Nicholas G. Maldonado, MD, FACEP
    Reviewed by Andrew J. Eyre, MD, MHPEd

Critical Cases in Orthopedics and Trauma — Orbital Compartment Syndrome Indicating
        Lateral Canthotomy and Cantholysis 18
    By Nneka Azih, MD; Ronya Silmi, MD; and Shama Patel, MD
    Reviewed by John Kiel, DO, MPH

The Critical Image — CT to Assess Urinary System Pathologies.................................20
    By Joshua S. Broder, MD, FACEP

CME Questions 30
    Reviewed by John Kiel, DO, MPH; and Wan-Tsu W. Chang, MD

Drug Box — Bebtelovimab 32
    By Amy Magdalany, PharmD; and Frank LoVecchio, DO, MPH, FACEP

Tox Box — Aliphatic Hydrocarbon Ingestion 32
    By Christian Tomaszewski, MD, MS, MBA, FACEP

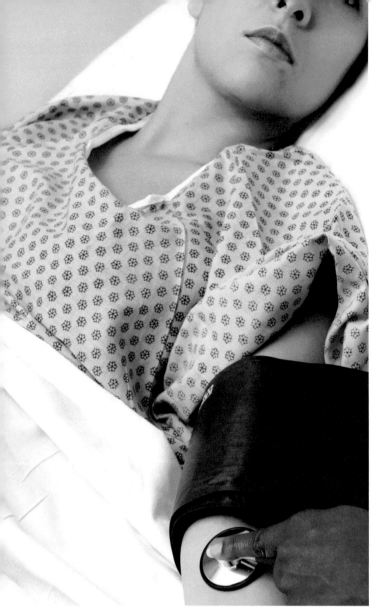

Born Yesterday

Postpartum Emergencies

LESSON **9**

By **Hunter Lively, DO**; and **Drew Clare, MD**
Dr. Lively is a resident and Dr. Clare is an assistant professor in the Department of Emergency Medicine at the University of Florida College of Medicine in Jacksonville.

Reviewed by **John Kiel, DO, MPH**

OBJECTIVES

On completion of this lesson, you should be able to:

1. Apply a stepwise approach to the treatment of postpartum hemorrhage.
2. Diagnose and manage postpartum preeclampsia, eclampsia, and HELLP syndrome.
3. Treat endometritis in an appropriate manner.
4. Recognize and manage an amniotic fluid embolism and postpartum cardiomyopathy.
5. Determine who is at risk for cerebral venous sinus thrombosis and how to diagnose it.

FROM THE EM MODEL

13.0 Obstetrics and Gynecology
       13.8 Postpartum Complications

■ CRITICAL DECISIONS ■

■ What is the initial management of postpartum hemorrhage?

■ How long after delivery can postpartum preeclampsia occur?

■ Who should be treated for endometritis?

■ What is the differential diagnosis for postpartum respiratory distress?

■ Who is at risk of cerebral venous sinus thrombosis, and how is it diagnosed?

Postpartum emergencies consist of a spectrum of potential complications that can occur in the days, weeks, and even months after childbirth. Because postpartum emergencies and pregnancy-related problems are often seen in the emergency department, physicians must be familiar with their management.

CASE PRESENTATIONS

■ CASE ONE

A 24-year-old gravida 3, para 3 woman at 38 weeks 6 days' gestation presents via EMS for evaluation of profuse vaginal bleeding. She gave birth at home via spontaneous vaginal delivery 25 minutes prior to arrival with the assistance of a midwife. The delivery was uncomplicated, followed by delivery of an intact placenta. Immediately after the placental delivery, a continuous flow of bright red blood from her vagina was observed. On arrival, the patient complains of mild abdominal pain and light-headedness. She received 1 L of IV fluids from EMS. Her vital signs are BP 89/66, P 117, R 20, and T 36.6°C (97.9°F); SpO$_2$ is 97% on room air.

■ CASE TWO

A 31-year-old gravida 1, para 1 woman presents with a headache and blurry vision 7 days after a normal spontaneous vaginal delivery. The symptoms began approximately 3 hours earlier and have been constant with no alleviating or exacerbating factors. She describes the pain as a dull ache located diffusely across the cranium. On physical examination, her vital signs are BP 162/92, P 92, R 12, and T 37°C (98.6°F); SpO$_2$ is 99% on room air. She has mild bilateral lower-extremity edema; otherwise, her examination is normal. Urinalysis reveals a 3+ protein reading.

■ CASE THREE

A 28-year-old gravida 2, para 2 woman presents 3 days after a caesarean delivery of a healthy baby, weighing 3,799 g. The patient was discharged from the hospital approximately 12 hours later, after an uneventful recovery. Once home, she began experiencing generalized malaise, subjective fevers, and nausea without vomiting. However, she began vomiting 10 hours later and had a temperature of 38.9°C (102°F). On arrival, her vitals are BP 110/78, P 118, R 14, and T 39.2°C (102.6°F); SpO$_2$ is 98% on room air. She has moderate periumbilical tenderness and malodorous lochia. The physical examination is otherwise noncontributory.

Annually, "problems of pregnancy" make up 1.3% of all emergency department visits for women aged 15 to 64 years.[1] Additionally, 25% of postpartum patients have at least one emergency department visit within 6 months of their deliveries.[2] These complications vary from mild discomfort to severe life-threatening illness. More than 60% of deaths related to pregnancy occur in the postpartum period.[3]

CRITICAL DECISION

What is the initial management of postpartum hemorrhage?

Postpartum hemorrhage (PPH) has the potential to cause massive blood loss that can lead to acute hemorrhagic shock and is associated with significant morbidity and mortality. Approximately 27% of all maternal deaths worldwide can be attributed to hemorrhage.[4] The initial approach to managing PPH is like any resuscitation, with a primary focus on circulation. Beyond airway, breathing, and circulation (the ABCs of resuscitation), correcting the underlying cause should be the goal. The four "Ts" of PPH — tone, trauma, tissue, and thrombin — can help identify its most common causes. Of the four, uterine atony (ie, tone) is the most common cause of PPH, resulting in 79% of all PPH cases.[5] With this in mind, initial management should be aimed at increasing uterine tone.

On examination, the uterus feels soft, often described as "boggy," and once uterine atony has been identified as the causative agent, treatment begins with bimanual uterine massage (*Figure 1*). This intervention is performed by inserting a hand inside the vagina and pressing against the body of the uterus. The other hand applies firm exterior pressure from the abdomen. This action compresses the uterine fundus between the two hands.[6]

This maneuver is often performed in tandem with administering oxytocin, which is a first-line uterotonic drug. Oxytocin is a hormone that acts on the myometrium, causing symmetric constriction of the hemorrhaging spiral arteries.[7,8] It can be administered intramuscularly (10 IUs) or intravascularly (20 IUs in 1 L of normal saline at 250 mL/hr). Second-line uterotonic agents that can be used next include methylergonovine, carboprost, and misoprostol.[9]

Methylergonovine is an ergot alkaloid that directly stimulates uterine smooth muscle. It can be given intramuscularly (0.2 mg) every 2 to 4 hours. It should not be given intravenously due to the risk of severe hypertension and cerebral ischemia. Because of the risk of acute blood pressure elevation, there is a relative contraindication in patients with hypertension or preeclampsia. Carboprost and misoprostol are both prostaglandin analogues that cause increased uterine tone and vasoconstriction. Carboprost

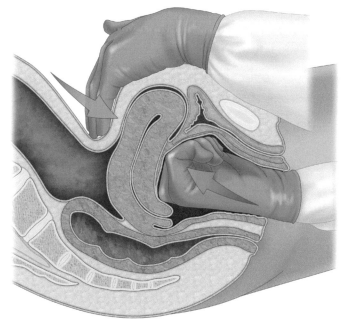

FIGURE 1. Bimanual uterine massage

Medication	Administration	Interval	Contraindications
Oxytocin	• 10 IUs IM • 20 IUs IV in 1 L of normal saline at 250 mL/hr)	• Once (IM) • Continuous infusion	None
Methylergonovine	• 0.2 mg IM	• Every 2-4 hrs	• Hypertension • Preeclampsia
Carboprost	• 250 µg IM	• Every 15 mins • Max 2 mg or 8 doses	Asthma
Misoprostol	• 1,000 µg rectally • 600 µg sublingually	• Once	None
Tranexamic acid	• 1-g dose intravascularly	• Over 10 mins with a second dose 30 mins later if bleeding continues	None

TABLE 1. Treatment for postpartum hemorrhage

is given intramuscularly (250 µg) and can be administered every 15 minutes. Because of carboprost's ability to cause acute smooth muscle constriction, it should be used with caution in asthmatic patients due to the risk of bronchoconstriction.[10] Misoprostol should be administered rectally (1,000 µg) or sublingually (600 µg).[9]

Tranexamic acid (TXA) decreases fibrinolysis by competitively inhibiting plasminogen activation.[9] Growing evidence supports its early use in PPH. The 2017 WOMAN trial is a large, randomized, double-blind, placebo-controlled trial that demonstrated that the use of TXA significantly reduces the number of deaths due to bleeding in women with PPH with no increase in adverse events when given early. TXA does not reduce the risk of hysterectomy or the requirement of blood transfusions.[11] It should be given in a 1-g dose, intravascularly, over 10 minutes with a second dose 30 minutes later if bleeding continues. It is not an FDA-approved drug for PPH, although it is widely used off label (*Table 1*).

CRITICAL DECISION

How long after delivery can postpartum preeclampsia occur?

The four major categories of pregnancy-related hypertensive disorders, as differentiated by the American College of Obstetrics and Gynecology (ACOG), include chronic hypertension, chronic hypertension with superimposed preeclampsia, preeclampsia-eclampsia, and gestational hypertension, which are commonly seen in the emergency department. Preeclampsia and eclampsia affect 6% to 8% of all pregnancies.[12] As such, this section covers the diagnosis and management of preeclampsia, eclampsia, and HELLP syndrome.

Preeclampsia is defined as a systolic blood pressure greater than or equal to 140 mm Hg or a diastolic pressure greater than or equal to 90 mm Hg on two separate occasions and proteinuria (or in the absence of proteinuria, in the presence of severe features) after 20 weeks' gestation.[13] Severe features are defined as signs and symptoms of end-organ damage. Severe hypertension (ie, ≥160 mm Hg systolic or ≥110 mm Hg diastolic) and severe proteinuria (ie, ≥5 g of protein in 24 hours) are both examples of symptoms indicating end-organ damage.[14] Additional evidence of end-organ damage includes altered mental status, vision changes, newly

elevated creatinine, oliguria, new transaminitis, thrombocytopenia, epigastric pain, right upper quadrant abdominal pain, and pulmonary edema. If seizures are present, the diagnosis changes from preeclampsia to eclampsia.

HELLP syndrome is a variant of severe preeclampsia. Its name serves as an acronym to define its features: hemolysis (H), elevated liver enzymes (EL), and low platelets (LP). HELLP syndrome is seen in 20% of pregnancies with severe preeclampsia, 30% of which occur postpartum.[15]

Of equal importance to these definitions and inclusion criteria is the chronology of the disease process. Preeclampsia and eclampsia can occur up to 6 weeks postpartum, although more than 90% of patients present to the emergency department within 7 days of delivery (*Table 2*).[16] Preeclampsia may also be diagnosed during a routine prenatal appointment, at which point the patient is often referred to the emergency department. When this occurs, the management is relatively straightforward. Mistakes or misdiagnoses are more likely to be made in postpartum preeclamptic patients, and these patients can deteriorate quickly into eclampsia. Quick recognition of the symptoms and initiation of antihypertensives and intravenous magnesium sulfate are critical.[17]

✔ Pearls

■ Preeclampsia and eclampsia are not only diseases of pregnancy; they are also seen during the postpartum period and should always be included in the differential diagnosis in women of child-bearing years.

■ Physicians should be mindful of contraindications and warnings for special populations associated with the second- and third-line uterotonic agents.

■ CT venography or MR venography is a necessary consideration in the differential diagnosis for pregnant or postpartum patients with headaches, especially if they have any neurologic deficits.

Patients often present with general malaise, abdominal pain, peripheral edema, dark or decreased urine output, or sometimes as referrals from clinics for an elevated blood pressure reading. In general, the differential diagnosis for hypertension and abdominal pain is extensive and expands when the patient is a woman of child-bearing age. The details of the history of present illness (HPI) should guide the workup. Patients may not always reveal that they recently delivered a baby, so it is crucial to ascertain a full obstetrics history for patients in this demographic. Risk factors noted in the HPI that should raise suspicion for preeclampsia include a history of prior preeclampsia, chronic hypertension, a primigravida, gestational diabetes, obesity, a twin pregnancy, and advanced maternal age. Any patient with an elevated blood pressure who is pregnant or recently delivered should immediately raise concern for preeclampsia.

Expectant management of mild preeclampsia at less than 37 weeks' gestation is acceptable, but patients must be managed in consultation with an obstetrician. Expectant management typically includes maternal monitoring (eg, bed rest, semiweekly blood pressure measurements, plus a complete blood count [CBC], platelet count, liver function test, creatinine level test, and urine protein measurement, all on a weekly basis) and fetal monitoring (eg, a semiweekly nonstress test, a weekly amniotic fluid index, and a weekly biophysical profile).[14]

Patients diagnosed with preeclampsia with severe features require admission to the hospital. If patients are preterm, efforts will be made to avoid delivery until 34 weeks; however, if they deteriorate, delivery is the treatment of choice regardless of gestational age.[17] Once admitted to the labor and delivery floor, patients are managed with maternal and fetal evaluations, magnesium sulfate, steroids for fetal lung development (if indicated), and antihypertensives.[14]

Delivery is the definitive treatment in antepartum patients with severe features at 34 weeks' gestation or more, or at 37 weeks' gestation or more for patients with mild preeclampsia (ie, without severe features). Management of eclampsia begins with resuscitation and stabilization, with a focus on airway management. Magnesium sulfate is the drug of choice for both the prevention and treatment of eclamptic seizures when compared to diazepam.[18,19] Magnesium should be administered as a 4-g to 6-g bolus over 15 minutes, followed by a continuous infusion of 2 g to 3 g every hour. Patients should be monitored for magnesium toxicity, including respiratory depression, hypotension, and loss of reflexes. There should also be an emergent consultation with obstetrics and gynecology.

CRITICAL DECISION

Who should be treated for endometritis?

Postpartum endometritis (PPE) is an infection of the endometrium that develops after giving birth. A caesarean section is the most significant risk factor for PPE. Incidence of PPE in vaginal deliveries is 1% to 3%, with a 5- to 20-fold increase following a caesarean section.[20,21] Other risk factors include prolonged labor, the use of an internal fetal or uterine monitor, an operative vaginal delivery, a group B *Streptococcus* infection, and the manual removal of the placenta.

Typically, abdominal pain and uterine tenderness are the first symptoms. Other signs and symptoms include fever, malodorous

Condition	Definition
Mild preeclampsia	• Systolic BP ≥140 mm Hg on two separate occasions • Diastolic BP ≥90 mm Hg on two separate occasions • Proteinuria • +20 weeks' gestation
Severe preeclampsia	Symptoms of mild preeclampsia, *plus* symptoms of end-organ damage (eg, severe hypertension, severe proteinuria, altered mental status, vision changes, newly elevated creatinine, oliguria, new transaminitis, thrombocytopenia, epigastric pain, right upper quadrant abdominal pain, and pulmonary edema)
Eclampsia	Symptoms of severe preeclampsia, *plus* seizures
HELLP syndrome	• Hemolysis • Elevated liver enzymes • Low platelets

TABLE 2. Preeclampsia, eclampsia, and HELLP syndrome

lochia, vaginal discharge, and leukocytosis. Some patients also have nausea and vomiting. Patients with advanced infections can be septic on presentation with pallor, tachycardia, and hypotension.

Emergency physicians should include tubo-ovarian abscess, ovarian torsion, and uterine rupture in the differential diagnosis. It is also important to include nonobstetric and gynecologic conditions. Pregnant and postpartum patients may develop cystitis, pyelonephritis, appendicitis, cholecystitis, and pancreatitis, which can present similarly. The workup for PPE includes a CBC, a complete metabolic panel, blood cultures if septic, and an evaluation for retained products in the uterus (eg, products of conception and surgical equipment) with pelvic ultrasound.

Most PPE infections are polymicrobial, including aerobic and anaerobic bacteria. These pathogens are typical vaginal flora that often ascend through the cervix into the uterus. Most patients require an obstetrics and gynecology consultation and admission for intravenous antibiotics. Treatment requires coverage against penicillin-resistant anaerobes and gram-positive skin flora like *Staphylococcus* and *Streptococcus* species. Intravenous clindamycin (900 mg every 8 hours) plus gentamicin (1.5 mg/kg every 8 hours) is considered first-line treatment because it is preferred over cephalosporins and penicillins.[20]

CRITICAL DECISION

What is the differential diagnosis for postpartum respiratory distress?

In the differential diagnosis for dyspnea, or shortness of breath, in postpartum patients, emergency physicians should consider typical causes of dyspnea (eg, myocardial infarction, pulmonary embolism, pneumonia, pneumothorax, and bronchospasm). However, two of the most concerning diagnoses specific to the postpartum period are amniotic fluid embolism (AFE) and postpartum cardiomyopathy (*Table 3*).

AFE is a catastrophic event where amniotic fluid (or other material such as hair or fetal cells) enters the maternal circulation and causes cardiovascular collapse. The incidence is between 1 in 8,000 and 1 in 80,000 live births; however, the mortality for mothers is as high as 61%, although only 15% of mothers have intact neurologic function. Fetuses in utero at the time of the embolic event have low survival rates as well.[22] Although previously thought to be more of an embolic disease, newer data suggests it is likely multifactorial and more of an immunological response and anaphylactoid-type reaction.

Patients typically present with sudden-onset dyspnea and tachypnea, which can rapidly progress to hypoxia, right ventricular failure, and cardiac arrest. Encephalopathy, coagulopathy, and hemorrhage are also seen. An elevated D-dimer level, low fibrinogen, and thrombocytopenia are key laboratory abnormalities. Chest x-ray may show dense bilateral infiltrates as AFE progresses. ECG often reveals sinus tachycardia or other dysrhythmias. TXA may be administered; otherwise, treatment is mainly supportive. Advanced therapies include exchange transfusions, uterine artery embolization, and venoarterial extracorporeal membrane oxygenation.[23]

Postpartum cardiomyopathy is a diagnosis of new-onset heart failure during or within 5 months of delivery.[24] It is a diagnosis of exclusion, applicable when no other alternative etiology of new left ventricular dysfunction can be identified. In the United States, the incidence is 10.3 cases per 10,000 births.[25,26] Risk factors include high gravidity or parity, poverty, hypertension, and cocaine abuse. Additionally, prolonged use of tocolytic medications (longer than 4 weeks) is thought to induce ischemia.[27] Other etiologies include viral, nutritional, ischemic, inflammatory, and hormonal causes.

Most patients present in the first week after delivery with typical symptoms of heart failure (eg, dyspnea on exertion,

Postpartum Respiratory Distress		
Amniotic fluid embolism	Amniotic fluid enters the maternal circulation, causing cardiovascular collapse	Sudden-onset dyspnea and tachypnea, which can rapidly progress to hypoxia, right ventricular failure, and cardiac arrest
Postpartum cardiomyopathy	New heart failure during or within 5 months of delivery	Diagnosis of exclusion, labeled only when there is no other alternative etiology of new left ventricular dysfunction

TABLE 3. Concerning causes of postpartum respiratory distress

paroxysmal nocturnal dyspnea, orthopnea, and bilateral lower-extremity edema). The initial workup also mirrors that of typical heart failure and includes basic laboratory tests as well as brain natriuretic peptide level, ECG, chest x-ray, and echocardiography to evaluate left ventricular function. Treatment is similar and includes diuresis, beta-blockers, and ACE-inhibitors, which are contraindicated in pregnancy. Although many patients may recover their ejection fraction, some may be left with permanent left ventricular dysfunction or require advanced therapies, such as assist devices.[28] Patients should be counseled regarding subsequent pregnancies, as

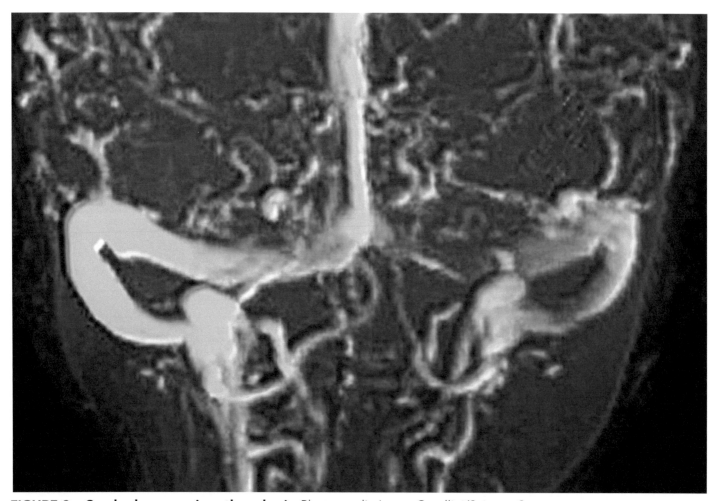

FIGURE 2. **Cerebral venous sinus thrombosis.** Photo credit James Cavallini/Science Source.

mortality can be up to 25% if entering the subsequent pregnancy with a persistent decreased ejection fraction.[29]

CRITICAL DECISION

Who is at risk of cerebral venous sinus thrombosis, and how is it diagnosed?

Cerebral venous sinus thrombosis (CVST) refers to a blood clot that forms in the venous sinuses of the brain that prevents outflow of blood from the brain's venous system, subsequently causing blood to leak out of vessels and resulting in cerebral hemorrhage (*Figure 2*). It is considered a stroke variant. CVST is a relatively understudied disease process due to its rarity. From 1985 to 2015, multiple studies from around the world reported incidences ranging from 12.3 to 15.7 cases per million per year.[30] Although the incidence of CVST is rising and is believed to be more common than originally thought, mortality rates are declining.[30] More than 50 years ago, a British journal reported a CVST mortality rate of greater than 50%.[31] A study published in 2004 reported a mortality rate of 4.3%.[32]

This decrease in mortality may be partly due to an increase in emergency physician awareness of the disease and improved diagnostic imaging modalities. Furthermore, the identification of key risk factors by emergency physicians may also be contributing to the decrease in mortality. It is widely accepted that patients who are pregnant or postpartum are at higher risk of stroke, likely due to relative hypercoagulability. A 2021 study looking at 88 cases of CVST from a neurology clinic from 2009 to 2020 reported 11.3% of all CVST cases occurred in women 6 weeks or less postpartum.[33]

These patients typically present with headache, seizures, papilledema, or focal neurologic deficits. Headache is by far the most common presenting factor; it is seen in 90% of CVST cases in postpartum women.[33] Unlike a subarachnoid hemorrhage, headaches associated with CVST often progress slowly over hours or days. Seizures are more commonly seen in the postpartum group when compared to nonpostpartum women (60% compared to 34.8%, respectively).[33]

CVST is a "can't miss" diagnosis in pregnant or postpartum women who present with a headache or neurologic deficits. Some other causes of headache in this population are benign migraine or tension-type headaches, dehydration, preeclampsia or eclampsia, meningitis, subarachnoid hemorrhage, neoplasm, carbon monoxide poisoning, giant cell arteritis, and post–epidural block headache.

The workup of CVST is centered around neuroimaging. There are no meaningful diagnostic laboratory studies; a negative D-dimer result does not rule out CVST.[34] Noncontrast CT of the head and lumbar puncture should be considered, depending on the patient. Overall, MRI — especially MR venography — is the single greatest-value modality for diagnosing CVST.[35] If there are contraindications to MRI, a CT venogram is a reasonable substitution. A direct comparison of CT venography to MR venography in the diagnosis of CVST has shown similar sensitivities.[36] MR venography is superior to CT venography in detecting parenchymal lesions, has a lower risk of contrast-related adverse reactions, and has no exposure to ionizing radiation.

Management includes initial anticoagulation with heparin followed by transition to oral anticoagulation for 3 to 6 months. The RE-SPECT CVT trial showed that use of warfarin and dabigatran have similar safety profiles and effectiveness. Seizure prophylaxis is only recommended for patients who present with seizures.[37] Patients who continue to decompensate despite maximal medical therapy may require endovascular therapy, including catheter-directed thrombolysis or mechanical thrombectomy.

CVST patients should always be admitted to an inpatient floor capable of frequent neurologic checks, and intracranial pressure monitoring with neurosurgical and hematological consultations are recommended.

Summary

Postpartum patients can be challenging, regardless of the chief complaint, as seemingly nonobstetric complaints can still be related to the recent delivery. To effectively care for these patients, emergency physicians must be familiar with the steps of PPH resuscitation and hemorrhage control. Headaches and hypertension in these patients require strong consideration to evaluate for preeclampsia and CVST. Postpartum infections are common and should be treated broadly. If there is concern for a postpartum patient, it is always appropriate to consult an obstetrician and gynecologist, in addition to either admitting the patient to the hospital or sending her home with strict return precautions and close follow-up care.

✖ Pitfalls

- Failing to initiate bimanual uterine massage for PPH, a temporizing measure while waiting for uterotonic drugs to be administered.
- Disregarding new-onset heart failure in an otherwise healthy young woman with shortness of breath after a recent delivery.
- Forgetting that most PPE cases are caused by polymicrobial infections and failing to provide broad-spectrum antibiotics that cover aerobic and anaerobic pathogens (clindamycin and gentamicin are first-line medications).

REFERENCES

1. National Center for Health Statistics. National Hospital Ambulatory Medical Care Survey: 2016 Emergency Department Summary Tables. Center for Disease Control and Prevention. Accessed March 2, 2022. https://www.cdc.gov/nchs/data/nhamcs/web_tables/2016_ed_web_tables.pdf
2. Harris A, Chang HY, Wang L, et al. Emergency room utilization after medically complicated pregnancies: a Medicaid claims analysis. *J Womens Health (Larchmt)*. 2015;24(9):745-754.
3. Li XF, Fortney JA, Kotelchuck M, Glover LH. The postpartum period: the key to maternal mortality. *Int J Gynaecol Obstet*. 1996;54(1):1-10.
4. Say L, Chou D, Gemmill A, et al. Global causes of maternal death: a WHO systematic analysis. *Lancet Glob Health*. 2014;2(6):e323-e333.
5. Bateman BT, Berman MF, Riley LE, Leffert LR. The epidemiology of postpartum hemorrhage in a large, nationwide sample of deliveries. *Anesth Analg*. 2010;110(5):1368-1373.
6. Anderson JM, Etches D. Prevention and management of postpartum hemorrhage. *Am Fam Physician*. 2007;75(6):875-82.
7. Parry Smith WR, Papadopoulou A, Thomas E, et al. Uterotonic agents for first-line treatment of postpartum haemorrhage: a network meta-analysis. *Cochrane Database Syst Rev*. 2020;11(11):CD012754.

CASE RESOLUTIONS

CASE ONE

The 24-year-old patient was immediately brought to a resuscitation bay. With airway and breathing intact, circulation was the first problem addressed. Frank blood soaked her clothes. Her uterus was soft and boggy. A second large-bore IV catheter was established, and bimanual uterine fundal massage was initiated. Two units of RBCs were crossmatched; obstetrics and gynecology were contacted; and 10 IUs oxytocin IM and 1g TXA IV were ordered. The oxytocin was more readily available and given almost immediately. Six minutes later, the TXA was administered. The patient's uterus then became firmer, her vital signs normalized, and the blood loss stopped. A CBC revealed a hemoglobin of 6.7 g/dL. One more unit of blood was transfused, and she was admitted to the obstetrics and gynecology service for further management.

CASE TWO

Due to a thorough history of the postpartum time frame, headache, hypertension, and proteinuria, the diagnosis of postpartum preeclampsia was made expeditiously. Intrave-nous access was established, and the patient was given a bolus of 4 g magnesium sulfate IV, followed by a 2 g/hour continuous infusion. She also received 40 mg labetalol IV. The patient was admitted to the obstetrics and gynecology service for further management. Her hypertension quickly resolved and did not progress to eclampsia. She was safely discharged home 1 week later.

CASE THREE

After seeing her initial triage vitals, the patient was placed in a resuscitation bay because she appeared ill. She was hooked up to a monitor and found to be hypotensive at 94/62 mm Hg. A sepsis alert was paged through the hospital's alert messaging system to mobilize resources. Within minutes, two large-bore IV catheters were established, and a 1-L bolus of sodium lactate was given. Blood was drawn for a variety of tests, including a venous blood gas with electrolytes. The patient had a pH of 7.21 and a lactic acid of 4.1. The decision to administer 900 mg clindamycin IV and 1.5 mg/kg of gentamicin was made. Antibiotics began shortly after collecting blood cultures. A second liter of sodium lactate was hung to work toward a goal of 30 mL/kg. The patient's vitals began to normalize, and she was admitted to a step-down unit for further management.

8. Soriano D, Dulitzki M, Schiff E, Barkai G, Mashiach S, Seidman DS. A prospective cohort study of oxytocin plus ergometrine compared with oxytocin alone for prevention of postpartum haemorrhage. *Br J Obstet Gynaecol*. 1996;103(11):1068-1073.

9. Hale K. Pharmacotherapeutic management of postpartum hemorrhage. *US Pharm*. 2019;44(9):HS-2–HS-10.

10. Hemabate. Package insert. Pfizer; 2017.

11. WOMAN Trial Collaborators. Effect of early tranexamic acid administration on mortality, hysterectomy, and other morbidities in women with post-partum haemorrhage (WOMAN): an international, randomised, double-blind, placebo-controlled trial. *Lancet*. 2017;389(10084):2105-2116.

12. National High Blood Pressure Education Program Working Group. Report on high blood pressure in pregnancy. *Am J Obstet Gynecol*. 2000;183(1):S1-S22.

13. America College of Obstetricians and Gynecologists' Task Force on Hypertension in Pregnancy. Hypertension in pregnancy. *Obstet Gynecol*. 2013;122(5):1122-1131.

14. Leeman L, Fontaine P. Hypertensive disorders of pregnancy. *Am Fam Physician*. 2008;78(1):93-100.

15. Sibai BM, Ramadan MK, Usta I, Salama M, Mercer BM, Friedman SA. Maternal morbidity and mortality in 442 pregnancies with hemolysis, elevated liver enzymes, and low platelets (HELLP syndrome). *Am J Obstet Gynecol*. 1993;169(4):1000-1006.

16. Al-Safi Z, Imudia AN, Filetti LC, Hobson DT, Bahado-Singh RO, Awonuga AO. Delayed postpartum preeclampsia and eclampsia: demographics, clinical course, and complications. *Obstet Gynecol*. 2011;118(5):1102-1107.

17. American College of Obstetrics and Gynecology Task Force on Hypertension in Pregnancy. Hypertension in Pregnancy. *ACOG Practice Guideline*. 2013:1-79.

18. Lucas MJ, Leveno KJ, Cunningham FG. A comparison of magnesium sulfate with phenytoin for the prevention of eclampsia. *N Engl J Med*. 1995;333(4):201-205.

19. Duley L, Henderson-Smart DJ, Walker GJ, Chou D. Magnesium sulphate versus diazepam for eclampsia. *Cochrane Database Syst Rev*. 2010;2010(12):CD000127.

20. Mackeen AD, Packard RE, Ota E, Speer L. Antibiotic regimens for postpartum endometritis. *Cochrane Database Syst Rev*. 2015;I2015(2):CD001067.

21. Conroy K, Koenig AF, Yu YH, Courtney A, Lee HJ, Norwitz ER. Infectious morbidity after cesarean delivery: 10 strategies to reduce risk. *Rev Obstet Gynecol*. 2012;5(2):69-77.

22. Clark SL, Hankins GD, Dudley DA, Dildy GA, Porter TF. Amniotic fluid embolism: analysis of the national registry. *Am J Obstet Gynecol*. 1995 Apr;172(4):1158-1169.

23. Durgam S, Sharma M, Dadhwal R, Vakil A, Surani S. The role of extra corporeal membrane oxygenation in amniotic fluid embolism: a case report and literature review. *Cureus*. 2021;13(2):e13566.

24. Sliwa K, Hilfiker-Kleiner D, Petrie, MC, et al. Current state of knowledge on aetiology, diag-nosis, management, and therapy of peripartum cardiomyopathy: a position statement from the Heart Failure Association of the European Society of Cardiology Working Group on peripartum cardiomyopathy. *Eur J Heart Fail*. 2010;12(8):767-778.

25. Kolte D, Khera S, Aronow WS, et al. Temporal trends in incidence and outcomes of peripartum cardiomyopathy in the United States: a nationwide population-based study. *J Am Heart Assoc*. 2014;3(3):e001056.

26. Isezuo SA, Abubakar SA. Epidemiologic profile of peripartum cardiomyopathy in a tertiary care hospital. *Ethn Dis*. 2007;17(2):228-233.

27. Bassett JM, Burks AH, Levine DH, Pinches RA, Visser GH. Maternal and fetal metabolic effects of prolonged ritodrine infusion. *Obstet Gynecol*. 1985;66(6):755-761.

28. Oosterom L, de Jonge N, Kirkels J, Klöpping C, Lahpor J. Left ventricular assist device as a bridge to recovery in a young woman admitted with peripartum cardiomyopathy. *Neth Heart J*. 2008;16(12):426-428.

29. Hilfiker-Kleiner D, Haghikia A, Masuko D, et al. Outcome of subsequent pregnancies in patients with a history of peripartum cardiomyopathy. *Eur J Heart Fail*. 2017;19(12):1723-1728.

30. Tatlisumak T, Jood K, Putaala J. Cerebral venous thrombosis: epidemiology in change. *Stroke*. 2016;47(9): 2169-2170.

31. Kalbag, RM. Cerebral venous thrombosis. *Br J Surg*. 1967:54(6):578.

32. Ferro JM, Canhão P, Stam J, Bousser, MG, Barinagarrementeria F; ISCVT Investigators. Prognosis of cerebral vein and dural sinus thrombosis: results of the international study on cerebral vein and dural sinus thrombosis (ISCVT). *Stroke*. 2004;35(3):664-670.

33. Bajko Z, Motataianu A, Stoian A, et al. Postpartum cerebral venous thrombosis — a single-center experience. *Brain Sci*. 2021;11(3):327.

34. Crassard I, Soria C, Tzourio C, et al. A negative D-dimer assay does not rule out cerebral venous thrombosis: a series of seventy-three patients. *Stroke*. 2005;36(8):1716-1719.

35. Rodallec MH, Krainik A, Feydy A, et al. Cerebral venous thrombosis and multidetector CT angiography: tips and tricks. *RadioGraphics*. 2006;26 (suppl 1):S5- S18.

36. Khandelwal N, Agarwal A, Kochhar R, et al. Comparison of CT venography with MR venography in cerebral sinovenous thrombosis. *AJR Am J Roentgenol*. 2006;187(6):1637-1643.

37. Ferro JM, Canhão P, Bousser MG, Stam J, Barinagarrementeria F; ISCVT Investigators. Early seizures in cerebral vein and dural sinus thrombosis: risk factors and role of antiepileptics. *Stroke*. 2008;39(4):1152-1158.

Ventricular Tachycardia

By Amal Mattu, MD, FACEP

Dr. Mattu is a professor, vice chair, and director of the Emergency Cardiology Fellowship in the Department of Emergency Medicine at the University of Maryland School of Medicine in Baltimore.

Objective

On completion of this article, you should be able to:

- Distinguish the features suggestive of ventricular tachycardia in a wide QRS complex tachycardia on ECG.

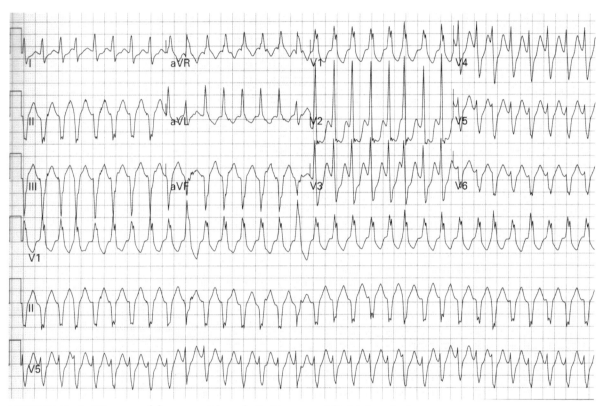

FIGURE 1. A 55-year-old man with palpitations and light-headedness

Ventricular tachycardia (VT), rate 190 (Figure 1). The differential diagnosis of a wide QRS complex tachycardia includes VT, supraventricular tachycardia (SVT) with aberrant conduction (eg, bundle branch block), and sinus tachycardia (ST) with aberrant conduction. In the absence of an obvious and repeating P-QRS pattern, ST can be excluded. This patient's ECG demonstrates several features that exclude the diagnosis of SVT and confirm VT: a taller left "rabbit ear" morphology of the QRS complex in lead V1, S > R in lead V6, atrioventricular dissociation, and the presence of fusion complexes (Figure 2). Even in the absence of these diagnostic features, however, VT should always be preferentially chosen and treated. Treating SVT as if it is VT is generally safe; however, if VT is mistakenly diagnosed and treated as SVT, the results can be deadly.

FIGURE 2. Features suggestive of VT in a wide QRS complex tachycardia.
A. Right bundle branch block–type of morphology with RsR' configuration.
B. The R wave is larger than the R' wave (taller left "rabbit ear") in the QRS complex, a finding that is consistent with VT.
C. Fusion beats (a combination of supraventricular and ventricular beats, indicated by the *arrows*) are also strongly suggestive of VT.

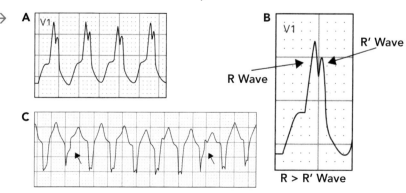

From **Mattu A, Brady W.** *ECGs for the Emergency Physician 2.* BMJ Publishing; 2008:11,23. Reprinted with permission.

Brain Abscess With Single Ventricle Anatomy Presenting as Stroke

By **Neehar Kundurti, MD, FAAP**; and
Jeffrey Bullard-Berent, MD, FAAP, FACEP
The University of New Mexico, Department of Emergency
Medicine, Division of Pediatric Emergency Medicine,
Albuquerque

Reviewed by **Sharon E. Mace, MD, FACEP**

Objective

On completion of this article, you should be able to:

■ Describe how congenital heart disease and heart surgery
affect pediatric stroke and abscess risk.

■ CASE PRESENTATION ■

A 2-year-old, 13.5-kg boy with a history of a double-inlet left ventricle with normally related great arteries
(DILV/NRGA) post bidirectional Glenn procedure (BDG), atrial septectomy with pulmonary artery banding (PAB),
and right pulmonary artery (RPA) plasty in infancy presents to the emergency department as a transfer from an urgent
care clinic with weakness and vomiting in the setting of a fall 2 nights ago. The patient's mother reports that he was in
his usual state of health 15 hours prior to presentation when she noticed that he was not using his right upper and lower
extremities as much as usual. He has had several episodes of nonbilious, nonbloody emesis and has increased fussiness.

Earlier that morning, he was unable to get himself out of bed. Two nights prior, he had an unwitnessed fall from a
2.5-foot-tall dining table. His mother heard him cry and then found him dangling upside down in between the dining
chairs. His head, however, was not touching the ground. She denied any loss of consciousness and was able to feed him
without emesis until the evening he arrived at the emergency department. There is no history of fever, headache, or
recent febrile illnesses.

Introduction

Pediatric patients who present with a history of
congenital heart disease and heart surgery are complex
cases. Younger patients with subtle signs and symptoms
can be especially challenging. In this case, a toddler with
congenital heart disease presents with signs of a stroke but is
found to have large intracranial abscesses.

Congenital heart disease is one of the most frequent
congenital disorders worldwide, affecting an estimated 0.8%
to 1.2% of all live births.[1] With the advancements in pediatric
cardiac surgery for critical congenital heart disease, survival has
increased. Premature mortality is estimated at 8.1%, and 3.4%
of these deaths are attributed to infections.[2] Pediatric patients
with congenital heart disease can present after surgery with
myriad issues that are complex to manage.

In young pediatric patients, intracranial pathology may
present with subtle neurologic findings, but it is critical that
emergency physicians recognize these signs. Intracardiac and
extracardiac right-to-left shunting allow microbes unfiltered
access to the brain, placing these patients at higher risk of
intracranial infection.[3] In this case, a toddler with single
ventricle anatomy and right-to-left shunt status after cardiac
surgeries presents with signs of a stroke but is found to have
a large brain abscess with midline shift.

Medical History

The patient was diagnosed prenatally with single
ventricle anatomy. An amniocentesis demonstrated 40 XY;
however, a microarray following delivery demonstrated
an 850-kb interstitial duplication at Xp25, a variant of

unknown significance and likely benign. A postnatal
echocardiogram demonstrated DILV/NRGA without
outflow obstruction. Within a few weeks of life, he
underwent atrial septectomy with PAB due to poor weight
gain and tachypnea related to congestive heart failure
without complications. He underwent an unremarkable
preoperative cardiac catheterization at 7 months, followed
by a routine bidirectional Glenn procedure, RPA plasty,
and PAB adjustment. He had postoperative hypertension
that was managed by enalapril. He was followed closely by
pediatric cardiology and pediatric cardiac surgery.

His last echocardiogram from 2 months ago showed DILV
with right ventricular hypoplasia, unrestrictive shunting
across a ventricular septal defect, atrial communication post
septectomy, patent superior vena cava–right pulmonary artery
(SVC-RPA) anastomosis, a normal left pulmonary artery
(LPA), a tight internal middle pulmonary artery (MPA)
band with a small amount of anterograde flow, trace mitral
regurgitation (MR), mild to moderate tricuspid regurgitation
(TR), a mildly dilated right atrium, a mildly dilated left
ventricle, and normal biventricular systolic function. His daily
medications include enalapril 0.75 mg twice per day and a
half tab (40.5 mg) of baby aspirin daily. His other pertinent
history includes a subdural hemorrhage after an accidental
fall in infancy, which was managed nonoperatively, and a
hypospadias repair at 18 months by pediatric urology.

Clinical Presentation, Evaluation, and Management

At the urgent care clinic, the mother relayed the history
of the fall, and the patient was fussy and weak on his right
side. He was transferred due to concerns of head trauma

and intracranial hemorrhage. On arrival at the emergency department, the patient is fussy and anxious. His vitals are BP (on the left upper extremity) 110/66 (mean arterial cuff pressure 81), P 111, R 36, and T 37.2°C (98.9°F); SpO_2 is 79% on room air (normal SpO_2 >75% per the mother's report). He has a 3/6 systolic ejection murmur heard best at the left mid and upper sternal border. While he is supine, he is anxious and moving his extremities. On initial assessment, he has decreased movement of the right upper and lower extremities compared to the left. As he cries, he has a noticeable left facial droop with forehead involvement. He also has hyperreflexia on the right brachioradialis and patellar reflexes compared to normal reflexes on the left. This presentation prompts an immediate pediatric stroke alert.

The differential diagnosis for a child with symptoms of a stroke are broad (*Table 1*).[4] This child also has a history of venovenous anastomosis and single ventricle anatomy, so a thrombotic event is possible. Given the absence of fever and the sudden, rapid onset of symptoms, a brain abscess has a lower likelihood.

Per the institutional pediatric stroke protocol, intravenous access is established on the nonaffected side, and blood work is obtained, including a complete blood count with differential, chemistries with renal function tests, a coagulation profile (prothrombin time with INR, activated partial thromboplastin time), and a point-of-care blood venous gas with electrolytes. An ECG, MRI brain, and MRA head and neck are ordered. In the meantime, the pediatric neurology stroke team comes to assess the patient and agrees with the plan. The patient is taken to MRI and provided sedation, using 0.1 mg/kg midazolam IV and 0.5 mg/kg ketamine IV (*Figure 1*).

Pathophysiology

In patients with single ventricle anatomy and physiology, a BDG procedure, followed by a Fontan procedure, creates superior cavopulmonary anastomosis. The BDG procedure helps eliminate volume load on the single

Differential Diagnosis of Pediatric Stroke

- Intracranial hemorrhage
- Venous sinus thrombosis
- Seizures with postictal paralysis
- Bell palsy
- Intracranial tumors
- Intracranial infections
- Complex or hemiplegic migraine
- Alternating hemiplegia of childhood
- Posterior reversible encephalopathy syndrome (PRES)
- Acute disseminated encephalomyelitis (ADEM)
- Idiopathic intracranial hypertension
- Acute cerebellar ataxia

TABLE 1. Differential diagnosis of pediatric stroke

ventricle. Patients who require BDG have complete mixing of systemic and pulmonary vascular beds in parallel. The BDG converts this circulation into a series circuit where pulmonary blood flow is based on systemic venous return (*Figure 2*).[5] As a result, venovenous collaterals create routes for bacteria to bypass the filtering effects of the lungs like adults with pulmonary arterio-venous malformations, which places patients at a higher risk of brain abscess by allowing pathogens direct access to the systemic vasculature.

Summary

Intracranial abscesses are an uncommon cause of pediatric stroke; however, they must be considered after

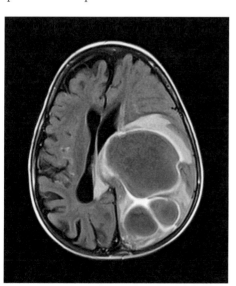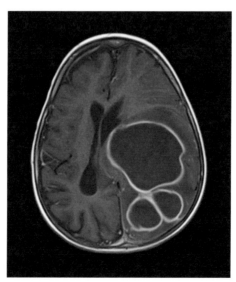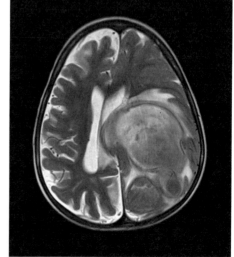

FIGURE 1. Initial MRI images showing multilocular diffusion restricting collection within the left frontoparietal region demonstrating a T2 double rim sign compatible with an abscess. The dominant abscess measures 6.2 × 5.1 × 4.7 cm with at least two adjacent daughter abscesses within the parietal lobe, likely contiguous with the parent abscess. There is extensive mass effect and ventricular entrapment.

cyanotic congenital heart disease surgery. Timely recognition of pediatric stroke is crucial for prompt imaging. Institutional protocols for pediatric stroke must be established to guide evidence-based evaluation and management strategies.

REFERENCES

1. Wu W, He J, Shao X. Incidence and mortality trend of congenital heart disease at the global, regional, and national level, 1990-2017. *Medicine* (Baltimore). 2020;99(23):e20593.

2. McCracken C, Spector LG, Menk JS, et al. Mortality following pediatric congenital heart surgery: an analysis of the causes of death derived from the National Death Index. *J Am Heart Assoc.* 2018;7(22):e010624.

3. Runkel BG, Drake WB, Raghuveer G. Brain abscess and the nonfenestrated Fontan circulation. *JACC Case Rep.* 2020;2(7):1029-1032.

4. Shellhaas RA, Smith SE, O'Tool E, Licht DJ, Ichord RN. Mimics of childhood stroke: characteristics of a prospective cohort. *Pediatrics.* 2006;118(2):704-709.

5. Salik I, Mehta B, Ambati S. Bidirectional Glenn procedure or hemi-Fontan. In: StatPearls. StatPearls Publishing. September 28, 2021.

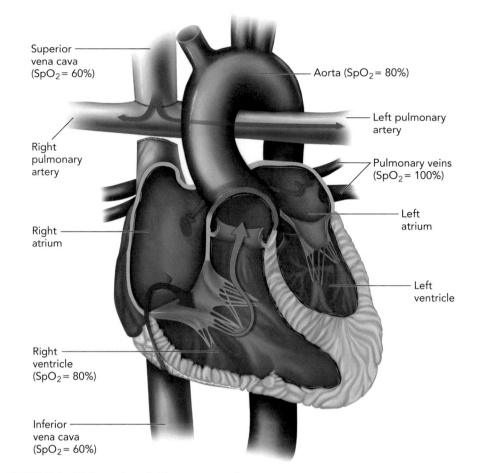

FIGURE 2. Bidirectional Glenn procedure

Superior vena cava (SpO$_2$ = 60%)

Aorta (SpO$_2$ = 80%)

Left pulmonary artery

Right pulmonary artery

Pulmonary veins (SpO$_2$ = 100%)

Right atrium

Left atrium

Left ventricle

Right ventricle (SpO$_2$ = 80%)

Inferior vena cava (SpO$_2$ = 60%)

CASE RESOLUTION

The pediatric neurology team was informed of the initial images, and the pediatric neurosurgery team was contacted. The patient required immediate operative intervention. The pediatric cardiologist was consulted for preoperative management, and an echocardiogram was performed, which demonstrated good ventricular function without evidence of vegetations. Intravenous fluids were started after an initial fluid bolus. On further assessment, the patient was noted to have poor dentition with a few cavities without signs of an abscess or infection. He was taken to the operating room, and the abscess was drained. Cultures from the abscess demonstrated moderate growth of *Streptococcus intermedius*, also known as *Streptococcus milleri*, which is normal flora in the oral cavity. He was treated empirically with vancomycin, ceftriaxone, and metronidazole until culture and susceptibility results were obtained. Antibiotics were subsequently switched to ceftriaxone and metronidazole per pediatric infectious disease recommendations. He also required re-exploration and washout. He remains in the hospital for neurological monitoring and completion of intravenous antibiotics but is now improving in the use of his right extremities.

Dental Fracture Dressing

By **Steven J. Warrington, MD, MEd**
MercyOne Siouxland, Sioux City, Iowa

Objective
On completion of this article, you should be able to:
- Apply dental cement to a fractured tooth with exposed dentin or pulp..

Introduction

Dental fractures vary in severity, but patients who have exposed dentin or pulp may need a dental dressing applied until follow-up and definitive care can be arranged. Calcium hydroxide dental cement can be used in such cases to protect the fractured tooth.

Contraindications

- Allergy to a component of the dressing materials

Benefits and Risks

The primary benefits of dressing a dental fracture that has exposed dentin or pulp include pain relief and a decreased risk of infection. Some patients may also benefit from having the sharp, exposed edges of a tooth covered to decrease discomfort and the risk of further injury.

Risks of the procedure are relatively minimal, but they include allergic reactions to the dressing materials and failure of the dressing to properly adhere to the tooth. Moreover, even with therapy, infection and pulp necrosis can occur. These possibilities should be discussed with patients, so they understand that the dressing may not prevent such complications.

Alternatives

The method described here uses calcium hydroxide dental cement as the dressing for a dental fracture; however, alternatives to its use in the emergency department include composites that require light curing and cyanoacrylate tissue adhesive. Some literature suggests that dentists prefer light-cured composites, but many emergency departments do not have such materials or equipment readily available.

Reducing Side Effects

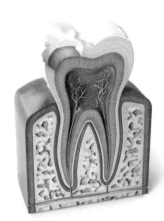

The potential side effects of using calcium hydroxide dental cement for dental fractures appear to be minimal. However, two conceivable risks, not explicitly found in the literature, include a piece of poorly secured dental cement breaking off and being aspirated or a sharp edge causing patient discomfort. Drying the outer tooth surface, ensuring good contact between the exposed area and the dental cement, and palpating the material after application to confirm it is stable and does not have sharp edges may be beneficial.

Special Considerations

When dispensing the materials, consider doing so one tube at a time to avoid mixing up the caps and inadvertently causing issues with future uses of the base or catalyst. Note that humidity around the calcium hydroxide mixture may cause it to harden. In some situations, gauze or a moist cotton roll can be placed near the mixture, but without making contact.

Dental injuries should also cause concern for potential abuse, especially in vulnerable populations such as those with developmental or cognitive delays, the elderly, and children.

TECHNIQUE

1. **Obtain** the patient's consent and obtain the materials and equipment for the procedure.
2. **Moisten** only the dentin- or pulp-exposed area by blotting it with wet or damp 2 × 2 gauze or cotton rolls.
3. **Place** 1 to 2 mm of base and 1 to 2 mm of catalyst slightly apart on a mixing pad. Wipe the nozzle of each tube and replace each cap on the correct tube.
4. **Mix** the two agents for approximately 15 seconds until the color is uniform.
5. **Apply** a thin layer (approximately 0.5-mm thickness) to the dentin- or pulp-exposed area.
6. **Hold** the lip and tongue away from the area with the dental cement, allowing it to dry for 30 to 60 seconds.
7. **Check** the area by palpating it with light pressure; there should be no significant indentation.

Cardioversion Strategies for Acute Uncomplicated Atrial Fibrillation

By **Megan J. Rivera, MD**; and
Nicholas G. Maldonado, MD, FACEP
University of Florida College of Medicine,
Department of Emergency Medicine, Gainesville

Reviewed by **Andrew J. Eyre, MD, MHPEd**

Objective

On completion of this article, you should be able to:

■ Determine the most appropriate cardioversion strategy for patients with acute uncomplicated atrial fibrillation.

Scheuermeyer FX, Andolfatto G, Christenson J, Villa-Roel C, Rowe B. A multicenter randomized trial to evaluate a chemical-first or electrical-first cardioversion strategy for patients with uncomplicated acute atrial fibrillation. *Acad Emerg Med.* 2019;26(9):969-981.

KEY POINTS

■ AF is a common, yet complex, dysrhythmia with multiple management strategies in the acute setting, depending on its classification and presentation.

■ In emergency department patients with first-onset or recurrent episodes of acute uncomplicated paroxysmal AF of less than 48 hours and a $CHADS_2$ score of 0 to 1, chemical-first and electrical-first cardioversion, using the alternative strategy if unsuccessful, are management options with similar discharge rates and conversion to sinus rhythm.

■ Electrical-first cardioversion results in a higher proportion of patients discharged within 4 hours, a shorter emergency department LOS, and higher rates of initial cardioversion compared to chemical-first cardioversion.

Atrial fibrillation (AF) is a common dysrhythmia and can be classified based on the duration of symptoms (ie, paroxysmal, persistent, long-standing, or permanent), the presence or absence of moderate-to-severe mitral stenosis or artificial heart valve (ie, valvular vs nonvalvular), the heart rate on presentation (ie, normal or rapid ventricular rate and response), and the level of stability (ie, stable versus unstable). Patients can also be categorized by their thromboembolic risk of cardioversion based on the timing of presentation after symptom onset (ie, less than or greater than 48 hours) in those with first-onset or recurrent episodes of acute paroxysmal AF as well as in all forms of AF based on previously studied risk factors.

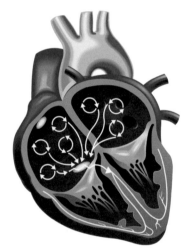

In the emergency department, presentations of first-onset or recurrent episodes of acute uncomplicated paroxysmal AF of less than 48 hours may be encountered. Rate- versus rhythm-control strategies for these cases have wide institutional and regional variability. For rhythm-control strategies, literature is emerging on whether a chemical or electrical cardioversion strategy should be used solely or in combination and, if combined, in what order. In this article, the authors sought to determine whether a cardioversion strategy using a chemical-first or electrical-first approach resulted in higher rates of sinus rhythm and faster disposition.

This multicenter randomized trial was conducted at six university-affiliated urban emergency departments in Canada. Patients included adults aged 18 to 75 years with AF of less than 48 hours as a primary diagnosis and a $CHADS_2$ score of 0 to 1. The study excluded patients who presented for other reasons and were incidentally found in AF; those with hemodynamic instability (defined as altered mental status, acute chest pain or heart failure, and systolic blood pressure <90 mm Hg); patients with atrial flutter; those having had a cardiac procedure within the last 2 weeks (ie, coronary artery bypass grafting, percutaneous coronary intervention, electrophysiologic ablation, or pacemaker or defibrillator insertion); and those acutely intoxicated or withdrawing from alcohol or illicit drugs.

With allocation concealment, patients were randomized to receive chemical-first cardioversion, followed by electrical cardioversion if unsuccessful, or to receive electrical-first cardioversion, followed by chemical cardioversion if unsuccessful. Although there was no standard treatment protocol in either group, the authors recommend that physicians manage the chemical-first cardioversion group with procainamidec 17 mg/kg IV (to a max of 1,500 mg) over 1 hour and the electrical-first cardioversion group with propofol sedation and a synchronized

Critical Decisions in Emergency Medicine's series of LLSA reviews features articles from ABEM's 2022 Lifelong Learning and Self-Assessment Reading List. Available online at acep.org/moc/llsa and on the ABEM website.

16 *Critical Decisions in Emergency Medicine*

biphasic waveform sequence of 100 to 150 to 200 J (to a maximum of 3 shocks).

The primary outcome was the difference in the number of patients discharged within 4 hours of arrival (defined as the time the patient registered at triage). Secondary outcomes included additional median time intervals (ie, randomization to conversion and randomization to discharge), emergency department–based adverse events (AEs), and 30-day patient-centered outcomes (physician or hospital visits and quality-of-life [QoL] assessment using the SF-8 at 3 and 30 days). Although it was unfeasible to blind physicians to the treatment arms, they were blinded to the study outcome measures.

Of the 135 eligible patients, 86 patients (63.7%) were enrolled. Although there was no loss to follow-up, one patient in each group withdrew; thus, 41 patients in the chemical-first group and 43 patients in the electrical-first group were analyzed with no significant between-group differences. Most patients were men (62%), aged 50 to mid-60 years, with a history of AF; more than half had a prior cardioversion of any type; and 44% were on aspirin. Few patients were on anticoagulation, nodal blocking agents, or antiarrhythmics.

There was a statistically significant difference in the proportion of patients discharged within 4 hours who were managed in the electrical-first group compared to the chemical-first group (67% vs 32%, a difference of 36% [95% CI = 16%-56%, $p < 0.001$]). With respect to secondary outcomes, the electrical-first group, compared to the chemical-first group, had a significantly shorter median emergency department length of stay (LOS) (3.5 hours versus 5.1 hours, a difference of 1.2 hours [95% CI = 0.4-2.0, $p < 0.001$]) and

higher rates of cardioversion with the initial method (88.4% vs 53.7% [$p < 0.001$]). All patients were discharged home, with 99% in sinus rhythm. AEs occurred in 25% of cases, all classified as minimal-risk outcomes with no difference between groups. At 30 days, there were no strokes or deaths in either group. Although no statistical analysis was performed, a higher number of patients in the chemical-first group represented to the emergency department at 3 and 30 days for recurrent AF and required admission compared to the electrical-first group. QoL scores were similar for both groups.

For patients with acute uncomplicated AF of less than 48 hours and a $CHADS_2$ score of 0 to 1, the results suggest that chemical-first and electrical-first cardioversion, using the alternative strategy if unsuccessful, are equally effective with respect to discharge rates in normal sinus rhythm, and both are well tolerated with minimal-risk AEs. Although no strokes occurred at 30 days in either group, this study was relatively small to detect this outcome in lower-risk populations. However, the results also suggest that electrical-first cardioversion results in a higher proportion of patients discharged within 4 hours, shorter emergency department LOS, and higher rates of initial cardioversion compared to chemical-first cardioversion. These results can be used to consider regional, institutional, and individual practice patterns and risk tolerance, for emergency department throughput decisions, in patient accessibility to close outpatient cardiology follow-up, and in shared decision-making in those who present with acute uncomplicated paroxysmal AF. If a rhythm-control strategy is considered appropriate in selected patients with AF, electrical-first cardioversion appears to be the optimal method with respect to throughput for these patients.

Orbital Compartment Syndrome Indicating Lateral Canthotomy and Cantholysis

By **Nneka Azih, MD**; **Ronya Silmi, MD**; and **Shama Patel, MD**
University of Florida College of Medicine – Jacksonville

Reviewed by **John Kiel, DO, MPH**

Objective

On completion of this article, you should be able to:
- Manage orbit compartment syndrome with lateral canthotomy and cantholysis..

CASE PRESENTATION

A 22-year-old man presents to the trauma center via ambulance after a possible gunshot wound (GSW) to the head. On arrival, the patient is confirmed to have a single round wound over the right temporal region and reports that the wound is self-inflicted with a small caliber pistol. Despite the mechanism of injury, he is in no apparent distress but has a severe headache and right eye pain. During the secondary survey, the patient's right eye is found to be proptotic with palpable firmness, periorbital swelling, and ecchymosis. Extraocular movement is restricted, and his pupil is dilated and nonreactive. The initial intraocular pressure of the right eye is 50 mm Hg (normal <20 mm Hg).

Imaging

An initial CT scan reveals a GSW to the calvarium with intracranial extension. Specifically, CT shows a calvarial entry wound with a comminuted displaced fracture at the anterior portion of the lateral wall of the right middle cranial fossa (*Figures 1* and *2*).

Clinical Considerations

Based on the mechanism of the GSW, a systematic and focused traumatic assessment must be completed on arrival to identify any life-threatening injuries. After an initial primary survey, a thorough secondary survey and pertinent history regarding the mechanism of injury should be conducted to

further identify and clarify injuries. In this case, knowing the type of gun, close-range approximation, and caliber of bullet can elucidate the extent of tissue damage. Combining anatomical knowledge with an estimation of the bullet trajectory may also help emergency physicians predict which structures are injured.

This patient reports eye pain and a severe headache. Given these complaints, the mechanism of injury, and the physical examination findings, there should be immediate concern for intracranial hemorrhage as well as the more clinically obvious ocular injury. Orbital compartment syndrome (OCS) is an ophthalmologic emergency that is a sight-threatening condition that requires prompt diagnosis and emergent treatment. This

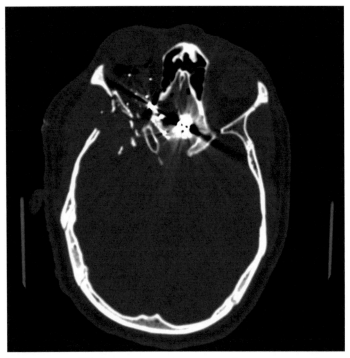

FIGURE 1. CT demonstrating extensive postseptal intraorbital emphysema and a high-attenuation intraluminal hemorrhage

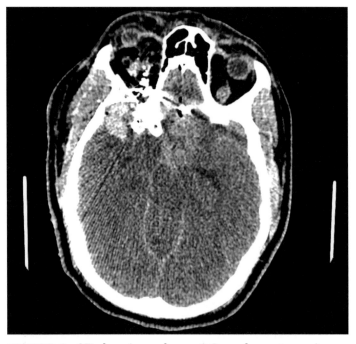

FIGURE 2. CT showing a large 2.3-cm hematoma in the anterior aspect of the right middle cranial fossa, which represents an epidural hematoma of likely venous origin

patient is experiencing many of the typical characteristics of OCS, including headache, ocular pain, blurred vision, reduced extraocular movements, proptosis, and vision loss. When there is an index of suspicion for OCS, emergency physicians should quickly assess for proptosis, ophthalmoplegia, visual acuity, an afferent pupillary defect, a tense globe resistant to retropulsion, and an elevated intraocular pressure. Variation in the physical examination findings may be due to the degree of the compartment syndrome. Note globe rupture must be excluded prior to measuring intraocular pressure. An elevated intraocular pressure is diagnostic of OCS.

Management

Emergent management of this condition includes lateral canthotomy and inferior cantholysis — a bedside procedure that aims to free the eye globe from its lateral attachment to the bony orbital wall and allow more eye protrusion. Release of the lateral canthus reduces tension on the optic nerve and retina, improves blood flow, and acts as a bridge procedure to definitive ophthalmological management.[1] One contraindication to lateral canthotomy is eye globe rupture, in which the affected eye shows clinical signs such as hyphema, subconjunctival hemorrhage, a misshapen pupil, enophthalmos, or exposed uveal tissue.[1]

Complications

Complications of lateral canthotomy and cantholysis include globe or lateral rectus injury, ptosis due to levator aponeurosis injury, injury to the lacrimal apparatus, ectropion due to excessive cantholysis, bleeding, infection, and cosmetic issues.[1]

REFERENCES

1. Amer E, El-Rahman Abbas A. Ocular compartment syndrome and lateral canthotomy procedure. *J Emerg Med.* 2019;56(3):294-297.
2. Rowh AD, Ufberg JW, Chan TC, Vilke GM, Harrigan RA. Lateral canthotomy and cantholysis: emergency management of orbital compartment syndrome. *J Emerg Med.* 2015;48(3):325-330.
3. Kam S, Wrenn JO, Valenzuela DA. Retrobulbar hematoma and orbital compartment syndrome requiring lateral canthotomy and cantholysis in patient with penetrating facial trauma. *Vis J Emerg Med.* 2021;24:101072.
4. Murali S, Davis C, McCrea MJ, Plewa MC. Orbital compartment syndrome: pearls and pitfalls for the emergency physician. *J Am Coll Emerg Physicians Open.* 2021;2(2):e12372.

KEY POINTS

- OCS is a medical emergency that is caused by an acute increase in intraocular pressure. The etiology can be traumatic, infectious, or any process that affects blood supply to the eye.

- A normal intraocular pressure is 10 to 20 mm Hg; concern for OCS should arise at an intraocular pressure of 40 mm Hg or greater.[2]

- Early recognition of OCS is critical, as a delay in treatment can cause optic nerve and retinal ischemia, which can result in permanent vision loss in as little as 60 to 100 minutes.[1,2,3,4]

TECHNIQUE

1. **Place** the patient in the supine position.

2. **Anesthetize** the lateral canthus with 1% lidocaine. The mixed form with epinephrine is preferred, as it can reduce bleeding, but it is not essential.[1]

3. **Place** a Kelly clamp across the lateral canthus for 1 to 2 minutes to minimize bleeding.

4. **Remove** the clamp and use sterile scissors to make a 1- to 2-cm lateral incision in the compressed tissue.

5. **Retract** the lower lid to expose the tendon of the lateral canthus.

6. **Direct** the scissors inferoposteriorly and cut the inferior crus of the lateral canthal tendon.

7. **Recheck** the intraocular pressure. If successful, the intraocular pressure should be less than 40 mm Hg, and visual acuity may improve. If the intraocular pressure remains elevated, the superior crus of the lateral canthus tendon can be cut.

CASE RESOLUTION

The patient was admitted to the trauma surgery service with neurology, neurosurgery, and ophthalmology consultations. Due to the mechanism of injury, the patient had a partially severed optic nerve, which resulted in permanent vision loss. Given the extent of the injury and embedded metallic fragments, the patient is expected to suffer from lifelong headaches.

The Critical Image

CT to Assess Urinary System Pathologies

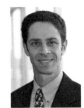

By Joshua S. Broder, MD, FACEP
Dr. Broder is a professor and the
residency program director in
the Department of Emergency
Medicine at Duke University
Medical Center in Durham,
North Carolina.

Objectives

On completion of this article, you should be able to:

■ Describe the appropriate use of CT with and without IV contrast as well as multiphase CT to assess urinary system pathologies.

CASE PRESENTATION

A 43-year-old woman presents with 1 month of dysuria and scant clear vaginal fluid leak. She denies fever, vomiting, and flank pain. The patient has a history of ectopic pregnancy and reports a hysterectomy and bilateral salpingo-oophorectomy more than 1 year prior. As a complication of that procedure, she had a ureteral injury and urinary/vaginal fistula, marked by vaginal urine output. She was treated with a temporary ureteral stent and improved. On arrival, her vital signs are BP 121/82, P 78, R 16, and T 36.1°C (97°F); SpO2 is 100% on room air. The patient appears comfortable and has no abdominal or costovertebral angle tenderness. Her urine hCG is negative. Urinalysis shows positive nitrites, leukocyte esterase, and greater than 50 bacteria. Blood urea nitrogen and creatinine are 23 mg/dL and 1.0 mg/dL, respectively. Her WBC count is 8.8. Multiphase CT to assess for a urinary fistula is ordered (*Figure 1*).

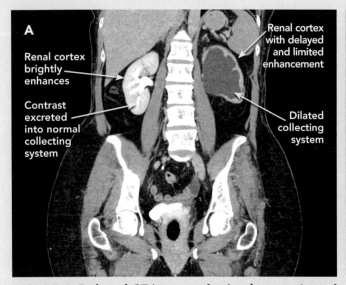
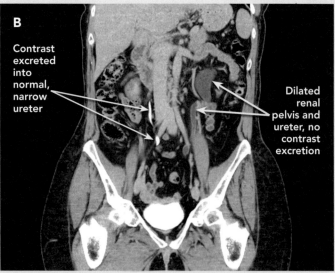

FIGURE 1. Delayed CT images obtained approximately 7 minutes after the injection of IV contrast

A. The obstructed left kidney shows delayed and reduced enhancement compared to the normal right kidney — a delayed nephrogram. The collecting system is markedly dilated, and no contrast has been excreted.
B. The obstructed left ureter is dilated compared to the normal right ureter and does not fill with contrast.

Emergency physicians must balance multiple factors when selecting an abdominal/pelvic CT protocol for a patient, including speed, diagnostic accuracy, radiation exposure, and contrast media risks. Noncontrast CT assesses a wide differential diagnosis with important exceptions, such as vascular dissections and occlusions, ischemic complications, and some neoplastic, infectious, and inflammatory conditions. Its benefits include relatively low radiation exposure (when tailored for nephrolithiasis), lack of exposure to iodinated contrast, and no requirement for intravenous (IV) access.[1] When IV contrast is given, multiple options exist for the timing of image acquisition relative to contrast injection.[2] Early image acquisition captures a contrast bolus in the arterial phase, optimized for arterial pathology, such as aortic dissection or superior mesenteric artery occlusion. Portal venous phase imaging is commonly used as a "standard" abdominal/pelvic CT with IV contrast and can detect a wide array of pathologies, as contrast is found within blood vessels and also enhances solid organs and bowel wall.

Additional delayed images are sometimes performed to observe the perfusion of organs or to track the progress of injected contrast as it is excreted by the kidneys. In most cases, additional contrast is not required, as the original contrast bolus can be followed over time. This diagnostic information, however, comes at the price of additional radiation exposure, imaging time, radiologist interpretation time, and financial cost. Sometimes, unenhanced CT is followed by a combination of contrast-enhanced images for comparison. Multiphase CT is unnecessary for most emergency diagnoses but can play an important role, as in this complex case; routine use is discouraged as a part of the *Choosing Wisely* campaign to limit radiation exposure.[3] When in doubt, discussion with a radiologist and specialist consultant about the patient presentation, differential diagnosis, and clinical information needed can help to tailor the imaging protocol.

A common scenario for emergency physicians is the patient with a differential diagnosis that includes both nephrolithiasis, for which IV contrast is unnecessary, and other conditions for which IV contrast is essential. A classic example is renal colic vs renal infarct, both of which share similar clinical presentations, but where the lack of perfusion of a renal segment is revealed by the difference in contrast enhancement of a normal and an infarcted kidney. A common concern when administering IV contrast is that kidney stones (intrarenal or within the renal collecting system) may be obscured by injected contrast, as both appear bright on CT. Fearing a missed diagnosis,

physicians may be tempted to perform all CTs without, and then with, contrast. The American College of Radiology rates CT without contrast as most appropriate, and CT with contrast as least appropriate, for suspected renal colic,[1] although this rating does not take into account the broad differential diagnosis that should be entertained for some patients.

Does CT with IV contrast obscure urinary stones? What about other findings of urinary obstruction? Compared with noncontrast CT, CT with portal venous phase IV contrast sensitivity is 88%, 95%, 99%, and 98% for stones ≥2, ≥3, ≥4, and ≥5 mm, respectively.[4] The negative predictive value of IV-contrast enhanced CT for obstructing ureteral calculi is 100%, compared to 99.5% for noncontrast CT.[5]

While small stones may not be recognized following IV contrast administration, other important findings of obstruction are identifiable or explicitly made evident by IV contrast.[4,5] Hydronephrosis and hydroureter are seen with high-grade obstruction, regardless of contrast use. With IV contrast, an obstructed kidney shows delayed parenchymal enhancement and delayed excretion of contrast — a "delayed nephrogram." In comparison to a contralateral normal kidney, the obstructed kidney appears less bright, and urine in the kidney and ureter is dark in appearance.

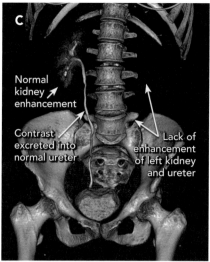

FIGURE 1 (*continued*).
Delayed CT images obtained approximately 7 minutes after the injection of IV contrast
C. This 3D reconstruction from the delayed CT images has the CT window adjusted to show only high-density materials (eg, contrast, bone). The right kidney is visible because of its contrast enhancement, as are the right ureter and bladder. Without contrast enhancement, the left kidney and ureter appear conspicuously absent.

CASE RESOLUTION

CT demonstrated high-grade obstruction of the left kidney and collecting system, presumably from stenosis or discontinuity following the earlier ureteral injury. No leak of urine or fistula was identified. The patient was admitted and underwent percutaneous nephrostomy to relieve her hydronephrosis, with plans for later ureteral reconstruction. Her urine culture grew greater than 100,000 colonies of *Escherichia coli*. She was treated with antibiotics with symptom resolution.

REFERENCES

1. American College of Radiology. ACR Appropriateness Criteria® acute onset flank pain—suspicion of stone disease (urolithiasis). Reviewed 2015. https://acsearch.acr.org/docs/69362/Narrative/
2. American College of Radiology. ACR–SABI–SAR–SPR practice parameter for the performance of computed tomography (CT) of the abdomen and computed tomography (CT) of the pelvis. Revised 2021. https://www.acr.org/-/media/ACR/Files/Practice-Parameters/ct-abd-pel.pdf
3. American College of Radiology. Don't routinely use a protocol for abdominal CT that includes a delayed post-contrast phase after the venous phase, except for the following indications: renal lesion characterization, hematuria work up, CT urogram, indeterminate adrenal nodule characterization, hepatocellular carcinoma and cholangiocarcinoma. Choosing Wisely. October 16, 2017. https://www.choosingwisely.org/clinician-lists/acr-abdominal-ct-with-delayed-post-contrast-phase-after-the-venous-phase/
4. Dym RJ, Duncan DR, Spektor M, Cohen HW, Scheinfeld MH. Renal stones on portal venous phase contrast-enhanced CT: does intravenous contrast interfere with detection? *Abdom Imaging*. 2014;39(3):526-532.
5. Lei B, Harfouch N, Scheiner J, Demissie S, Hayim M. Can obstructive urolithiasis be safely excluded on contrast CT? A retrospective analysis of contrast-enhanced and noncontrast CT. *Am J Emerg Med*. 2021;47:70-73.

Feature Editor: **Joshua S. Broder, MD, FACEP.** See also *Diagnostic Imaging for the Emergency Physician* (Winner of the 2011 Prose Award in Clinical Medicine, the American Publishers Award for Professional and Scholarly Excellence) and *Critical Images in Emergency Medicine* by Dr. Broder.

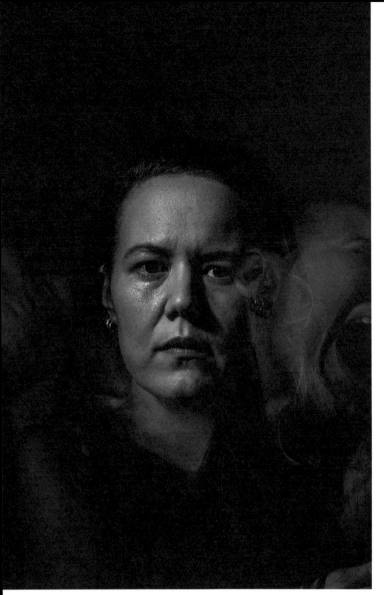

Warning Signs
Identifying Intimate Partner Violence

LESSON **10**

By **Heather V. Rozzi, MD, FACEP**; and **Lisa E. Smale, DO**
Dr. Rozzi is an emergency physician at WellSpan York Hospital in York, Pennsylvania. Dr. Smale is an emergency physician at Beebe Healthcare in Rehoboth Beach, Delaware.

Reviewed by **Wan-Tsu W. Chang, MD**

OBJECTIVES

On completion of this lesson, you should be able to:

1. Recognize warning signs that should raise suspicion for IPV.

2. Understand and use effective screening tools for IPV.

3. Identify the important elements in a safety plan for victims of domestic violence.

4. Describe how IPV affects special populations, including pregnant patients and those in same-sex relationships.

FROM THE EM MODEL

14.0 Psychobehavioral Disorders
    14.6 Patterns of Violence/Abuse/Neglect
        14.6.1.2 Intimate Partner

■ CRITICAL DECISIONS ■

■ How should the terms intimate partner and intimate partner violence be defined in the acute setting?

■ How and when should patients be screened for IPV?

■ What clues in a patient's history and physical examination should raise suspicion for IPV?

■ What can be done to better understand and help patients who will not leave an abusive relationship?

■ How should IPV be documented?

■ What special considerations must be addressed when managing pregnant victims of IPV?

■ What unique concerns should be addressed when managing patients in abusive same-sex relationships?

Intimate partner violence (IPV) affects millions of people each year, regardless of gender, age, race, and socioeconomic status. IPV can masquerade as a host of common complaints, including chronic pain, substance abuse, and depression. Consequently, this potentially lethal cycle can be particularly difficult to identify and address in a busy emergency department, where it can be hard to find a quiet moment to connect with reluctant or frightened patients.

CASE PRESENTATIONS

■ CASE ONE

A 26-year-old woman presents with nausea, headache, and blurred vision. On examination, she has periorbital ecchymoses, a bruise to the left lateral aspect of the neck, and bruising of both upper extremities. She is hesitant to describe how these injuries occurred, and she repeatedly checks her cell phone during the examination.

■ CASE TWO

A 43-year-old woman presents with vaginal bleeding, headache, and pain with swallowing. She states that her husband became enraged and choked her when she declined to have sex with him. She recalls thinking that he was going to kill her before she passed out. While she was unconscious, he raped her.

■ CASE THREE

A 60-year-old man presents with injuries to his right ear, left shoulder, and back. He states that he was intoxicated and must have fallen down the steps, but he does not recall the event. He is accompanied by his husband, who is very attentive and answers most of the questions asked of the patient.

Introduction

In the United States alone, it is estimated that 10 million people experience physical violence each year at the hands of a current or former intimate partner.[1] However, the individual biases of medical professionals can inadvertently limit screening efforts to patients with a perceived high risk of IPV — an oversight that can result in missed opportunities for critical interventions. It is vital to remember that IPV can affect anyone, including particularly vulnerable populations such as pregnant patients, same-sex couples, and the elderly.[2]

Unfortunately, many clinicians are uncomfortable addressing this sensitive, emotionally loaded topic due to limited education and experience. Nevertheless, it is crucial for frontline physicians to know which local resources are available for victims and to actively seek out additional education on IPV, just as they would for any other disease process.

CRITICAL DECISION

How should the terms intimate partner and intimate partner violence be defined in the acute setting?

To properly identify victims of IPV, it is important to understand the relevant terminology. An intimate partner is one with whom a patient has a close personal relationship. This dynamic can be characterized by one or more of the following traits: emotional connectedness, regular contact, ongoing physical contact and sexual behavior, identity as a couple, and familiarity and knowledge about the other's life.[3] IPV includes physical, sexual, economic, emotional, or psychological abuse by a current or former intimate partner.[3]

Most cases of IPV are never reported, so the incidence is difficult to determine. In 2011, an anonymous telephone survey found that 32% of women and 28% of men reported having experienced rape, physical violence, or stalking by an intimate partner; rates of psychological violence were much higher.[1]

IPV is part of a spectrum of family violence that includes intimate partner abuse, child abuse, elder abuse, and animal abuse. Unfortunately, particular forms of family violence rarely occur in isolation. An abuser often harms not only the intimate partner, but also other members of the household, including children and even pets. An estimated 50% to 70% of abuse victims own pets that also have been abused or killed.[4]

Type of Abuse	Characteristics
Physical abuse	Hitting, slapping, shoving, grabbing, pinching, biting, and hair pulling are examples of physical abuse. Physical abuse also includes denying a partner medical care or forcing them to use alcohol or drugs.
Sexual abuse	Sexual abuse includes coercing or attempting to coerce any sexual contact or behavior — without consent. Sexual abuse includes — but is not limited to — marital rape, attacks on sexual parts of the body, forcing sex after physical violence has occurred, or treating a partner in a sexually demeaning manner.
Emotional abuse	Emotional abuse includes undermining an individual's sense of self-worth or self-esteem. This behavior may include — but is not limited to — constant criticism, diminishing a partner's abilities, name calling, or damaging a partner's relationship with their children.
Economic abuse	Economic abuse is defined as making or attempting to make an individual financially dependent by maintaining total control over financial resources, withholding a partner's access to money, or forbidding a partner's attendance at school or employment.
Psychological abuse	Elements of psychological abuse include — but are not limited to — causing fear by intimidation; threatening physical harm to self, partner, children, or a partner's family or friends; harming pets; damaging property; and forcing isolation from family, friends, school, or work.

TABLE 1. Types of IPV as defined by the US Department of Justice[6]

Most clinicians have a good understanding of what constitutes physical and sexual harm, but emotional, psychological, and economic abuse can be more difficult to define and recognize. These latter forms of maltreatment can include threats of suicide or abandonment, threats to children, blackmail, social isolation from friends and family, control of money and resources, and other manipulative behaviors (*Table 1*).[5,6,7]

Screening Tool	Questions
Universal Violence Prevention Screening Protocol[9]	Have you been in a relationship with a partner in the past year? If yes, within the past year, has a partner: • Slapped, kicked, pushed, choked, or punched you? • Forced or coerced you to have sex? • Threatened you with a knife or gun to scare or hurt you? • Made you afraid that you could be physically hurt? • Repeatedly used words, yelled, or screamed in a way that frightened you, threatened you, put you down, or made you feel rejected?
Partner Violence Screen[10]	• Have you been hit, kicked, punched, or otherwise hurt by someone in the past year? If so, by whom? • Do you feel safe in your current relationship? • Is there a partner from a previous relationship who is making you feel unsafe now?

TABLE 2. Common IPV screening questions

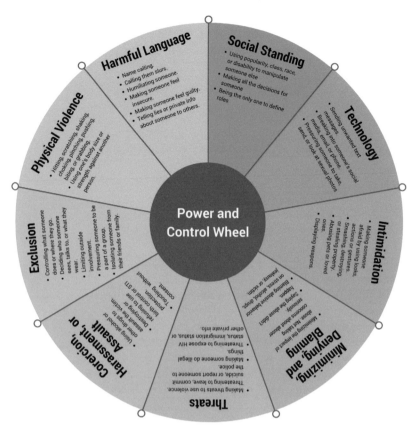

FIGURE 1. Power and control wheel

The power and control wheel illustrates the experience of individuals who live with abusive intimate partners (*Figure 1*). Battering is the pattern of actions used to intentionally control or dominate one's partner. "Power and control" constitute the center of the wheel. The spokes, which contain the behaviors used to instill fear in the partner, include specific threats, intimidation, and coercions.[7] Physical and sexual violence are rarely isolated and are often part of this dysfunctional dynamic.

CRITICAL DECISION

How and when should patients be screened for IPV?

In some emergency departments, IPV screening begins with the nursing staff; however, it is important to note that IPV can be missed during triage for a multitude of reasons, including severe medical illness necessitating immediate stabilization, altered mental status, intoxication, or the presence of visitors during the triage process. If suspicion of IPV persists despite a negative initial screening, physicians should conduct a secondary screening during the visit. If this is impossible due to ongoing medical or social issues, it is critical to relay the need for IPV screening to the subsequent treating physician during handoff; it may also be beneficial to involve other staff members, such as social workers. Physicians should remain attuned to aspects of the history and physical examination that increase the potential for domestic abuse.[8]

There are multiple tools that can guide the secondary screening, but clinicians should develop their own set of questions tailored to fit the specific concerns of each case (*Table 2*).[9,10] A positive answer to any screening question should

prompt the development of a patient safety plan prior to discharge.[2]

Ideally, IPV screening should be conducted in a private setting in the absence of visitors. To help gain the patient's trust, physicians should refrain from using judgmental or condescending tones and body language. Physicians should be mentally prepared for a positive screening result and be ready to offer a comforting response, such as "I'm sorry this happened to you, and I'm glad you shared this with me," or "This is not your fault."[2,8]

✔ Pearls

- All patients should be screened for IPV.

- A secondary screening should be performed if a patient's history or physical examination is suspicious for signs of abuse.

- Be prepared with an appropriate response and management plan in the event a victim of IPV is identified in the emergency department.

- Prior to discharge, IPV victims should receive information about local emergency shelters and identify a point person who can be called if they feel endangered.

What clues in a patient's history and physical examination should raise suspicion for IPV?

Warning signs that may indicate potential IPV include a delay in seeking care (eg, a patient who reports falling a week prior to their emergency department visit), multiple visits for chronic or seemingly minor complaints, and trauma during pregnancy.[2] Emergency physicians should note whether patients seem apprehensive about speaking in front of their partner; a dominating partner who attempts to control the visit or consistently speaks for the patient should raise concerns about potential IPV.[2]

IPV victims may present with complications from chronic illnesses or demonstrate nonadherence with medications and office visits. For example, patients who present in diabetic ketoacidosis may have had difficulty remembering to take insulin due to safety concerns for themselves or loved ones. It is important to recognize that nonadherent patients may be prevented from taking proper care of themselves and their children.[2,5]

During the physical examination, it is important to note injury patterns that may suggest IPV, including defensive wounds to the forearms or patterned injuries such as ligature marks, linear markings from a broom handle (*Figure 2*), marks from handcuffs (*Figure 3*), or imprints from the sole of a shoe. Contusions, which are among the most common manifestations of abuse, can be used to help determine the mechanism of injury but should not be used to estimate the age or force of the injury. Bruising is unique to each patient; multiple variables can influence the appearance of bruises, including location on the body and overall health status.

Lacerations, slicing or cutting wounds, and penetrating wounds can also suggest the mechanism of injury (*Figure 4*). Any injury that appears to have been caused by a wielded object should be examined closely (*Figure 5*). The hand, which is the most commonly used weapon in IPV, has a

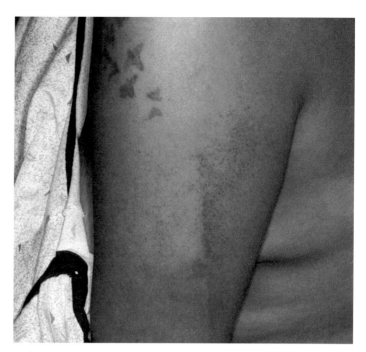

FIGURE 2. Bruising caused by a broom handle. *Credit:* Photo courtesy of Elizabeth Jenkins, BSN, RN, SANE-A, SANE-P.

distinct injury pattern that is usually evidenced by linear contusions with central areas of clearing. Bites and burns can also be identified by their characteristic appearance. A human bite wound may contain saliva that could be useful in later legal proceedings (*Figure 6*).[5]

The majority of injuries incurred during an intimate partner assault are craniofacial (*Figure 7*). Blunt force trauma to the face can result in characteristic injuries secondary to the patient's own accessories; for example, periorbital contusions or lacerations can result from contact with the victim's eyeglasses.[5] Patients who experience IPV are at high risk of traumatic brain injury (TBI) and, ultimately, chronic traumatic encephalopathy, which may occur in the absence of obvious facial or head trauma. In addition to the physical symptoms of TBI (eg, headaches and visual changes), these patients may experience personality changes; have difficulty with organization and memory processing; and develop sleep dysfunction, depression, or anxiety. These symptoms may interfere with the ability to obtain appropriate follow-up care or to appropriately care for themselves and their children. All patients who have experienced IPV should be screened for TBI.[11]

Strangulation (*Figure 8*) can result in subconjunctival hemorrhages and petechiae around the eyes, nose, mouth, and oral mucosa. Patients may present with abrasions, erythema, ligature marks to the chin or neck, or subcutaneous emphysema; however, a normal examination does not rule out a serious injury, such as carotid artery dissection.[5] Positive examination findings, in addition to other factors (eg, dysphonia, difficulty swallowing, dyspnea, positive loss of consciousness, and visual changes), should prompt further imaging to assess the structures of the neck. CT angiography of the neck is the gold standard for evaluation of cervical vessels and bony or cartilaginous structures.[12]

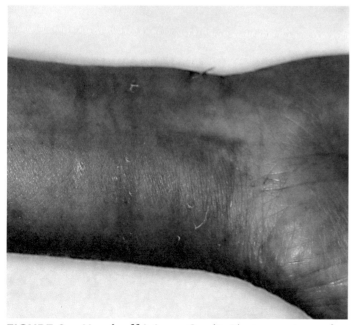

FIGURE 3. Handcuff injury. *Credit:* Photo courtesy of Elizabeth Jenkins, BSN, RN, SANE-A, SANE-P.

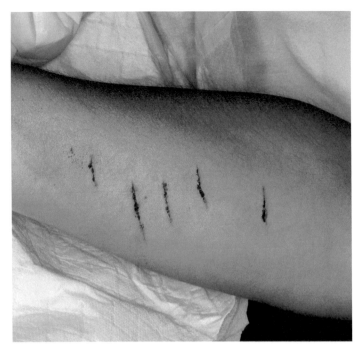

FIGURE 4.   Linear lacerations from a box cutter.
Credit: Photo courtesy of Tracy Hunter, RN, SANE-A, SANE-P.

Although craniofacial trauma is the most common injury in cases of domestic violence, it is crucial to have the patient undress fully and examine the entire body for additional wounds. Frequently, injuries are discovered in regions separate from those specific to the patient's complaints.[5]

CRITICAL DECISION

What can be done to better understand and help patients who will not leave an abusive relationship?

It can be very difficult for those who have not experienced IPV to understand why victims choose not to disclose the abuse, decline help, or return to their abusers. This frequent reality can frustrate caregivers, but the goal should be to work with the patient to develop a safety plan, regardless of whether that plan includes leaving the abuser.

Victims of IPV choose to remain in the abusive relationship for many reasons, and it is important to understand that any patient seeking help for IPV is taking a significant risk. According to the Bureau of Justice Statistics, one-third of female murder victims are killed by their intimate partners, and these homicides often occur after the victim attempts to leave the relationship.[2] Additionally, patients may fear for the well-being of their children, pets, or other family members. Oftentimes, the victim of homicide is not the intimate partner, but rather a family member, friend, neighbor, intervening person, first responder, or bystander.[13,14]

Patients may also choose to remain in abusive relationships out of economic concern. They may fear homelessness or the inability to provide for themselves and their children. Immigrant patients may be unsure of their legal rights or fear deportation. Moreover, patients may feel pressure from family, peers, religious beliefs, or cultural norms to remain with their abusive partners. Some victims simply choose to stay because they are still in love with

their abusers and harbor hope that things will change. Because many victims feel that these forces outweigh the danger of staying in the relationship, a safety plan must be put into place.[2,5,8]

A social worker or advocate from an IPV organization should be involved if the patient's domestic abuse screen is positive or if obvious signs of abuse are revealed during the examination. A social worker is essential to the safety planning process and will help ensure that the patient has support following the emergency department visit. The social worker can help arrange emergency shelter, assist with services for children, and provide resources for legal advocacy and emotional support. If the patient refuses to leave the abuser, the physician or social worker can help to develop a simple safety plan. The plan should start with identifying a point person that the patient can call in the event of danger, such as a relative, friend, or other close contact; importantly, this individual should be aware that they may need to contact law enforcement. The victim should have a hidden emergency bag containing extra clothes, necessary keys, and an accessible source of money. Important phone numbers and documents should also be readily available, including the patient's social security card, birth certificate, driver's license, bank account information, insurance policies, and immunization records.[2,5]

CRITICAL DECISION

How should IPV be documented?

If a patient discloses IPV, this should be documented in the medical record. However, in the era of electronic medical records, it is imperative that sensitive information such as disclosures and safety plans not be available for the patient's abuser to view via the patient portal. Most electronic medical records have a function that permits a note to be hidden in order to protect the patient's safety.

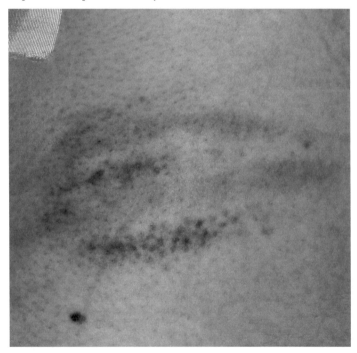

FIGURE 5.   Patterned injury caused by an unknown wielded object. *Credit:* Photo courtesy of Michelle Frey, RN-BC.

Reporting laws pertaining to IPV vary from state to state; it is important for physcians to understand the requirements of the jurisdictions in which they practice. Mandatory reporting of IPV is controversial. If victims know their physician is required to report, they may be less likely to seek health care. Victims may also fear retaliation by the perpetrator.

Patients who show signs of abuse but do not admit to being in danger should be reminded to return to the emergency department at any time for help. This information can be conveyed in statements like "Should your situation ever change, I want you to know that we'll always be available to talk with you about it."[2,5] This conversation should be documented in the medical record and hidden from the patient portal.

CRITICAL DECISION

What special considerations must be addressed when managing pregnant victims of IPV?

Homicide is a frequent cause of traumatic death among pregnant and postpartum patients in the United States.[2,15] Abusers may attempt to induce miscarriage by inflicting direct trauma to the abdomen or genitalia. Fathers of newborn children may harbor jealousy or resentment that can result in physical violence to the mother or child. When the relationship is abusive, the stress of pregnancy can exacerbate an already tenuous situation.[2,16] Nearly 90% of patients who suffer abuse during pregnancy have a history of IPV prior to becoming pregnant.[5]

IPV is associated with direct fetal injury, placental abruption, premature labor, and stillbirth. Life-threatening maternal trauma results in fetal loss in 40% to 50% of cases;

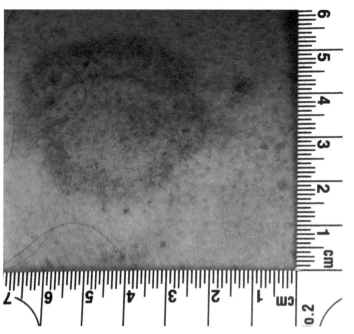

FIGURE 6. Bite wound. *Credit:* Photo courtesy of Brandi Castro, BSN, RN, SANE-A, SANE-P.

non–life-threatening trauma results in fetal loss in 1% to 5% of patients.[5] The physiological changes in pregnancy demand special considerations when managing patients with traumatic injuries. Heart rate increases by 15% in normal pregnancy; due to expanded maternal blood volume, patients can tolerate about 1,500 mL of blood loss before becoming hypotensive. These changes make it difficult to use vital signs as a predictor of shock. Moreover, acute blood loss is disproportionately detrimental to the fetus. In cases of hemorrhage, maternal blood pressure is maintained by shunting blood away from the fetus, a process that results in fetal hypoxia.[5,17]

By the second trimester, the uterus has risen into the abdominal cavity, and minor blows to the abdomen can cause uterine rupture or abruption. The enlarging uterus further displaces intra-abdominal structures, and bowel injuries are more common with penetrating trauma to the upper abdomen. Slowed gastric emptying and increased intra-abdominal pressure confers an increased risk of aspiration.[5,17]

Maternal stabilization takes precedence and follows the normal trauma mantra of airway, breathing, circulation, disability, and environment. Pregnant patients should be placed in the left lateral decubitus position to maintain venous return and prevent uterine compression of the inferior vena cava. Fetal evaluation should occur after the patient has been stabilized, but it is important to note that significant fetal injury can be present even with only minor injuries.

Complaints of extreme uterine tenderness or vaginal bleeding may be signs of uterine rupture or abruption. The fetal heart rate should be obtained as a general indicator of fetal well-being. If the fetus has reached at least 20 weeks' gestation, the patient should undergo contraction monitoring for a minimum of 4 to 6 hours. Kleihauer-Betke testing may be helpful to detect concealed maternal-fetal bleeding. In such cases, rho(D) immune globulin should be administered.[5,17,18]

As with any other type of IPV, appropriate follow-up and safety planning should be arranged, and the patient's safety should be evaluated by a social worker. Resources for housing

---

✖ Pitfalls

- Assuming patients do not need to be screened for IPV based on gender, race, age, or socioeconomic status.

- Failing to address concerns for IPV with patients due to a personal discomfort with discussing the topic of abuse.

- Becoming frustrated with patients who will not leave their abusers and failing to provide them with appropriate resources.

- Failing to use ancillary staff to help patients develop an individualized safety plan.

- Sharing notes with information regarding a patient's experience of abuse and safety plans through the patient portal.

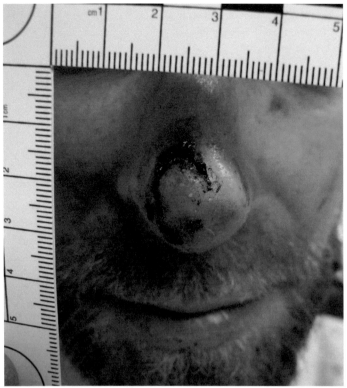

FIGURE 7. Facial injury. *Credit:* Photo courtesy of York Hospital Forensic Examiner Team.

What unique concerns should be addressed when managing patients in abusive same-sex relationships?

Although heterosexual women are most likely to be the target of IPV screening in the emergency department, it is vitally important to consider the possibility of relationship violence when assessing lesbian, gay, bisexual, and transgender (LGBT) patients. A study comparing lesbian and heterosexual women showed that lesbians are more likely to experience nonsexual physical violence.[2,19] Unlike the heterosexual community, in which women are victimized far more often than men, victims in the LGBT community are equally likely to be men.[5]

It can be particularly difficult for LGBT patients to discuss IPV with health care professionals. Patients may not have disclosed their sexual orientation to friends and family; homophobia and a lack of family and community support can result in severe feelings of isolation and a reluctance to seek help. Furthermore, LGBT patients who do reach out for help may have difficulty finding resources that include same-sex relationships. For example, many shelters segregate by gender — a dynamic that poses a unique risk of further abuse to members of the LGBT community. In such cases, same-sex abusers could potentially gain entry to the shelter.[5]

Summary

IPV includes any behavior that is used to control or manipulate a partner, and it affects all genders, races, ages, sexual orientations, and socioeconomic statuses. Special

and shelter should be discussed, and information about advocacy groups specific to pregnant patients should be provided prior to discharge.[2,5]

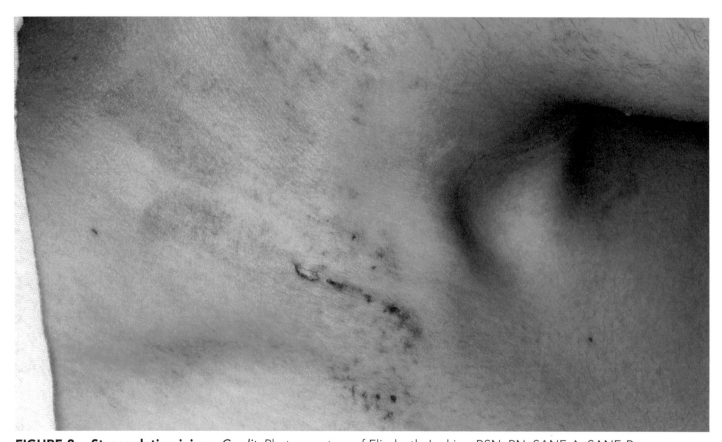

FIGURE 8. Strangulation injury. *Credit:* Photo courtesy of Elizabeth Jenkins, BSN, RN, SANE-A, SANE-P.

CASE RESOLUTIONS

CASE ONE

Although the IPV screening from triage was negative, upon gentle questioning by the physician, the 26-year-old woman disclosed that she had been assaulted by her fiancé. She stated that this only happens when he is intoxicated, and she showed text messages in which he promised to quit drinking. She declined to speak with the advocate from the local IPV organization. The emergency department social worker provided resources, including phone numbers for the IPV hotline, and worked with the patient to develop a safety plan that included strategies to escape the house and a list of safe places to go.

CASE TWO

Because the 43-year-old woman's strangulation resulted in loss of consciousness and pain with swallowing, CT angiography of the neck was performed. Luckily, CT did not reveal any acute injuries. Gynecology was consulted for extensive lacerations of the lateral and posterior vaginal walls. The IPV advocate assisted with arranging safe housing and obtaining an emergency protection from abuse order.

CASE THREE

Because the 60-year-old man's history was vague and he had several injuries, an emergency department clinician followed the patient to the radiology suite to speak with him without his husband present. The patient disclosed a long history of emotional abuse by his husband, which had recently progressed to physical abuse. The patient expressed a desire to leave his husband but was worried about where he would live and what would happen to his dog if he left the home he shared with his husband. The local IPV organization assisted with placing the patient in a local hotel suite and arranged for the patient's dog to be boarded in a nearby kennel until more permanent housing could be found.

consideration should be given when screening pregnant patients for IPV because they are at particular risk. IPV can be an uncomfortable topic to discuss with patients, but it is the duty of emergency physicians to help protect this vulnerable population. Active screening, education, and preparation for a positive IPV screen are key. The effective use of ancillary staff is crucial when managing and developing a safety plan for any suspected victim of IPV.

REFERENCES

1. Breiding MJ, Smith SG, Basile KC, Walters ML, Chen J, Merrick MT. Prevalence and characteristics of sexual violence, stalking, and intimate partner violence victimization – national intimate partner and sexual violence survey, United States, 2011. *MMWR Surveil Summ.* 2014 Sep 5;63(8):1-18.

2. Kaplan C, Lovelace D, Pittard A, Lewis D, Corcoran C, Martin ML. Domestic violence and intimate partner violence. *Emerg Med Reports.* 2006 Nov 12.

3. Breiding M, Basile K, Smith S, Black MC, Mahendra R. *Intimate Partner Violence Surveillance Uniform Definitions and Recommended Data Elements Version 2.0.* National Center for Injury Prevention and Control of the Centers for Disease Control and Prevention; 2015. https://www.cdc.gov/violenceprevention/pdf/intimatepartnerviolence.pdf

4. Ascione FR, Weber CV, Wood DS. The abuse of animals and domestic violence: a national survey of shelters for women who are battered. *Society and Animals.*1997;5(3):205-218.

5. Markowitz J, Polsky S. *Color Atlas of Domestic Violence.* Mosby; 2004.

6. Domestic violence. The United States Department of Justice. October 31, 2016. https://www.justice.gov/ovw/domestic-violence

7. Power and control wheel. Domestic Abuse Intervention Project. http://www.ncdsv.org/images/powercontrolwheelnoshading.pdf

8. Choo EK, Houry DE. Managing intimate partner violence in the emergency department. *Ann Emerg Med.* 2015 Apr;65(4):447-451.

9. Heron SL, Thompson MP, Jackson E, Kaslow NJ. Do responses to an intimate partner violence screen predict scores on a comprehensive measure of intimate partner violence in low income black women? *Ann Emerg Med.* 2003 Oct;42(4):483-491.

10. Feldhaus KM, Koziol-McLain J, Amsbury HL, Norton IM, Lowenstein SR, Abbott JT. Accuracy of 3 brief screening questions for detecting partner violence in the emergency department. *JAMA.* 1997 May 7;277(17):1357-1361.

11. McAfee RE. Physicians and domestic violence: can we make a difference? *JAMA.* 1995 Jun 14;273:1790-1791.

12. Recommendations for the medical radiographic evaluation of acute adult, non-fatal strangulation. The Training Institute for Strangulation Prevention. https://www.strangulationtraininginstitute.com/wp-content/uploads/2015/07/Recommendations-for-Medical-Radiological-Eval-of-Non-Fatal-Strangulation-v17.9.pdf

13. National statistics. National Coalition Against Domestic Violence. http://ncadv.org/learn-more/statistics

14. Smith SG, Fowler KA, Niolon PH. Intimate partner homicide and corollary victims in 16 states: National Violent Death Reporting System, 2003-2009. *Am J Public Health.* 2014 March;104(3):461-466.

15. Chang J, Berg CJ, Saltzman LE, Herndon J. Homicide: a leading cause of injury deaths among pregnant and postpartum women in the United States, 1991-1999. *Am J Public Health.* 2005 March;95(3):471-477.

16. Bacchus L, Bewley S, Mezey G. Domestic violence in pregnancy. *Fetal Matern Med Rev.* 2001 Nov;12(4):249-271.

17. Lavin JP Jr, Polsky SS. Abdominal trauma during pregnancy. *Clin Perinatol.* 1983 Jun;10(2):423-428.

18. Coleman MT, Trianfo VA, Rund DA. Nonobstetric emergencies in pregnancy: trauma and surgical conditions. *Am J Obstet Gynecol.* 1997 Sep;177(3):497-50.

19. Baum R, Moore K. Lesbian, gay, bisexual and transgender domestic violence: 2003 supplement. National Coalition of Anti-Violence Programs; 2004:42. ACCESS. Assault Care Center Extending Shelter and Support. www.assaultcarecenter.org

CME Questions

Reviewed by John Kiel, DO, MPH; and Wan-Tsu W. Chang, MD

Qualified, paid subscribers to *Critical Decisions in Emergency Medicine* may receive CME certificates for up to 5 ACEP Category I credits, 5 *AMA PRA Category 1 Credits*™, and 5 AOA Category 2-B credits for completing this activity in its entirety. Submit your answers online at acep.org/cdem; a score of 75% or better is required. You may receive credit for completing the CME activity any time within 3 years of its publication date. Answers to this month's questions will be published in next month's issue.

1 **What is the first-line uterotonic drug for postpartum hemorrhage after uterine massage has been initiated?**
   A. Carboprost
   B. Methylergonovine
   C. Misoprostol
   D. Oxytocin

2 **What are the four Ts of postpartum hemorrhage?**
   A. Tension, torsion, trauma, thrombin
   B. Tone, torsion, tissue, thrombin
   C. Tone, trauma, tissue, thrombin
   D. Trauma, tension, thrombin, tamponade

3 **What is the mechanism of action for oxytocin?**
   A. Competitive and reversible inhibitor of plasminogen activation that decreases fibrinolysis
   B. Ergot alkaloid that directly stimulates uterine smooth muscle
   C. Hormone that acts on the myometrium, causing symmetric constriction of the hemorrhaging spiral arteries
   D. Prostaglandin analogue that causes increased uterine tone and vasoconstriction

4 **What is the postpartum period in which preeclampsia or eclampsia can occur?**
   A. Up to 7 days postpartum
   B. Up to 2 weeks postpartum
   C. Up to 6 weeks postpartum
   D. Up to 6 months postpartum

5 **What symptom falls short of the "severe feature" classification in preeclampsia?**
   A. Altered mental status
   B. Diarrhea
   C. Newly elevated creatinine
   D. Vision changes

6 **What is the correct treatment approach for postpartum preeclampsia?**
   A. Intravenous rehydration and seizure prevention
   B. Lowering blood pressure and seizure prevention
   C. Pain control and increasing urine output
   D. Pain control and nausea control

7 **What is the most common risk factor for postpartum endometritis?**
   A. Caesarean delivery
   B. History of a sexually transmitted infection
   C. Maternal tobacco use during pregnancy
   D. Preterm premature rupture of membranes

8 **What is the recommended first-choice treatment for postpartum endometritis?**
   A. Ampicillin and clindamycin
   B. Ceftriaxone and doxycycline
   C. Clindamycin and gentamicin
   D. Vancomycin and piperacillin-tazobactam

9 **What is the image modality of choice for diagnosis of cerebral venous sinus thrombosis?**
   A. CT venography
   B. MR venography
   C. Noncontrast CT of the head
   D. X-ray

10 **Venoarterial extracorporeal membrane oxygenation is most likely to be used as an advanced therapy in which cause of shortness of breath in postpartum patients?**
   A. Amniotic fluid embolism
   B. COVID-19
   C. Pneumonia
   D. Pneumothorax

11 **Which question is least appropriate to ask when screening a patient for IPV?**
   A. Do you feel safe in your current relationship?
   B. Has your current partner ever forced or coerced you to have sex?
   C. Have you been hit, kicked, punched, or otherwise hurt by someone in the last year?
   D. How many sexual partners have you had in the past year?

12 What is the best approach when discharging an IPV victim who refuses help and intends to return to their abuser?

A. Encourage them to "be strong" and reiterate that they are taking an unnecessary risk by staying in the abusive relationship
B. Inform the patient that you will be contacting the authorities for their protection
C. Reassure the patient that help is always available in the emergency department and encourage them to return at any time if they feel unsafe
D. Respect the patient's privacy and discharge them without further comment

13 A 23-year-old man presents with multiple contusions and a wound that appears to be caused by a wielded object. He claims his injuries are the result of a fall, and his initial IPV screen is negative. Despite these findings, abuse is suspected. What is an appropriate next step?

A. Call the patient's bluff and privately contact the authorities
B. Conduct a secondary IPV screen, express concern for his safety, and offer to help develop a safety plan
C. Men are unlikely to be victims of abuse; no further questioning is required
D. Reveal your suspicions and advise the patient to leave his abusive relationship immediately

14 Which injury is most commonly seen in victims of IPV?

A. Abdominal injuries
B. Bite marks
C. Craniofacial trauma
D. Strangulation

15 What should be considered when managing a pregnant victim of abuse?

A. Even minor trauma during the second trimester can cause uterine rupture or abruption
B. Life-threatening maternal trauma results in fetal loss in about 85% to 95% of cases
C. Significant fetal trauma is unlikely in pregnant patients with only minor injuries
D. Vital signs remain the most reliable predictor of shock in pregnant patients

16 What should be considered when reporting a case of IPV?

A. IPV reporting is mandated in every state
B. Reporting requirements vary from jurisdiction to jurisdiction
C. Retaliation is unlikely when IPV is documented in the electronic patient portal
D. There are no reporting requirements for IPV

17 What is a common direct sequela of IPV?

A. Diabetes
B. Hypertension
C. Stroke
D. Traumatic brain injury

18 What is an appropriate step when managing a victim of IPV?

A. Advise the patient to leave the abuser
B. Confront the abuser and report the case to law enforcement
C. Enlist ancillary resources to assist with safety planning
D. Never report IPV to the authorities due to HIPAA regulations

19 What is a characteristic of IPV?

A. 50% to 70% of victims have pets that also have been mistreated or killed by their abusers
B. IPV, child abuse, elder abuse, and animal abuse are unrelated
C. It is always safest for a victim of IPV to leave the relationship
D. Patients in same-sex relationships are not at risk of IPV

20 What is the best imaging modality for the evaluation of a strangulation injury?

A. Carotid ultrasonography
B. CT angiography
C. No imaging is required
D. X-ray

ANSWER KEY FOR APRIL 2022, VOLUME 36, NUMBER 4

1	2	3	4	5	6	7	8	9	10	11	12	13	14	15	16	17	18	19	20
B	C	C	A	C	C	D	B	B	D	A	D	C	D	C	B	C	B	C	D

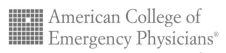

American College of Emergency Physicians®

ADVANCING EMERGENCY CARE

Post Office Box 619911
Dallas, Texas 75261-9911

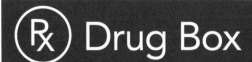

Drug Box

Bebtelovimab

By Amy Magdalany, PharmD; and Frank LoVecchio, DO, MPH, FACEP
St. Joseph's Hospital and Medical Center; and Valleywise Health, ASU, University of Arizona, Phoenix

OBJECTIVE
On completion of this column, you should be able to:
■ Describe the use of bebtelovimab to treat COVID-19.

The FDA issued an EUA for bebtelovimab to treat mild to moderate COVID-19 in positive patients of direct SARS-CoV-2 testing at high risk for progression to severe disease (ie, hospitalization, death) when alternative treatments are inaccessible or clinically inappropriate.

Mechanism of Action
Recombinant human IgG1k monoclonal antibody that binds SARS-CoV-2 spike protein and blocks attachment to human ACE2 receptor

Indications
Bebtelovimab is active against all circulating Omicron sublineages; based on lab data, it works against the BA.2 variant. Bebtelovimab is not authorized for use in patients who are hospitalized, require oxygen therapy or respiratory support, or require an increase in baseline oxygen flow rate or respiratory support due to COVID-19 or those on chronic oxygen therapy or respiratory support due to an underlying non–COVID-19-related comorbidity.

Dosage and Administration
Administer ASAP after a positive test, within 7 days of symptom onset.
Adult: 175 mg IV, single dose. No dosage adjustment recommended for kidney or hepatic impairment.
Pediatric: 175 mg IV, single dose. In clinical trials, only three adolescents received bebtelovimab; EUA is based on likelihood of similar exposure in patients aged ≥12 years weighing ≥40 kg.

Common Adverse Effects
Rare infusion related reactions, altered mental status, angioedema, asthenia, bronchospasm, cardiac arrhythmia (atrial fibrillation, sinus tachycardia, bradycardia), chest pain or discomfort, chills, diaphoresis, dizziness, dyspnea, fatigue, fever, headache, hypertension, hypotension, myalgia, nausea, pruritus, rash (urticaria), reduced oxygen saturation, throat irritation, and vasovagal reactions (presyncope, syncope) with infusion-related reactions

Warnings and Precautions
Pregnancy: Reproductive toxicity has not been evaluated; effects of in utero exposure are unknown. In general, COVID-19 treatment is the same as in nonpregnant patients. Consider in nonhospitalized, COVID-19–positive, pregnant patients with mild to moderate symptoms, especially those with one or more risk factors (eg, BMI >25, cardiovascular disease, chronic kidney disease, diabetes mellitus). No dose adjustments recommended.
Hypersensitivity: If serious hypersensitivity reactions (anaphylaxis) occur, immediately discontinue and initiate appropriate medications and supportive care. Adverse effects can occur up to 24 hours after infusion. Monitor patients for ≥1 hour; if a reaction occurs, slow or stop the infusion and administer appropriate medications or supportive care.
Contraindications: None listed.

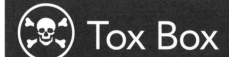

Tox Box

Aliphatic Hydrocarbon Ingestion

By **Christian Tomaszewski, MD, MS, MBA, FACEP**
University of California San Diego Health

OBJECTIVE
On completion of this column, you should be able to:
■ Describe the management of aliphatic hydrocarbon ingestions.

Aliphatic hydrocarbons include a variety of petroleum distillates, including gasoline, and are present in many household cosmetics and chemicals (eg, lamp oils, furniture polish, paint thinner). Most ingestions are unintentional pediatric exposures that can result in life-threatening pulmonary complications, especially if accompanied by vomiting. In addition, halogenated hydrocarbons (eg, chloroform, trichloroethylene), which are usually inhaled, can lead to sudden death.

Mechanism
■ Aspiration of low-viscosity agents leading to surfactant destruction
■ General anesthetic effects on the CNS
■ Increased myocardial sensitivity to epinephrine (halogenated)

Clinical Manifestations
■ CNS — slurred speech, disorientation, dizziness, ataxia
■ Cardiac — dysrhythmias (halogenated)
■ GI — nausea, vomiting, abdominal pain, diarrhea
■ Pulmonary — cough, dyspnea
■ Dermal (spill) — irritation, defatting, full-thickness burns

Diagnostics
■ Chest x-ray (may not show changes until ~6 hours)
■ Pulse oximetry
■ ECG (optional)
■ Acetaminophen level in intentional ingestions
■ Rule out life-threatening coingestants (camphor, halogenated or aromatic hydrocarbons, metals, or pesticides) and treat accordingly.

Treatment
■ Avoid activated charcoal because of vomiting and aspiration risk.
■ Administer supplementary oxygen or intubate as needed.
  ● Steroids and antibiotics are routinely unhelpful.
  ● Bronchoalveolar lavage is controversial.
  ● Instillation of surfactant or ECMO may help severe cases.
■ Short-acting beta-blockers for ventricular dysrhythmias

Disposition
■ If asymptomatic, patients may be observed at home.
■ Evaluate deliberate ingestions or symptomatic cases.
  ● Discharge asymptomatic cases at 6 to 8 hours.
  ● Admit if persistent pulmonary or CNS symptoms.

Critical decisions
in emergency medicine

Volume 36 Number 6: **June 2022**

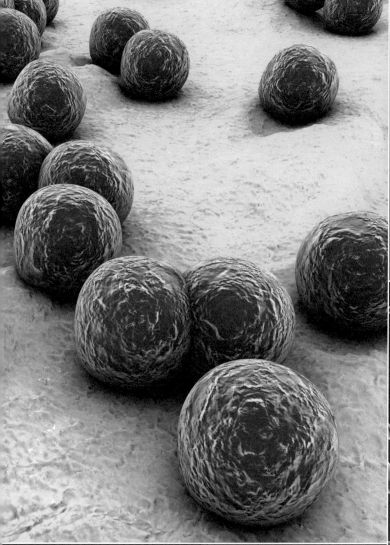

Under the Skin

Necrotizing fasciitis, a life-threatening condition with high rates of morbidity and mortality, is much less common than cellulitis. However, because surgical exploration is the only way to confirm or exclude the diagnosis of necrotizing fasciitis, emergency physicians must keep a high index of suspicion and advocate for patients early in the hospital course to ensure the best outcomes.

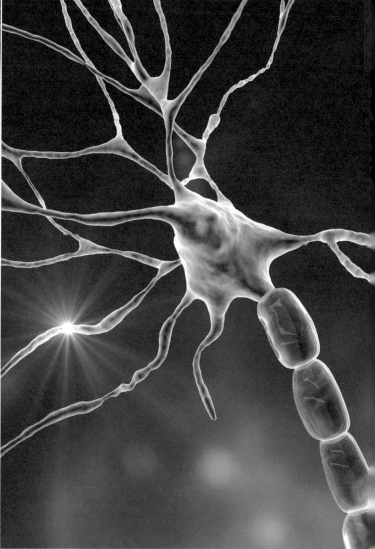

Breathing Room

Neuromuscular disorders like myasthenia gravis can lead to rapidly progressive paresis, paralysis of respiratory and oropharyngeal muscles, and the inability to manage oral secretions. Because delayed intervention can lead to disastrous consequences, emergency physicians must be able to quickly recognize the features of impending respiratory failure that can arise from a myasthenic crisis.

THE OFFICIAL CME PUBLICATION OF THE AMERICAN COLLEGE OF EMERGENCY PHYSICIANS

Contributor Disclosures. In accordance with the ACCME Standards for Commercial Support and policy of the American College of Emergency Physicians, all individuals with control over CME content (including but not limited to staff, planners, reviewers, and authors) must disclose whether they have any relevant financial relationship(s) to learners prior to the start of the activity. These individuals have indicated that they have a relationship which, in the context of their involvement in the CME activity, could be perceived by some as a real or apparent conflict of interest (eg, ownership of stock, grants, honoraria, or consulting fees), but these individuals do not consider that it will influence the CME activity. Joshua S. Broder, MD, FACEP, is a founder and president of OmniSono Inc, an ultrasound technology company. Sharon E. Mace, MD, FACEP, performs contracted research funded by Biofire Corporation, Genetesis, Quidel, and IBSA Pharma. Elizabeth DeVos, MD, MPH, performs contracted research for Inflammatix, and payment is made to the emergency department related to sepsis. All remaining individuals with control over CME content have no significant financial interests or relationships to disclose.

This educational activity consists of two lessons, eight feature articles, a post-test, and evaluation questions; as designed, the activity should take approximately 5 hours to complete. The participant should, in order, review the learning objectives for the lesson or article, read the lesson or article as published in the print or online version until all have been reviewed, and then complete the online post-test (a minimum score of 75% is required) and evaluation questions. Release date June 1, 2022. Expiration date May 31, 2025.

Accreditation Statement. The American College of Emergency Physicians is accredited by the Accreditation Council for Continuing Medical Education to provide continuing medical education for physicians.

The American College of Emergency Physicians designates this enduring material for a maximum of 5 *AMA PRA Category 1 Credits™*. Physicians should claim only the credit commensurate with the extent of their participation in the activity.

Each issue of *Critical Decisions in Emergency Medicine* is approved by ACEP for 5 ACEP Category I credits. Approved by the AOA for 5 Category 2-B credits.

Commercial Support. There was no commercial support for this CME activity.

Target Audience. This educational activity has been developed for emergency physicians.

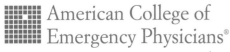

American College of Emergency Physicians®

ADVANCING EMERGENCY CARE

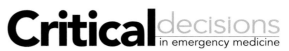

Contents

Lesson 11 4
Under the Skin
Necrotizing Fasciitis and Cellulitis
By Jeremy Riekena, MD; Sonya Naganathan, MD, MPH;
and Faroukh Mehkri, DO
Reviewed by Walter L. Green, MD, FACEP

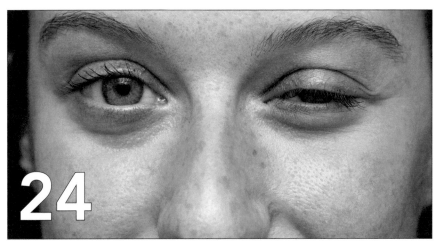

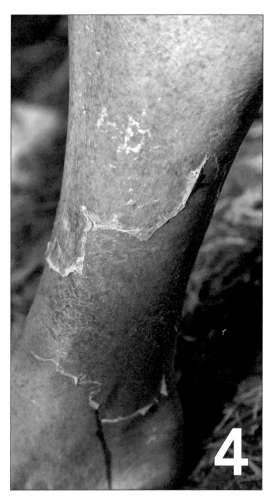

Lesson 12 24
Breathing Room
Respiratory Failure in a Myasthenic Crisis
By Zackary M. Funk, MD; Elizabeth L. DeVos, MD, MPH; and Adnan Javed, MD
Reviewed by John Kiel, DO, MPH

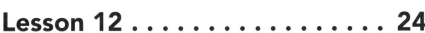

FEATURES

Clinical Pediatrics — Spontaneous Splenic Rupture in Infectious Mononucleosis 12
By Sarah Young, MD
Reviewed by Sharon E. Mace, MD, FACEP

The LLSA Literature Review — Pulmonary Embolism..14
By Lachlan Driver, MD; and Andrew J. Eyre, MD, MSHPEd

The Critical Procedure — Negative Pressure Wound Therapy Application 16
By Steven J. Warrington, MD, MEd, MS

Critical Cases in Orthopedics and Trauma — Pelvic Fractures With Urethral Injury 18
By William Perkins, MD; and Victor Huang, MD, CAQ-SM
Reviewed by John Kiel, DO, MPH

The Critical Image — Chest Pain and Imaging for Cardiac Ischemia..20
By Joshua S. Broder, MD, FACEP

The Critical ECG — Myocardial Infarction or Hyperkalemia..22
By Amal Mattu, MD, FACEP

CME Questions 30
Reviewed by Walter L. Green, MD, FACEP; and John Kiel, DO, MPH

Drug Box — Capsaicin for CHS 32
By Frank LoVecchio, DO, MPH, FACEP

Tox Box — Xylazine Toxicity 32
By Christian Tomaszewski, MD, MS, MBA, FACEP

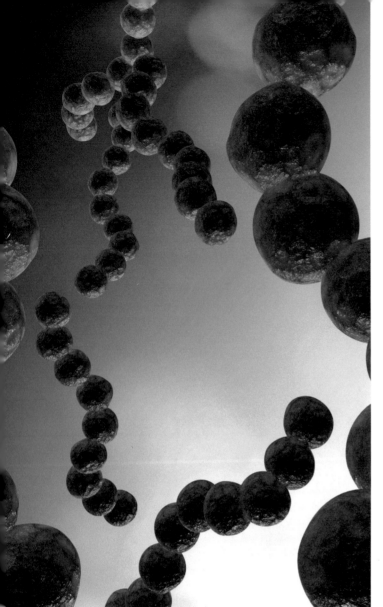

Under the Skin

Necrotizing Fasciitis and Cellulitis

LESSON 11

By Jeremy Riekena, MD; Sonya Naganathan, MD, MPH;
and Faroukh Mehkri, DO

Dr. Riekena is a simulation-based education fellow and an assistant instructor of emergency medicine. Dr. Naganathan is an assistant professor of emergency medicine for the Emergency Disaster and Global Health Division, and Dr. Mehkri is an assistant professor of emergency medicine for the Division of Prehospital Medicine and Emergency Medical Services at the University of Texas Southwestern Medical Center in Dallas. Dr. Mehkri is also the deputy medical director for the City of Dallas and Dallas Fire-Rescue Department.

Reviewed by Walter L. Green, MD, FACEP

Objectives

On completion of this lesson, you should be able to:

1. Define cellulitis and differentiate it from other SSTIs.
2. Integrate laboratory and imaging studies to determine the severity of SSTIs.
3. Use evidence-based guidelines to select the best treatment for NF and cellulitis.
4. Dispel common dogma regarding the treatment of SSTIs using emerging evidence and guidelines.

From the EM Model

4.0 Cutaneous Disorders
    4.4 Infections
        4.4.1 Bacterial
            4.4.1.2 Cellulitis
            4.4.1.5 Necrotizing Infection

■ CRITICAL DECISIONS ■

- What are the subtypes of cellulitis, and how do their treatment regimens differ?

- What are the types of NF, and when should NF be suspected?

- How can physical examination and imaging findings be used to evaluate SSTIs and NF?

- What are the optimal treatment options for NF?

- What are some commonly held myths and practice patterns with SSTIs?

Necrotizing fasciitis (NF) is a life-threatening condition with high morbidity and mortality. Fortunately, NF is much less common than simple cellulitis, which is regularly seen by emergency physicians. However, NF requires a high index of suspicion since surgical exploration is the only way to confirm or exclude the diagnosis. Advocacy for patients early in their hospital course can help ensure the best outcomes.

CASE PRESENTATIONS

■ CASE ONE

An ill-appearing elderly man from a nearby skilled nursing facility presents via EMS. The patient was in his usual state of health before he slowly became more lethargic and confused until he was no longer speaking coherently. Upon review of his records, the patient has a history of insulin-dependent type 2 diabetes mellitus complicated by bilateral below-knee amputations, hypertension, and coronary artery disease with cardiac stents. His vital signs are notable for tachycardia, hypotension, and confusion. While beginning initial resuscitation with crystalloids and broad-spectrum antibiotics, the secondary survey of the fully undressed patient reveals warm, necrotic-appearing tissue with crepitus in the perineum.

■ CASE TWO

A 32-year-old woman presents with a 1-week history of an increasingly painful and enlarging patch of redness on her lower left leg. She has no significant medical history but is concerned because her leg started to swell. She asks for antibiotics because she is concerned about an infection. Her examination reveals normal vital signs and a warm, poorly demarcated 4 × 5 cm area of erythema on her lower left leg without fluctuance. Subcutaneous "cobblestoning" is noted on bedside ultrasound without any focal hypoechoic or anechoic region.

■ CASE THREE

A 25-year-old man presents with complaints of severe lower right leg pain but is still able to ambulate. He has no significant medical history and is angry about his long wait time. He states that he took several tablets of acetaminophen and codeine from a friend, which has not helped his symptoms. The physical examination of his lower extremities is unrevealing, but needle marks are noted on the patient's arms. When questioned, he admits to frequent intravenous drug use.

Introduction

Skin and soft tissue infections (SSTIs) contribute to more than 2 million emergency department visits annually.[1] SSTIs encompass a spectrum of conditions, ranging from simple abscesses to NF.[2] The 2014 practice guidelines from the Infectious Diseases Society of America (IDSA) help to categorize these conditions into two major categories — purulent and nonpurulent infections. Purulent infections include a range of abscesses, but this lesson instead focuses on the nonpurulent infections cellulitis and NF.[3] Given the frequency and potential severity of these conditions, it is of the utmost importance for emergency physicians to recognize cellulitis and NF and respond appropriately.

NF is a rarer illness to encounter in the emergency department, but it has a much higher mortality and morbidity in comparison to other SSTIs, with mortality rates exceeding 30%.[4-6] NF affects about 0.4 in every 100,000 people per year in the United States; in some areas of the world, NF is as common as 1 in every 100,000 people.[7,8] Thus, diligent physicians must maintain a high index of suspicion for patients presenting with findings concerning for NF, and they must be acutely aware of the immediate steps to care for these patients.

CRITICAL DECISION

What are the subtypes of cellulitis, and how do their treatment regimens differ?

Cellulitis is a nonpurulent bacterial infection of the skin involving the dermis and subcutaneous layers.[3,9] More than 14 million cases of cellulitis are seen annually.[10] The most recent available data from 2005 show nearly 3.5 million emergency department visits for cellulitis.[11] Cellulitis commonly presents with erythema, swelling, warmth, and tenderness over the affected area (*Figure 1*). The culprit bacteria often enter the skin at areas of compromised integrity. The lower legs are commonly affected.[3] Nonpurulent SSTIs are categorized as mild, moderate, and severe. The treatment for each category ranges from oral to varying degrees of parenteral antibiotics.

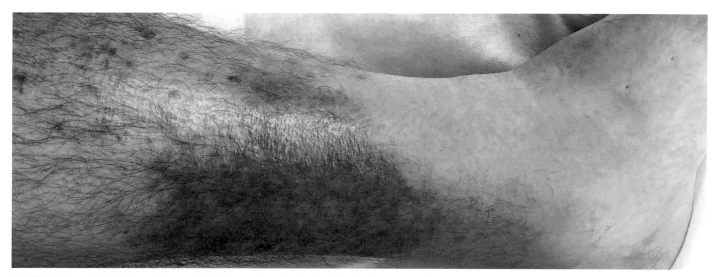

FIGURE 1. Cellulitis at lower left leg. *Credit:* TisforThan/Shutterstock.com.

MRSA

Despite the increase of methicillin-resistant *Staphylococcus aureus* (MRSA) infections in the United States in the late 1990s to the early 2000s, MRSA-related infections, while still present, have trended downward.[12,13] A 2017 study by Moran et al demonstrated no increased clinical cure rate when trimethoprim-sulfamethoxazole (TMP-SMX) was added to a 7-day regimen of cephalexin.[14] When certain risk factors (eg, known nasal colonization, history of MRSA infection, concurrent MRSA infection from another source, hospitalization, or recent antibiotics) are present, it is appropriate to consider the addition of MRSA coverage.[3]

Mild Cellulitis

Mild, uncomplicated cellulitis can be treated with a course of oral antibiotics. These patients often do not require hospitalization. Most uncomplicated cases are caused by group A *Streptococcus* (GAS), so many of the initial antibiotic therapies are targeted toward these bacteria.[3] Penicillins, cephalosporins, and clindamycin are the mainstays of treatment (*Table 1*). Suggested oral regimens for adults include penicillin VK 250 to 500 mg every 6 hours plus cephalexin 500 mg every 6 hours. A 5- to 7-day course is generally sufficient for the typical patient.[3] It may be worthwhile to consider methicillin-susceptible *S. aureus* (MSSA) and MRSA as possible culprits of mild cellulitis, although evidence suggests this is unnecessary since MSSA and MRSA are generally associated with purulent SSTIs.[3,15,16]

Moderate and Severe Cellulitis

The IDSA defines a moderate nonpurulent SSTI as a "typical cellulitis with systemic signs of infection." Generally, these are patients who meet Systemic Inflammatory Response Syndrome (SIRS) criteria and can be managed with parenteral antibiotics targeted at the most likely causative agent. Since GAS is still the most common pathogen, treatment regimens without MRSA coverage are reasonable (see *Table 1*). Suggested intravenous medications include penicillin (2-4 million units every 4 to 6 hours), clindamycin (600-900 mg every 8 hours), cefazolin (1 g every 8 hours), and in certain cases, nafcillin (1-2 g every 4 to 6 hours).[3]

Patients that are refractory to outpatient oral therapy, show signs of sepsis, have concern for deeper infection, or have risk factors for MRSA colonization warrant the addition of broad-spectrum antibiotics that include MRSA coverage. Vancomycin, linezolid, and in rarer cases (in the United States), daptomycin are indicated.[3]

CRITICAL DECISION

What are the types of NF, and when should NF be suspected?

Patients often have inconspicuous injuries with no recollection of the inciting event that becomes the nidus for the NF infection. In the vast majority of NF cases, skin tissue is compromised with direct seeding of bacteria that leads to a deeper infection (*Figure 2*).

Generally, patients with deep-space infections suggestive of NF complain of pain out of proportion to the physical examination when compared to simple cellulitis or a small abscess. Any patient with significant tenderness to the site of

Condition	Antibiotic	Dosage
Cellulitis (mild)	Penicillin VK	250-500 mg PO every 6 hours
	Cephalexin	500 mg PO every 6 hours
	Dicloxacillin	250 mg PO every 6 hours
	Clindamycin	300-400 mg PO every 6 hours
	Amoxicillin-clavulanate	875/125 mg PO every 12 hours
Cellulitis with MRSA (mild)	TMP-SMX	One to two double-strength tablets PO every 12 hours
	Doxycycline	100 mg PO every 12 hours
	Clindamycin	450 mg PO every 6 hours
	Linezolid	600 mg PO every 12 hours
Cellulitis (moderate and severe)	Penicillin	2-4 million units IV every 4-6 hours
	Ceftriaxone	1 g IV every 24 hours
	Cefazolin	1 g IV every 8 hours
	Nafcillin	1-2 g IV every 4-6 hours
Cellulitis with MRSA (moderate and severe)	Vancomycin	30 mg/kg/day IV in two divided doses
	Daptomycin	4 mg/kg IV every 24 hours
	Linezolid	600 mg IV every 12 hours
	Clindamycin	600-900 mg IV every 8 hours
Necrotizing fasciitis	Linezolid	600 mg IV every 12 hours
	Vancomycin	30 mg/kg/day IV in two divided doses
	Piperacillin-tazobactam	4 g/500 mg IV every 6 hours
	Clindamycin	900 mg IV every 8 hours
	Meropenem	1 g IV every 8 hours

TABLE 1. **Antibiotic selection by SSTI.** Adapted from IDSA guidelines.

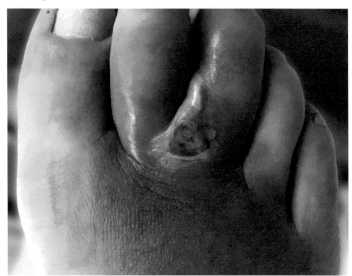

FIGURE 2. **NF at right foot in a diabetic patient.**
Credit: TisforThan/Shutterstock.com.

pain, crepitus, or skin changes (eg, bullae or ecchymoses) should be treated for NF. Emphysema and crepitus are sometimes present because there are gas-forming bacteria.[17]

Patients often have a medical history that is consistent with diabetes or alcoholism, both of which can contribute to the development of NF. Other forms of immunocompromise may lead to increased risk of NF as well. Increased awareness of the various subtypes of NF may help physicians recognize risk factors for NF development and understand the nuances of NF treatment.

Type 1: Polymicrobial

Polymicrobial infection is the most common bacterial pathology in NF. These infections are typically seen in patients who are at risk of infections, such as patients with diabetes, postoperative status, and organ dysfunction. These patients are more likely to have malodorous gas-forming infections. Anaerobic coverage is particularly important when initiating treatment.

Type 2: Group A *Streptococcus*

GAS infections may be seen in younger or healthier patients, but they can also be present in more classically at-risk patients (eg, patients with immunocompromise, intravenous drug use, organ failure, or postoperative status). These infections may also occur at typical sites (eg, extremities or wounds) or less commonly through hematogenous spread. Patients may present with toxic shock syndrome. Notably, clindamycin has been shown to be superior to penicillin in treating GAS infections.[3,18]

Type 3: Clostridial

Clostridium perfringens is often introduced through skin penetration, but it may also be introduced through hematogenous seeding or GI routes (eg, immunocompromised individuals and GI cancers). Consequently, *C. perfringens* can present in a variety of locations. This category of NF is characterized by a high occurrence of gas formation, which may be evident during the physical examination or through advanced imaging. Clindamycin has also demonstrated antitoxin effects in clostridial infections.[19,20]

Other

Less commonly, NF infections may be caused by *Vibrio vulnificus* or *Aeromonas hydrophila*. These infections may occur in patients who are exposed to seawater or fresh water during trauma, consume contaminated seafood, or have liver disease.

CRITICAL DECISION

How can physical examination and imaging findings be used to evaluate SSTIs and NF?

Physical Examination

Cellulitis

Cellulitis is hallmarked by a poorly demarcated, erythematous cutaneous eruption with swelling, palpable tenderness, and warmth. Patients may demonstrate systemic symptoms, such as fever, tachycardia, chills, and rigors.

NF

When considering NF, skin and other physical examination findings may not be evident early in the disease course because the fascial layers are deep; however, serial examinations demonstrating rapidly changing symptoms may aid in diagnosis. These patients are generally toxic appearing. Vital sign abnormalities (eg, fever [45% sensitive] and tachycardia) and septic shock with hypotension (21% sensitive) may be evident as well as systemic toxicity.[8]

Care must be taken to perform a thorough skin and soft tissue examination. Infection may be associated with skin breakdown from traumatic or surgical wounds, ulcerations, and injection sites. It is also possible to have hematogenous spread into many locations. Extremities often represent areas at risk of skin violation, but examination should also include less visible areas, such as the genitals, skinfolds, and areas commonly covered by clothing.

NF can be incredibly difficult to diagnose. A hallmark of NF is subjective pain out of proportion to the physical examination (90% sensitivity) with rapidly progressing symptoms since the infection spreads through the fascial plane and subcutaneous tissue. Similar to cellulitis, NF may display soft tissue swelling with poorly demarcated erythema, along with the presence of "skip lesions" (ie, patches of erythema) representing spread through tissue planes. The skin may be tender to palpation, and there may be minimal pain elicited on physical examination since severe tissue destruction may lead to insensate tissue. Other examination features include bullae, which may be hemorrhagic (25.3% sensitivity) or violaceous, and crepitus due to gas-forming pathogens and underlying tissue necrosis.[8]

The hallmark sign of the physical examination — and the only way to truly diagnose or rule out NF — is to directly visualize the fascial layer with surgical exploration.[8] After skin incision, the fascia may be explored by bluntly dissecting it with a finger or probe. Findings of NF include "dishwater-like" drainage, poor fascial layer integrity with a necrotic appearance,

✔ Pearls

- The only way to rule out NF is through surgical exploration of the fascia; no imaging modality or laboratory test has enough negative predictive value.
- In simple cellulitis without MRSA risk factors, there is no clinical benefit in supplementing standard streptococcal coverage with the addition of TMP-SMX.
- NF may present in a variety of patient populations, ranging from young and healthy to elderly with comorbidities, especially given the range of causative bacteria and routes of introduction.
- The mainstay of NF treatment is appropriate broad-spectrum antibiotic coverage, including clindamycin for toxin suppression, linezolid for toxin synthesis, or vancomycin for MRSA, and piperacillin-tazobactam.

and minimal bleeding. Although classically performed by a surgeon, emergency physicians and intensivists may perform a fascial cutdown in resource-limited settings.

Imaging

Although imaging may help differentiate SSTIs from other possible diagnoses, imaging is not required to make the diagnosis. Of particular importance is the use of imaging modalities to help with the diagnosis of life-threatening infections such as NF. However, definitive diagnosis or treatment should not be delayed while awaiting advanced imaging modalities since NF is a surgical diagnosis.

X-rays

Plain x-rays can demonstrate gas within soft tissues with a poor sensitivity of 48.9% and specificity of 94.0% (*Figure 3*).[8]

Ultrasound

A diagnosis of cellulitis may be supported with visualization of a "cobblestoning" appearance of subcutaneous tissue on ultrasound. An abscess may also be recognized with the identification of a hypoechoic or anechoic region, representing a fluid collection with swirling material contained within.

A diagnosis of NF can also be supported with ultrasound imaging. Fascial planes may appear thickened or irregular. There may also be fluid identified between the planes or "dirty shadowing," representing free air in subcutaneous tissues. The "champagne sign" demonstrates air bubbling in subcutaneous tissue from gas-forming infections.[21]

CT

CT imaging is likely the most useful imaging modality if it is immediately available and does not delay definitive treatment. However, even CT cannot be used to rule out NF, since it carries a sensitivity of 88.5% and specificity of 93.3%. CT may help surgical teams focus on areas of fascial exploration by identifying involved tissue (*Figures 4* and *5*).[8] Gas within soft tissues (as well

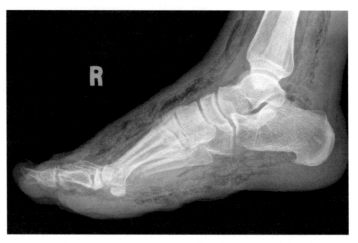

FIGURE 3. Lateral x-ray showing NF in a diabetic foot. *Credit:* Copyright 2022 Dr. Matt Skalski. Image courtesy of Dr. Matt Skalski and Radiopaedia.org, rID: 25026. Used under license.

as subcutaneous fluid, fat stranding, and fascial thickening) may be identified. Contrast-enhanced CT may aid in identification with lack of fascial enhancement due to tissue destruction.

MRI

From a radiographic standpoint, MRI is the gold standard imaging modality for NF because it is more sensitive (93%) than CT.[22,23] Although MRI may perform better than CT, it is clinically impractical and would likely lead to delays in timely patient care.

CRITICAL DECISION

What are the optimal treatment options for NF?

Standard Treatment Options

The mainstay of NF treatment is early and complete surgical debridement combined with antimicrobial therapy, close monitoring, and physiologic support.[5] Repeat

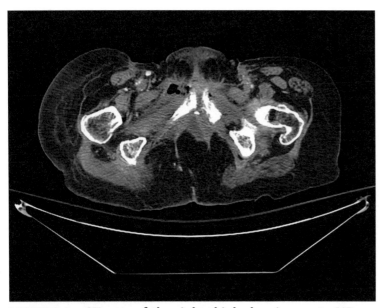

FIGURE 4. CT scan of the right thigh showing acute NF. Copyright 2022 Dr. Maxime St-Amant. Image courtesy of Dr. Maxime St-Amant and Radiopaedia.org, rID: 20377. Used under license.

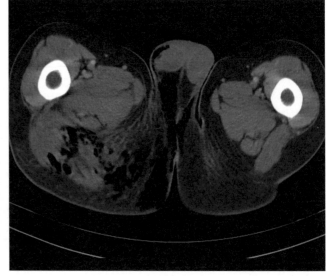

FIGURE 5. CT scan of the right thigh and perineum showing swelling and cellulitis. Copyright 2022 Dr. Chris O'Donnell. Image courtesy of Dr. Chris O'Donnell and Radiopaedia.org, rID: 16849. Used under license.

debridements may be necessary until all nonviable tissue has been resected (*Figure 6*). Any delay in treatment may cause extensive soft tissue loss and loss of limb. Amputation may be required to preempt further spread of the infection. Mortality rates can exceed 30% even with aggressive surgical treatment.

Broad-spectrum antibiotic coverage is also necessary for treating NF, including anaerobic coverage (see *Table 1*). A suggested approach is:

1. Linezolid 600 mg every 12 hours, **and** *either*

2. Piperacillin-tazobactam 4 g/500 mg IV every 6 hours or as an initial loading dose followed by 16 g/2 g over 24 hours as a continuous infusion and daptomycin 6 mg/kg per 24 hours, *or*

3. Piperacillin-tazobactam 4 g/500 mg IV every 6 hours or as an initial loading dose followed by 16 g/2 g over 24 hours as a continuous infusion and clindamycin 900 mg every 8 hours.[24]

Nonstandard Treatment Options

IVIG

Poly-specific intravenous immune globulin (IVIG) contains toxin-neutralizing antibodies. IVIG may be useful in type 2 NF because it has previously shown trends toward decreased mortality for GAS toxic shock syndrome and multisystem organ failure.[25,26] Literature suggests its utility in the treatment of NF by reducing the need for aggressive operative debridement and amputations.[27]

Hyperbaric Oxygen

Hyperbaric oxygen is theoretically helpful for anaerobically driven infections since oxygen is toxic to these categories of bacteria.[28] Hyperbaric oxygen is difficult to access and lacks good evidence for treatment benefit, but it can be considered in select patient populations.[29] A more feasible alternative for increased oxygen would be delivery with high FiO_2 on a ventilator, high-flow nasal cannula, or a nonrebreather mask paired with nasal cannula.

CRITICAL DECISION

What are some commonly held myths and practice patterns with SSTIs?

Vancomycin should always be given for MRSA coverage

Although vancomycin is effective and useful in a variety of roles, including coverage of MRSA SSTIs, other drugs

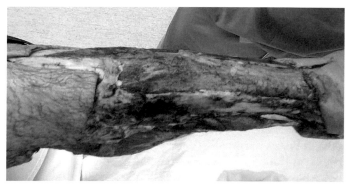

FIGURE 6. Lower leg after serial debridements of skin and fascia in NF. Contributed by Mark A. Dreyer, DPM, FACFAS. Manna B, Nahirniak P, Morrison CA. Wound debridement. In: *StatPearls [Internet]*. StatPearls Publishing; 2022.

may be more effective and should at least be considered based on the clinical context.

- **Vancomycin:** Vancomycin is effective against MRSA, especially with SSTIs. However, it is nephrotoxic, and higher levels require frequent monitoring of drug levels.

- **Linezolid:** Linezolid has benefits of toxin suppression for community-acquired MRSA and toxic shock syndrome, and it may be more effective than vancomycin. Additionally, there is no nephrotoxicity since it is hepatically cleared, in contrast to vancomycin. Linezolid may also have an increasing role as vancomycin resistance builds.[30,31]

- **Daptomycin:** Daptomycin is particularly effective in bacteremia as well as in SSTIs. It can be used for MRSA endocarditis but is ineffective against pneumonia.

- **Clindamycin:** Clindamycin can be used for MRSA coverage in addition to GAS and *Clostridium* toxin suppression.

- **TMP-SMX:** TMP-SMX is effective for skin-based MRSA infections but is less effective than vancomycin for MRSA bacteremia.[32]

- **Doxycycline:** Doxycycline is effective in community-acquired pneumonia with MRSA and atypical coverage in addition to staphylococcal SSTIs.

- **Rifampin and tigecycline are less commonly indicated for MRSA coverage.**

All uncomplicated cellulitis requires MRSA coverage

Although the utility of local antibiograms and resistance patterns should always be kept in mind, individual patient risk for MRSA should be considered, rather than covering every patient for MRSA. Studies have shown that uncomplicated cellulitis does not have higher rates of clinical resolution when comparing cephalexin to cephalexin plus TMP-SMX.[3] However, when dealing with small, simple abscesses (purulent SSTI) with overlying cellulitis, the addition of oral antibiotics with MRSA coverage after incision and drainage should be considered to improve cure rates.[33]

✖ Pitfalls

- Failing to perform an extensive skin examination, including the sacrum and perineum, especially on altered or sick patients exhibiting appropriate concern for pain out of proportion to examination.

- Believing that all simple cellulitis requires MRSA coverage, even if the patient lacks specific risk factors or signs of systemic illness.

- Relying on laboratory work, imaging studies, or physical examination findings to rule out NF.

A single dose of vancomycin IV should be given to patients discharged on oral antibiotics

Many emergency physicians continue to administer a single dose of vancomycin IV prior to discharging a patient home with oral antibiotics for cellulitis. However, there is no evidence of any benefit to this practice, and it is not recommended by the IDSA. Within 12 hours of a normal loading dose of 15 mg/kg or 1 g, serum vancomycin levels remain subtherapeutic in 97% of patients.[34] Administration could easily lead to patient harm in the form of increased bacterial resistance to vancomycin, prolonged emergency department stays, and increased health care costs.

The LRINEC score can be used to distinguish NF from other SSTIs

The Laboratory Risk Indicator for Necrotizing Fasciitis (LRINEC) scoring tool has been widely used; however, its use can be dangerous because it may give false reassurance and inappropriately rule out a life- and limb-threatening diagnosis. Studies have shown that as many as 63.8% of patients with known NF had a LRINEC score ≤5 (a cutoff of 6 is recommended to rule in NF).[35] Additionally, a LRINEC score ≥6 (the cutoff recommended to rule in NF) had a sensitivity of only 68.2%, and a score ≥8 showed only 40.8% sensitivity.[8]

Use single-dose intravenous antibiotics for cellulitis

Although prior studies have debunked the myth that one dose of vancomycin IV is beneficial for patients discharged on oral antibiotics for cellulitis, recent literature suggests decreased patient hospitalization rates after a single dose of dalbavancin IV (a long-acting antibiotic, unlike vancomycin) in the emergency department.[36] Use of dalbavancin IV may be appropriate in emergency departments with an established clinical pathway, including close patient follow-up after its administration. However, it is not currently a widely accessible medication.

Summary

Cellulitis and NF refer to a broad spectrum of illnesses. The diagnosis of these conditions is greatly aided by careful physical examination, appropriate imaging, and clinical gestalt to guide appropriate treatment options and disposition. Given the high mortality for NF, expedited diagnosis, treatment, and disposition should be prioritized as much as possible. If the patient's history, physical examination, and risk factors are highly suspicious for NF, then rapid support of the patient with early broad-spectrum antibiotics and surgical consultation for operating room exploration and ICU monitoring are warranted.

REFERENCES

1. May L, Klein EY, Martinez EM, Mojica N, Miller LG. Incidence and factors associated with emergency department visits for recurrent skin and soft tissue infections in patients in California, 2005–2011. *Epidemiol Infect.* 2017;145(4):746-754.

2. Long B, Gottlieb M. Diagnosis and management of cellulitis and abscess in the emergency department setting: an evidence-based review. *J Emerg Med.* 2022;62(1):16-27.

3. Stevens DL, Bisno AL, Chambers HF, et al; Infectious Diseases Society of America. Practice guidelines for the diagnosis and management of skin and soft tissue infections: 2014 update by the Infectious Diseases Society of America [published correction appears in *Clin Infect Dis.* 2015;60(9):1448]. *Clin Infect Dis.* 2014;59(2):e10-e52.

4. Puvanendran R, Huey JC, Pasupathy S. Necrotizing fasciitis. *Can Fam Physician.* 2009;55(10):981-987.

5. Hussein QA, Anaya DA. Necrotizing soft tissue infections. *Crit Care Clin.* 2013;29(4):795-806.

6. Magala J, Makobore P, Makumbi T, Kaggwa S, Kalanzi E, Galukande M. The clinical presentation and early outcomes of necrotizing fasciitis in a Ugandan tertiary hospital—a prospective study. *BMC Res Notes.* 2014 Jul 28;7(1):476.

7. Khalid M, Junejo S, Mir F. Invasive community acquired methicillin-resistant Staphylococcal aureus (CA-MRSA) infections in children. *J Coll Physicians Surg Pak.* 2018;28(09):S174-S177.

8. Fernando SM, Tran A, Cheng W, et al. Necrotizing soft tissue infection: diagnostic accuracy of physical examination, imaging, and LRINEC score: a systematic review and meta-analysis. *Ann Surg.* 2019;269(1):58-65.

9. Sullivan T, de Barra E. Diagnosis and management of cellulitis. *Clin Med (Lond).* 2018;18(2):160-163.

10. Raff AB, Kroshinsky D. Cellulitis: a review. *JAMA.* 2016;316(3):325-327.

11. Pallin DJ, Camargo CA, Schuur JD. Skin infections and antibiotic stewardship: analysis of emergency department prescribing practices, 2007–2010. *West J Emerg Med.* 2014;15(3):282-289.

12. Klein E, Smith DL, Laxminarayan R. Community-associated methicillin-resistant *Staphylococcus aureus* in outpatients, United States, 1999-2006. *Emerg Infect Dis.* 2009;15(12):1925-1930.

13. Kourtis AP, Hatfield K, Baggs J, et al. Vital signs: epidemiology and recent trends in methicillin-resistant and in methicillin-susceptible Staphylococcus aureus bloodstream infections — United States. *MMWR Morb Mortal Wkly Rep.* 2019;68(9):214-219.

14. Moran GJ, Krishnadasan A, Mower WR, et al. Effect of cephalexin plus trimethoprim-sulfamethoxazole vs cephalexin alone on clinical cure of uncomplicated cellulitis: a randomized clinical trial. *JAMA.* 2017;317(20):2088-2096.

15. McCreary EK, Heim ME, Schulz LT, Hoffman R, Pothof J, Fox B. Top 10 myths regarding the diagnosis and treatment of cellulitis. *J Emerg Med.* 2017;53(4):485-492.

16. Pulia MS, Calderone MR, Meister JR, Santistevan J, May L. Update on management of skin and soft tissue infections in the emergency department. *Curr Infect Dis Rep.* 2014;16(9):418.

17. Erichsen Andersson A, Egerod I, Knudsen VE, Fagerdahl AM. Signs, symptoms and diagnosis of necrotizing fasciitis experienced by survivors and family: a qualitative Nordic multi-center study. *BMC Infect Dis.* 2018;18(1):429.

18. Zimbelman J, Palmer A, Todd J. Improved outcome of clindamycin compared with beta-lactam antibiotic treatment for invasive *Streptococcus pyogenes* infection. *Pediatr Infect Dis J.* 1999;18(12):1096-1100.

19. Bryant AE, Stevens DL. Clostridial myonecrosis: new insights in pathogenesis and management. *Curr Infect Dis Rep.* 2010;12(5):383-391.

20. Stevens DL, Maier KA, Mitten JE. Effect of antibiotics on toxin production and viability of *Clostridium perfringens. Antimicrob Agents Chemother.* 1987;31(2):213-218.

CASE RESOLUTIONS

■ CASE ONE

In addition to empiric linezolid and piperacillin-tazobactam, clindamycin was ordered along with an immediate urology and surgery consultation due to high clinical concern for Fournier gangrene. The elderly man remained hypotensive and encephalopathic after fluid resuscitation, and he required vasopressors for hemodynamic support. Due to the extent of tissue necrosis throughout the perineum, he was immediately taken to the operating room for surgical exploration and debridement. After a prolonged ICU stay requiring repeated debridements, the patient was able to return to his skilled nursing facility after 3 weeks.

■ CASE TWO

The 32-year-old woman's examination findings were concerning for simple cellulitis. Upon further discussion, she revealed that she frequently shaves her legs and often gets small cuts and abrasions from her razor. Given her lack of medical comorbidities and normal vital signs, neither laboratory studies nor additional imaging was indicated. She was discharged home with a 5-day course of cephalexin and instructions to follow-up with her primary care physician that week. Ultimately, she demonstrated improvement and resolution without any further issues.

■ CASE THREE

Due to concern for drug-seeking behavior and malingering, the 25-year-old man was discharged without any further workup or treatment. Approximately 5 hours later, the same man presented via EMS after being found unresponsive on a sidewalk 1 mile from the hospital. EMS did not notice anything suspicious at the scene but states that he groaned whenever they tried to stimulate him. His vital signs were notable for tachycardia, hypotension, and a Glasgow coma scale score of 8. Due to his rapid clinical decline, the man was intubated, resuscitated, and stabilized, and broad-spectrum antibiotics were given.

While performing the secondary survey, the nurse noted scattered bullae throughout his lower right extremity and edema that was not present on his prior presentation. The patient was not deemed stable enough for imaging studies, and surgery was consulted due to concern for NF. He was immediately taken to the operating room for debridement. In the operating room, the diagnosis of NF was confirmed. During the next week, the patient required prolonged intubation due to vasopressor requirements and septic shock, and the decision was eventually made to amputate his leg given the extensive tissue loss. After a 4-week hospital stay, he was discharged to a rehabilitation facility.

21. Castleberg E, Jenson N, Dinh VA. Diagnosis of necrotizing fasciitis with bedside ultrasound: the STAFF Exam. *West J Emerg Med.* 2014;15(1):111-113.

22. Kim KT, Kim YJ, Won Lee J, et al. Can necrotizing infectious fasciitis be differentiated from nonnecrotizing infectious fasciitis with MR imaging? *Radiology.* 2011;259(3):816-824.

23. Tso DK, Singh AK. Necrotizing fasciitis of the lower extremity: imaging pearls and pitfalls. *Br J Radiol.* 2018;91(1088):20180093.

24. Wallace HA, Perera TB. Necrotizing fasciitis. In: *StatPearls [Internet].* StatPearls Publishing, 2021 Jul 27. https://www.ncbi.nlm.nih.gov/books/NBK430756/

25. Darenberg J, Söderquist B, Normark BH, Norrby-Teglund A. Differences in potency of intravenous polyspecific immunoglobulin G against streptococcal and staphylococcal superantigens: implications for therapy of toxic shock syndrome. *Clin Infect Dis.* 2004;38(6):836-842.

26. Stevens DL, Bryant AE, Goldstein EJ. Necrotizing soft tissue infections. *Infect Dis Clin North Am.* 2021;35(1):135-155.

27. Norrby-Teglund A, Muller MP, Mcgeer A, et al. Successful management of severe group A streptococcal soft tissue infections using an aggressive medical regimen including intravenous polyspecific immunoglobulin together with a conservative surgical approach. *Scand J Infect Dis.* 2005;37(3):166-172.

28. Eckmann C, Montravers P. Current management of necrotizing soft-tissue infections. *Curr Opin Infect Dis.* 2021;34(2):89-95.

29. Levett D, Bennett MH, Millar I. Adjunctive hyperbaric oxygen for necrotizing fasciitis. *Cochrane Database Syst Rev.* 2015;1(1):CD007937.

30. Yue J, Dong BR, Yang M, Chen X, Wu T, Liu GJ. Linezolid versus vancomycin for skin and soft tissue infections. *Cochrane Database Syst Rev.* 2013;(1):CD008056.

31. Tessier JM, Sanders J, Sartelli M, et al. Necrotizing soft tissue infections: a focused review of pathophysiology, diagnosis, operative management, antimicrobial therapy, and pediatrics. *Surg Infect (Larchmt).* 2020;21(2):81-93.

32. Goldberg E, Paul M, Talker O, et al. Co-trimoxazole versus vancomycin for the treatment of methicillin-resistant Staphylococcus aureus bacteraemia: a retrospective cohort study. *J Antimicrob Chemother.* 2010;65(8):1779-1783.

33. Gottlieb M, DeMott JM, Hallock M, Peksa GD. Systemic antibiotics for the treatment of skin and soft tissue abscesses: a systematic review and meta-analysis. *Ann Emerg Med.* 2019;73(1):8-16.

34. Rosini JM, Laughner J, Levine BJ, Papas MA, Reinhardt JF, Jasani NB. A randomized trial of loading vancomycin in the emergency department. *Ann Pharmacother.* 2015;49(1):6-13.

35. Neeki MM, Dong F, Au C, et al. Evaluating the laboratory risk indicator to differentiate cellulitis from necrotizing fasciitis in the emergency department. *West J Emerg Med.* 2017;18(4):684-689.

36. Talan DA, Mower WR, Lovecchio FA, et al. Pathway with single-dose long-acting intravenous antibiotic reduces emergency department hospitalizations of patients with skin infections. *Acad Emerg Med.* 2021;28(10):1108-1117.

ADDITIONAL REFERENCE

1. LRINEC score for necrotizing soft tissue infection. MDCalc. https://www.mdcalc.com/lrinec-score-necrotizing-soft-tissue-infection

Spontaneous Splenic Rupture in Infectious Mononucleosis

By Sarah Young, MD
Prisma Health, University of South Carolina
College of Medicine, Greenville

Reviewed by Sharon E. Mace, MD, FACEP

Objective

On completion of this article, you should be able to:

- Determine how to manage pediatric patients with splenomegaly in infectious mononucleosis.

CASE PRESENTATION

A 14-year-old girl presents with generalized abdominal pain and nonbloody, nonbilious vomiting for the last 18 hours. She has no preceding illnesses, fever, symptoms of upper respiratory infection, or diarrhea. She is currently menstruating but denies menorrhagia. She also knows of no exposures to sick contacts. Initially, she presented to an outside hospital and was diagnosed with a mild transaminitis and new anemia at 8.2 g/dL (down from 12 g/dL 3 months ago). She was transferred to the pediatric emergency department for evaluation of biliary pathologies, including cholecystitis.

Her vital signs are BP 104/60, P 88, R 18, and T 36.7°C (98.1°F) orally; SpO_2 is 98% on room air. Her abdomen is soft and mildly tender to palpation in the bilateral lower quadrants and epigastric region with no peritoneal signs. CBC shows a hemoglobin level of 6.7 g/dL and leukocytosis at 13.7 with 78% lymphocytes. Ultrasound of the right upper quadrant, appendix, and pelvis is notable for a large amount of free fluid and an enlarged spleen (*Figure 1*). The patient's repeat vital signs on return from ultrasound include BP 100/69, P 94, and R 23; SpO_2 is 98% on room air. Pediatric surgery is consulted due to concern for splenic rupture, and Epstein-Barr virus (EBV) testing is added. CT of the abdomen and pelvis confirm a ruptured spleen (*Figure 2*). Monospot results are positive.

Discussion

The most common cause of splenomegaly in children is infection, particularly infectious mononucleosis (IM). IM is most often caused by an EBV infection. The incidence of EBV infection is high across the population, although it is often seen with no signs or symptoms, as in this case. Approximately 90% to 95% of adults test EBV seropositive, with the incidence of IM highest in patients aged 15 to 24 years. Only 10% of children with an EBV infection are symptomatic.[1]

Classic signs and symptoms of IM are fever, fatigue, pharyngitis, and lymphadenopathy.[2] Common laboratory abnormalities are atypical lymphocytosis with an overall leukocytosis and a benign limited transaminitis. Splenomegaly is seen in approximately 50% to 60% of patients with IM. Splenomegaly can be seen as early as day 4 and as late as 8 weeks from infection, but it most commonly occurs about 14 days after symptom onset.[3] Treatment for IM is the same as for other viral respiratory illnesses, with the primary focus on supportive care and symptom management.

Splenic rupture is a feared complication of splenomegaly in IM. Rupture occurs spontaneously (ie, with no identifiable trauma to the abdomen) in approximately half of all cases.[3] About 70% of all splenic rupture cases occur in men.[4] As in other splenic injuries, management favors supportive care and close observation. In rare cases, a splenectomy is required. Although potentially life-threatening, fatalities are quite rare.[5] These patients require serial abdominal examinations and trending of hemoglobin and hematocrit (H/H). They may require blood transfusions and should be monitored and treated in close consultation with surgical colleagues.

After identification of IM with or without splenomegaly, education and instruction to the patient and family on

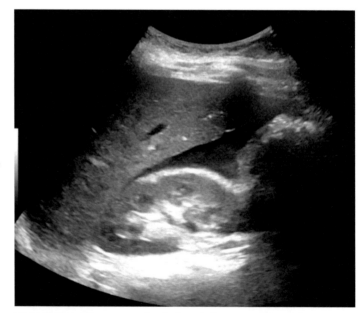

FIGURE 1. Ultrasound of the right upper quadrant showing an anechoic fluid collection in the hepatorenal recess and at the liver tip, which is consistent with a positive FAST examination and free fluid in the abdomen

activity restriction is crucial. Because most IM cases are seen in teenagers and young adults, these patients are commonly involved in sports and strenuous activities. All patients should refrain from activities during the early stages of the illness. Because splenic rupture is most common in the first 4 weeks after symptom onset, avoidance of all sports is recommended until at least 3 to 4 weeks have passed. At that time, consideration can be given to a gradual resumption of lower-impact, noncontact sports, with a return to contact sports and other strenuous activity after a minimum of 4 weeks.[6] Chronic fatigue noted by these patients can also limit their ability to perform physical activities, and it is recommended that activities advance slowly as tolerated by the patient. This process may take 3 to 4 months for competitive and elite athletes.[7]

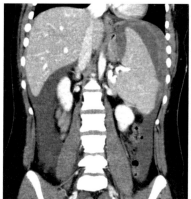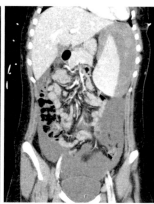

FIGURE 2. Coronal CT views of the abdomen and pelvis demonstrating hemoperitoneum (grade 3), an enlarged spleen at 14 cm, and an acute subcapsular splenic hematoma from the grade 2 splenic laceration

CASE RESOLUTION

The patient was admitted to the pediatric ICU for serial abdominal examinations and trending of her H/H. She received two total units of packed RBCs. She was monitored closely for hemodynamic decompensation for approximately 72 hours with serial abdominal examinations that were reassuring. Her H/H remained stable with no further transfusions required. At discharge, she had minimal abdominal pain, and her primary symptom was fatigue. She was seen in the pediatric surgery clinic 2 weeks after discharge. She had persistent fatigue and pallor but no recurrence of her abdominal pain. She had one final repeat hemoglobin check that was stable. She was started on an iron-containing multivitamin and discharged from the surgery clinic with routine primary care follow-up.

REFERENCES

1. Macsween KF, Johannessen I. Epstein-Barr virus (EBV): infectious mononucleosis and other nonmalignant EBV-associated diseases. In: Kaslow RA, Stanberry LR, Le Duc JW, eds. *Viral Infections of Humans: Epidemiology and Control.* 5th ed. Springer;2014:867-896.
2. Luzuriaga K, Sullivan JL. Infectious mononucleosis. *N Engl J Med.* 2010;362(21):1993-2000.
3. Gayer G, Zandman-Goddard G, Kosych E, Apter, S. Spontaneous rupture of the spleen detected on CT as the initial manifestation of infectious mononucleosis. *Emerg Radiol.* 2003;10(1):51-52.
4. Bartlett A, Williams R, Hilton M. Splenic rupture in infectious mononucleosis: a systematic review of published case reports. *Injury.* 2016;47(3):531-538.
5. Asgari MM, Begos DG. Spontaneous splenic rupture in infectious mononucleosis: a review. *Yale J Biol Med.* 1997;70(2):175-182.
6. Auwaerter PG. Infectious mononucleosis: return to play. *Clin Sports Med.* 2004;23(3):485-497.
7. Noffsinger J. Physical activity considerations in children and adolescents with viral infections. *Pediatr Ann.* 1996;25(10):585-589.

The Literature Review
Pulmonary Embolism

By Lachlan Driver, MD;
and Andrew J. Eyre, MD, MSHPEd
Harvard Affiliated Emergency Medicine Residency,
Boston, Massachusetts

Objective

On completion of this article, you should be able to:

■ Interpret D-dimer and Wells score results to determine when patients need further testing for a pulmonary embolism.

Kearon C, de Wit K, Parpia S, et al. Diagnosis of pulmonary embolism with D-dimer adjusted to clinical probability. *N Eng J Med.* 2019 Nov 28;381(22):2125-2134.

KEY POINTS

■ D-dimer testing can be used in combination with the Wells score risk stratification tool to differentiate patients in need of testing to rule out PE.

■ This prospective study of 2,017 outpatients in Canada showed that there were no VTEs during a 3-month follow-up period for participants with a low or medium risk of PE per the Wells score, with D-dimer levels less than 1,000 ng/mL for low-risk patients and 500 ng/mL for medium-risk patients, who did not receive CTPA or AC therapy.

■ This strategy resulted in a small reduction in the use of chest imaging as compared to the strategy used in the YEARS study and a greater reduction in chest imaging as compared to the age-adjusted cutoff strategy, with an average of 17.6% fewer CTPAs in the low-risk and low–D-dimer category compared to the standard approach.

D-dimer diagnostic tests can be used to determine which patients require further testing, such as CT pulmonary angiography (CTPA), to evaluate for the presence of a pulmonary embolism (PE). Past retrospective studies have shown that a D-dimer level under 1,000 ng/mL is sufficient to rule out a PE in those with a low clinical pretest probability (C-PTP), while a D-dimer level under 500 ng/mL is sufficient to rule out a PE in those with a moderate C-PTP.

This prospective study enrolled 2,017 adult outpatients from Canadian emergency departments or clinics who had a history concerning for PE. Subsequently, physicians used the Wells clinical prediction rule to categorize patients into low-, moderate-, and high-risk C-PTP categories. Those patients with a low or moderate C-PTP underwent D-dimer serum testing. If patients had a low C-PTP with a D-dimer level less than 1,000 ng/mL or if patients had a medium C-PTP with a D-dimer level less than 500 ng/mL, no further testing was performed, and these patients did not receive anticoagulation (AC) therapy. Otherwise, all other patients (ie, those with elevated D-dimers for their risk categories and those with a high C-PTP) underwent CTPA. Patients only received AC therapy if a PE was found on CTPA. All patients in the study were followed for 3 months to evaluate for further venous thromboembolisms (VTEs).

In total, 7.4% of the 2,017 patients enrolled in this Pulmonary Embolism Graduated D-Dimer (PEGeD) diagnostic strategy had a PE on initial testing and thus received AC therapy. A total of 1,285 patients had a low C-PTP with a D-dimer level less than 1,000 ng/mL, and 40 patients had a moderate C-PTP with a D-dimer level less than 500 ng/mL. None of these patients had a VTE during the 3-month follow-up period (95% confidence interval [CI], 0.00 to 0.29). By contrast, of the 1,863 patients who did not have a PE on initial workup, only one subsequently had a VTE (0.05%; 95% CI, 0.01 to 0.30).

Using the PEGeD diagnostic strategy for outpatient encounters, 34.3% of patients received CTPA. Using the standard approach, where a PE is ruled out using a combination of a low C-PTP and a D-dimer level less than 500 ng/mL, would have resulted in using CTPA in 51.9% of patients (a difference of –17.6 percentage points; 95% CI, –19.2 to –15.9). Additionally, the PEGeD strategy resulted in a small decrease in the use of CT imaging compared to the YEARS strategy (–2.0 percentage points; 95% CI, –2.8 to –1.2), while the PEGeD strategy resulted in a somewhat greater reduction in CTPA as compared to the age-adjusted cutoff strategy (–8.6 percentage points; 95% CI, –10.0 to –7.2).

In summary, with CTPAs having associated risks, including contrast reactions, increased radiation exposure, increased cost, and increased lengths of stay, multiple decision-making tools can be used to evaluate patients who are at low risk of PE. The PEGeD strategy uses a combination of the Wells score and specific D-dimer cutoffs for low- and medium-risk patients and resulted in no VTEs in these patients during a 3-month follow-up period. Additionally, it resulted in less imaging compared to both the age-adjusted cutoff strategy and the YEARS strategy as well as compared to the standard approach of using a low C-PTP and a D-dimer level less than 500 ng/mL.

Critical Decisions in Emergency Medicine's series of LLSA reviews features articles from ABEM's 2022 Lifelong Learning and Self-Assessment Reading List. Available online at acep.org/moc/llsa and on the ABEM website.

14 *Critical Decisions in Emergency Medicine*

Negative Pressure Wound Therapy Application

By Steven J. Warrington, MD, MEd, MS
MercyOne Siouxland, Sioux City, Iowa

Objective

On completion of this article, you should be able to:

■ Apply a new negative pressure wound therapy dressing for patients with existing devices and dressings.

Introduction

It is not uncommon to see patients with negative pressure wound therapy (NPWT) devices, or vacuum-assisted devices, in the emergency department (*Figure 1*). At times, these patients present solely for issues with these dressings. Understanding how to apply a new NPWT dressing for patients with existing devices and dressings can lead to quick visits for patients and less stress for emergency physicians.

Contraindications
■ Thick exudates
■ Purulent drainage
■ Necrotic wounds
■ Visible large vascular structures or viscera

Benefits and Risks

The benefits of NPWT relate to expediting and improving wound healing. Exactly how NPWT improves wound healing is undergoing active research, and multiple mechanisms have been

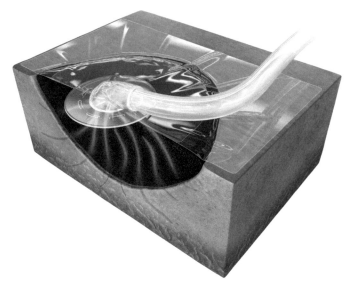

FIGURE 1. Negative pressure wound therapy setup. *Credit:* ACEP.

TECHNIQUE

1. **Obtain** the materials, such as the reticulated foam sponge, occlusive dressing material, vacuum or suction tubing, scissors to trim the sponge to size, and any saline, cleansers, or personal protective equipment required.
2. **Consider** instilling saline through the tubing if there is concern the sponge removal may be difficult.
3. **Remove** the existing dressing. If the sponge is adhered to tissue, apply saline and allow it to sit for 5 to 10 minutes.
4. **Cleanse** the wound bed and surrounding tissue. Consider gentle irrigation and wiping with gauze. Tweezers may be beneficial if small pieces of sponge need to be removed from the wound.
5. **Cleanse** and dry the periwound area.
6. **Consider** applying an initial layer of adhesive occlusive dressing trimmed to the healthy tissue surrounding the wound. This may take multiple pieces of dressing. Doing so can help protect the healthy tissue and provide a better seal.
7. **Cut** the foam into the shape of the wound. If the wound is deep, multiple pieces of foam may be required; when the vacuum is applied to the top of the foam, it should be approximately level with the periwound area. Consider basing the number of foam pieces on how many pieces were just removed from the previous dressing.
8. **Place** the cut foam into the wound.
9. **Place** the adherent occlusive dressing over the sponge and wound. It should extend past all edges of the wound margin by a half inch.
10. **Cut** a 1- to 2-cm hole in the top adhesive dressing over the middle of the foam.
11. **Apply** the vacuum tubing over the hole that was just created.
12. **Connect** the vacuum tubing to the system and activate it to ensure a seal.
13. **Label** the dressing with the date, time, and number of foam pieces. Document details of the wound and dressing as indicated.

suggested, such as increasing perfusion, decreasing bacterial rate, and altering the wound environment. Risks are relatively minimal if contraindications are noted.

A primary risk is that the sponge placed over regular tissue may cause maceration and weaken or damage the periwound area. Risks associated with application when there is thick exudate, purulent drainage, or necrotic tissue are related to the sponge becoming clogged and the device not functioning as intended. Finally, the most severe risk is adhesion of the sponge to vascular structures or viscera, if present, which can remove layers of tissue and cause hemorrhage and trauma.

Delay in changing the sponge can also result in risks to patients. The risks range from toxic shock syndrome to tissue growth adhering to the sponge and creating trauma to the wound when it is eventually changed.

Alternatives

The procedure suggested is to replace the dressing, including the sponge, adhesive occlusive dressing, and appropriate connection with the vacuum tubing. The primary alternatives include turning the task over to someone with more experience (eg, some institutions have dedicated nursing staff available), admitting the patient for replacement and additional needs, or discharging them to have the dressing replaced at another location.

Reducing Side Effects

Cleansing the wound when changing the dressing may help wound healing and can be done with saline, wound cleanser, or gentle wiping with gauze. Ensuring the wound has been adequately prepped and the sponge is the appropriate size for the wound can reduce the risk of injuring the periwound area. Using appropriate personal protective equipment may help reduce the risk of pathogen exposure to physicians.

Special Considerations

Different types of sponges are available for use, but black reticulated polyurethane ether foam sponges are the most common. A denser white foam made of polyvinyl alcohol is also available and can be used when tougher sponges are required, such as when there is tunneling present. Additionally, sponges impregnated with silver are available when there is concern for bacterial counts.

If the existing dressing is difficult to remove, moisten the foam and allow it to sit for 5 to 10 minutes. Alternatively, consider instilling saline through the tubing while the existing dressing is present and allowing it to sit.

In wounds with vascular structures or viscera exposed, apply a petroleum gauze over the structure to create a barrier between the structure and the sponge.

Pelvic Fractures With Urethral Injury

By William Perkins, MD; and Victor Huang, MD, CAQ-SM
NewYork-Presbyterian Queens

Reviewed by John Kiel, DO, MPH

Objective

On completion of this article, you should be able to:
- Assess and manage a pelvic fracture with a urethral injury.

CASE PRESENTATION

A 45-year-old man presents with severe suprapubic pain after being thrown from a forklift at work. On examination, he is hemodynamically stable, and his pelvis is stable. However, there is significant pelvic tenderness to palpation and blood at the urethral meatus.

Introduction

The bony pelvis is composed of five main elements: the ilium, ischium, pubis, sacrum, and coccyx. These are held together by strong ligaments. Fractures or ligamentous disruptions indicate a high-energy mechanism of injury. Mortality for pelvic fractures is around 10% to 13% and, if unstable, up to 50%.[1]

Pelvic fractures can be broken down into three different types: single bone fractures, acetabular fractures, and pelvic ring fractures. Single bone fractures are most common, particularly pubic rami fractures. Acetabular fractures are less common overall, but most likely involve the posterior wall. Meanwhile, pelvic ring fractures have the highest mortality and are often associated with venous plexus or arterial injury.[2]

The Young-Burgess classification system differentiates types of pelvic ring fractures based on the primary mechanism as well as the extent of injury and instability. The three main patterns of injury by mechanism are lateral compression (LC), anterior-posterior compression (APC), and vertical shear (VS). LC and APC are further subdivided into three classes based on the severity of the injury.[1]

Mechanism of Injury

Pelvic fractures are seen in a bimodal distribution. Young men are more likely to suffer from high-energy trauma, such as a motor vehicle crash, and elderly women predisposed to osteoporosis are more likely to suffer pelvic fractures after a low-energy mechanism, such as a fall from standing.[3]

Common mechanisms associated with pelvic ring fractures can be delineated by fracture pattern. LC and APC fractures are commonly seen in rollover motor vehicle crashes or in pedestrians struck by motor vehicles. VS is more common with motor vehicle crashes or falls from a height where a significant force is transmitted upward through the lower extremities to the pelvis.[4]

Physical Examination

Tenderness to palpation of the pelvis and hips is expected. Pelvic stability should be evaluated with manual compression to the bilateral iliac crests. The abdomen and perineum should be examined for ecchymosis and associated injuries. A rectal examination is important to check for gross blood, tone, and sensation to assess for visceral and neurologic injury. Although patients often have pain or difficulty moving one or both lower extremities, each lower limb should be thoroughly inspected to identify other possible associated fractures or neurovascular injuries.[5]

Imaging

In a critical trauma setting, there may only be time for a portable anterior-posterior (AP) pelvic x-ray, which reveals 90% of pelvic injuries (*Figure 1*).[5] It is important to look for any discontinuity in the "rings and lines" to assess for fractures, including the three pelvic rings; the iliopectineal, ilioischial, Shenton, and arcuate lines; the anterior and posterior walls; and the roof of the acetabulum. Other views can be used to isolate different parts of the bony pelvis, including inlet, outlet, and Judet views.[2]

Because the pelvis is a complicated three-dimensional structure, CT is often preferred over multiple x-rays to better identify bony injuries and to aid in operative planning. CT can also be used to evaluate for associated injuries like retroperitoneal and intraperitoneal injuries.[5]

A retrograde urethrogram should be performed in men with pelvic trauma and blood at the urethral meatus, gross hematuria, difficulty voiding, perineal bruising, or a boggy prostate (*Figures 2* and *3*). A cystogram should be performed after ruling

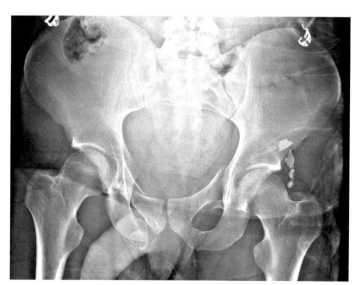

FIGURE 1. AP view of the pelvis demonstrating bilateral pubic rami fractures. *Credit:* Copyright 2022 Dr. Andrew Dixon. Image courtesy of Dr. Andrew Dixon and Radiopaedia.org, rID: 31674. Used under license.

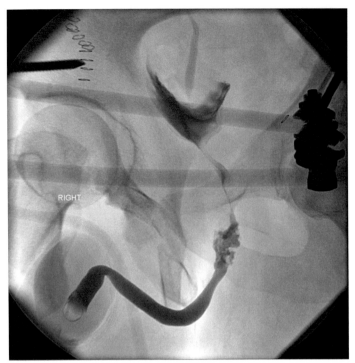

FIGURE 2. Retrograde urethrogram demonstrating urethral disruption and contrast extravasation at the posterior urethra. *Credit:* Copyright 2022 Dr. Andrew Dixon. Image courtesy of Dr. Andrew Dixon and Radiopaedia.org, rID: 31648. Used under license.

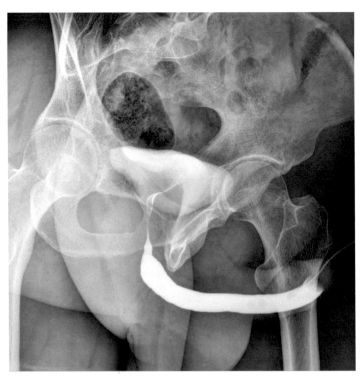

FIGURE 3. Retrograde urethrogram without extravasation. *Credit:* Copyright 2022 Dr. MT Niknejad. Image courtesy of Dr. MT Niknejad and Radiopaedia.org, rID: 92046. Used under license.

out a urethral injury. Extravasation of contrast during these studies is suggestive of a urethral or bladder injury, and urology should be consulted.[6]

Emergency Department Management

Physicians should start with advanced trauma life support and remember that pelvic fractures are indicative of a high-energy mechanism that necessitates a systematic evaluation for other injuries. A pelvic binder should be placed at the level of the greater trochanters for hypotensive pelvic fractures, particularly APC injuries. LC injuries have the potential to be exaggerated

if a pelvic binder is placed too tightly.[2,7] VS injuries can be stabilized with skeletal traction.[5] Many of these patients require resuscitation with blood products, angiography and embolization with interventional radiology, or external fixation.[2,5]

Definitive Management

Stable fractures, including pubic rami fractures, APC I, and LC I injuries, may be treated nonoperatively with protected weight bearing and physical therapy. Unstable fracture patterns such as APC II-III, LC II-III, and VS require surgical management with open reduction and internal fixation.[2]

CASE RESOLUTION

In addition to bilateral pubic rami fractures, a posterior urethral injury was identified on retrograde urethrogram. CT imaging was performed, and it ruled out any additional injuries. The patient was taken to the operating room by orthopedics and urology. He underwent open reduction and internal fixation for the pubic rami fractures. Urology initially placed a suprapubic catheter but was subsequently able to insert a Foley catheter over a guidewire.

REFERENCES

1. Manson T, O'Toole RV, Whitney A, Duggan B, Sciadini M, Nascone J. Young-Burgess classification of pelvic ring fractures: does it predict mortality, transfusion requirements, and non-orthopaedic injuries? *J Orthop Trauma.* 2010;24(10):603-609.
2. Perry K, Mabrouk A, Chauvin BJ. Pelvic ring injuries. In: *StatPearls [Internet].* StatPearls Publishing; 2021. Accessed May 17, 2022. https://www.ncbi.nlm.nih.gov/books/NBK544330/
3. Wong JML, Bucknill A. Fractures of the pelvic ring. *Injury.* 2017;48(4):795-802.
4. Griffin DR, Starr AJ, Reinert CM, Jones AL, Whitlock S. Vertically unstable pelvic fractures fixed with percutaneous iliosacral screws: does posterior injury pattern predict fixation failure? *J Orthop Trauma.* 2006;20(suppl 1):S30-S36.
5. Davis DD, Foris LA, Kane SM, Waseem M. Pelvic fracture. In: *StatPearls [Internet].* StatPearls Publishing; 2021. Accessed May 17, 2022. https://www.ncbi.nlm.nih.gov/books/NBK430734/
6. Uehara DT, Eisner RF. Indications for retrograde cystourethrography in trauma. *Ann Emerg Med.* 1986;15(3):270-272.
7. Ghaemmaghami V, Sperry J, Gunst M, et al. Effects of early use of external pelvic compression on transfusion requirements and mortality in pelvic fractures. *Am J Surg.* 2007;194(6):720-723.

Chest Pain and Imaging for Cardiac Ischemia

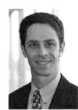

By Joshua S. Broder, MD, FACEP
Dr. Broder is a professor and the residency program director in the Department of Emergency Medicine at Duke University Medical Center in Durham, North Carolina.

Objectives

On completion of this article, you should be able to:

■ Discuss the sensitivity and specificity of nuclear medicine myocardial perfusion imaging.
■ Identify some causes of false-negative stress testing.
■ Describe the role of CT as an adjunct to nuclear perfusion cardiac stress testing.

CASE PRESENTATION

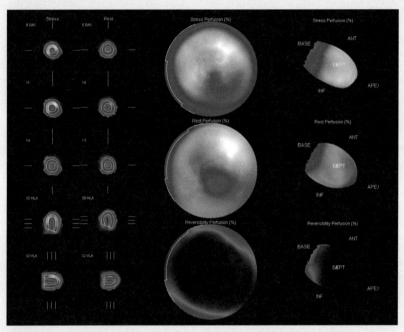

FIGURE 1. Prior myocardial perfusion SPECT/CT. SPECT images reveal no reversible perfusion abnormalities.

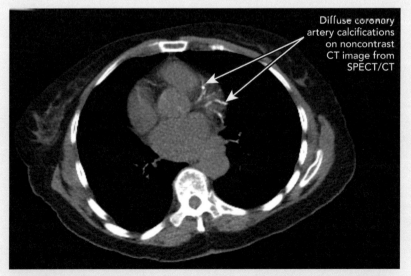

FIGURE 2. Noncontrast CT image from the patient's SPECT/CT myocardial perfusion stress test reveals diffusely calcified coronary arteries.

A 78-year-old woman with hypertension and peripheral vascular disease presents with episodic chest pain and dyspnea over the past month. She describes symptoms as now occurring with minimal exertion and increasingly while at rest. She thinks nitroglycerin alleviates the pain. She was evaluated in the emergency department 1 week prior for these concerns and discharged. Her vital signs are BP 189/81, P 65, R 18, and T 36.7°C (98.1°F); SpO_2 is 100% on room air.

The patient appears comfortable and denies any current symptoms. Her heart is regular and without murmurs. Her lung examination is clear. She has no peripheral edema. Her ECG is unchanged from baseline, showing normal sinus rhythm with ST depressions in leads I, II, aVF, and V_3 through V_6. She has normal posterior-anterior and lateral chest x-rays. Her initial high sensitivity troponin T level is 37 ng/L.

A non–ST-elevation myocardial infarction is suspected, aspirin is administered, and heparin and nitroglycerin infusions are initiated. A cardiologist is consulted, and all prior imaging studies are reviewed. The patient's stress nuclear medicine myocardial perfusion single-photon emission computed tomography (SPECT)/CT scan, performed with regadenoson, from the earlier visit shows no evidence of inducible myocardial ischemia (*Figure 1* and *2*).

Myocardial nuclear perfusion stress testing compares the distribution of an injected radiopharmaceutical agent on rest and physiologic stress images.[1] Physiologic stress can be induced by exercise or by pharmacologic means, either increasing myocardial workload (eg, dobutamine) or increasing myocardial blood flow by pharmacologically dilating coronary arteries (eg, regadenoson, an adenosine receptor agonist).

Defects present on stress images that are absent on rest images are interpreted to represent inducible ischemia. Fixed defects, present on both rest and stress images, may represent areas of prior infarction or artifacts from attenuation by overlying tissues. Imaging is accomplished by the detection of emitted radiation by a variety of techniques, such as scintigraphy, positron emission tomography (PET), or SPECT.

Although SPECT includes the term "computed tomography," this scintigraphic technology uses an external gamma camera to detect emitted radiation and should not be confused with CT scans, which apply an external x-ray source through a patient to a series of detectors. Hybrid scanners combining CT and SPECT offer precise anatomic localization (from CT) of physiologic nuclear medicine data (from SPECT).[1] In addition, CT allows quantitative attentuation correction of nuclear medicine data, helping to address attenuation artifacts.

A meta-analysis found SPECT myocardial perfusion imaging to have a sensitivity of 85% and specificity of 85% for obstructive coronary artery disease (CAD).[2] Another meta-analysis found that nuclear perfusion imaging with dobutamine as the pharmacologic stress agent had a sensitivity of 88% and specificity of 74%; sensitivity for multivessel disease was as low as 44%.[3]

False-negative stress testing can result from a variety of factors, including inadequate stress, variable definitions or thresholds for a positive test, the radiopharmaceutical agent used, the imaging technique, collateral circulation, and human error in interpretation.[3] An important patient factor

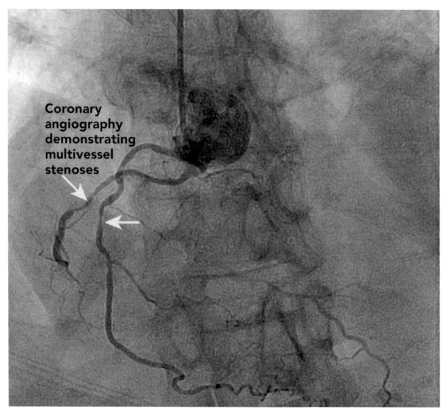

FIGURE 3. Coronary angiogram showing multivessel high-grade stenoses

in false-negative perfusion imaging is balanced ischemia in the setting of diffuse or multivessel CAD.[3-5] For example, in the case of diffuse CAD with heavily calcified coronary arteries, administration of a vasodilator may fail to alter blood flow compared to the preceding rest images, and blood flow is uniformly decreased on both rest and stress images. In this case, stress images may show no change, falsely ascribed to the absence of flow-limiting CAD.

While the final interpretation of a nuclear stress test is important, emergency physicians should be attentive to the techniques used and findings noted because additional diagnostic information may be derived, as in this case. Given this patient's risk factors, typical angina presentation, and the presence of diffuse coronary artery calcifications on the CT portion of the SPECT/CT stress test, the stress test result was determined to be falsely negative.

CASE RESOLUTION

The patient was admitted, and cardiac catherization was performed, which demonstrated diffuse highly calcified native CAD, including 100% stenosis of the right coronary artery, 95% stenosis of the left main coronary artery, and 99% occlusion of the left circumflex coronary artery (*Figure 3*). Thus, the patient underwent coronary artery bypass grafting.

REFERENCES

1. Patton JA, Turkington TG. SPECT/CT physical principles and attenuation correction. *J Nucl Med Technol.* 2008;36(1):1-10.
2. Mc Ardle BA, Dowsley TF, deKemp RA, Wells GA, Beanlands RS. Does rubidium-82 PET have superior accuracy to SPECT perfusion imaging for the diagnosis of obstructive coronary disease?: a systematic review and meta-analysis. *J Am Coll Cardiol.* 2012;60(18):1828-1837.
3. Geleijnse ML, Elhendy A, Fioretti PM, Roelandt JRTC. Dobutamine stress myocardial perfusion imaging. *J Am Coll Cardiol.* 2000;36(7):2017-2027.
4. Leibzon R, Arbit B. False negative nuclear stress test. *Proceedings of UCLA Healthcare.* 2020;24. https://proceedings.med.ucla.edu/wp-content/uploads/2020/09/Leibzon-A200623RL-BLM-formatted.pdf
5. Baqi A, Ahmed I, Nagher B. Multi vessel coronary artery disease presenting as a false negative myocardial perfusion imaging and true positive exercise tolerance test: a case of balanced ischemia. *Cureus.* 2020;12(11):e11321.

Feature Editor: Joshua S. Broder, MD, FACEP. See also *Diagnostic Imaging for the Emergency Physician* (Winner of the 2011 Prose Award in Clinical Medicine, the American Publishers Award for Professional and Scholarly Excellence) and *Critical Images in Emergency Medicine* by Dr. Broder.

The Critical ECG

Myocardial Infarction or Hyperkalemia

By Amal Mattu, MD, FACEP
Dr. Mattu is a professor, vice chair, and director of the Emergency Cardiology Fellowship in the Department of Emergency Medicine at the University of Maryland School of Medicine in Baltimore.

Objective

On completion of this article, you should be able to:

- Recognize how a patient's history and examination can aid in resolving a confusing ECG.

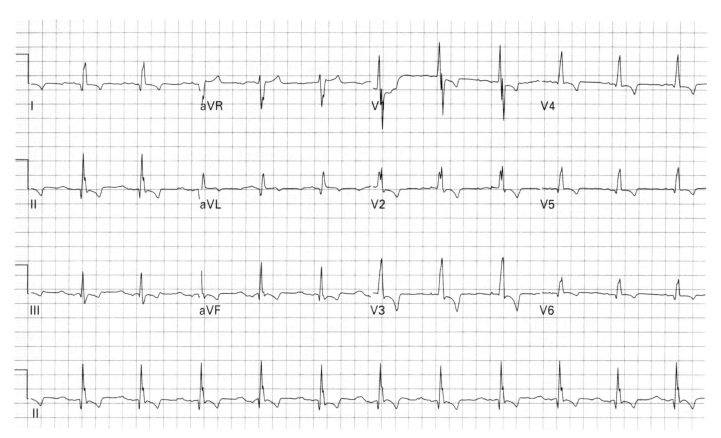

FIGURE 1. A 59-year-old man with dyspnea after missing his last hemodialysis session for renal failure

Sinus rhythm with first-degree atrioventricular (AV) block, rate 70, possible inferior-posterior-lateral myocardial infarction (MI) of undetermined age, nonspecific intraventricular conduction delay, T-wave abnormality suggestive of hyperkalemia (*Figure 1*).

In the absence of further clinical information, this ECG is confusing. A prominent R wave is present in lead V1, and the QRS progression across the precordium is unusual. The differential diagnosis for this finding includes Wolff-Parkinson-White syndrome, posterior MI, right bundle branch block (RBBB) (or incomplete RBBB), ventricular ectopy, right ventricular hypertrophy, acute right ventricular dilatation (right ventricular "strain" such as a massive pulmonary embolism), hypertrophic cardiomyopathy, progressive muscular dystrophy, dextrocardia, and misplaced precordial electrodes. Small Q waves are present in the inferior and lateral leads, which

is suggestive of a prior MI; these findings lend credence to the possibility that the prominent R wave in lead V1 represents the posterior extension of an MI. However, the Q waves are smaller and narrower than normal infarction-induced Q waves — infarction Q waves are expected to be at least 40 msec in duration and at least 25% of the amplitude of the entire QRS complex. Further history and examination solved the puzzle. The patient had a history of dextrocardia. When the ECG leads were repositioned to account for this, the small Q waves "disappeared," and the QRS progression "normalized." The prolonged PR interval and the "peaked" T waves in the precordial leads suggest hyperkalemia. This patient's serum potassium level was 7.9 mEq/L (normal 3.5-5.3 mEq/L). It is important to remember that the peaked T waves of hyperkalemia can be upright or inverted, depending on the patient's baseline T-wave morphology.

From Mattu A, Brady W. *ECGs for the Emergency Physician 2*. BMJ Publishing. Reprinted with permission.

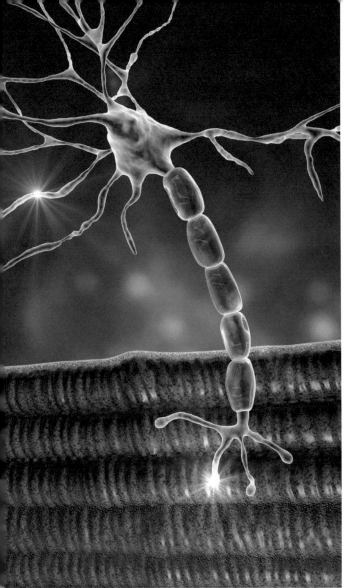

Breathing Room

Respiratory Failure in a Myasthenic Crisis

LESSON 12

By Zackary M. Funk, MD; Elizabeth L. DeVos, MD, MPH; and Adnan Javed, MD

Dr. Funk is a resident in the Department of Emergency Medicine; Dr. DeVos is a board-certified emergency physician, an associate professor of emergency medicine, and medical director of International Emergency Medicine Education; and Dr. Javed is a board-certified emergency physician and an assistant professor of emergency medicine at the University of Florida College of Medicine in Jacksonville. Dr. Javed also holds a subspecialty certification in anesthesiology critical care medicine.

Reviewed by John Kiel, DO, MPH

Objectives

On completion of this lesson, you should be able to:

1. Distinguish important features in the initial assessment of patients with impending respiratory failure.
2. Recognize how the pathophysiology of neuromuscular disorders can impact the effects of neuromuscular blockade agents.
3. Design a basic framework to select appropriate equipment and medications for patients in myasthenic crisis.
4. Evaluate potential problems that may arise related to disease processes or iatrogenic complications.

From the EM Model

12.0 Nervous System Disorders
    12.7 Neuromuscular Disorders
        12.7.2 Myasthenia Gravis

■ CRITICAL DECISIONS ■

- In patients with underlying neuromuscular disorders, which aspects of the presentation and physical examination indicate an urgent need for airway management and ventilatory support, and what tools can assess respiratory status?
- What indicates the need for intubation in patients with acute respiratory failure due to a neuromuscular disorder?
- Which patients may benefit from noninvasive positive-pressure ventilation?
- How should neuromuscular disorders like MG affect the choice and dosing of paralytics in patients needing rapid-sequence intubation?
- Is the early use of pyridostigmine or other cholinergic agents beneficial in patients in myasthenic crisis?
- What is the proper disposition of patients exhibiting pathology on the spectrum of respiratory compromise?

Neuromuscular disorders like myasthenia gravis (MG) can lead to rapidly progressive paresis, paralysis of respiratory and oropharyngeal muscles, and the inability to manage oral secretions. Because delayed intervention can lead to disastrous consequences, emergency physicians must be able to quickly recognize this condition and the features of impending respiratory failure.

■ CASE ONE

A 21-year-old man presents with increasing ptosis and diplopia. He has also experienced increased difficulty swallowing his medications over the last several days. He was recently diagnosed with MG by his neurologist and was prescribed pyridostigmine and prednisone, which were increased without relief. He exhibits ptosis at rest that obstructs the bilateral visual fields and diplopia at rest; however, he is tolerating his oral secretions, speaks in complete sentences, and walks without assistance. He exhibits unlabored breathing and can recite a 50-word script in one breath. His NIF is consistently less than –40 cm H_2O on serial examinations.

■ CASE TWO

A 40-year-old woman with a previous diagnosis of MG and a recent diagnosis of COVID-19 (7 days prior to presentation) arrives via EMS with concern for increasing drowsiness, dyspnea at rest that worsens on mild exertion, and a recurrence of her previously well-controlled symptoms of ptosis, diplopia, and dysphagia. Due to her symptoms, she is sleeping more and is unable to take her prescribed medications on her usual schedule. On initial presentation, she is hypoxic at 88% on room air, is tachypneic at 40 breaths per minute, and has frequent episodes of a productive cough. Her NIF is –7 cm H_2O, although the respiratory therapist notes frequent and prolonged coughing episodes that could have confounded the test.

Introduction

MG is an autoimmune neuromuscular disorder characterized by fluctuating muscle weakness. In MG, IgG autoantibodies are produced against nicotinic acetylcholine receptors (n-AChRs) and related proteins in the postsynaptic myoneural junction (eg, muscle-specific tyrosine kinase, also referred to as MuSK). These autoantibodies lead to receptor internalization and, therefore, a reduction in the number of receptors available to transmit a signal to skeletal muscles (*Figure 1*).[1] The disease often presents with the hallmark feature of muscle weakness that worsens with repeated use. About 50% of patients with MG initially present with ocular symptoms such as ptosis or diplopia.[2] For patients in whom the disease progresses, it enters a "generalized" phase that can involve the bulbar muscles and proximal muscle groups.[2] Weakness progresses to eventually involve other muscle groups, including the muscles of respiration, such as the diaphragm and intercostal muscles.[3] The prevalence of MG is estimated at approximately 14 to 40 per 100,000 individuals in the United States, with similar figures seen in the global population (approximately 12.4 per 100,000).[4-6]

Classic teaching is that MG is more commonly diagnosed in females, with a bimodal distribution peaking at approximately 20 to 29 years of age and 60 to 79 years of age. In a meta-analysis of several large population-based studies, however, only 5 out of the 14 studies showed this distribution. Thus, a high index of suspicion should be maintained for individuals of any sex, age, or racial or ethnic background.[6]

Several outpatient treatment modalities range from symptomatic management with acetylcholinesterase inhibitors (eg, pyridostigmine) to long-term immunosuppression using regimens that contain a combination of glucocorticoids, azathioprine, or mycophenolate, if patients remain or become symptomatic on first-line therapy.[1,7-8] For severe or refractory cases

not in acute myasthenic crisis, intravenous immune globulin and plasma exchange (PLEX) are two mainstays of therapy, in addition to further escalation of immunosuppression with agents such as cyclophosphamide or rituximab. When these patients present to the emergency department, it is essential to consider that they could be on aggressive immunosuppressive regimens. Further attenuation of the patients' immune responses can be accomplished with thymectomy, which can be considered if the treating neurologist determines that the patient meets specific criteria.[8]

If the condition is untreated or patients exhibit increased resistance to treatment, they can develop a myasthenic crisis. A myasthenic crisis is characterized by a rapidly progressive paresis or paralysis of respiration and oropharyngeal muscles, leading to respiratory failure that can be further complicated by the inability to manage oral secretions.[3]

In undiagnosed patients with signs and symptoms concerning for MG, emergency physicians can perform an ice pack test to help confirm the diagnosis (*Figure 2*). The ice pack test is conducted by placing an ice pack on the eye for 2 to 5 minutes.

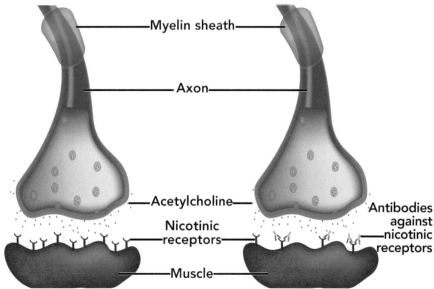

FIGURE 1. Normal myoneural junction (*left*) versus MG (*right*)

Patients with ptosis from MG exhibit improvement after applying ice to the periorbital region for as few as 2 minutes. It is thought that, by cooling the tissues, the activity of local acetylcholinesterases is inhibited, thereby providing temporary improvement in muscle strength.[9]

Other forms of testing, (eg, serologic testing and electromyography) have excellent test characteristics for making a definitive diagnosis of MG; however, such testing methods are not widely available in the emergency department. Thus, the time to obtain results makes their use impractical in the acute setting.

Although edrophonium testing has historically been used as a diagnostic tool for MG, it is no longer available in the United States. The FDA discontinued the drug in 2018 due to concerns regarding a high false-positive rate and the paradigm shift toward relying on serologic testing for a more definitive diagnosis.[10]

CRITICAL DECISION

In patients with underlying neuromuscular disorders, which aspects of the presentation and physical examination indicate an urgent need for airway management and ventilatory support, and what tools can assess respiratory status?

History and Physical Examination

Respiratory failure in MG patients is usually caused by infection, surgery, or the rapid tapering of immunosuppressive drugs. Features that should alert clinicians to possible impending respiratory failure in a myasthenic crisis include evident dyspnea, either reported by the patient or apparent on examination; difficulty handling oral secretions; hypophonia (reduced speech intensity); accessory muscle usage; and paradoxical breathing. Early in the disease course, patients may be able to compensate for a decreased ability to generate tidal volumes with tachypnea; however, their ability to generate frequent respirations is likely to decline. As the disease progresses, these findings may become less pronounced because the developing weakness limits the patient's ability to initiate these movements. Of note, patients

with evolving diaphragmatic weakness may exhibit orthopnea. The hypothesis is that the assistance gravity provides the diaphragm when upright is removed when lying down.

It is also important to note that antibiotics can worsen MG symptoms and consequently further compromise a patient's ability to breathe without intervention. Aminoglycosides (eg, gentamicin), quinolones (eg, ciprofloxacin), and macrolides (eg, azithromycin) can all inhibit transmission at the presynaptic terminal, inhibiting binding with the postsynaptic acetylcholine receptor, or alter postsynaptic ion permeability. Ceftriaxone, a cephalosporin, is a safer choice for MG patients because it is less likely to affect synaptic transmission.

Bedside Quantitative Measures of Respiratory Muscle Function

Assessment of the patient's forced vital capacity (FVC) and negative inspiratory force (NIF), also known as maximal inspiratory pressure, are critical in the initial assessment of a patient's respiratory status and for monitoring disease progression in the acute setting.[3] Because neither measurement is superior, the two measurements are often analyzed in combination. If such testing is not readily available, however, single breath counting (SBC), where patients speak as many words as they can after one inhalation, is a potentially useful surrogate measure for FVC and NIF until other evaluation methods become available.[11] It is important to note that assessment of FVC, NIF, or SBC can lead to more rapid fatigue due to the necessary patient effort involved in this testing.

Laboratory Evaluation

Multiple measures (eg, NIF, FVC, SBC, and point-of-care blood gas analysis) should be obtained early when there is possible respiratory compromise due to progressive muscle weakness. They should be repeated often while closely monitoring the patient's overall clinical status. Given the time delay, even in the case of point-of-care studies, priority should be given to assessing the bedside quantitative measures such as FVC and NIF. If time and resources permit, it may be useful

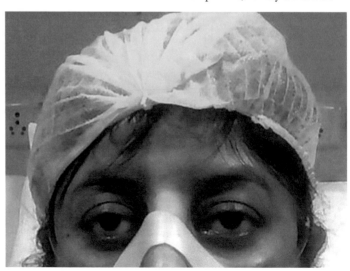

FIGURE 2. Ice pack test. A. Ptosis can be seen before the test. B. Resolution occurs after the test.
Credit: Dave H, Desai R, Checker S, et al. Selective type 2 respiratory failure followed by ocular myasthenia gravis diagnosed by ice pack test: a case report. *Cureus.* 2019;11(6):e4927.

to trend the patient's acid-base status to determine the timing of elective versus emergent intubation, as discussed in the next section.

CRITICAL DECISION

What indicates the need for intubation in patients with acute respiratory failure due to a neuromuscular disorder?

The methods of assessment outlined in this article are best used to supplement and inform clinical judgment; physiologic parameters should be evaluated in the context of each patient's overall presentation. Measures concerning for impending respiratory failure include the patient's FVC measuring or approaching less than 10 to 20 mL/kg of ideal body weight or NIF measuring or trending to less negative than −20 to −30 cm H_2O. Most literature indicates that elective intubation is warranted at these thresholds to prevent an emergent intubation and its complications after an anticipated decline in respiratory status.[3] Regarding SBC, uncompromised patients can typically speak 40 to 50 words after a single forced inspiration. Evolving trends in the literature suggest that patients who can speak fewer than 15 to 20 words are more likely to require ventilatory support.[11]

The presence or development of respiratory acidosis in conjunction with the patient's clinical status should prompt clinicians to strongly consider intubation. Extrapolating from the teachings from obstructive lung pathologies such as asthma or COPD exacerbations, even a PCO_2 that is within the reference range despite patient tachypnea is likely to be an ominous sign of imminent failure of a patient's compensatory mechanisms.

CRITICAL DECISION

Which patients may benefit from noninvasive positive-pressure ventilation?

Patients who are alert and oriented and present early in a myasthenic crisis, without having yet progressed to respiratory failure, may benefit from a trial of noninvasive positive-pressure ventilation. In a retrospective study of 60 patients in myasthenic crisis, the use of bilevel positive airway pressure (BiPAP) was found to be associated with fewer days on a ventilator and a shorter time in the ICU compared to patients who were initially intubated.[12] However, patients who were already hypercapnic when BiPAP was initiated failed the trial of noninvasive ventilation and required endotracheal intubation.

In another cohort of 9 patients, BiPAP helped avoid endotracheal intubation, but hypercapnia ($PaCO_2$ >50 mm Hg) was predictive of the need for invasive mechanical ventilation.[13] This data may indicate that noninvasive ventilation such as BiPAP may provide the most benefit to patients who have mild respiratory compromise.

Lastly, the use of BiPAP in patients experiencing a myasthenic crisis requires frequent monitoring and clinical reassessment to evaluate the patient's response to therapy and to avoid the complications of a potential decline (eg, aspiration in a patient on BiPAP who now has worsening

mental status). BiPAP may also serve as a bridge to intubation.

CRITICAL DECISION

How should neuromuscular disorders like MG affect the choice and dosing of paralytics in patients needing rapid-sequence intubation?

The pathophysiology of neuromuscular disorders plays a crucial role in understanding patients' responses to paralytic agents. In MG, fewer postsynaptic acetylcholine receptors are present, so depolarizing agents (namely, succinylcholine) are less potent, theoretically necessitating higher doses. Due to observations of significant variation and unpredictability in patient responses, some professional societies discourage using succinylcholine in this setting.[14]

Thus, when indicated, nondepolarizing neuromuscular blocking agents (eg, rocuronium and vecuronium) are preferred. Because these agents act as direct competitors for acetylcholine in the fewer-than-normal postsynaptic receptor binding sites in MG, lower doses should be used to prevent unnecessarily prolonged neuromuscular blocking and its associated complications.[15]

CRITICAL DECISION

Is the early use of pyridostigmine or other cholinergic agents beneficial in patients in myasthenic crisis?

Medications, such as pyridostigmine (most commonly used) and neostigmine (less commonly used), are the mainstay of treatment for MG because they act as cholinergic agents by increasing the amount of acetylcholine available to the reduced number of postsynaptic receptors. Pyridostigmine has a rapid onset of 15 to 30 minutes and peak action at about 2 hours; its effects last for approximately 3 to 4 hours. Pyridostigmine is available in tablet, liquid, or intravenous preparations.

✔ Pearls

- The ice pack test can help diagnose patients with signs and symptoms of MG.

- When evaluating patients with possible respiratory compromise due to progressive muscle weakness, measures such as NIF, FVC, SBC, and point-of-care blood gas analysis should be obtained early and repeated often while closely monitoring the patient's overall clinical status.

- FVC measurements of 10 to 20 mL/kg of ideal body weight, NIF measurements less negative than −20 to −30 cm H_2O, and SBC results of fewer than 15 to 20 words after one forced inspiration may indicate an impending need to intubate and to provide ventilatory support.

- Noninvasive ventilation such as BiPAP may provide the most benefit to patients who have mild respiratory compromise.

A common starting dose for adults is 30 mg PO 3 times a day; however, most adults respond to 60 to 90 mg PO every 4 to 6 hours while awake, with a maximum of 120 mg every 3 hours and total dose of 960 mg every 24 hours. A common starting dose for children is 0.5 to 1 mg/kg every 4 to 6 hours, with a maximum dose of 7 mg/kg every 24 hours. Dosing regimens are individualized to increase symptomatic benefit while limiting cholinergic side effects.

Medications like pyridostigmine may have a role in the myasthenic crisis, as they can contribute to mucous plugging, aspiration pneumonitis, or difficulties with laryngoscopy due to bronchorrhea caused by their muscarinic effects. The toxidrome of cholinergic overdose is well described and can be remembered by using several mnemonics. One commonly used mnemonic is DUMBELS, which stands for diarrhea/diaphoresis, urination, miosis/muscle weakness/muscle fasciculations, bronchorrhea/bradycardia/bronchospasm, emesis, lacrimation, and salivation/sweating (*Table 1*). Also useful is the mnemonic SLUDGE, which stands for salivation, lacrimation, urination, diaphoresis/diarrhea, gastrointestinal distress, and emesis (*Table 2*).

While administration of therapeutic doses of pyridostigmine is unlikely to result in a florid presentation of this toxidrome, the treatment can cause increased airway secretions. Because its onset is typically about 15 minutes from administration, pyridostigmine is unlikely to sufficiently improve respiratory mechanics to outweigh the risks or prevent intubation for patients already in the beginning stages of respiratory failure.[16]

✖ Pitfalls

- Overlooking conditions that predispose patients to respiratory failure or delaying preparation for elective intubation. Close monitoring and frequent reassessment of patients with compromised respiratory statuses can prevent disastrous complications.

- Neglecting to use FVC, NIF, SBC, and other data points to assess patients' overall clinical appearance, which can provide false reassurance and delay preparation for elective intubation.

- Failing to recognize and prepare for the reality that assessment of FVC, NIF, or SBC may lead to more rapid fatigue due to the necessary patient effort involved in testing.

- Ignoring the role neuromuscular disorders play in the effects of neuromuscular blocking agents, confounding post-intubation assessment and care.

- Forgetting that medications such as pyridostigmine, which have a role in the management of a myasthenic crisis, may contribute to mucous plugging, aspiration pneumonitis, or difficulties with laryngoscopy due to bronchorrhea caused by their muscarinic effects.

CRITICAL DECISION

What is the proper disposition of patients exhibiting pathology on the spectrum of respiratory compromise?

Patients in respiratory failure requiring intubation and mechanical ventilation require ICU level of care due to the need for experienced physicians and staff to closely monitor and titrate settings and intervene should complications arise. Determining an appropriate disposition may be more challenging for patients who display a reassuring examination but are at risk of catastrophic and sometimes unpredictable deterioration if sufficient observation and swift intervention are unavailable. For these patients, emergency physicians should discuss these risks with the inpatient team and, if any concern for potential decline exists, strongly consider advocating for a higher level of care.

In addition to discussion of the patient's anticipated course with the neurology and critical care teams, consideration must be given to each institution's guidelines regarding acceptable levels of respiratory support for each level of care. For example, does the institution allow for patients on high-flow nasal cannula to be on the general floor service and, if so, is there an FiO_2 or flow threshold? Such parameters may influence the proper disposition.

Summary

Managing the airway and supporting patients' breathing are essential in the initial stabilization and management of those who present in extremis. For many patients, immediate life-threatening pathology is apparent in the primary survey.

DUMBELS	
D	Diarrhea/diaphoresis
U	Urination
M	Miosis/muscle weakness/muscle fasciculations
B	Bronchorrhea/bradycardia/bronchospasm
E	Emesis
L	Lacrimation
S	Salivation/sweating

TABLE 1. DUMBELS mnemonic for the toxidrome of cholinergic overdose

SLUDGE	
S	Salivation
L	Lacrimation
U	Urination
D	Diaphoresis/diarrhea
G	Gastrointestinal distress
E	Emesis

TABLE 2. SLUDGE mnemonic for the toxidrome of cholinergic overdose

N CASE ONE

The neurology team arrived at the patient's bedside shortly after consultation. After a shared decision-making discussion with the teams involved and the patient, prednisone 60 mg PO was administered, and the patient was admitted to the neurology floor service for further observation and optimization of therapy. The patient had significant improvement in reported symptom severity after the initial dose of prednisone and an increase in his maintenance prednisone dosing. Serial NIF measurements were consistently reassuring and unchanged throughout his admission, and he was able to be discharged after 48 hours with outpatient follow-up.

■ CASE TWO

The patient was admitted to the neuro-ICU and remained intubated for 5 days. NIF improved after initiation of methylprednisolone and three rounds of PLEX, allowing for an uneventful extubation and a swift wean to room air. Of note, her urine culture revealed an *Escherichia coli* infection, which was treated with ceftriaxone. She was then downgraded to the neurology floor service on inpatient day 7, where she received continued intravenous steroids and two additional rounds of PLEX. Afterward, the patient chose to leave against medical advice, and refills of her immunosuppressant medications were sent to her pharmacy.

For those who may develop respiratory failure but do not present with obvious primary survey findings that necessitate intervention, physicians must be attuned to often subtle findings. Familiarity with such presentations and the methods of evaluating and monitoring disease progression in the acute setting is of the utmost importance in avoiding or preempting emergent situations.

REFERENCES

1. Schneider-Gold C, Gajdos P, Toyka KV, Hohlfeld RR. Corticosteroids for myasthenia gravis. *Cochrane Database Syst Rev.* 2005;2005(2):CD002828.

2. Grob D, Arsura EL, Brunner NG, Namba T. The course of myasthenia gravis and therapies affecting outcome. *Ann N Y Acad Sci.* 1987;505(1):472-499.

3. Roper J, Fleming ME, Long B, Koyfman A. Myasthenia gravis and crisis: evaluation and management in the emergency department. *J Emerg Med.* 2017;53(6):843-853.

4. Myasthenia Gravis. National Organization of Rare Disorders. Accessed January 27, 2022. https://rarediseases.org/rare-diseases/myasthenia-gravis/

5. Salari N, Fatahi B, Bartina Y, et al. Global prevalence of myasthenia gravis and the effectiveness of common drugs in its treatment: a systematic review and meta-analysis. *J Transl Med.* 2021;19(1):516.

6. Carr AS, Cardwell CR, McCarron PO, McConville J. A systematic review of population based epidemiological studies in myasthenia gravis. *BMC Neurol.* 2010;10(1):46. https://bmcneurol.biomedcentral.com/articles/10.1186/1471-2377-10-46

7. Maggi L, Mantegazza R. Treatment of myasthenia gravis: focus on pyridostigmine. *Clin Drug Invest.* 2011;31(10):691-701.

8. Sanders DB, Wolfe GI, Benatar M, et al. International consensus guidance for management of myasthenia gravis: executive summary. *Neurology.* 2016;87(4):419-425. https://n.neurology.org/content/87/4/419

9. Kearsey C, Fernando P, D'costa D, Ferdinand P. The use of the ice pack test in myasthenia gravis. *JRSM Short Rep.* 2010 Jun 30;1(1):1-3. https://journals.sagepub.com/doi/full/10.1258/shorts.2009.090037

10. Naji A, Owens ML. Edrophonium. In: *StatPearls [Internet].* StatPearls Publishing; 2022. Accessed January 27, 2022. https://www.ncbi.nlm.nih.gov/books/NBK554566/

11. Elsheikh B, Arnold WD, Gharibshahi S, Reynolds J, Freimer M, Kissel JT. Correlation of single-breath count test and neck flexor muscle strength with spirometry in myasthenia gravis. *Muscle Nerve.* 2016;53(1):134-136.

12. Seneviratne J, Mandrekar J, Wijdicks, EFM, Rabinstein AA. Noninvasive ventilation in myasthenic crisis. *Arch Neurol.* 2008;65(1):54-58. https://jamanetwork.com/journals/jamaneurology/fullarticle/795076

13. Rabinstein A, Wijdicks EFM. BiPAP in acute respiratory failure due to myasthenic crisis may prevent intubation. *Neurology.* 2002;59(10):1647-1649.

14. Ammundsen HB, Sørensen MK, Gätke MR. Succinylcholine resistance. *Brit J Anaesth.* 2015;115(6):818-821. https://academic.oup.com/bja/article/115/6/818/241002?login=true

15. Caro D. Neuromuscular blocking agents (NMBAs) for rapid sequence intubation in adults outside of the operating room. UpToDate. Accessed January 27, 2022. https://www.uptodate.com/contents/neuromuscular-blocking-agents-nmbas-for-rapid-sequence-intubation-in-adults-outside-of-the-operating-room

16. Punga AR, Stålberg E. Acetylcholinesterase inhibitors in MG: to be or not to be? *Muscle Nerve.* 2009;39(6):724-728.

CME Questions

Reviewed by Walter L. Green, MD, FACEP; and John Kiel, DO, MPH

Qualified, paid subscribers to *Critical Decisions in Emergency Medicine* may receive CME certificates for up to 5 ACEP Category I credits, 5 *AMA PRA Category 1 Credits*™, and 5 AOA Category 2-B credits for completing this activity in its entirety. Submit your answers online at acep.org/cdem; a score of 75% or better is required. You may receive credit for completing the CME activity any time within 3 years of its publication date. Answers to this month's questions will be published in next month's issue.

1 Although the diagnosis of necrotizing fasciitis can only be confirmed with surgical exploration, what is the gold standard imaging study for investigating the condition?

- A. CT
- B. MRI
- C. Ultrasound
- D. X-ray

2 What is the most common bacterial pathology associated with necrotizing fasciitis?

- A. Anaerobic organisms
- B. Group A *Streptococcus*
- C. Polymicrobial organisms
- D. *Staphylococcus aureus*

3 Which antibiotic is given for toxin suppression in necrotizing fasciitis?

- A. Clindamycin
- B. Piperacillin-tazobactam
- C. Trimethoprim-sulfamethoxazole
- D. Vancomycin

4 In a patient with a high clinical suspicion for necrotizing fasciitis based on the initial presentation, what is the next best step in evaluation to expedite care and maximize the patient outcome?

- A. Bedside ultrasound of the affected area
- B. CT scan of the affected region
- C. Early surgical consultation
- D. LRINEC score calculation

5 What is considered the standard of care for treating necrotizing fasciitis?

- A. Intravenous antibiotics, IVIG, hyperbaric oxygen therapy, and surgical debridement
- B. Intravenous broad-spectrum antibiotics alone
- C. Intravenous broad-spectrum antibiotics and surgical debridement
- D. IVIG and hyperbaric oxygen therapy

6 Which finding may be encountered on bedside ultrasound when investigating for necrotizing fasciitis?

- A. Dirty shadowing
- B. Fascial plane thickening
- C. Subcutaneous cobblestoning
- D. All of these

7 In which patient is a treatment regimen of oral cephalexin paired with trimethoprim-sulfamethoxazole most appropriate?

- A. 23-year-old woman with no significant medical history who presents with a 3-day history of a 2 × 2 cm area of cellulitis on her shin
- B. 43-year-old woman with a history of hypertension and a short hospitalization 1 week ago for a cardiac workup who presents with a 3- to 4-cm buttock abscess that requires incision and drainage
- C. 57-year-old man with a history of hypertension and type 2 diabetes mellitus with cellulitis from his right knee to his right ankle, which spread over 2 days while on 1 day of cephalexin, who now presents with fever and malaise
- D. 60-year-old woman with active breast cancer who complains of severe leg pain that has spread rapidly over the past day, who is toxic appearing and uncomfortable, and who has a normal physical examination of her lower extremities

8 What findings are considered risk factors for MRSA?

- A. History of breast cancer, known nasal colonization, and concurrent or previous MRSA infection
- B. Known nasal colonization, age >65 years, concurrent MRSA infection, and hospitalization
- C. Known nasal colonization, concurrent or previous MRSA infection, hospitalization, and recent antibiotic use
- D. Recent antibiotic use, known nasal colonization, history of MRSA infection, and concurrent hypertension

9 What is the recommended treatment for simple cellulitis in a hemodynamically stable patient without obvious risk factors for MRSA?

- A. Inpatient admission for intravenous clindamycin
- B. Inpatient observation for empiric antibiotics, including vancomycin
- C. Outpatient treatment with cephalexin for 5 days
- D. Outpatient treatment with trimethoprim-sulfamethoxazole for 10 days

10 A patient who was treated for simple cellulitis 5 days ago presents with a failed outpatient course, worsening symptoms, and new-onset fever and tachycardia. What is the next best step in management?

- A. Administer clindamycin 600 mg IV 3 times daily and place in the observation unit overnight
- B. Change the outpatient regimen to trimethoprim-sulfamethoxazole for another 3 days and discharge home
- C. Initiate a new regimen of antibiotics (nafcillin PO and cefazolin IV) and admit the patient for treatment and continued monitoring
- D. Initiate broad-spectrum antibiotics, including MRSA coverage with vancomycin and piperacillin-tazobactam, and admit the patient for treatment and continued monitoring

11 Which physical examination finding most suggests impending respiratory failure in a patient with a neuromuscular disease?

A. Diplopia
B. Hypophonia
C. Lower-extremity weakness
D. Ptosis

12 Which quantitative finding is most concerning for impending respiratory failure in a patient with a suspected neuromuscular disorder?

A. FVC <10-20 mL/kg
B. FVC = 20-30 mL/kg
C. FVC = 30-40 mL/kg
D. FVC >40 mL/kg

13 What is the pathophysiology of the most common variant of myasthenia gravis?

A. Autoantibodies against voltage-gated calcium channels
B. Autoantibodies directed against acetylcholine receptors at the postsynaptic end plate
C. Autoantibodies that are cross-reactive to gangliosides and other antigens on peripheral nerves
D. Cellular internalization of an exogenous toxin directed against intracellular proteins needed for neurotransmitter release

14 What mediates both the therapeutic and adverse effects of pyridostigmine?

A. Acting as a direct agonist to postsynaptic acetylcholine receptors
B. Increasing the availability of acetylcholine in synapses
C. Lowering a neuron's threshold potential by stimulating sodium-potassium ATPase
D. Potentiating voltage-gated calcium channels on the postsynaptic neuron

15 A 70-kg patient presents with complaints of diplopia, dysphagia, and increasing dyspnea. On examination, the patient is somnolent, has bilateral ptosis and hypophonia, and is tachypneic to 30 breaths per minute with shallow respirations. NIF is −30 cm H_2O, FVC is 1,000 mL, SBC is 35 words, and ABG is 7.46/30/90. Given this data, what is most concerning for impending respiratory compromise in this patient?

A. ABG
B. Clinical status
C. NIF
D. SBC

16 What is a potential pitfall of pyridostigmine for patients with respiratory distress?

A. Increased respiratory secretions that complicate intubation
B. Muscle fatigue and bronchospasm in overdose
C. Onset of action of approximately 15 minutes
D. All of these

17 Which patient with respiratory compromise due to a myasthenic crisis is most likely to benefit from a trial of BiPAP?

A. Alert patient who is spitting up oral secretions but has a normal SpO_2 on 2 L of supplemental oxygen via nasal cannula and an end-tidal reading of 35 mm Hg
B. Alert patient with a PaO_2 of 80 mm Hg on 4 L of supplemental oxygen via nasal cannula and a $PaCO_2$ of 40 mm Hg
C. Somnolent patient with a normal SpO_2 on room air and a respiratory rate of 10 breaths per minute
D. Tachypneic patient who is agitated and refusing IV placement

18 Which antibiotic is least likely to exacerbate muscle weakness in a patient with myasthenia gravis?

A. Azithromycin
B. Ceftriaxone
C. Ciprofloxacin
D. Gentamicin

19 A patient with myasthenia gravis presents in respiratory distress and requires rapid-sequence intubation. IV access is obtained, and ketamine 1 mg/kg IV and succinylcholine 1.5 mg/kg IV are administered. After 60 seconds, no fasciculations are perceived. The physician attempts to open the patient's mouth but has significant difficulty and cannot adequately open the mouth to introduce the laryngoscope blade. This difficulty persists even at 120 seconds. Assuming the IV was intact, what most likely explains what happened?

A. An error occurred, and rocuronium 1.5 mg/kg IV was administered instead
B. The dose of ketamine was insufficient to achieve adequate sedation
C. The dose of succinylcholine was insufficient to achieve adequate paralysis
D. The patient suffered a masseter spasm after succinylcholine administration

20 In an undifferentiated patient with signs and symptoms concerning for myasthenia gravis, which available test is most likely to provide information useful to emergency physicians?

A. Antibody test
B. Edrophonium test
C. Electromyography
D. Ice pack test

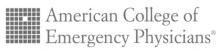

American College of Emergency Physicians®

ADVANCING EMERGENCY CARE

Post Office Box 619911
Dallas, Texas 75261-9911

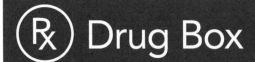

CAPSAICIN For CHS

By Frank LoVecchio, DO, MPH, FACEP
Valleywise Health and ASU, Phoenix, Arizona

Objective
On completion of this column, you should be able to:
- Describe the use of capsaicin to treat cannabinoid hyperemesis syndrome.

Cannabinoid hyperemesis syndrome (CHS) — cyclic or intractable episodes of nausea, vomiting, and abdominal pain — is associated with chronic cannabis abuse and resolves with its cessation. Capsaicin is a naturally occurring component of several Capsicum chili peppers that can be used for CHS.

Mechanism of Action
Capsaicin, a transient receptor potential vanilloid 1 (TRPV1) receptor agonist, activates TRPV1 ligand-gated cation channels on nociceptive nerve fibers, resulting in depolarization, initiation of action potentials, and pain signal transmission to the spinal cord. Capsaicin exposure desensitizes the sensory axons and inhibits pain transmission initiation. In arthritis, capsaicin induces release of substance P, the principal chemomediator of pain impulses from the periphery to the CNS; after repeated application, capsaicin depletes the neuron of substance P and prevents reaccumulation. The functional link between substance P and the capsaicin receptor, TRPV1, is not well understood.

Research
In a retrospective review of 43 emergency department patients treated for CHS, use of capsaicin cream decreased total medications administered and reduced opioid requirements; most patients (67%) had no further treatment prior to discharge. In a retrospective study of 201 patients with CHS, capsaicin cream was associated with greater efficacy for symptom relief than other treatments but was not associated with lower rates of admission or return visits within 24 hours. Thus, capsaicin may be useful in the acute treatment of CHS. Patients may not tolerate the discomfort of capsaicin use at home.

Adult Dosing
Topical cream, gel, liquid, or lotion: Apply a thin film to the affected areas 3 to 4 times daily.
For CHS (off label): Apply capsaicin cream (0.075%) to a 15 × 25 cm area in the periumbilical region, with reapplications every 4 hours until symptoms resolve.

Precautions
Adverse reactions with topical use:
- ***Local:*** Erythema (63%), pain (42%), pruritus (6%), edema (4%), swelling (2%)
- ***Cardiovascular:*** Hypertension (2%; transient)
- ***Dermatologic:*** Papule (6%), local dryness (2%), pruritus (2%)
- ***Gastrointestinal:*** Nausea (5%), vomiting (3%)
- ***Respiratory:*** Nasopharyngitis (4%), sinusitis (3%), bronchitis (2%)
Pregnancy: Category B

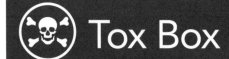

XYLAZINE TOXICITY

By Christian Tomaszewski, MD, MS, MBA, FACEP
University of California San Diego Health

Objective
On completion of this column, you should be able to:
- Recognize xylazine toxicity in recreational drug overdoses.

Xylazine, the "horse tranquilizer," is an unscheduled veterinary medication increasingly found as an adulterant to enhance euphoria in commonly injected drugs (ie, fentanyl and cocaine). It is increasingly implicated in overdose deaths and should be suspected in any symptomatic opioid overdoses unresponsive to naloxone.

Mechanism
- Alpha-2 adrenergic agonist (eg, clonidine)
- Centrally mediated decrease in sympathetic tone

Kinetics
- Usually injected (as little as ~10 mg can cause symptoms)
- Absorbed well with ingestion or insufflation
- Half-life ~5 hours post injection

Clinical Manifestations
- ***CNS:*** miosis, sedation
- ***Cardiac:*** bradycardia, hypotension (can be preceded by hypertension)
- ***Pulmonary:*** respiratory depression
- ***Metabolic:*** mild hyperglycemia
- ***Dermal:*** ulcerations at injection sites

Diagnostics
- Serum and urine levels generally unavailable
- Acetaminophen level in intentional ingestions
- BMP in symptomatic cases to check for acidosis or hypoglycemia
- ECG

Treatment
- Consider activated charcoal within an hour of massive ingestions, if awake
- Liberal naloxone if suspicion of opioid coingestant
- Supplementary oxygen or intubation as needed
- Atropine for symptomatic bradycardia
- Fluids and norepinephrine as needed for hypotension
- Amiodarone or lidocaine for threatening ventricular dysrhythmias

Disposition
- If asymptomatic at 4 to 6 hours, patients may be medically cleared.
- Symptomatic bradycardia or hypotension requires admission.

Critical decisions
in emergency medicine

Volume 36 Number 7: **July 2022**

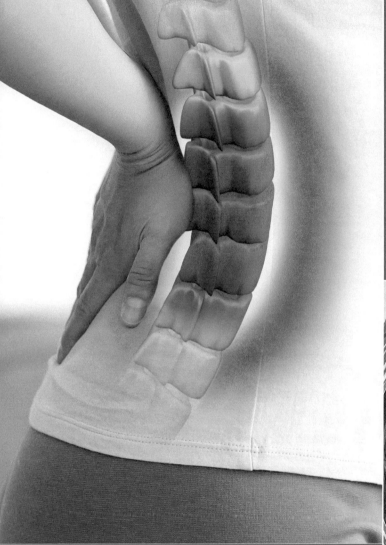

Watch Your Back

Most cases of back pain have a mechanical musculoskeletal etiology, but back pain can also be the harbinger of a life-threatening or paralyzing disease process. No emergency physician wants to miss a diagnosis, especially when the consequences are so dire, so a systematic approach to evaluating back pain and understanding the risk factors and warning signs are essential.

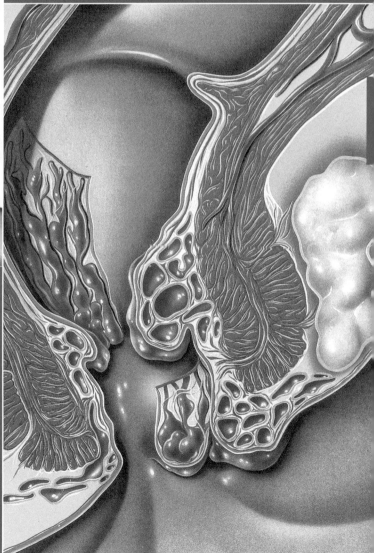

Bringing Up the Rear

Abscesses in the anorectal region are common complaints that may cause localized, compressive, or systemic symptoms; however, perirectal, perianal, and pilonidal abscesses can be difficult to differentiate. Emergency physicians must be able to rapidly identify and correctly treat these divergent disease processes to prevent complications.

THE OFFICIAL CME PUBLICATION OF THE AMERICAN COLLEGE OF EMERGENCY PHYSICIANS

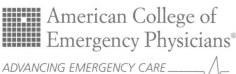

American College of Emergency Physicians®

ADVANCING EMERGENCY CARE

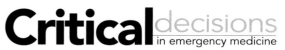

Critical**decisions**
in emergency medicine

Critical Decisions in Emergency Medicine is the official CME publication of the American College of Emergency Physicians. Additional volumes are available.

EDITOR-IN-CHIEF

Michael S. Beeson, MD, MBA, FACEP
Northeastern Ohio Universities,
Rootstown, OH

SECTION EDITORS

Joshua S. Broder, MD, FACEP
Duke University, Durham, NC

Andrew J. Eyre, MD, MS-HPEd
Brigham and Women's Hospital/
Harvard Medical School, Boston, MA

John Kiel, DO, MPH, FACEP, CAQSM
University of Florida College of Medicine,
Jacksonville, FL

Frank LoVecchio, DO, MPH, FACEP
Valleywise, Arizona State University, University of Arizona,
and Creighton Colleges of Medicine, Phoenix, AZ

Sharon E. Mace, MD, FACEP
Cleveland Clinic Lerner College of Medicine/
Case Western Reserve University, Cleveland, OH

Amal Mattu, MD, FACEP
University of Maryland, Baltimore, MD

Christian A. Tomaszewski, MD, MS, MBA, FACEP
University of California Health Sciences,
San Diego, CA

Steven J. Warrington, MD, MEd, MS
MercyOne Siouxland, Sioux City, IA

ASSOCIATE EDITORS

Tareq Al-Salamah, MBBS, MPH, FACEP
King Saud University, Riyadh, Saudi Arabia/
University of Maryland, Baltimore, MD

Wan-Tsu Chang, MD
University of Maryland, Baltimore, MD

Ann M. Dietrich, MD, FAAP, FACEP
University of South Carolina School of Medicine,
Greenville, SC

Kelsey Drake, MD, MPH, FACEP
St. Anthony Hospital, Lakewood, CO

Walter L. Green, MD, FACEP
UT Southwestern Medical Center, Dallas, TX

John C. Greenwood, MD
University of Pennsylvania, Philadelphia, PA

Danya Khoujah, MBBS, MEHP, FACEP
University of Maryland, Baltimore, MD

Nathaniel Mann, MD
University of South Carolina School of Medicine,
Greenville, SC

George Sternbach, MD, FACEP
Stanford University Medical Center, Stanford, CA

EDITORIAL STAFF

Suzannah Alexander, Editorial Director
salexander@acep.org

Joy Carrico, JD
Managing Editor

Alex Bass
Assistant Editor

Kel Morris
Assistant Editor

ISSN2325-0186 (Print)   ISSN2325-8365 (Online)

Contents

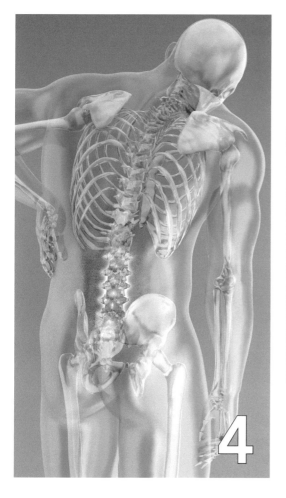

Lesson 13............................**4**

Watch Your Back
Back Pain as a Red-Flag Symptom
By Nikki Cali, MD; and Michael C. Bond, MD, FACEP
Reviewed by Tareq Al-Salamah, MBBS, MPH, FACEP

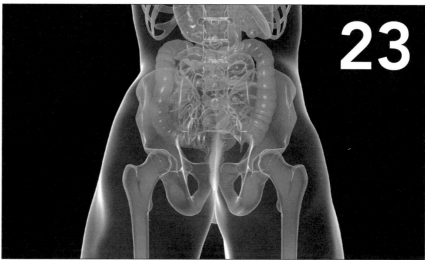

Lesson 14..........................**23**

Bringing Up the Rear
Perirectal, Perianal, and Pilonidal Abscesses
By Matthew Sherman, MD; Dalbir Bahga, MD; and Vietvuong Vo, MD
Reviewed by Walter L. Green, MD, FACEP

FEATURES

Clinical Pediatrics — Peritonsillar Abscesses and Deep Space Neck Infections.............................12
By Sarah Guess, MD; and Mark Pittman, MD
Reviewed by Sharon E. Mace, MD, FACEP

The Critical Procedure — Reduction of Rectal Prolapse 15
By Steven J. Warrington, MD, MEd, MS

The LLSA Literature Review — Cerebral Intraparenchymal Hemorrhage..................................16
By Paula N. Kreutzer, MD, MPH; and Nicholas G. Maldonado, MD, FACEP
Reviewed by Andrew J. Eyre, MD, MSHPEd

Critical Cases in Orthopedics and Trauma — Patella Fracture With Traumatic Arthrotomy..........18
By John Kiel, DO, MPH

The Critical Image — Right Lower Quadrant Pain in Pregnancy 20
By Joshua S. Broder, MD, FACEP

The Critical ECG — Signs of Hypothermia...22
By Amal Mattu, MD, FACEP

CME Questions 30
Reviewed by Tareq Al-Salamah, MBBS, MPH, FACEP; and Walter L. Green, MD, FACEP

Drug Box — Giapreza 32
By Frank LoVecchio, DO, MPH, FACEP

Tox Box — Acute Oral Methotrexate Overdose 32
By Christian Tomaszewski, MD, MS, MBA, FACEP

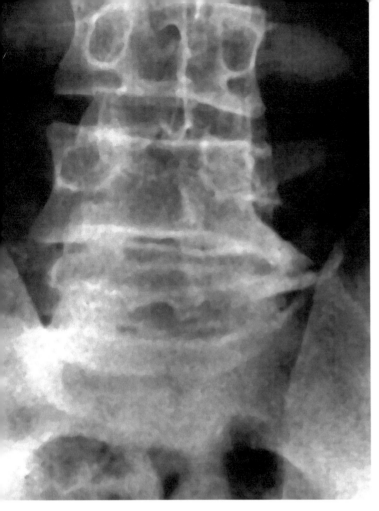

Watch Your Back

Back Pain as a Red-Flag Symptom

LESSON 13

By Nikki Cali, MD; and Michael C. Bond, MD, FACEP
Dr. Cali is a resident at University of Maryland Medical Center in Baltimore, and Dr. Bond is a professor of emergency medicine at the University of Maryland School of Medicine in Baltimore.
Reviewed by Tareq Al-Salamah, MBBS, MPH, FACEP

Objectives

On completion of this lesson, you should be able to:

1. Describe the diagnostic accuracy of red-flag symptoms in low back pain and associated diagnoses.
2. Compare and contrast the various imaging studies used to evaluate back pain.
3. Explain the appropriate medical treatment options for patients who present with back pain.
4. Distinguish back pain patients who require admission from those who require outpatient follow-up.
5. Discuss cost-effective evaluation options and workup for back pain.

From the EM Model

1.0 Signs, Symptoms, and Presentations
    1.2 Pain
        1.2.7 Back Pain

■ CRITICAL DECISIONS ■

■ What critical information from a patient's history and physical examination should prompt laboratory tests and imaging?

■ What imaging best elicits alarming back pain conditions?

■ What are the medical treatment options for patients with acute and chronic back pain?

■ Which back pain patients are high risk to discharge, and who should be admitted?

■ How can emergency physicians effectively and safely reduce costs in evaluating back pain patients?

Back pain is one of the most common symptom-related complaints in the emergency department, with up to 90% of adults experiencing back pain at some time in their lives. Most cases have a mechanical musculoskeletal etiology, but back pain can also be the harbinger of a life-threatening or paralyzing disease process.

Often these patients are triaged to lower-acuity areas, which can introduce additional biases that influence the approach to treatment. No emergency physician wants to miss a diagnosis, especially when the consequences are so dire, so a systematic approach to evaluating back pain patients and understanding the risk factors and warning signs are essential.

CASE ONE

A 73-year-old woman presents with acute-onset low back pain. When she got out of bed to use the bathroom the night before, she slipped and fell backward onto the tile floor. She required significant assistance from her husband to get back into bed due to back pain when trying to walk. When she awoke, she experienced excruciating back pain that prevented her from getting out of bed. She tried acetaminophen and a heating pad without significant relief.

On examination, she is comfortable and in no acute distress while lying still. She is thin appearing and has midline spinal tenderness to palpation in the thoracolumbar region without any palpable step-offs or deformities. She has normal rectal tone, and her sensation and strength are grossly intact in all four extremities. She can ambulate a few steps but is limited secondary to her back pain.

CASE TWO

A 35-year-old man with a past medical history notable for polysubstance abuse presents with persistent back pain for the past week and a half. He reports a history of intravenous drug use and last injected drugs into his groin earlier in the morning. He complains of diffuse myalgias, middle back pain, and urinary incontinence. He also reports difficulty walking because his legs feel weak. He was seen at an outside hospital 1 week ago for his back pain and was discharged with a diagnosis of musculoskeletal pain. Today, he presents because his back pain has worsened and he has developed new urinary symptoms and weakness in his legs.

His vital signs include BP 106/72, P 112, R 16, and T 37.9°C (100.2°F). On physical examination, he has track marks on his bilateral upper extremities and right groin. His right groin appears to be erythematous and warm to touch without evidence of a pulsatile mass, hematoma, or area of fluctuance. On neurologic examination, he has tenderness to palpation overlying the T10 spinous process without external signs of injury. He has 2/5 strength and absent deep tendon reflexes in his bilateral lower extremities. He has decreased rectal tone and decreased perineal sensation. He cannot ambulate, which is a progressive decline from when he presented at triage a few hours earlier.

CASE THREE

A 27-year-old man presents with right-sided low back pain. He is otherwise healthy and follows up regularly with his primary care physician. He works in a warehouse, and his job is labor intensive, requiring frequent heavy lifting. As he was lifting a box at work 2 days ago, he felt a "twinge" in his low back. Initially, he could not stand up straight because of the pain and had to leave work. Since the incident, he has been in bed resting. The pain is intermittent and associated with spasms; sometimes, the pain radiates down the side of his right thigh. It worsens with specific twisting movements, and he took 1,000 mg of acetaminophen once yesterday without improvement.

On examination, he has limited range of motion with lumbar flexion in a standing position due to pain. The pain is reproduced with lateral extension to the left and improves with lateral extension to the right. On palpation of the right lumbar region, no overlying ecchymoses, rashes, or signs of trauma are noted. He has tenderness to palpation in the right lumbar paraspinal region with palpable muscle contracture when compared to the left lumbar paraspinal region. Straight leg raise testing is positive on the right and negative on the left. Crossed leg testing is negative bilaterally. His sensation and strength are grossly intact in his lower extremities. He has 5/5 strength with hip flexion and extension, knee flexion and extension, ankle dorsiflexion and plantar flexion, great toe extension, and ankle eversion. His patellar and Achilles reflexes are intact. He ambulates with a steady gait and has no difficulty with toe walking or heel walking.

Introduction

Back pain is the fifth most common reason for all physician office visits and a common symptomatic complaint in the emergency department.[1,2] Back pain often contributes to lost work days, disability, and health care utilization. Because most cases of back pain are caused by a musculoskeletal disorder, it can be easy to become complacent in the evaluation of these patients and, thus, overlook patients whose symptoms indicate a dangerous disease process.

CRITICAL DECISION

What critical information from a patient's history and physical examination should prompt laboratory tests and imaging?

Low back pain (LBP) accounts for over 2.63 million visits to the emergency department annually, and emergency physicians are responsible for differentiating "can't miss" diagnoses from more commonly benign complaints.[2] Many guidelines suggest red-flag screening questions to detect serious back pain pathologies. Although guidelines fail to provide supporting evidence behind red-flag screening questions and symptoms, classically taught risk factors are extremes of age, trauma, a history of cancer, unexplained weight loss, pain that is worse at night, fever, and bowel or bladder incontinence. These questions are focused on eliciting alarming back pain diagnoses, such as malignancy, fracture, infection, cauda equina syndrome, and spinal epidural abscesses or osteomyelitis. Screening tools and assessments can assist the diagnostic process but are less valuable when disease prevalence is low and sensitivity is compromised. These red flags should supplement, not replace, clinician judgment. Basing a diagnostic workup solely on the presence of a "red flag" can lead to unnecessary diagnostic evaluations.[3] Physicians should consider these risk factors in the total assessment and use them to ensure performance of detailed histories and physical examinations and then order appropriate diagnostic studies as needed.

Physicians should conduct and document detailed physical examinations that include an assessment of gait, strength, sensation, and deep tendon reflexes. Functional strength testing is also helpful to elicit perceived weakness from a patient's positioning when sitting down. Perceived weakness when a patient is seated can be secondary to pain, which functional testing will not demonstrate. Functional strength documentation includes a patient's ability to squat, stand on their toes, rock back on their heels, and flex their back anteriorly,

Medical Conditions	Potential Sources of Bacteremia
• Abnormality of the vertebral column • AIDS • Alcoholism • Diabetes mellitus • Immunosuppressive therapy • Intravenous drug use • Local spine risk factor (ie, degenerative disc disease or osteophytes) • Malignancy • Steroid use • Trauma of the spine	• Recent infection (eg, UTI, endocarditis, or dental abscess) • Epidural anesthesia • Hemodialysis • Recent bone or soft tissue infection • Recent spinal instrumentation • Sepsis • Skin ulcers

TABLE 1. Risk factors for SEA

posteriorly, and laterally. Functional testing is also helpful when a patients overpower examiners but still have weakness when compared to their normal baseline.

Malignancy

Guidelines that discuss how back pain arises from malignancy almost always include two red flags: a history of cancer and unexplained or unintentional weight loss.[4] Physicians should always avoid applying red-flag symptoms in isolation; clinical context is important in light of red-flag symptoms. For example, a history of recent breast, lung, prostate, renal, gastrointestinal, or thyroid cancer is more concerning than a remote history of squamous cell carcinoma of the skin, considering the metastatic properties of cancers.[5]

Fractures

Vertebral compression fractures occur in almost 25% of postmenopausal women, with the prevalence linearly increasing with advanced age.[4] The additional red-flag symptom of trauma should exponentially heighten clinical suspicion for a fracture and the need for diagnostic imaging. Some guidelines lack

precision in their definition of trauma, including severe or major as the criteria. However, minimal trauma like a ground-level fall can have a similar, if not more significant, impact on an 80-year-old woman as a high-speed motor vehicle crash on a 40-year-old man. Physicians should evaluate the mechanism of injury when assessing the risk of vertebral fracture.

Infection

When a patient presents with back pain in the setting of a current fever, a history of intravenous drug use, or recent spinal surgery or spinal manipulation, a spinal infection should undoubtedly be included in the differential diagnosis. Patients with a more indolent infectious presentation (eg, borderline elevation in temperature and mild leukocytosis) are especially challenging to diagnose.

Patient risk factors for postoperative spinal infections include advanced age, a higher American Society of Anesthesiologists (ASA) physical status score, diabetes mellitus, cardiovascular disease, obesity, smoking, malignancy, steroid use, prior lumbar surgery, nutritional status, chronic obstructive pulmonary disease, and immunologic competency. Surgery-related risk factors include the duration of the surgery, blood loss, use of instrumentation, the number of levels fused, the surgical approach, and a prolonged preoperative hospital stay.[6]

Spinal epidural abscesses (SEAs) are often missed on the first presentation and are usually not diagnosed until symptoms develop. The classic symptoms of fever, back pain, and neurologic manifestations are only seen in 10% of cases. Patient risk factors include diabetes, intravenous drug use, long-term corticosteroid use, spinal abnormalities from recent trauma or surgery, epidural anesthesia, or a recent bacterial infection (*Table 1*).[7] Patients with these risk factors warrant an infectious workup, including a complete blood count and inflammatory markers (ie, erythrocyte sedimentation rate [ESR] and C-reactive protein [CRP]). If the WBC, ESR, and CRP levels are normal, the risk of an

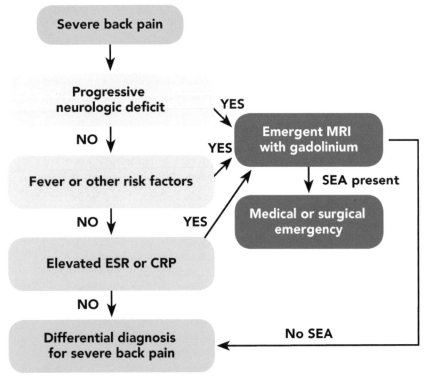

FIGURE 1. Evaluation of patients at risk of SEA

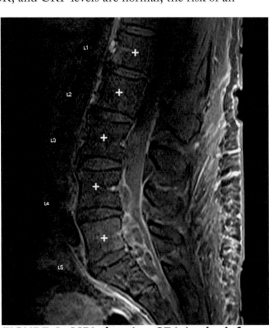

FIGURE 2. MRI showing SEA in the left anterior epidural space. Copyright 2022 Dr. Chris O'Donnell. Image courtesy of Dr. Chris O'Donnell and Radiopaedia.org, rID: 29169. Used under license.

SEA is exceedingly low, and further evaluation is unwarranted (*Figure 1*). In cases where the WBC, ESR, or CRP levels are elevated, the patient should be considered for a whole spine (ie, cervical, thoracic, and lumbar) MRI with gadolinium or a CT myelogram to exclude osteomyelitis or SEAs (*Figure 2*).

Staphylococcus aureus (>50% of cases) is the leading pathogen in both SEAs and vertebral osteomyelitis. Therefore, empiric antibiotics should include coverage for methicillin-resistant *S. aureus*. Other pathogens include *Streptococcus* species, coagulase-negative staphylococci associated with spinal surgery and foreign bodies, enteric gram-negative bacilli (eg, *Escherichia coli* in the setting of a UTI), *Candida* species in immunocompromised patients and those with recent spinal surgery, and *Pseudomonas aeruginosa* in intravenous drug use.[3]

Cauda Equina Syndrome

Cauda equina syndrome (CES) is a constellation of symptoms that occurs when there is compression of multiple lumbar and sacral nerve roots at the caudal end of the spinal cord (*Figure 3*). There are multiple causes of CES, including a herniated disc, spinal stenosis, trauma, infection, a tumor, spinal hemorrhage, or postoperative complications, which can make the diagnosis challenging. In fact, no sign or symptom combination can reliably diagnose or exclude CES. As proof of how challenging the diagnosis can be, one study showed that senior neurosurgical residents were only able to accurately identify 56% of patients with MRI-proven CES.[8]

The classic features of CES include bilateral radiculopathy, perineal numbness (ie, saddle anesthesia), altered bladder function, loss of rectal tone, and sexual dysfunction.[9] Loss of bladder or bowel control and saddle anesthesia are common red-flag symptoms seen in the emergency department. Physical examinations must include an assessment of perineal sensation; one study determined that saddle sensory deficits were the only clinical feature associated with a positive MRI finding of CES.[10] Although the loss of bladder or bowel control in a patient experiencing LBP is suspicious for CES, studies show that this combination of symptoms is not highly predictive of the diagnosis.[11] What "loss of bladder control" means can vary. It can mean urinary retention, incontinence, or generic dysfunction. Obtaining a postvoid residual volume is helpful with inconsistent patient descriptions of urinary symptoms and should be performed in a comprehensive physical examination where CES is suspected.

Aortic Aneurysm

It is important to remember that other serious disease processes outside the spine can elicit back pain and warrant further evaluation. The combination of hypotension, back or flank pain, and a pulsatile mass are highly concerning for a ruptured abdominal aortic aneurysm (AAA), although the presentation of the classic triad is uncommon. Risk factors include age older than 65 years, male sex, Caucasian, a history of smoking, a family history of aneurysms, and a personal history of a known aneurysm. "Renal colic" in older individuals who have never had kidney stones is also suspicious for an acute aortic pathology. AAAs can sometimes be seen on plain x-rays of the lumbar spine obtained in older patients with LBP (*Figure 4*). Vascular calcifications anterior to the lumbar spine are often seen on lateral x-rays and can help drive physicians to the correct diagnosis.

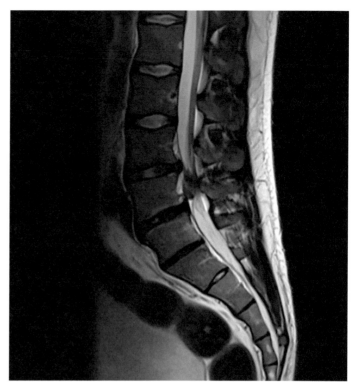

FIGURE 3. MRI of cauda equina syndrome. Copyright 2022 Dr. Henry Knipe. Image courtesy of Dr. Henry Knipe and Radiopaedia.org, rID: 53615. Used under license.

CRITICAL DECISION

What imaging best elicits alarming back pain conditions?

Most patients do not require imaging for back pain. Imaging should only be obtained when physicians determine a patient may have a pathologic cause of pain or a neurologic deficit is noted on physical examination. However, many imaging options are available to evaluate back pain when needed. According to a study conducted in the early 2000s, approximately one-third of all patients who present with back pain receive diagnostic imaging.[2] When choosing what imaging study to order, it is essential to consider what resources are available because many emergency departments do not have around-the-clock MRI capabilities or in-house sonographers for formal ultrasound studies. It is important to consider not only what is appropriate for patient care, but also what is possible.

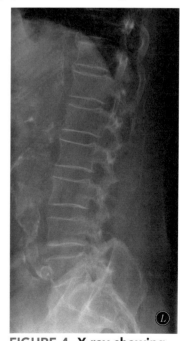

FIGURE 4. X-ray showing AAA. Copyright 2022 Dr. Boris Schulz. Image courtesy of Dr. Boris Schulz and Radiopaedia.org, rID: 24449. Used under license.

Plain X-rays

Routine x-ray imaging is not indicated for most

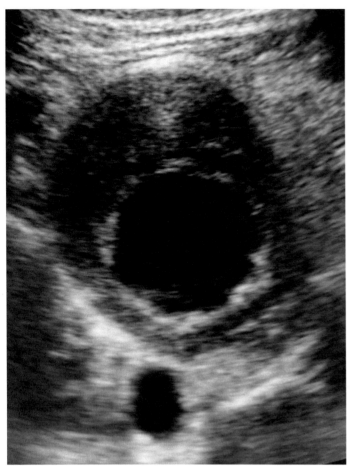

FIGURE 5. Ultrasound showing AAA. DrCHAMPGO/
Shutterstock.com.

patients with uncomplicated acute LBP; however, plain x-rays are suggested as the first-line evaluation for patients with red-flag symptoms, including patients older than age 50 years when a fracture or cancer is suspected and patients with a history of osteoporosis, immunosuppression, chronic oral steroid use, intravenous drug use, substance abuse, or failure to improve after 6 weeks of conservative therapy.[12] Obtaining plain x-rays without a clear indication in an effort to reassure the physician, reassure the patient, or meet patient expectations has risks. Obtaining plain x-rays early is associated with worse overall outcomes because they are likely to identify minor abnormalities in asymptomatic patients or label patients with an anatomic diagnosis that is not causing the symptoms.[12,13]

Plain x-rays should also be avoided as a screening test when a more serious pathology is suspected. X-rays are insensitive in many spinal pathologies. Use of more advanced imaging at the initial presentation of back pain is appropriate when serious etiologies, such as CES, SEA, or a tumor, are suspected. Additionally, osteoporosis decreases the sensitivity of plain x-rays, making them less useful in older patients.

CT and MRI

When suspicion is high for a serious underlying back pain pathology, it may be appropriate to proceed directly to advanced imaging. One of the more apparent indications is in the setting of neurologic symptoms, such as progressive motor or sensory deficits, saddle anesthesia, bilateral sciatica or leg weakness, difficulty urinating, or fecal incontinence. MRI is

the recommended diagnostic study of choice if any of these symptoms are present and should be obtained emergently when there is concern for CES.[12] MRI with intravenous gadolinium contrast is the preferred imaging modality when the suspected etiology of back pain is infection, malignancy, or postoperative sequelae.[14] Noncontrast CT scans are often obtained in the setting of a suspected fracture, whether it is traumatic or pathologic. Due to the widespread availability of CTs, plain x-rays of the spine are typically bypassed in polytrauma patients. Reconstructions of the spine can easily be accomplished with the chest and abdominal-pelvic CTs that these patients usually receive. MRIs should follow CT scans in the setting of traumatic injuries with neurologic deficits, regardless of the CT findings. CT is extremely limited in evaluating intervertebral discs or the epidural space that may contain a hematoma or abscess.

CT Myelogram and Ultrasound

In patients who cannot safely undergo MRI, CT with or without myelography can be considered as a less sensitive diagnostic imaging tool. CT myelography has drastically fallen out of favor with the increasing accessibility of MRI. Still, it is a valuable alternative for patients with MRI-incompatible implanted devices, a large body habitus, claustrophobia, or an inability to stay still for an extended period of time. Patients with significant back pain often find it extremely difficult to lie still long enough to render optimal MRI images.

Another imaging modality is ultrasound. It is important to remember that not all back pain originates from the spine, and other deadly pathologies (eg, ruptured AAAs) can present with back pain (*Figure 5*). Many emergency departments have easily accessible ultrasound machines that can be used at the bedside to evaluate an enlarged aorta. Although it is difficult to assess if the aorta is ruptured on ultrasound, a cross-sectional diameter can be obtained to help determine the need for an expedited CT angiogram of the abdomen.

✔ Pearls

- Red flags should supplement rather than replace a physician's decision about whether advanced imaging or laboratory tests are needed.

- NSAIDs are first-line therapy in patients with acute LBP.

- If there is concern for SEA, a whole spine MRI with gadolinium should be obtained because skip lesions are common in this condition.

- Severe spinal pathology can be missed on the initial emergency department visit, so special attention should be paid to repeat visits within a short period of time.

- Back pain in the absence of red flags typically does not warrant imaging or laboratory tests unless it persists beyond 6 weeks with conservative measures.

CRITICAL DECISION

What are the medical treatment options for patients with acute and chronic back pain?

Most back pain improves regardless of the treatment rendered; therefore, treatment should be optimized to minimize harm and help return patients to their normal activity level as quickly as possible. NSAIDs have the best efficiency and should be the first-line treatment for back pain. A Cochrane review of 51 trials found that NSAIDs are superior to placebo for global improvement and for not requiring additional analgesics after 1 week of therapy.[15] Regularly scheduled NSAIDs (eg, ibuprofen and naproxen) are an effective option for treating back pain. Although acetaminophen in combination with ibuprofen is an effective treatment option for those with acute fractures, acetaminophen use has little benefit in treating back pain whether used in conjunction with NSAIDs or alone.[16,17]

Muscle relaxants (eg, cyclobenzaprine, carisoprodol, baclofen, and tizanidine) are often prescribed for patients who have muscle spasms or moderate to severe pain. Their use should be limited to those with acute back pain because there is insufficient evidence to show their effectiveness in patients with chronic back pain.[18] Most trials restrict the use of muscle relaxants to 2 weeks or less. Muscle relaxants are associated with adverse effects (eg, drowsiness, sedation, and dizziness) that should limit their use, especially in older patients who are at increased risk of delirium and falls.[19] Benzodiazepines have also been used to treat back pain; however, they also have not been shown to have any benefit over NSAIDs used alone at 1 week or 3 months after emergency department discharge.[20,21]

Opiates should be reserved for those who cannot take NSAIDs or have severe pain that NSAIDs cannot control. The early use of opiates has been shown to increase long-term opioid use, medical costs, and disability in patients with acute occupational LBP.[22] Opiates should only be prescribed for a short period of time and ideally in conjunction with NSAIDs. Lidocaine patches are a topical option for those with paraspinal muscle pain and may be effective in limiting the use of opiates.

There is no evidence to support the role of systemic corticosteroids in the treatment of nonradicular or radicular acute LBP.[23,24] While one study showed a small short-term benefit in emergency department patients with cervical and lumbar radiculopathy who were given a single parenteral dose of dexamethasone,[25] numerous other studies have not demonstrated any clinically significant benefit over placebo when given parenterally or as a short oral course.[23,26-28] Finally, combination therapy is no better than monotherapy with NSAIDs. Adding an opiate or muscle relaxants has no effect on functional outcomes at 3 months.[17,29-33]

CRITICAL DECISION

Which back pain patients are high risk to discharge, and who should be admitted?

The incidence of serious pathology exists in only a small fraction of patients who present with back pain, so most patients can be discharged. Although studies note trends of women and the elderly being at greater risk of hospital admission, this is not necessarily indicative of women being at greater risk of developing clinically significant back pain than men.[34]

Before discharging any patient, emergency physicians should follow a methodical approach to the discharge process. First, the patient must be reassessed before discharge. This process includes documenting the latest vital signs and reviewing all laboratory and imaging results, if obtained. If patients present with abnormal vital signs, the discharge process is an opportunity to ensure any abnormalities have been addressed, improved, or documented in the patient's medical chart if alternative reasoning explains their presence.

Predischarge review of vital signs also provides an opportunity to observe trends and see if a patient is decompensating and no longer safe for discharge. It is crucial to personally view all plain x-rays and read the fine print of radiology imaging reports (if available at the time of the visit). Treating physicians know exactly where patients have pain and may notice subtle fractures or findings that the radiologist may miss. Special attention should be paid to patients who have a repeat visit for their back pain within a relatively short period of time because many cases of severe spinal pathology are missed on the first emergency department visit.

If abnormalities such as fractures, metastases, or abscesses are noted on imaging studies, patients must be informed of the finding, and the appropriate follow-up care must be arranged. Most abscesses and many fractures warrant admission; however, some fractures and metastatic lesions can be treated as an outpatient. Speaking to the appropriate specialist while the patient is still in the emergency department can help ensure that the proper treatment plan and follow-up care are coordinated. For metastases or abscesses with neurologic deficits, immediate consultation with a spine surgeon for operative intervention is warranted. If a patient presents to a free-standing emergency department, this often necessitates emergent transfer to a center that can provide the patient with comprehensive surgical and medical care.

After all the objective data is reviewed, a reassessment of the patient should be performed before discharge. In a patient with back pain, evaluation of pain and mobility is necessary for discharge planning to help determine if a patient needs a prescription for medication on discharge or if they need medical equipment such as a cane or walker to help with ambulation. Patients who cannot ambulate safely should be admitted or have a physical therapy evaluation before discharge.

✖ Pitfalls

- Failing to consider the diagnosis of SEA because there is no neurologic deficit noted on physical examination.

- Ordering diagnostic studies indiscriminately in acute LBP. They increase costs with little benefit to the patient.

- Starting opiates early in the treatment of LBP, without a trial of NSAIDs.

- Neglecting to provide return precautions and timely follow-up recommendations.

If the patient is deemed safe for discharge, the patient should be provided with a follow-up plan and informative discharge instructions with return precautions. If the patient has a primary care physician, set a defined time frame of 1 to 2 days to call and schedule a follow-up appointment. All patients should be told to return if they develop neurologic symptoms, increasing pain, an inability to ambulate, or have bladder or bowel incontinence.

CRITICAL DECISION

How can emergency physicians effectively and safely reduce costs in evaluating back pain patients?

Most patients with back pain have pain due to a musculoskeletal cause, so a detailed assessment (ie, history and physical examination) is often all that is needed. Laboratory tests and x-rays should not be a standard part of these evaluations. Laboratory studies are rarely required for the assessment of back pain unless there is concern for infection or malignancy. This strategy alone can significantly reduce costs. Obtaining unnecessary laboratory tests and x-rays is also potentially harmful, as incidental findings, laboratory test errors, and artifacts on imaging can cause anxiety and lead to additional testing that is of no benefit to the patient.

Unless there are red-flag signs or the pain lasts for more than 6 weeks, imaging is not required. About 95% of patients with back pain experience a complete resolution of their symptoms within 6 weeks regardless of the treatment provided. Obtaining MRIs in patients before 6 weeks may identify herniated disks, degenerative disc disease, arthritis, or other incidental pathologies that are not the cause of their pain, but these findings may make them believe they need steroid injections or surgery. MRIs do not reduce return visits. Patients in the emergency department who receive an MRI are just as likely to return within 1 week as those who do not receive an MRI.[35] Conservative treatment with heat, range-of-motion exercises, and massage, plus physical therapy, is often the most cost-effective strategy in treating patients with back pain.

Summary

Most emergency department visits for back pain are for benign musculoskeletal complaints. To help identify those patients with serious underlying pathologies that cause back pain, physicians should use red-flag symptoms in conjunction with clinical judgment to help guide diagnostic testing. Although most patients do not require laboratory or imaging tests during their visit, they are necessary for the diagnosis of malignancies, fractures, infection, CES, and SEA or osteomyelitis. If clinical suspicion is high for a serious underlying back pain pathology, it is appropriate to order advanced imaging such as CTs and MRIs.

When treating musculoskeletal back pain, NSAIDs are the first-line treatment and early opioid use should be used sparingly because opioids increase medical costs and disability in patients with acute back pain. It is important to perform thorough neurologic examinations on all patients with back pain. A comprehensive history and physical examination can help in the early diagnosis of a serious life-threatening pathology and can help prevent long-term neurologic disability and mortality.

REFERENCES

1. Hart LG, Deyo RA, Cherkin DC. Physician office visits for low back pain. Frequency, clinical evaluation, and treatment patterns from a U.S. national survey. *Spine (Phila Pa 1976)*. 1995;20(1):11-19.
2. Friedman BW, Chilstrom M, Bijur PE, Gallagher EJ. Diagnostic testing and treatment of low back pain in United States emergency departments: a national perspective. *Spine (Phila Pa 1976)*. 2010;35(24):E1406-E1411.
3. Corwell BN, Davis NL. The emergent evaluation and treatment of neck and back pain. *Emerg Med Clin North Am*. 2020;38(1):167-191.
4. Verhagen AP, Downie A, Maher CG, Koes BW. Most red flags for malignancy in low back pain guidelines lack empirical support: a systematic review. *Pain*. 2017;158(10):1860-1868.
5. Ziu E, Viswanathan VK, Mesfin FB. Spinal metastasis. In: *StatPearls [Internet]*. StatPearls Publishing; 2022. https://www.ncbi.nlm.nih.gov/books/NBK441950/
6. Schömig F, Putzier M. Clinical presentation and diagnosis of delayed postoperative spinal implant infection. *J Spine Surg*. 2020;6(4):772-776.
7. Tetsuka S, Suzuki T, Ogawa T, Hashimoto R, Kato H. Spinal epidural abscess: a review highlighting early diagnosis and management. *JMA J*. 2020;3(1):29-40.
8. Bell DA, Collie D, Statham PF. Cauda equina syndrome: what is the correlation between clinical assessment and MRI scanning? *Br J Neurosurg*. 2007;21(2):201-203.
9. Todd NV. Guidelines for cauda equina syndrome. Red flags and white flags. Systematic review and implications for triage. *Br J Neurosurg*. 2017;31(3):336-339.
10. Balasubramanian K, Kalsi P, Greenough CG, Kuskoor Seetharam MP. Reliability of clinical assessment in diagnosing cauda equina syndrome. *Br J Neurosurg*. 2010;24(4):383-386.
11. Premkumar A, Godfrey W, Gottschalk MB, Boden SD. Red flags for low back pain are not always really red: a prospective evaluation of the clinical utility of commonly used screening questions for low back pain. *J Bone Joint Surg Am*. 2018;100(5):368-374.
12. Kinkade S. Evaluation and treatment of acute low back pain. *Am Fam Physician*. 2007;75(8):1181-1188.
13. Chou R. Low back pain. *Ann Intern Med*. 2021;174(8):ITC113-ITC128.
14. Rao D, Scuderi G, Scuderi C, Grewal R, Sandhu SJ. The use of imaging in management of patients with low back pain. *J Clin Imaging Sci*. 2018;8:30.
15. Roelofs PDDM, Deyo RA, Koes BW, Scholten RJ, van Tulder MW. Non-steroidal anti-inflammatory drugs for low back pain. *Cochrane Database Syst Rev*. 2008;(1):CD000396.
16. Saragiotto BT, Machado GC, Ferreira ML, Pinheiro MB, Abdel Shaheed C, Maher CG. Paracetamol for low back pain. *Cochrane Database Syst Rev*. 2016;(6):CD012230.
17. Friedman BW, Irizarry E, Chertoff A, et al. Ibuprofen plus acetaminophen versus ibuprofen alone for acute low back pain: an emergency department-based randomized study. *Acad Emerg Med*. 2020;27(3):229-235.
18. Abdel Shaheed C, Maher CG, Williams KA, McLachlan AJ. Efficacy and tolerability of muscle relaxants for low back pain: systematic review and meta-analysis. *Eur J Pain*. 2017;21(2):228-237.
19. van Tulder MW, Touray T, Furlan AD, Solway S, Bouter LM; Cochrane Back Review Group. Muscle relaxants for nonspecific low back pain: a systematic review within the framework of the Cochrane collaboration. *Spine (Phila Pa 1976)*. 2003;28(17):1978-1992.
20. Friedman BW, Irizarry E, Solorzano C, et al. Diazepam is no better than placebo when added to naproxen for acute low back pain. *Ann Emerg Med*. 2017;70(2):169-176.e1.
21. Hingorani K. Diazepam in backache. A double-blind controlled trial. *Ann Phys Med*. 1966;8(8):303-306.
22. Lee SS, Choi Y, Pransky GS. Extent and impact of opioid prescribing for acute occupational low back pain in the emergency department. *J Emerg Med*. 2016;50(3):376-384.e1-2.
23. Friedman BW, Holden L, Esses D, et al. Parenteral corticosteroids for emergency department patients with non-radicular low back pain. *J Emerg Med*. 2006;31(4):365-370.
24. Eskin B, Shih RD, Fiesseler FW, et al. Prednisone for emergency department low back pain: a randomized controlled trial. *J Emerg Med*. 2014;47(1):65-70.

CASE RESOLUTIONS

CASE ONE

Due to multiple risk factors, including advanced age, female sex, and acute trauma, there was high clinical suspicion for a fracture. CT of the thoracic spine was obtained and notable for an acute compression fracture at the level of T11. The fracture was stable, and the case was discussed with a spine surgeon who recommended conservative management and outpatient follow-up in the spine clinic.

The patient's pain was acutely controlled in the emergency department with ibuprofen, acetaminophen, and a lidocaine patch to the point that she could ambulate with a walker. Acetaminophen was given in the acute phase due to its added benefits in pain control for fractures. She was advised to continue with scheduled ibuprofen and lidocaine patches at home. The patient also disclosed a history of several falls over the past 6 months, typically tripping over objects in her house and when using steps, so muscle relaxants were avoided. She followed up with her primary care physician within 3 weeks of her emergency department visit, and her pain improved. She began doing physical therapy as an outpatient and made changes in her home to help prevent falls. Her spine surgeon recommended a nonoperative approach to her stable compression fracture, because her pain improved with conservative measures.

CASE TWO

After the initial evaluation, an infectious workup was pursued. Laboratory tests were obtained and were notable for leukocytosis to 19.4 with a left shift. Inflammatory markers, including ESR and CRP, were significantly elevated. Due to the patient's acute neurologic deficits, neurosurgery was consulted, and broad-spectrum antibiotics were administered.

MRI of the cervical, thoracic, and lumbar spine with gadolinium contrast was obtained to ensure no skip lesions were missed. MRI showed soft tissue swelling from T9 to L1 with evidence of cord compression and abscess formation, consistent with SEA. The patient went for emergent surgical decompression and drainage. Cultures obtained were positive for *S. aureus*, and the patient's antibiotics were tailored to sensitivities obtained with the cultures.

Postoperatively, the patient was discharged from the hospital to subacute rehabilitation. After extensive rehabilitation with physical therapy, his strength improved to 4/5 in his lower extremities, and he could ambulate with a cane.

CASE THREE

This young, otherwise healthy man's history and physical examination findings indicated that he was likely suffering from acute lumbar radiculopathy, which was evident by the paraspinal muscle spasm and positive straight leg raise test on the right. His pain radiated down the side of his thigh, which is most consistent with an L2-L3 or L3-L4 disc level injury.

The patient was informed that his injury pattern was suspicious for acute lumbar radiculopathy and that imaging was unnecessary because it would not change the recommended management for his symptoms but instead prolong his time in the emergency department and increase costs. The patient was treated conservatively with ibuprofen and a short course of nocturnal cyclobenzaprine. He was advised to limit his lifting at work and gradually return to his full duties as tolerated. He was also advised to schedule a follow-up with his primary care physician, who could refer him to physical therapy if needed. Upon discharge, it was explained that conservative management and a tincture of time could improve his symptoms.

He was given strict return precautions to return to the emergency department if he developed new weakness or numbness in his legs, urinary or bowel incontinence, difficulty walking, or if his pain persisted for more than 6 weeks because these symptoms can indicate the need for further workup and imaging.

25. Balakrishnamoorthy R, Horgan I, Perez S, Steele MC, Keijzers GB. Does a single dose of intravenous dexamethasone reduce symptoms in emergency department patients with low back pain and radiculopathy (SEBRA)? A double-blind randomised controlled trial. *Emerg Med J.* 2015;32(7):525-530.

26. Finckh A, Zufferey P, Schurch MA, Balague F, Waldburger M, So AKL. Short-term efficacy of intravenous pulse glucocorticoids in acute discogenic sciatica. A randomized controlled trial. *Spine (Phila Pa 1976).* 2006;31(4):377-381.

27. Haimovic IC, Beresford HR. Dexamethasone is not superior to placebo for treating lumbosacral radicular pain. *Neurology.* 1986;36(12):1593-1594.

28. Porsman O, Friis H. Prolapsed lumbar disc treated with intramuscularly administered dexamethasonephosphate. A prospectively planned, double-blind, controlled clinical trial in 52 patients. *Scand J Rheumatol.* 1979;8(3):142-144.

29. Friedman BW, Cisewski D, Irizarry E, et al. A randomized, double-blind, placebo-controlled trial of naproxen with or without orphenadrine or methocarbamol for acute low back pain. *Ann Emerg Med.* 2018;71(3):348-356.e5.

30. Friedman BW, Dym AA, Davitt M, et al. Naproxen with cyclobenzaprine, oxycodone/acetaminophen, or placebo for treating acute low back pain: a randomized clinical trial. *JAMA.* 2015;314(15):1572-1580.

31. Friedman BW, Irizarry E, Solorzano C, et al. A randomized, placebo-controlled trial of ibuprofen plus metaxalone, tizanidine, or baclofen for acute low back pain. *Ann Emerg Med.* 2019;74(4):512-520.

32. Khwaja SM, Minnerop M, Singer AJ. Comparison of ibuprofen, cyclobenzaprine or both in patients with acute cervical strain: a randomized controlled trial. *CJEM.* 2010;12(1):39-44.

33. Turturro MA, Frater CR, D'Amico FJ. Cyclobenzaprine with ibuprofen versus ibuprofen alone in acute myofascial strain: a randomized, double-blind clinical trial. *Ann Emerg Med.* 2003;41(6):818-826.

34. Waterman BR, Belmont PJ Jr., Schoenfeld AJ. Low back pain in the United States: incidence and risk factors for presentation in the emergency setting. *Spine J.* 2012;12(1):63-70.

35. Aaronson EL, Yun BJ, Mort E, et al. Association of magnetic resonance imaging for back pain on seven-day return visit to the emergency department. *Emerg Med J.* 2017;34(10):677-679.

ADDITIONAL REFERENCE

ASA Physical Status (PS) Classification System. American Society of Anesthesiologists. Accessed July 7, 2022. https://www.asahq.org/standards-and-guidelines/asa-physical-status-classification-system

Peritonsillar Abscesses and Deep Space Neck Infections

By Sarah Guess, MD; and Mark Pittman, MD
Prisma Health — Upstate, Greenville, South Carolina

Reviewed by Sharon E. Mace, MD, FACEP

Objective

On completion of this article, you should be able to:

■ Determine how to manage pediatric patients with a peritonsillar abscess.

CASE PRESENTATION

A 6-year-old boy with no significant past medical history presents to the pediatric emergency department after multiple previous presentations to his local emergency department. His mother contacted his pediatrician on day 1 of his illness for medication due to a nocturnal cough. They were sent a prescription for brompheniramine and counseled to follow up as needed. He presented to the emergency department on day 2. He was diagnosed with a viral upper respiratory illness. Neck pain was reported with no peritonsillar exudate and no documentation of meningismus. Influenza testing was negative. He then presented on day 3 to a different outlying emergency department and remained febrile following acetaminophen administration. Testing included a negative rapid throat culture and a respiratory pathogen panel positive for rhinovirus and enterovirus. He received a dose of dexamethasone during this visit. Subsequently, a throat culture came back positive for group A *Streptococcus*, although antibiotics were not started. The patient was seen in the pediatrician's office on day 4 with ongoing neck and head pain. Guarding of the neck when looking up was present. No tonsillar asymmetry was noted. A CT scan of the soft tissue of the neck, mononucleosis test, throat culture, and COVID-19 test were ordered. CT noted "asymmetric soft tissue swelling of the left nasopharynx and oropharynx, highly worrisome for a large peritonsillar abscess (PTA). This communicates with the retropharyngeal and dangerous spaces and tracks inferiorly into the lower neck. This is a potential rate of communication with the mediastinum, although there is no evidence for mediastinal extension at this point." The patient was then sent to the pediatric emergency department for further evaluation.

Pathophysiology

Patients commonly develop tonsilitis, which has the potential to progress to cellulitis and eventually develop into a PTA.[1,2] PTA is defined as a collection of purulent materials between the tonsillar capsule and pharyngeal constrictor muscle (*Figure 1*). The development of an abscess from cellulitis is more common in young adults and less so in young children or the elderly.[2] PTA occurs from necrosis of tissue and pus development between the tonsillar capsule and lateral pharyngeal wall.[2] The bacteriology of these infections is complex, and a culture often results in mixed aerobes and anaerobes. Some well-described aerobic pathogens include *Streptococcus pyogenes* and *Staphylococcus aureus*.[3-5] Anaerobic pathogens include *Peptostreptococcus* and *Prevotella*.[3-5] In many cases, the isolate is simply mixed flora.[2,4]

Complications

Airway compromise is the primary initial concern in a patient with a PTA. Signs of impending airway compromise include intolerance of secretions (including drooling), trismus, sniffing position, stridor, voice changes, and changes in vital signs.[1,5] Oropharyngeal edema can make it difficult to intubate these patients. If time allows, the ideal management includes intubation in the operating room with anesthesia and otolaryngology (ENT) present. If this is not possible, and there is pending airway compromise, physicians should consider the possibility of pus in the airway caused by a rupture of the abscess. Use of other methods, such as fiberoptics or nasopharyngeal intubation may be needed in these scenarios. As with any

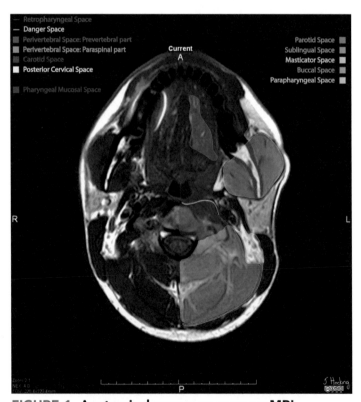

Retropharyngeal Space
Danger Space
Perivertebral Space: Prevertebral part
Perivertebral Space: Paraspinal part
Carotid Space
Posterior Cervical Space

Pharyngeal Mucosal Space

Parotid Space
Sublingual Space
Masticator Space
Buccal Space
Parapharyngeal Space

Current
A

R

L

P

FIGURE 1. Anatomical spaces as seen on MRI.

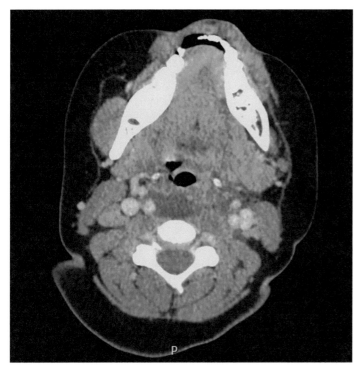

FIGURE 2. Large peritonsillar abscess, measuring 1.6 × 3.1 cm in (anteroposterior) AP and transverse dimensions. The main portion of the collection extends over 2.5 cm inferiorly, beginning almost at the skull base.

difficult intubation, the most experienced physician should perform the procedure. Where possible, the patient should be seated in an upright position, and as much intervention as possible should be performed while the patient is awake.[1,5,6]

Descending necrotizing mediastinitis is one of the more common complications of PTA.[7] A 2020 article cited a review of 334 patients, with 113 patients developing this complication (approximately one-third). Descending necrotizing mediastinitis occurs as the result of an extension of the infection into the "danger space," traversing into the mediastinum (*Figure 2*). The so-called danger space, which is synonymous with the alar space, allows for direct access from the neck to the mediastinum. This is a concerning complication because there is a high rate of mortality, approximately 40% as determined by a 2018 article.[8] Delayed diagnosis leads to worse outcomes and more extensive surgical intervention.

The infection travels first to the parapharyngeal space.[8] The parapharyngeal space is defined superiorly by the base of the skull and extends downward to the lesser cornua of the hyoid. The lateral margin is defined by the superficial layer of the deep cervical fascia, and the medial margin is defined by the visceral division of the middle layer of the deep cervical fascia. The retropharyngeal space is deep to the parapharyngeal space, and the danger space is deep to the retropharyngeal space.[9] The parapharyngeal space itself is not directly connected to the danger space; infection must travel through the retropharyngeal or vascular space. Once infection reaches the retropharyngeal or vascular space, it can travel into the mediastinal space and cause mediastinitis. The primary vascular access in the parapharyngeal space is the carotid vessels because the carotid sheath passes through this space.

Lemierre syndrome, also known as postanginal sepsis, is a potential complication of PTA caused by *Fusobacterium necrophorum*, an aerobic bacterium that is part of the normal flora

of the human body. It can lead to extensive infection involving the tonsillar and internal jugular vein.[10,11] It is associated with septic emboli and was first described by André Lemierre in 1936.[10,11] While this condition is not strictly defined, there is a generally accepted set of symptoms. Typically, affected patients are otherwise healthy prior to infection.[11] Internal jugular venous thrombosis forms due to the bacterium causing platelet aggregation without lysis.[10] Septic emboli within the lungs are frequently seen, and infiltrates can be seen on x-ray, often associated with pleural effusion. A Lemierre syndrome diagnosis can be confused with a mononucleosis infection, resulting in a delay in diagnosis.[10] Management of Lemierre syndrome consists of antibiotics, including metronidazole; drainage of abscesses; and other supportive care.[10]

Diagnosis

Although feared, deep space neck infections are rare. A preceding untreated or incompletely treated oropharyngeal infection is a risk factor. Worrisome presenting symptoms include trismus, decreased range of motion of the neck, the inability to tolerate oral secretions, and a muffled voice often described as a "hot potato" voice.

A physical examination finding of pain with posterior extension of the neck is more consistent with a retropharyngeal abscess. Alternatively, patients with meningitis resist flexion at the neck because flexion induces stretching of the meninges, causing severe pain. Physical examination findings often include exudate on the tonsils due to the common precursor tonsillitis.[5]

Imaging modalities used to characterize the extent of the infection include ultrasound, CT, and MRI. On contrast-enhanced CT, an abscess is visible as a central hypodense mass surrounded by a hyperdense rim.[5,12] In children, low-voltage CT can be used to lower radiation exposure and can provide clearer images for diagnosis.[5,12] Ultrasound can play a role in both bedside drainage and intraoperative management of PTAs; however, accuracy is user dependent. Ultrasound does not characterize the deep spaces of the neck well. MRI remains a valid diagnostic tool without radiation exposure, although pediatric patients may require sedation.[13] In a patient with concern for airway compromise or where rapid diagnosis is vital, other imaging modalities should be pursued.

Care should be taken to assess for complications, including mediastinitis and Lemierre syndrome. Patients with these conditions tend to present more ill appearing because of the systemic spread of these infections. Advanced imaging is useful for identifying the extent of the infection. As is the case with any septic patient, resuscitation is a mainstay of management, along with early antibiotic administration.

Management

The management of PTAs and deep space neck infections begins with the ABCs — airway, breathing, and circulation. Because the disease process affects the oropharynx, the airway is a primary concern. Initial evaluation should focus on the patient's ability to protect the airway, and airway intervention should be approached cautiously. Adjunct equipment should be readily available, and back-up physicians should be alerted. Unless emergent intervention is indicated, airway intervention should be undertaken in the operating room with anesthesia and ENT present. If emergently needed, the intubating physician

On evaluation, the patient presented with ongoing neck pain, difficulty swallowing, and drooling. No airway compromise or meningismus was noted. He was resistant to turning his head and experienced pain while looking up, although he was able to tuck his chin to his chest. Laboratory results included a C-reactive protein level of 133 mg/L, an erythrocyte sedimentation rate of 49, and a WBC count of 26. Blood cultures were also obtained.

ENT was consulted and evaluated the patient with a plan for operative management based on CT imaging. The patient was taken to the operating room approximately 2 hours after presentation. Antimicrobial administration included vancomycin, metronidazole, and cefepime due to allergies to erythromycin, azithromycin, and penicillin. In the operating room, the patient underwent a 1-cm lateral pharyngeal wall vertical incision with the expression of copious purulent material. Irrigation was performed. The patient was subsequently extubated with no significant laryngeal edema noted. He received intraoperative dexamethasone.

Postoperatively, the patient did well. Wound cultures grew gram-positive cocci and coccobacilli. The intraoperative aerobic culture ultimately demonstrated light growth of beta-hemolytic *Streptococcus* group A, and blood cultures were negative. On postoperative day 1, his neck pain was improving, and he started on a regular diet with overall improvement in symptoms. On postoperative day 2, he showed increased range of motion of the neck and was eating well. He was subsequently transitioned to cefdinir after clindamycin resulted in emesis. On postoperative day 3, the patient was discharged home.

---

should use the most facile method of intubation — direct or video-assisted laryngoscopy. If time and expertise permit, awake fiberoptic intubation allows for preservation of airway reflexes.

For a deep space neck infection, surgical intervention is primary, and a specialist should be consulted as soon as possible.[4,13] Often this is ENT, although the specialty managing these infections may vary in some locations. In uncomplicated PTAs, bedside drainage may be performed by an emergency physician.[1]

Management, including antibiotic coverage, should be administered swiftly if a high clinical suspicion is present. Simple infections in well-appearing patients may respond to antibiotics alone; however, these patients should be closely monitored for signs of disease progression.[4,13] The primary microbial concerns include common skin microbes such as *S. aureus* and *S. pneumoniae*, in addition to less commonly isolated bacteria such as *Prevotella*, *Porphyromonas*, *Fusobacterium*, and *Peptostreptococcus*.[1,4,6] If, however, *Fusobacterium* is suspected as the pathogen, as in Lemierre syndrome, macrolides should be avoided because resistance has been noted with this bacterium.[12] Often, isolates demonstrate polymicrobial flora, without specific speciation. Patients, especially those who present as critically ill, should receive broad-spectrum coverage with piperacillin-tazobactam or clindamycin. Ampicillin-sulbactam is also a viable option for these patients because it covers most of the pathogens.

REFERENCES

1. Galioto NJ. Peritonsillar abscess. *Am Fam Physician.* 2017;95(8):501-506.
2. Passy V. Pathogenesis of peritonsillar abscess. *Laryngoscope.* 1994;101(2):185-190.
3. Klug TE. Peritonsillar abscess: clinical aspects of microbiology, risk factors, and the association with parapharyngeal abscess. *Dan Med J.* 2017;64(3);B5333.
4. Brook I. Microbiology and management of peritonsillar, retropharyngeal, and parapharyngeal abscesses. *J Oral Maxillofac Surg.* 2004;62(12):1545-1550.
5. Steyer TE. Peritonsillar abscess: diagnosis and treatment. *Am Fam Physician.* 2002;65(1):93-96.
6. Beriault M, Green J, Hui A. Innovative airway management for peritonsillar abscess. *Can J Anaesth.* 2006;53(1):92-95.
7. Klug TE, Greve T, Hentze M. Complications of peritonsillar abscess. *Ann Clin Microbiol Antimicrob.* 2020;19(1):32.
8. Jiwangga D. Clinical characteristic and management of descending necrotizing mediastinitis: a retrospective study, Dr. Soetomo hospital, Surabaya. *J Vis Surg.* 2018;4:246.
9. St-Amant M, Jones J. Danger space. Radiopaedia. Reviewed September 26, 2021. Accessed June 16, 2022. https://radiopaedia.org/articles/danger-space?lang=us
10. Riordan T, Wilson M. Lemierre's syndrome: more than a historical curiosa. *Postgrad Med J.* 2004;80(944):328-334.
11. Lemierre A. On certain septicaemias due to anaerobic organisms. *Lancet.* 1936;227(5874):701-703.
12. Hochstim CJ, Messner AH. Pediatric inflammatory neck mass. *Curr Treat Options Pediatr.* 2016;2(3):216-223.
13. Herzon FS, Martin AD. Medical and surgical treatment of peritonsillar, retropharyngeal, and parapharyngeal abscesses. *Curr Infect Dis Rep.* 2006;8(3):196-202.

The Critical Procedure
Reduction of Rectal Prolapse

By Steven J. Warrington, MD, MEd, MS
MercyOne Siouxland, Sioux City, Iowa

Objective

On completion of this article, you should be able to:

- Perform a reduction on a patient experiencing rectal prolapse.

Introduction

Rectal prolapse most often occurs in pediatric and elderly patients and presents with complaints ranging from discomfort to blood or masses coming from the rectum. Prompt recognition and reduction can help mitigate risks to the tissue and sphincter.

Contraindications

- Necrosis of tissue

Benefits and Risks

The primary benefits of reduction in the emergency department are preventing further delay and damage or breakdown of tissue and avoiding operative care.

Risks include failure of the procedure (ie, incarcerated prolapse), ulceration, bleeding, and discomfort.

Alternatives

In the event a patient's rectal prolapse is very edematous, granulated sugar (not a substitute sweetener) applied to the mucosa can aid in reducing edema of the tissue, which may then allow for manual reduction. Additionally, the patient may need an anxiolytic or sedative.

Aside from various alternatives to reduce mucosal edema and ensure patient relaxation, the primary alternative to the procedure is operative care with a consultant.

Reducing Side Effects

Recognition of an incarcerated rectal prolapse and early consultation avoids unnecessary delays and expedites care, reducing the risk of necrosis. Additionally, delay in reduction increases risks of incontinence and decreased sphincter tone.

Special Considerations

While rectal prolapse may occur for many reasons, the need for close follow-up care should be discussed with patients due to the potential of a malignancy being the causative agent. Many individuals with a nonmalignant etiology are managed conservatively, so the discussion should also convey this information.

Moreover, the discussion should include actions the patient can take to help prevent and manage a recurrence, such as bowel regimens and pelvic floor exercises. Additionally, some professionals suggest discussing methods of self-reduction with patients, including the use of topical granulated sugar to help with reduction. Finally, discussion about risks of prolonged prolapses (eg, necrosis and ulceration) may be indicated.

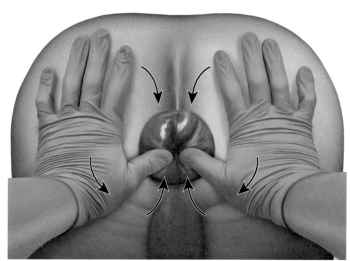

FIGURE 1. Technique for reduction of rectal prolapse

TECHNIQUE

1. **Obtain** the patient's consent and determine if an anxiolytic or sedative is needed.

2. **Consider** having an assistant who may also serve as a chaperone.

3. **Position** the patient in a lateral decubitus or prone position.

4. **Apply** granulated sugar or a gauze soaked in sugar water over the prolapsed mucosa if significant edema may make the reduction difficult. Allow 10 to 20 minutes for the sugar to have an effect.

5. **Instruct** the patient to relax and have the assistant help retract the cheeks. Alternatively, tape can be used to help retract the cheeks.

6. **Place** the thumbs of both hands towards the central opening with the rest of the fingers positioned circumferentially. The thumbs should apply constant, gentle pressure, while the rest of the fingers apply circumferential pressure to roll the tissue towards the opening. This process may take several minutes, depending on variables such as the amount of edema, relaxation level of the patient, and underlying sphincter tone.

7. **Apply** a pressure dressing against the anus to help prevent short-term recurrence. Some physicians use gauze with a lubricant.

Cerebral Intraparenchymal Hemorrhage

By Paula N. Kreutzer MD, MPH; and
Nicholas G. Maldonado MD, FACEP
Department of Emergency Medicine, University of Florida
College of Medicine, Gainesville
Reviewed by Andrew J. Eyre, MD, MSHPEd

Objective

On completion of this article, you should be able to:
■ Describe the essential elements of diagnosis and treatment of intraparenchymal hemorrhage.

Gross BA, Jankowitz BT, Friedlander RM. Cerebral intraparenchymal hemorrhage: a review. *JAMA*. 2019;321(13):1295-1303.

KEY POINTS

■ IPH comprises up to 20% of all strokes and has a 40% chance of survival within 1 year.
■ A patient presenting with acute-onset headache, seizure, or focal neurologic deficit should be evaluated for IPH.
■ Rapid CT or MRI is required for diagnosis, and a baseline IPH severity score should be assessed.
■ Neurosurgery should be consulted early to evaluate the need for surgical intervention.
■ Aggressively lower systolic blood pressure greater than 220 mm Hg with continuous infusion.
■ Correct initial systolic blood pressure of 150 mm Hg to 220 mm Hg to below 140 mm Hg.
■ In patients with a high international normalized ratio due to vitamin K antagonists, prothrombin complex concentrates are preferred over fresh frozen plasma.
■ Patients should be managed in a dedicated stroke or neurosurgery unit with experienced nursing.

Introduction

Stroke is an essential diagnosis of emergency medicine in which early recognition and management are paramount. Intraparenchymal hemorrhage (IPH) accounts for 6.5% to 19.6% of all stroke cases and has a 1-year survival rate of 40%. This article provides an overview of IPH, including its epidemiology, pathophysiology, diagnosis, and treatment.

Epidemiology and Pathophysiology

IPH can be classified into two categories: primary and secondary. Primary IPH accounts for nearly 90% of all cases and refers to the rupture of damaged small vessels, mostly secondary to hypertension or cerebral amyloid angiopathy (CAA). Hypertension induces degenerative changes in small arterial perforating vessels, whereas CAA results from the accumulation of ß-amyloid in cortical vessels causing weakening, with both mechanisms risking vessel rupture and associated IPH. The location of affected vasculature helps explain the tendency for IPH to occur in characteristic locations, with hypertensive IPH commonly occurring in the basal ganglia, thalamus, brainstem, and cerebellum and IPH due to CAA occurring in lobar locations. Hypertension is the most significant risk factor for primary IPH, and other notable risk factors include smoking and heavy alcohol use (ie, more than 30 drinks per month or binge drinking). Secondary IPH can be the result of multiple causes, including hemorrhagic conversion of ischemic stroke, coagulopathy, vascular malformation rupture, cerebral venous thrombosis, moyamoya, tumors, mycotic aneurysm rupture, or vasculitis. Knowledge and identification of the cause of secondary IPH is important, as it impacts surgical options for therapy.

Clinical Presentation and Diagnosis

IPH from any cause should be suspected in patients who present with acute-onset headache, nausea or vomiting, seizures, or focal neurologic deficits, and it may resemble an ischemic stroke–like presentation. In those who present with stroke-like symptoms, signs such as severe hypertension or depressed mental status should increase suspicion for IPH. Common deficits seen in patients with primary IPH include arm or leg paralysis, dysphasia, or aphasia. Within one of the reviewed studies, 60% of patients presented with a Glasgow Coma Scale (GCS) score of 12 or below. Nearly half of all patients with IPH deteriorate during transport to the hospital or in the emergency department, highlighting the urgency of diagnosis. Thus, a rapid neurologic examination with GCS assessment should be part of the initial evaluation when IPH is suspected. In taking a history, it is important to elicit the time of symptom onset, a history of hypertension, and anticoagulation use. Rapid CT or MRI is the imaging of choice for diagnosis. CT angiography and venography can identify specific causes of secondary IPH, and a "spot sign" on CT angiography suggests the presence of active contrast extravasation and is predictive of hematoma expansion. Once IPH is diagnosed, the American Heart Association/American Stroke Association (AHA/ASA) guidelines recommend calculating a baseline severity score as part of the initial assessment, of which the article recommends the Intracerebral Hemorrhage Score, given its ease of use and prediction of mortality. Neurosurgical consultation should also be rapidly obtained.

Treatment

A summary approach to the initial emergency management of IPH, using information present in the article and clinical practice recommendations from the AHA/ASA, is provided (*Table 1*). Mainstays of treatment include emergency stabilization with airway management when indicated, blood pressure control, reversal of anticoagulation, treatment of seizures, and neurosurgical consultation for surgical management.

Critical Decisions in Emergency Medicine's series of LLSA reviews features articles from ABEM's 2022 Lifelong Learning and Self-Assessment Reading List. Available online at acep.org/moc/llsa and on the ABEM website.

16   *Critical Decisions in Emergency Medicine*

STEP 1

Early Recognition	Symptoms of IPH	Patient presentation of acute-onset headache, nausea or vomiting, seizure, or stroke symptoms
	Signs of IPH	Presence of severe hypertension, focal neurologic deficit, or depressed mental status

STEP 2

Emergency Stabilization	Assess ABCs	Manage airway, if indicated, to reduce the risk of secondary injury from aspiration or hypoxia
	Bedside assessment	Obtain history with emphasis on time of onset, anticoagulant use, and neurologic or stroke examination

STEP 3

Rapid Diagnostic Workup and Neurosurgical Consultation	Laboratory and ancillary testing	Obtain early fingerstick glucose, routine laboratory tests (eg, complete blood count, prothrombin time, partial thromboplastin time, international normalized ratio) as well as troponin and ECG for screening
	Neuroimaging	Obtain rapid CT head/MRI and consider more advanced imaging (ie, CT angiography)
	Interpret IPH severity	Assess intracerebral brain hemorrhage location, volume, and "spot sign," and calculate Intracerebral Hemorrhage Score
	Early consultation	Obtain neurosurgical consultation to assess the need for surgical management

STEP 4

Medical Management	Blood pressure control	Reduce SBP to <140 mm Hg, using rapid acting (ie, labetalol) or titratable medications (ie, nicardipine or clevidipine)
	Hemostasis and coagulopathy reversal	Administer repletion for coagulation factor deficiency or thrombocytopenia
	Seizure control	Manage seizures with antiepileptics (AEDs); however, prophylactic AEDs are not recommended

STEP 5

Surgical Management Options	Ventricular drainage	Ventricular drainage for hydrocephalus
	Surgical drainage	Surgical drainage for hydrocephalus, worsening cerebellar IPH, or clinical deterioration
	Craniectomy	Craniectomy for coma, large hematomas with shift, or refractory high intracranial pressure

STEP 6

Disposition	Admit to ICU	Admit or transfer for initial management in ICU or dedicated stroke unit with neurologic expertise

TABLE 1. Summary approach to the emergency management of IPH

STEP 1 PEARLS

Risk Factors for Primary IPH
- Hypertension (significant)
- Smoking
- Heavy alcohol intake
- High HDL cholesterol
- Low total cholesterol
- Low non-HDL cholesterol

STEP 3 PEARLS

Neuroimaging in IPH
- CT angiography/venography can identify secondary causes of IPH.
- A "spot sign" suggests the presence of contrast extravasation and is predictive of hematoma expansion.
- The Intracerebral Hemorrhage Score includes GCS score, age, IPH location, IPH volume, and presence of intraventricular hemorrhage and predicts mortality. A baseline severity score is recommended and should be obtained.

STEP 4 PEARLS

Coagulopathy	Reversal Agent
Severe thrombocytopenia	Platelets
Heparins	Protamine sulfate
Vitamin K antagonists (warfarin)	Vitamin K Prothrombin complex concentrate (PCC)*
Direct thrombin inhibitors (dabigatran)	Idarucizumab
Factor Xa inhibitors (apixaban, rivaroxaban)	Andexanet alpha

*PCCs are preferred over fresh frozen plasma.

Not recommended: Empiric recombinant factor VIIa, tranexamic acid, or platelet transfusion for antiplatelet agents (ie, clopidogrel)

STEP 5 PEARLS

Secondary IPH	Surgical Options
Hemorrhagic brain tumor or metastasis	Surgical resection
Arteriovenous malformations or fistulas	Excision, embolization, or radiosurgery
Cavernous malformations	Excision
Distal or mycotic aneurysms	Embolization or surgery
Cerebral venous thrombosis	Anticoagulation/ thrombectomy
Moyamoya	Revascularization
Vasculitis	Immunomodulatory agents

Patella Fracture With Traumatic Arthrotomy

By John Kiel DO, MPH
Assistant Professor of Emergency Medicine and Sports Medicine,
University of Florida Jacksonville College of Medicine

Objective

On completion of this article, you should be able to:
- Describe the management of patellar fractures.

CASE PRESENTATION

A 25-year-old woman presents following a motor vehicle collision (MVC). The patient states that she was in a front-end collision at an unknown speed. She was restrained. She complains primarily of right knee pain. She is diagnosed with a right patella fracture with pneumarthrosis.

Discussion

Patella fractures are relatively uncommon, representing less than 1% of all fractures. They most commonly occur after an MVC but can also be seen in work-related accidents, domestic incidents, and sports and recreation injuries.[1] In these cases, direct trauma to a flexed knee leads to a patella fracture. Less commonly, rapid knee flexion against an eccentrically contracting quadriceps muscle can result in an indirect patella fracture. Patella fractures are often associated with osteochondral defects. In high-force mechanisms, other traumatic injuries to the affected limb, such as a femur fracture or a hip or knee dislocation, can cause patella fractures.[2]

Patients tend to present with a chief complaint of knee pain. In the setting of polytrauma, a thorough physical examination is necessary when the patient may be distracted or unable to direct the physician to the knee. On examination, there is typically a palpable defect in the bone. Any breaks in the skin suggesting a traumatic arthrotomy or "open fracture" should be noted. It is critical to evaluate whether the knee extensor mechanism is intact.

X-rays are typically sufficient to make the diagnosis (*Figures 1* and *2*). The presence of a patella alta (high-riding) or patella baja (low-riding) fracture suggests an injury to the patellar or quadriceps tendon, respectively.

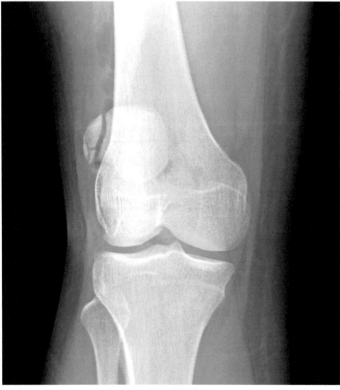

FIGURE 1. Posteroanterior (PA) knee x-ray showing a lateral patella fracture with pneumarthrosis

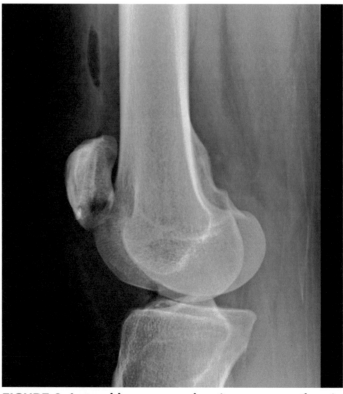

FIGURE 2. Lateral knee x-ray showing pneumarthrosis with fracture not well visualized

The patient was seen and evaluated by orthopedic surgery for her patella fracture and traumatic arthrotomy. She was given antibiotics and a tetanus booster on the day of admission. The following day, she was taken to the operating room for joint irrigation and debridement and bone irrigation and debridement without excision. She had persistent pain postoperatively and subsequently underwent excision of fragments due to nonunion about 5 months after the initial injury. During her last outpatient follow-up visit, approximately 16 months after the MVC, she had persistent lateral knee pain and had been unable to return to work.

Bipartite patella represents a congenital ossification center that failed to fuse and can easily be confused with a fracture on x-ray. It occurs in about 2% of individuals and is bilateral 50% of the time. CT may be indicated for surgical planning; MRI is useful to evaluate soft tissue structure, such as the patellar articular cartilage.

In the emergency department, the key is to evaluate the extensor mechanism. If it is intact, a trial of nonoperative management may be possible. Vertical fracture patterns are more likely to maintain the extensor mechanism than horizontal fracture patterns, which are likely to displace from the tension of the quadriceps and patellar tendons. These patients should be placed in a knee immobilizer, crutches, restricted to non–weight bearing, and referred for outpatient follow-up care with an orthopedic surgeon. Patients without an intact extensor mechanism can also likely be discharged with orthopedic surgery follow-up; however, since they require surgery, it is prudent to consult the orthopedic surgeon in the emergency department.

Traumatic arthrotomy, or an open fracture, is an indication to emergently consult orthopedic surgery. In some cases, this may be subtle, requiring either a saline load test (SLT) or, based on more recent literature, CT scan. The current literature states that a CT scan without contrast is both more sensitive and specific (100% and 100%) than the SLT (92% and 92%) at detecting traumatic arthrotomy of the knee.[3] In cases where the traumatic arthrotomy is obvious, either clinically or radiographically, CT or SLT may be unnecessary. In all cases, patients should be given antibiotics and a tetanus booster; orthopedic surgery generally takes these patients to the operating room.

REFERENCES

1. Nummi J. Fracture of the patella. A clinical study of 707 patellar fractures. *Ann Chir Gynaecol Fenn Suppl.* 1971;179:1-85.
2. Catalano JB, Iannacone WM, Marczyk S, et al. Open fractures of the patella: long-term functional outcome. *J Trauma.* 1995;39(3):439-444.
3. Konda SR, Davidovitch RI, Egol KA. Computed tomography scan to detect traumatic arthrotomies and identify periarticular wounds not requiring surgical intervention: an improvement over the saline load test. *J Orthop Trauma.* 2013;27(9):498-504.

Right Lower Quadrant Pain in Pregnancy

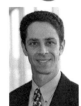

By Joshua S. Broder, MD, FACEP
Dr. Broder is a professor and the residency program director in the Department of Emergency Medicine at Duke University Medical Center in Durham, North Carolina.

Objectives

On completion of this article, you should be able to:

- Select appropriate imaging for right lower quadrant pain with suspected appendicitis in pregnancy.

- Describe cautions about gadolinium-based contrast agents and ionizing radiation from CT.

CASE PRESENTATION

A 35-year-old woman presents at 17 weeks' gestation with right lower abdominal pain that woke her up around 2 AM. The pain has been intermittently severe, and the patient noted increased pain while riding in a car on a bumpy road. She denies fever, nausea, vomiting, diarrhea, urinary complaints, and vaginal bleeding. She has received prenatal care and is known to have an intrauterine pregnancy based on ultrasound.

Her vital signs are BP 93/60, P 57, R 16, and T 36.4°C (97.5°F); SpO$_2$ is 98% on room air. The patient is in no distress, noting only mild pain at rest. With palpation, she has significant right lower quadrant tenderness, without rebound or guarding. Her WBC count is 10.7. Liver function tests and urinalysis are within normal limits. Ultrasound is performed but fails to definitively identify the appendix. An MRI of the abdomen and pelvis is obtained (*Figure 1*).

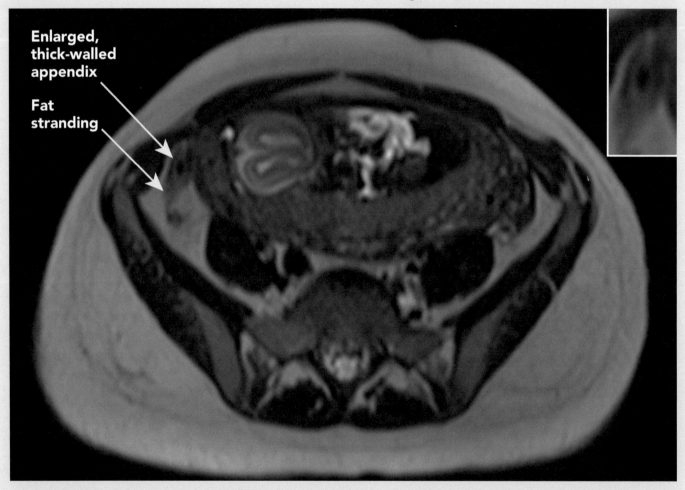

Enlarged, thick-walled appendix

Fat stranding

FIGURE 1. MRI without contrast, HASTE sequence. HASTE is a rapid T2-weighted technique. Images are acquired in less than 1 second and, therefore, are unaffected by breathing. The appendix is enlarged (1 cm, with normal <6 mm) and thick-walled. Fat stranding is visible.

The American College of Radiology (ACR) rates noncontrast MRI of the abdomen and pelvis as a "usually appropriate" initial imaging modality in pregnant patients with suspected appendicitis.[1,2] Unlike CT, MRI does not use ionizing radiation, and no adverse fetal effects of MRI have been described. As with CT, MRI findings of appendicitis include increased appendiceal diameter (≥6 mm), increased wall thickness (≥2 mm), and periappendiceal fat stranding or fluid.[3]

Emergency physicians accustomed to ordering CT with intravenous (IV) contrast in nonpregnant patients should note the *lack of contrast use* for MRI. A meta-analysis found no difference in accuracy between MRI with and without contrast.[4] Although no teratogenic fetal effects of gadolinium-based contrast agents (GBCAs) are known, well-controlled studies are lacking. Some GBCAs cross the placenta and are renally excreted by the fetus into the amniotic fluid, where they may be swallowed again by the fetus. Clearance rates for GBCAs from amniotic fluid are unknown and may vary among specific contrast agents.[5,6] The ACR and the American College of Obstetricians and Gynecologists (ACOG) recommend against GBCAs in pregnancy unless the clinical information required cannot otherwise be obtained, will affect the care of the patient or fetus, and cannot safely be deferred until the patient is no longer pregnant.[6,7]

A meta-analysis found the sensitivity and specificity of MRI for appendicitis in pregnancy to be 94% (95% CI, 87% to 98%) and 97% (95% CI, 96% to 98%).[4] Multiple MRI techniques can be used for the evaluation of appendicitis; MRI sequences are often proprietary to particular manufacturers, although similar

CASE RESOLUTION

The patient underwent a laparoscopic appendectomy, which confirmed appendicitis, and recovered uneventfully.

techniques available with other vendors will likely yield similar results. MRI may also provide alternative diagnoses. Studies point to differences in diagnostic performance when MRI is interpreted by MR-expert versus MR-nonexpert radiologists, so local experience should be considered. In one study, sensitivity for appendicitis was 89% for MR-nonexpert radiologists and 97% for experts. Specificity was 83% and 93%, respectively.[8]

Ultrasound is also rated by the ACR as "usually indicated" in pregnant patients with right lower quadrant pain and suspected appendicitis.[1] Ultrasound for appendicitis in pregnancy can have a sensitivity as low as 18% due largely to the high frequency of nonvisualization of the appendix, while specificity remains high (99%).[9] For this reason, some authors have recommended MRI as the first-line imaging modality for appendicitis in pregnancy.

In pregnant patients with suspected appendicitis, CT of the abdomen and pelvis with IV contrast is rated by the ACR as "may be appropriate."[1] Low-osmolality iodinated contrast media used in CT have no known mutagenic or teratogenic effects.[6] A single CT of the abdomen and pelvis confers a fetal ionizing radiation dose below the exposure known to cause teratogenic effects, but ultrasound or MRI is recommended when available because there is no ionizing radiation exposure from these modalities.[7,10]

REFERENCES

1. American College of Radiology. ACR Appropriateness Criteria® right lower quadrant pain. Accessed June 17, 2022. https://acsearch.acr.org/docs/69357/Narrative/
2. Garcia EM, Camacho MA, Smith MP, et al; Expert Panel on Gastrointestinal Imaging. ACR Appropriateness Criteria® right lower quadrant pain-suspected appendicitis. *J Am Coll Radiol.* 2018;15(suppl 11):S373-S387.
3. Spalluto LB, Woodfield CA, DeBenedectis CM, Lazarus E. MR imaging evaluation of abdominal pain during pregnancy: appendicitis and other nonobstetric causes. *Radiographics.* 2012;32(2):317-334.
4. Duke E, Kalb B, Arif-Tiwari H, et al. A systematic review and meta-analysis of diagnostic performance of MRI for evaluation of acute appendicitis. *AJR Am J Roentgenol.* 2016;206(3):508-517.
5. Kodzwa R. ACR manual on contrast media: 2018 updates. *Radiol Technol.* 2019;91(1):97-100.
6. 2022 ACR Committee on Drugs and Contrast Media. ACR Manual on Contrast Media. Accessed June 17, 2022. https://www.acr.org/-/media/ACR/files/clinical-resources/contrast_media.pdf
7 Committee on Obstetric Practice. Committee opinion No. 723: guidelines for diagnostic imaging during pregnancy and lactation. *Obstet Gynecol.* 2017;130(4):e210-e216.
8. Leeuwenburgh MMN, Wiarda BM, Jensch S, et al; OPTIMAP Study Group. Accuracy and interobserver agreement between MR-non-expert radiologists and MR-experts in reading MRI for suspected appendicitis. *Eur J Radiol.* 2014;83(1):103-110.
9. Konrad J, Grand D, Lourenco A. MRI: first-line imaging modality for pregnant patients with suspected appendicitis. *Abdom Imaging.* 2015;40(8):3359-3364.
10. American College of Radiology. ACR–SPR practice parameter for imaging pregnant or potentially pregnant adolescents and women with ionizing radiation. Revised 2018 (Resolution 39). Accessed June 20, 2022. https://www.acr.org/-/media/acr/files/practice-parameters/pregnant-pts.pdf

Feature Editor: Joshua S. Broder, MD, FACEP. See also *Diagnostic Imaging for the Emergency Physician* (Winner of the 2011 Prose Award in Clinical Medicine, the American Publishers Award for Professional and Scholarly Excellence) and *Critical Images in Emergency Medicine* by Dr. Broder.

Signs of Hypothermia

By Amal Mattu, MD, FACEP

Dr. Mattu is a professor, vice chair, and director of the Emergency Cardiology Fellowship in the Department of Emergency Medicine at the University of Maryland School of Medicine in Baltimore.

Objective

On completion of this article, you should be able to:

■ Identify ECG findings of hypothermia.

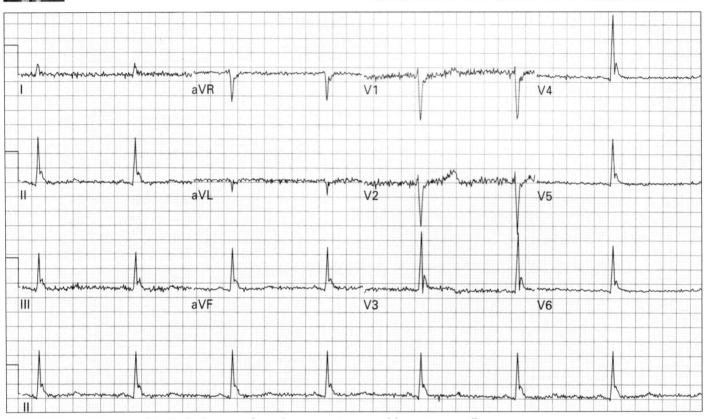

FIGURE 1. A 49-year-old alcoholic man found unconscious and lying in an alley

Probable sinus bradycardia (SB), rate 45, Osborne waves consistent with hypothermia, nonspecific T-wave flattening. Significant artifact (due to shivering) is present, which somewhat obscures the rhythm interpretation. However, there appear to be upright P waves preceding the QRS complexes, best noted in the rhythm strip, consistent with SB. Sizeable upward deflections occur just after the QRS complexes. These are referred to as Osborne waves, or J waves, and are most notably found in cases of hypothermia. They tend to be most prominent in the precordial leads, and they gradually reduce in size and eventually disappear with rewarming.

FIGURE 2.
The electrocardiographic triad of hypothermia: Osborne wave, bradycardia, and artifact.

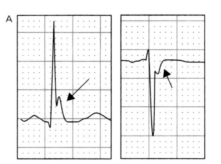
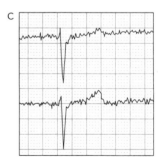
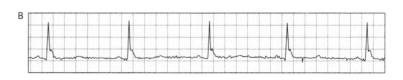

A. The Osborne wave, also known as the J wave (*arrow*), is highly suggestive of significant hypothermia. The J wave is a terminal slurring of the QRS complex; the J wave can be either upright (positive polarity) or inverted (negative polarity).
B. Sinus bradycardia.
C. Muscle tremor artifact.

This patient's core body temperature was 29°C (84.2°F). Typical ECG abnormalities associated with hypothermia include Osborne waves, sinus bradycardia or atrial fibrillation with slow ventricular response, and prolongation of all the intervals (PR, QRS, and QT).

From Mattu A, Brady W. *ECGs for the Emergency Physician 2*. BMJ Publishing. Reprinted with permission.

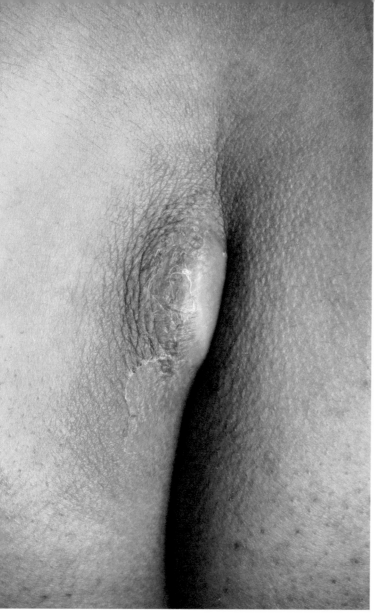

Bringing Up the Rear

Perirectal, Perianal, and Pilonidal Abscesses

LESSON 14

By Matthew Sherman, MD; Dalbir Bahga, MD; and Vietvuong Vo, MD
Dr. Sherman, Dr. Bahga, and Dr. Vo are assistant professors at the University of Texas Southwestern Medical Center in Dallas.

Reviewed by Walter L. Green, MD, FACEP

Objectives

On completion of this lesson, you should be able to:

1. Identify the anatomic landmarks and relative locations of perianal, perirectal, and pilonidal abscesses.
2. Recognize when to obtain a CT scan for deep abscess involvement.
3. Determine which abscess cases may be managed at the bedside and which cases necessitate surgical consultation for operative management.
4. Demonstrate proper incision and drainage techniques for perianal, perirectal, and pilonidal abscesses.
5. Distinguish when antibiotics should be started for perianal, perirectal, and pilonidal abscesses.

From the EM Model

2.0 Abdominal and Gastrointestinal Disorders
    2.10 Rectum and Anus
        2.10.1 Infectious Disorders
            2.10.1.1 Perianal/Anal Abscess
            2.10.1.2 Perirectal Abscess
            2.10.1.3 Pilonidal Cyst and Abscess

CRITICAL DECISIONS

- How can anorectal abscesses be differentiated?

- When should anorectal abscesses be suspected, and how should they be managed?

- Where should incision and drainage be performed for different anorectal abscesses?

- What is a pilonidal abscess, and how should it be treated?

- How should perianal abscesses be diagnosed and managed?

Abscesses in the anorectal region are common complaints that may cause localized, compressive, or systemic symptoms. However, perirectal, perianal, and pilonidal abscesses can be difficult to differentiate. Emergency physicians must be able to rapidly identify and correctly treat these divergent disease processes to prevent complications.

CASE ONE

A 20-year-old woman presents with a 2-day history of painful swelling between her buttocks that is worse when she sits down. She denies fevers, chills, bloody stool, abdominal pain, nausea, and vomiting and states that she has no issues with bowel movements. When questioned, she reports that this has happened to her two times before. During the prior two incidents, she states that an emergency physician "did something" that made it better. She was told to follow up with a surgeon both times but was unable to do so.

Her vital signs are BP 132/89, P 95, R 16, and T 37.0°C (98.6°F); SpO$_2$ is 98% on room air. A focused examination of her gluteal cleft shows a large area of swelling. This area is tender to palpation, is indurated, and has mild hyperemia without fluctuance. It appears to have maximal tenderness about 4 cm superior to the anus, and there are no findings along the anal verge.

CASE TWO

A 35-year-old diabetic man presents with a painful mass on his right buttock that started 3 days ago. The patient reports that he has been experiencing worsening pain with movement, sitting, and defecation. He denies fevers, fatigue, abdominal pain, nausea, vomiting, trauma, and a history of prior episodes.

His vital signs are BP 112/78, P 99, R 14, and T 37.1°C (98.8°F); SpO$_2$ is 99% on room air. On physical examination, the patient is noted to have a 3 × 4 cm erythematous mass with center fluctuance and surrounding erythema to the right perineal area just lateral to the anus without drainage.

CASE THREE

A 45-year-old man presents with a 2-week history of worsening, insidious-onset, dull, and poorly localized pain in his lower abdomen. He also reports associated progressive urinary retention, nausea without vomiting, and tenesmus; he sought a medical evaluation after developing a fever and chills. He denies dysuria, blood in his urine and stool, and diarrhea. The patient has a history of diabetes, constipation, and diverticulitis that was treated with resolution of symptoms about 1 month ago. Since his last hospital encounter, the patient reports consistency with lifestyle changes, including increased exercise and a healthier diet, and he no longer experiences constipation.

His vital signs are BP 145/85, P 102, R 18, and T 38.4°C (101.1°F); SpO$_2$ is 97% on room air. The physical examination reveals an uncomfortable man with diffuse lower abdominal tenderness to palpation but no distension, guarding, or rigidity. There is mild suprapubic fullness. The genitourinary examination is unrevealing, and the anorectal examination reveals no acute skin lesions. The digital rectal examination reveals a normal-sized and nontender prostate as well as no significant tenderness, induration, or fluctuance of the anorectal canal. Brown stool without blood is seen on the gloved finger.

A bedside ultrasound reveals a postvoid residual of 500 mL but no hydronephrosis bilaterally. Treatment with a urinary catheter relieves some pain. However, he still appears uncomfortable, and he reports severe pain. Laboratory work reveals leukocytosis (WBC 15) and elevated C-reactive protein. The remainder of his laboratory work, including urinalysis, lipase, and a metabolic panel, is unremarkable.

Introduction

Anorectal abscesses include a broad spectrum of diseases that can be classified in different categories depending on the location. Perirectal, perianal, and pilonidal abscesses can range from simple local infections to markers of systemic disease or causes of severe infection. Understanding the anatomy of the perineum is vital to the appropriate diagnosis and subsequent treatment of anorectal abscesses. Differentiating these processes allows for improved treatment and outcomes for patients.

The incidence of anorectal infections is more than 100,000 cases per year in the United States, but this incidence is likely underestimated since patients with anorectal symptoms may not seek medical attention and may misdiagnose themselves with a more benign process, such as hemorrhoids. Anorectal abscesses are typically present in patients aged 20 to 60 years, with the average age being 40 years. Notably, men are twice as likely to develop anorectal abscesses and associated complications compared to women.[1,2]

Most anorectal abscesses originate from a blocked anal crypt gland.[3] Other conditions that are associated with the occurrence of anorectal abscesses include Crohn disease, radiation fibrosis, diabetes, chronic steroid use, an immunocompromised state, malignancy, and trauma. The anorectal anatomy is complex and contains multiple tissue planes and potential spaces in which an abscess can arise. The treatment of perianal, perirectal, and pilonidal abscesses usually involves prompt incision and drainage, but the location of the abscess dictates the surgical approach. Some anorectal abscesses may be drained at the bedside, while others require general anesthesia and surgical drainage in the operating room.

Untreated anorectal abscesses can lead to significant morbidity, including fecal incontinence, chronic pain, constipation, and recurrence. Complications of untreated anorectal abscesses include further expansion, fistula formation, and systemic illness. Notably, up to 70% of anorectal abscesses are associated with concomitant anorectal fistulas.[2,4]

CRITICAL DECISION

How can anorectal abscesses be differentiated?

Anorectal abscesses (including perianal and perirectal abscesses) generally arise from obstructed anal crypt gland ducts, which allows for bacterial growth, inflammation, and eventually, abscess formation. Approximately 10 anal glands (believed to be rudimentary in function) occur at the dentate line (*Figure 1*). The dentate line divides the embryogenically distinct portions of the anal canal: the upper intestinal columnar epithelium and lower squamous epithelium. The anal

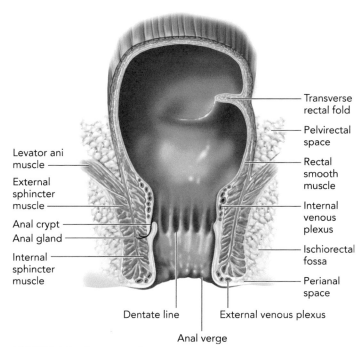

FIGURE 1. Anorectal anatomy.
Elise Walmsley-MacWha/Stocktrek Images.

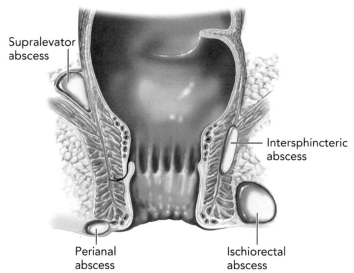

FIGURE 2. Anorectal abscess locations.
Elise Walmsley-MacWha/Stocktrek Images.

glands are arranged circumferentially and penetrate through the internal anal sphincter to the intersphincteric plane (ie, the potential space between the internal and external anal sphincters).

Perianal abscesses, which are the most common anorectal abscesses, arise when infections spread distally through the intersphincteric groove to the perianal skin, usually leading to a superficial, tender, fluctuant, and erythematous mass near the anal verge. *Perirectal abscesses* occur when the infection travels to other deep spaces, including the intersphincteric, ischiorectal, or supralevator spaces, and they are classified based on the anatomical location (*Figure 2*).

Ischiorectal abscesses (also known as ischioanal abscesses) occur when abscesses develop in the adipose-tissue–filled ischiorectal fossa, which is bound by the obturator internus muscle laterally, the pelvic diaphragm superiorly, and the external anal sphincter muscles medially (see *Figure 2*). The lateral portions of the ischiorectal fossa communicate posteriorly. Ischiorectal abscesses present as deeper, fluctuant masses, usually with diffuse tenderness and induration within the buttocks.

Intersphincteric abscesses occur in the intersphincteric groove. Without extension to the perianal area, there may be no appreciable skin changes during external examination, but a fluctuant and tender mass may be palpated during digital rectal examination.

Supralevator abscesses may form when infection tracks superiorly from the typical cryptoglandular source to the supralevator space via the intersphincteric groove (see *Figure 2*). These abscesses may also arise from an intra-abdominal source, such as a perforated colon, or from inflammatory bowel disease. Supralevator abscesses account for less than 5% of total anorectal abscesses.[5]

Patients with supralevator abscesses may present with pain during defecation, systemic symptoms of infection, and urinary complaints, especially urinary retention due to local tissue compression. A supralevator abscess may also present with neurologic symptoms due to local compression of adjacent nerves, including the sacral nerves. Symptoms vary depending on the nerves being compressed. Since these infections occur above the pelvic floor muscles, external examination is usually unrevealing. However, a digital rectal examination may reveal a fluctuant and tender mass above the level of the anorectal ring. Suspicion of a supralevator abscess requires further diagnostic studies; CT is usually the first-line imaging study.

A *horseshoe abscess* is a distinct and complex type of perirectal abscess. It is bound by the pelvic floor muscles superiorly, the anococcygeal ligament inferiorly, the coccyx posteriorly, and the anal canal anteriorly. These borders form a tight and unyielding space, so further expansion of this abscess usually extends into the ischiorectal space either unilaterally or bilaterally, giving it a U-shaped appearance — hence the name horseshoe abscess.

CRITICAL DECISION

When should anorectal abscesses be suspected, and how should they be managed?

Symptoms

Patients with anorectal abscesses usually present with severe, constant anorectal pain that may or may not be associated with defecation. Patients may have systemic symptoms of infection, including fever, chills, malaise, nausea, and vomiting. Patients may notice purulent rectal drainage if spontaneous drainage occurs. An expanding abscess may cause neurologic and local compressive symptoms, including urinary retention, sciatica, constipation, and pressure-like pain.

Clinical Examination

Depending on the anatomical location, external signs of anorectal abscesses may be absent. Perianal abscesses are superficial and often present as a raised, erythematous, tender, fluctuant mass at the anal verge. Deeper perirectal abscesses, however, may be appreciated as a tender, fluctuant, or indurated mass only on digital rectal examination, or they may not be appreciated at all.

Anorectal abscesses may be diagnosed via direct visualization or with palpation during digital rectal examination; however, high suspicion without definitive examination findings should prompt further imaging studies, including CT (typically first line), pelvic MRI, and endorectal ultrasound.

Differential Diagnosis

Anorectal abscesses should be suspected whenever patients present with anorectal pain. The differential diagnosis includes other entities affecting this region, such as a buttock skin abscess, internal hemorrhoid, external hemorrhoid (thrombosed or nonthrombosed), anal fissure, anal fistula, pilonidal disease, vulvar cyst or abscess (Bartholin abscess), and hidradenitis suppurativa.

Management

Once an anorectal abscess is diagnosed, physicians should act quickly to drain it because untreated abscesses can lead to complications and significant morbidity and mortality. Surgical drainage approaches depend on the anatomical location. Superficial perianal abscesses may be drained at the bedside, but perirectal abscesses are usually deeper, are more complex, and have a higher risk of fistulization. Therefore, they usually require management in the operating room with a surgical team and varying levels of anesthesia.

Regardless of the surgical approach, complete evacuation of the abscess cavity is necessary for proper management, which includes breaking up all loculations and removing all purulent content. Sterile rinses may be used, but wound packing has not been shown to be beneficial. All patients should receive a 4- to 5-day course of empiric antibiotics after incision and drainage of anorectal abscesses because this approach can reduce the rate of fistula formation. The antibiotic choice should cover intra-abdominal sources. A routine wound culture is usually unhelpful for selecting an antibiotic, as abscesses are typically polymicrobial. Generally, postprocedural care includes taking frequent warm sitz baths, keeping the area clean and dry, and following up closely for wound healing.

CRITICAL DECISION

Where should the incision and drainage be performed for different anorectal abscesses?

The incision for *perianal abscesses* should be made as close to the anal verge as possible to minimize the length of potential fistula formation (*Figure 3*). *Ischiorectal abscesses* usually require drainage through a skin incision after local anesthetic infiltration. As with perianal abscesses, potential fistula formation is a concern, so the incision should be made as close to the anal verge as possible. All abscess content should be thoroughly evacuated, and any loculations should be broken up. The wound may be irrigated with sterile saline. No wound packing is necessary, but a clean dressing should be placed.

Intersphincteric abscesses require surgical management. An internal sphincterotomy should be performed, which involves going through the anal mucosa under regional or general anesthesia.

There are generally two approaches to the incision and drainage of *supralevator abscesses*, depending on the originating abscess. Supralevator abscesses that originate from ischiorectal abscesses and extend upward into the supralevator area should be treated in the same fashion as other ischiorectal abscesses: with incision and drainage through the skin. Supralevator abscesses that originate from intersphincteric abscesses and spread upward into the supralevator space should be treated in the same manner as other intersphincteric abscesses: with surgical incision through the anorectal mucosa and drainage into the rectum.

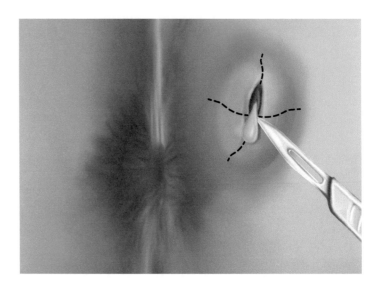

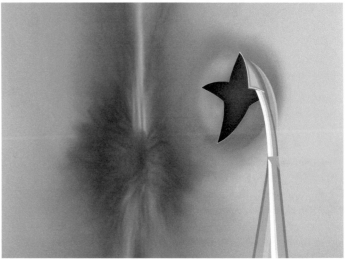

FIGURE 3. Incision and drainage procedure

Horseshoe abscesses usually require a complex operative course under general anesthesia because they typically involve a posterior incision between the coccyx and the anus. *Anal fistulas* may be present in up 70% of anorectal abscesses. Generally, it is more favorable to perform a delayed fistulotomy after any inflammation and edema have subsided. A primary fistulotomy may be performed for simple anal fistulas or when there is a high risk of recurrence, such as with horseshoe abscesses.

CRITICAL DECISION

What is a pilonidal abscess, and how should it be managed?

Introduction

Pilonidal abscesses originate in the upper natal cleft (*Figure 4*). They are caused by the development of a pilonidal sinus with subsequent blockage that is followed by a purulent infection. Pilonidal abscesses are like most cutaneous abscesses, in that damage to the skin barrier is the initial cause of infection. Skin flora is the normal causative organism. Pilonidal abscesses present and are managed similarly to other cutaneous abscesses.

There is some debate about the origin of the pilonidal sinus that subsequently becomes blocked and infected. The most supported explanation is that the sinus develops from an ingrown hair causing a local reaction that leads to a tract capable

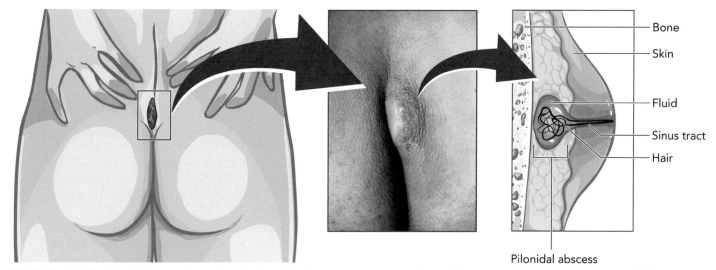

FIGURE 4. Pilonidal abscess location. Pilonidal abscesses occur in the midline near the superior aspect of the gluteal cleft. *Credit: Illustration: corbac40/iStock/Getty Images Plus; photo: Alan Nissa/Shutterstock.com.*

of becoming blocked and infected. Repeated infections and ingrown hairs worsen the issue. However, there is some thought that the tract development is caused by local trauma, and it has been considered that embryogenesis may predispose some individuals to future problems. The most current hypothesis, however, is that this is an acquired condition, not a congenital disease.[5]

Clinical Examination

Patients with pilonidal abscesses usually present with painful swelling in the intergluteal cleft (classically in the superior gluteal cleft). The swelling should overlie the sacrum and coccyx at the upper portion of the gluteal cleft distant from the anus. Painless presentations with just swelling are possible but are less common. Generally, the abscess is tender when palpated and, depending on body habitus, may have palpable fluctuance; however, palpable induration is more common than fluctuance. Classically, patients present with overlying erythema.[6] Systemic symptoms are rare but can occur if the abscess is the source of bacteremia.

Patients typically present in their late teens to early 20s. Initial occurrence is markedly rare after age 40 years. Pilonidal cysts are also more common among Caucasians than Asians or Blacks, and men are affected about three times more often than women.[7] The at-risk population is more likely to have obesity, local trauma, and increased hair density in the gluteal cleft.

Because pilonidal abscesses are caused by blockage of a sinus tract, recurrence is a fairly common problem (10%-55%).[6] It is not uncommon for patients to present multiple times with abscess formation in the same location. Those who suffer from recurrent pilonidal abscesses may develop fistula tracts from prior drainages. These will not communicate with the anorectal area. Definitive care requires surgical removal of this tract.

Diagnosis

Pilonidal abscesses are usually easy to identify. The diagnosis is made by identifying an abscess in the superior gluteal cleft. The differential diagnosis is narrow, and the physical examination is usually sufficient to differentiate a pilonidal abscess from other anorectal causes. First, pilonidal abscesses can exist as simple cysts that are uninfected. Commonly, they are painful or uncomfortable and require similar management. Gluteal cleft cellulitis without abscess formation presents similarly and has a comparable appearance.

Ultrasound does not typically play a large role in the diagnosis, given the usually clear clinical picture, but it could be used should there be difficulty in determining the presence of fluid collection.[5] Overall, imaging is only required to make the diagnosis in rare instances (eg, when there is a concern for atypical large size, immunocompromise, deeper spread, or anorectal disease with fistulation).

It is important to recognize the potential for mistaking a pilonidal abscess for a perirectal abscess. A large perirectal abscess tracking superiorly or a large pilonidal abscess with spread towards the rectum could enter the same anatomic areas. However, the pilonidal abscess' site of maximal fluctuance, the overall location in relation to the midline, and a patient history of prior incidents should help separate these two processes. Tracts developed from prior pilonidal drainage

✔ Pearls

- Neurologic complaints (eg, neurogenic bladder and sciatica), infectious symptoms, and lower abdominal or pelvic pain should raise suspicion for a perirectal abscess with nerve compression.

- The treatment approach for anorectal abscesses depends strongly on the anatomical location.

- Incisions for simple perianal abscesses should be made through the skin and as close to the anal verge as possible to minimize the length of a potential fistula tract.

- For recurrent cases of anorectal abscesses, etiologies such as Crohn disease should be considered, and a referral for follow-up care with a general surgeon should be ordered.

do not involve the rectum. Perirectal abscesses with horseshoe-type fistulas have the potential to appear like a pilonidal abscess, but these abscesses are most commonly located off the midline, differentiating them from pilonidal abscesses.

Other differential diagnoses are rare causes of the clinical findings most consistent with pilonidal abscesses, including abnormal fistula tracts from other anorectal abscesses, simple cutaneous boils or abscesses, fungal infections, and atypical presentations of sacral osteomyelitis.[7] Simple cutaneous abscesses may be similar and therefore difficult to differentiate, but they would be treated in a similar manner. Finally, it is important to be aware that a rare squamous cell carcinoma can arise from chronic recurrent pilonidal abscesses.[6]

Management

Incision and drainage in the emergency department is the key management step for pilonidal abscesses. This procedure is best performed with the patient in a prone position. An extra set of hands may be required to separate the buttocks and allow access to the abscess. Standard abscess incision and drainage techniques can be performed to treat this condition. It is ideal to prepare the area with a cleansing agent, preferably povidone-iodine, and to drape the area with sterile towels. Wearing a mask and eye protection during the procedure is strongly encouraged because these abscesses are often under pressure and tend to expel their contents rapidly.

As with all procedures, sedation may be required, depending on the specific patient characteristics and magnitude of the drainage required. Local anesthesia (with lidocaine or a similar analog) is commonly sufficient for these drainages. The ideal infiltration of the agent should occur in the subcutaneous tissue over the abscess in the same area that the physician plans to incise to minimize the sensation of the scalpel.[8] Standard abscess management applies. Start with incision followed by drainage; then, probe with hemostats to break any loculations. Generally, a No. 11 or No. 15 blade is preferred.

An interesting 2018 study attempted needle aspiration with antibiotics instead of incision and drainage on 100 patients, with an 83% first aspiration success rate in the resolution of the acute episode without requiring open incision and drainage.[8] Although it was a small study without a control group for comparison, it does raise an interesting potential for an alternative to standard incision and drainage.[9]

There is continued controversy regarding packing or not packing pilonidal abscesses. UpToDate still recommends packing pilonidal wounds, in particular, because of the recurrence rate and to encourage slow secondary healing, with removal in 24 to 48 hours.[6] A bulky dressing should be placed over top.[7] A short review of recent articles about packing looks to exclude pilonidal abscesses from their inclusion criteria. Overall, the trend for packing abscesses is moving away from packing small abscesses, but there does not seem to be conclusive evidence one way or the other specifically regarding pilonidal abscesses.

Antibiotics are unnecessary in most pilonidal abscess cases. Antibiotics should only be considered in cases of immunocompromised patients or if there is a concerning amount of surrounding cellulitis. After discharge, patients should be educated to begin taking sitz baths 24 hours after the abscess is drained to assist with adequate perineal hygiene. Given the risk of recurrence, patients should be given referrals to a surgeon for follow-up care and definitive management.[7]

CRITICAL DECISION

How should perianal abscesses be diagnosed and managed?

Diagnosis

Perianal abscesses are located the closest to the anal verge, often in the posterior midline (*Figure 5*). They usually present as a tender superficial mass that is often palpable close to the anal verge. Patients with perianal abscesses typically have a painful mass that is worse with movement and sitting and is often not accompanied by systemic features, such as fever or leukocytosis.

Management

Due to its superficial nature, an isolated perianal abscess is safe to be incised and drained in the emergency department; however, if there is any concern for the extent of involvement or for deeper involvement, advanced imaging and surgical management should be considered. Physicians should consider deeper involvement when patients present with significant pain that is out of proportion to the physical examination findings. Deep anal abscesses may present with rectal pain and tenderness without obvious cutaneous findings.

To perform an incision and drainage of a perianal abscess, the patient should be positioned adequately, and proper local anesthetic (ie, lidocaine with epinephrine) should be injected around the painful area of the abscess. Usually, local anesthetics are adequate for simple incisions, but procedural sedation can be considered for some cases. A linear or cruciate incision should be made over the fluctuant part of the abscess. If a linear incision is used, ensure that there is enough space to keep the skin edges open for drainage. The skin flaps could be trimmed to prevent skin closure, which would interfere with adequate drainage. After successful incision and drainage of a perianal abscess, it is important to refer the patient for a surgical follow-up because fistulas commonly develop afterward.

✕ Pitfalls

- Excluding deep space infections based on the absence of external findings of infection.

- Treating anorectal abscesses without complete radiographic or surgical evaluation.

- Managing all patients with anorectal abscesses with antibiotics alone.

- Failing to consider large pilonidal abscesses in patients with a history of prior fistulization from anorectal disease.

CASE RESOLUTIONS

CASE ONE

The examination of the 20-year-old woman was consistent with a pilonidal cyst. The patient was educated on her disease and the importance of follow-up care to avoid recurrence. After appropriate pain control and local anesthetics were administered, the abscess was drained using the standard technique.

CASE TWO

The 35-year-old man's laboratory studies revealed mild hyperglycemia at 210 mg/dL without leukocytosis. CT imaging showed a superficial 2.6 × 2.0 × 2.2 cm abscess posterior and lateral of the anus, with no deep involvement or subcutaneous air. The emergency physician anesthetized the area with lidocaine (with epinephrine) and performed a simple cruciate inclusion that resulted in moderate purulent drainage. The patient tolerated the procedure without any complications. He was sent home on amoxicillin-clavulanic acid for 1 week with surgery follow-up.

CASE THREE

The 45-year-old man was suspected to have sepsis secondary to an intra-abdominal source. Blood cultures were collected, and he was treated with broad-spectrum antibiotics, pain medications, and intravenous fluids while awaiting further investigations. A CT scan revealed a large supralevator abscess. Other findings included diverticulosis without any signs of diverticulitis, perforation, or fistula formation. A distended bladder, but no prostate enlargement or hydronephrosis, was also noted.

General surgery evaluated the patient and recommended urgent surgical management in the operating room. The supralevator abscess was completely evacuated. He had an uncomplicated postoperative course, was discharged, and completed a course of antibiotics. The patient had complete resolution of his urinary retention and had no further complications.

Summary

Abscesses in the anorectal region may cause localized, compressive, or systemic symptoms. Prompt management is necessary because delayed diagnosis and treatment can result in complications and cause significant morbidity and mortality, such as fecal incontinence, chronic pain, fistula formation, and sepsis. Definitive treatment usually requires incision and drainage, but the approaches vary based on anatomical location. Generally, superficial purulent infections may be managed with skin incisions and drainage, but deeper space infections generally require operative management. All patients with anorectal abscesses should complete a course of antibiotics, but antibiotics are generally unwarranted for pilonidal infections. Close follow-up care is crucial to ensure proper wound healing and to assess for complications.

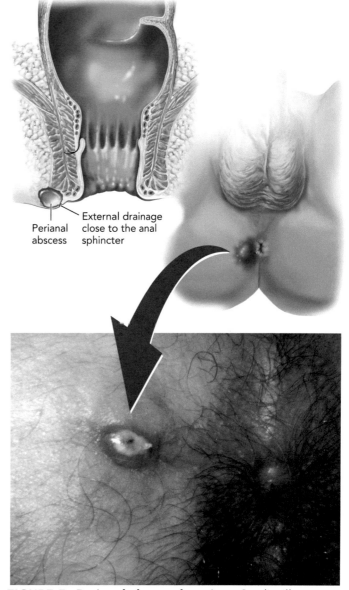

FIGURE 5. Perianal abscess location. *Credit: Illustration: Elise Walmsley-MacWha/Stocktrek Images; photo: BSIP SA/Alamy Stock Photo.*

REFERENCES

1. Nelson RL, Abcarian H, Davis FG, Persky V. Prevalence of benign anorectal disease in a randomly selected population. *Dis Colon Rectum.* 1995;38(4):341-344.
2. Abcarian H. Anorectal infection: abscess-fistula. *Clin Colon Rectal Surg.* 2011;24(1):14-21.
3. Rizzo JA, Naig AL, Johnson EK. Anorectal abscess and fistula-in-ano: evidence-based management. *Surg Clin North Am.* 2010;90(1):45-68.
4. Aggarwal P, Ternent CA, Thorson AG. Anal fistula management. In: Yeo CJ, DeMeester SR, McFadden DW, Matthews JB, Fleshman JW, eds. *Shackelford's Surgery of the Alimentary Tract.* Vol 2. 8th ed. Elsevier 2007:1871-1887.
5. Femling J. Soft tissue infections. In: Cydulka RK, Fitch MT, Joing SA, Wang VJ, Cline DM, Ma OJ, eds. *Tintinalli's Emergency Medicine Manual.* 8th ed. McGraw-Hill Education; 2017:491-496.
6. Johnson EK. Pilonidal disease. UpToDate. Updated October 20, 2021. https://www.uptodate.com/contents/pilonidal-disease
7. Berberian JG, Burgess BE. Anorectal disorders. In: Tintinalli JE, Ma OJ, Yealy DM, et al, eds. *Tintinalli's Emergency Medicine: A Comprehensive Study Guide.* 9th ed. McGraw-Hill Education; 2020:536-551.
8. Lasithiotaks K, Aghahoseini A, Volanaki D, Peter M, Alexander D. Aspiration for acute pilonidal abscess-a cohort study. *J Surg Res.* 2018;223:123-127.
9. Chooljian C. Pilonidal abscess or cyst incision and drainage. In: Reichman EF, ed. *Emergency Medicine Procedures.* 3rd ed. McGraw-Hill Education; 2019:1126-1130.

CME Questions

Reviewed by Tareq Al-Salamah, MBBS, MPH, FACEP; and Walter L. Green, MD, FACEP

Qualified, paid subscribers to *Critical Decisions in Emergency Medicine* may receive CME certificates for up to 5 ACEP Category I credits, 5 *AMA PRA Category 1 Credits*™, and 5 AOA Category 2-B credits for completing this activity in its entirety. Submit your answers online at acep.org/cdem; a score of 75% or better is required. You may receive credit for completing the CME activity any time within 3 years of its publication date. Answers to this month's questions will be published in next month's issue.

1   What is the first-line therapy for patients with back pain?
   A.   Benzodiazepines
   B.   Muscle relaxants
   C.   NSAIDs
   D.   Opiates

2   In patients suspected of having a spinal epidural abscess, what is the preferred imaging modality?
   A.   CT
   B.   CT myelogram
   C.   MRI with gadolinium
   D.   MRI without gadolinium

3   In patients with a fever and back pain, what testing can help risk stratify the patient to determine if an MRI with gadolinium is needed to exclude a spinal epidural abscess?
   A.   Blood cultures
   B.   Erythrocyte sedimentation rate and C-reactive protein
   C.   Lumbar puncture
   D.   Procalcitonin level

4   Which condition can decrease the sensitivity of plain x-rays in identifying spinal fractures?
   A.   Diabetes
   B.   Obesity
   C.   Osteophytes
   D.   Osteoporosis

5   Which treatment option has been associated with increased medical costs and disability in patients with acute occupational low back pain?
   A.   Acetaminophen
   B.   Muscle relaxants
   C.   NSAIDs
   D.   Opiates

6   What causative organisms are most common in patients with a spinal epidural abscess?
   A.   Enteric gram-negative bacilli
   B.   *Pseudomonas aeruginosa*
   C.   *Staphylococcus aureus*
   D.   *Streptococcus* species

7   In which situation should emergency physicians refrain from ordering advanced imaging?
   A.   18-year-old with a history of intravenous drug use who complains of weakness in the left leg and back pain
   B.   22-year-old who developed back pain that shoots down the left leg 3 days ago after lifting a box at work who has a normal neurologic examination
   C.   50-year-old with a history of recently treated infected olecranon bursitis who presents with a fever and back pain and has elevated C-reactive protein and erythrocyte sedimentation rate levels
   D.   67-year-old with a fever and back pain after lumbar discectomy

8   In the setting of back pain, what additional clinical feature requires further diagnostic evaluation?
   A.   Pain refractory to NSAIDs for 3 days
   B.   Paraspinal muscle spasm
   C.   Unilateral back pain
   D.   Urinary incontinence

9   A 72-year-old man presents with acute-onset severe back pain that radiates to his groin. He has no history of trauma. He has a history of hypertension and tobacco use. His vital signs include BP 75/40 and P 115. What is the best initial imaging study to obtain?
   A.   CT abdomen/pelvis
   B.   Lumbar x-ray
   C.   MRI with gadolinium
   D.   Ultrasound

10   When cauda equina syndrome is suspected in a patient who has an MRI-incompatible implanted device, what is the next best diagnostic imaging study of choice?
   A.   CT myelogram
   B.   CT with IV contrast
   C.   Plain x-ray
   D.   Ultrasound

11 Which statement regarding perirectal abscesses is true?
  A. Antibiotic treatment alone may be adequate
  B. Bedside incision and drainage are usually definitive
  C. External signs of infection may be absent
  D. Fistula formation is a rare complication

12 Which isolated purulent abscess may present with compressive neurologic symptoms (ie, urinary retention, fecal incontinence, and sciatica)?
  A. Intersphincteric
  B. Perianal
  C. Pilonidal
  D. Supralevator

13 Which statement regarding the anatomical considerations of anorectal abscesses is false?
  A. Anorectal abscesses are usually caused by obstruction of anal crypt glands
  B. Intestinal columnar epithelium lies below the dentate line
  C. Supralevator abscesses may originate from more inferior infections
  D. The lateral portions of the ischiorectal fossa communicate posteriorly

14 What is the most common anatomic location for a pilonidal abscess?
  A. Anal verge
  B. In the buttocks
  C. Lateral to the rectum
  D. Superior gluteal cleft

15 After incision and drainage of a pilonidal abscess, what is the best disposition?
  A. Admission for intravenous antibiotics
  B. Discharge home with follow-up as needed
  C. Discharge home with primary care follow-up
  D. Discharge home with referral to a surgeon

16 When is it appropriate to start outpatient oral antibiotics for pilonidal abscesses?
  A. For all pilonidal abscesses
  B. For large pilonidal abscesses
  C. For marked overlying cellulitis with induration beyond the abscess cavity
  D. For pilonidal abscesses with a large amount of fluctuance

17 Which abscess location is most likely to require surgical drainage?
  A. Intersphincteric
  B. Ischiorectal
  C. Perianal
  D. Pilonidal

18 Which statement about perirectal abscess fistulas is true?
  A. About 70% of anorectal abscesses are complicated by fistula formation
  B. Fistula formation is a rare complication
  C. Fistula repair should not be considered for horseshoe abscesses
  D. Primary fistula repair is superior to delayed fistula repair after inflammation resolution in almost all cases

19 For perianal abscesses, how should the incision be made to minimize the potential for fistula tract formation?
  A. As small as possible
  B. Through the skin as close to the anal verge as possible
  C. Through the skin elliptically
  D. Through the skin longitudinally

20 What statement regarding antibiotics is true when managing anorectal abscesses?
  A. All pilonidal abscesses require antibiotics
  B. It is reasonable in a conservative management approach of perirectal abscesses to use antibiotics alone without drainage
  C. Perianal abscesses typically respond to antibiotics without procedural intervention
  D. Those with large amount of cellulitis, diabetes, sepsis, or immunocompromise should be given antibiotics for perirectal abscesses

ANSWER KEY FOR JUNE 2022, VOLUME 36, NUMBER 6

1	2	3	4	5	6	7	8	9	10	11	12	13	14	15	16	17	18	19	20
B	C	A	C	C	D	B	C	C	D	B	A	B	B	B	D	B	B	C	D

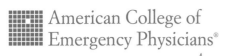
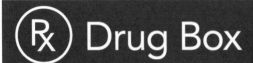

Drug Box

GIAPREZA

By Frank LoVecchio, DO, MPH, FACEP
Valleywise Health and ASU, Phoenix, Arizona

Objective
On completion of this column, you should be able to:
■ Describe the use of Giapreza and its adverse reactions.

Giapreza (angiotensin II) is used to increase blood pressure (BP) in adults with septic or other distributive shock. In a clinical trial of 321 patients with shock and a critically low BP, significantly more patients responded to treatment with Giapreza than a placebo. Giapreza effectively increased BP when added to conventional treatments used to raise BP.

Dosage
Adults: Giapreza is administered by IV infusion at an initial dose of 20 ng/kg/min. Titration occurs every 5 minutes by increments of up to 15 ng/kg/min as needed based on BP response, with a maximum dose of 80 ng/kg/min during the first 3 hours of treatment. A maintenance dose is a maximum of 40 ng/kg/min. Doses as low as 1.25 ng/kg/min may be used. Once sufficiently improved, down-titration should occur every 5 to 15 minutes by increments of up to 15 ng/kg/min based on the patient's BP. The half-life elimination of Giapreza is less than 1 minute, and the time to peak is 5 minutes.
Children: Giapreza's use in children has not been established.

Contraindications
None

Warnings and Precautions
Giapreza's safety was evaluated in a randomized, double-blind, placebo-controlled study of 321 adults with septic or other distributive shock, called ATHOS-3. There was a higher incidence of arterial and venous thrombotic and thromboembolic events in patients who received Giapreza compared to placebo-treated patients (13% [21/163 patients] versus 5% [8/158 patients]). Deep venous thromboses showed the greatest imbalance between Giapreza-treated patients and those receiving a placebo. Use of a concurrent venous thromboembolism prophylaxis is therefore recommended.

Adverse Reactions
Thromboembolic events were the most common adverse reactions reported (greater than 10% in Giapreza-treated patients). Adverse reactions in the ATHOS-3 study (occurring in ≥4% of Giapreza-treated patients and occurring ≥1.5% more often than in placebo-treated patients) were thromboembolic events, thrombocytopenia, tachycardia, fungal infection, delirium, acidosis, hyperglycemia, and peripheral ischemia.

Drug Interactions and Metabolism
Angiotensin-converting enzyme inhibitors may increase a patient's response to Giapreza, and angiotensin II receptor blockers may reduce the response to Giapreza. Giapreza is metabolized by aminopeptidase A and angiotensin-converting enzyme 2 to angiotensin–(2-8), also known as angiotensin III, and angiotensin–(1-7), respectively in plasma, erythrocytes, and many of the major organs.

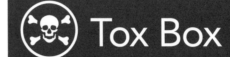

Tox Box

ACUTE ORAL METHOTREXATE OVERDOSE

By Christian Tomaszewski, MD, MS, MBA, FACEP
University of California San Diego Health

Objective
On completion of this column, you should be able to:
■ Manage patients suffering a methotrexate overdose.

Methotrexate (MTX) treats a variety of cancers as well as rheumatoid arthritis. It is the most common antineoplastic agent involved in oral overdoses. Although bone marrow suppression can be delayed, larger oral overdoses saturate absorption and do not cause toxicity unless they are massive, occur repeatedly, or occur in combination with renal failure.

Mechanism of Action
■ Folate antimetabolite that inhibits dihydrofolate reductase
■ Decreases tetrahydrofolate production needed for DNA synthesis and repair

Pharmacokinetics
■ Oral bioavailability about 60%, but variable
■ 1 to 3 hours to peak blood concentration
■ Dose cutoffs tolerated well
  ● Children ≤20 mg
  ● Adults ≤60 mg
■ Effective half-life of 8 hours

Clinical Manifestations
■ *Gastrointestinal:* nausea, vomiting, diarrhea, stomatitis, hepatitis
■ *Blood:* pancytopenia delayed days to 1 week (rare with oral)
■ *Metabolic:* renal failure (decreases MTX excretion)

Diagnostics
■ Daily CBC and CMP for large oral ingestions
■ Acetaminophen level in intentional ingestions
■ Serum MTX concentration to help dictate treatment

Treatment
■ Activated charcoal if caught early (multiple doses if renal failure is present)
■ IV hydration with sodium bicarbonate solution to enhance elimination
■ Leucovorin rescue if patient is symptomatic, the dose is greater than 1,000 mg, or renal failure is present
  ● 40 mg oral to start
  ● 10 mg/m² (or mg ≥50% of MTX dose taken) IV over 15 minutes, with dosing every 3 hours dictated by MTX level (stop when MTX level is <0.01 µmol/L)
■ Glucarpidase is usually reserved for intrathecal or massive IV overdose.
■ Hemodialysis is of questionable benefit unless renal injury is a factor.

Disposition
■ Symptomatic exposures require observation and treatment (MTX goal <0.01 µmol/L).
■ If asymptomatic at 6 hours post ingestion, the patient can be medically cleared.

Critical decisions
in emergency medicine

Volume 36 Number 8: **August 2022**

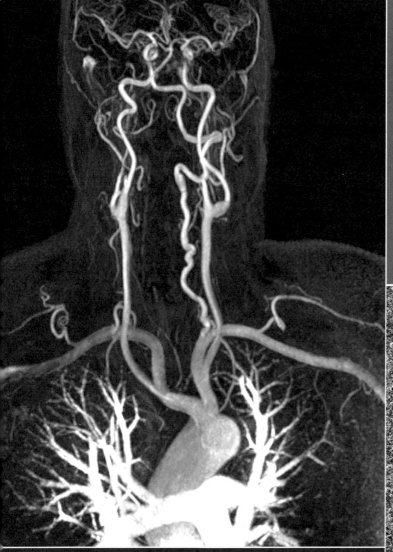

Neck Deep

Although the overall incidence is low, cervical artery dissection can cause up to 20% of acute strokes in patients younger than 45 years. Cervical artery dissection can occur spontaneously or with trauma. Emergency physicians must diagnose and treat it early to prevent thromboembolic events and other complications.

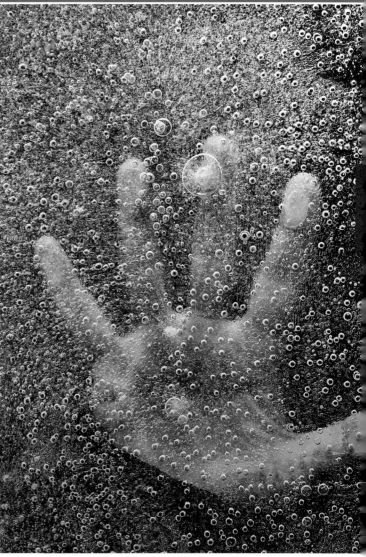

Going Under

Emergency departments incur roughly 8,000 annual visits for drownings, typically from freshwater bodies, swimming pools, bathtubs, or buckets. As such, emergency physicians must properly manage patients to avoid complications like hypoxemia, acidosis, and structural insult to the lungs, which can increase morbidity and mortality.

THE OFFICIAL CME PUBLICATION OF THE AMERICAN COLLEGE OF EMERGENCY PHYSICIANS

Contributor Disclosures. In accordance with the ACCME Standards for Commercial Support and policy of the American College of Emergency Physicians, all individuals with control over CME content (including but not limited to staff, planners, reviewers, and authors) must disclose whether they have any relevant financial relationship(s) to learners prior to the start of the activity. These individuals have indicated that they have a relationship which, in the context of their involvement in the CME activity, could be perceived by some as a real or apparent conflict of interest (eg, ownership of stock, grants, honoraria, or consulting fees), but these individuals do not consider that it will influence the CME activity. Joshua S. Broder, MD, FACEP, is a founder and president of OmniSono Inc, an ultrasound technology company. Sharon E. Mace, MD, FACEP, performs contracted research funded by Biofire Corporation, Genetesis, Quidel, and IBSA Pharma. All remaining individuals with control over CME content have no significant financial interests or relationships to disclose.

This educational activity consists of two lessons, eight feature articles, a post-test, and evaluation questions; as designed, the activity should take approximately 5 hours to complete. The participant should, in order, review the learning objectives for the lesson or article, read the lesson or article as published in the print or online version until all have been reviewed, and then complete the online post-test (a minimum score of 75% is required) and evaluation questions. Release date August 1, 2022. Expiration date July 31, 2025.

Accreditation Statement. The American College of Emergency Physicians is accredited by the Accreditation Council for Continuing Medical Education to provide continuing medical education for physicians.

The American College of Emergency Physicians designates this enduring material for a maximum of 5 *AMA PRA Category 1 Credits™*. Physicians should claim only the credit commensurate with the extent of their participation in the activity.

Each issue of *Critical Decisions in Emergency Medicine* is approved by ACEP for 5 ACEP Category I credits. Approved by the AOA for 5 Category 2-B credits.

Commercial Support. There was no commercial support for this CME activity.

Target Audience. This educational activity has been developed for emergency physicians.

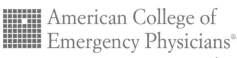
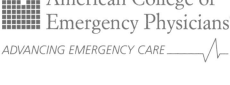

American College of Emergency Physicians®

ADVANCING EMERGENCY CARE

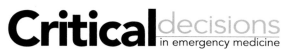

Critical **decisions** in emergency medicine

Critical Decisions in Emergency Medicine is the official CME publication of the American College of Emergency Physicians. Additional volumes are available.

EDITOR-IN-CHIEF
Michael S. Beeson, MD, MBA, FACEP
Northeastern Ohio Universities, Rootstown, OH

SECTION EDITORS
Joshua S. Broder, MD, FACEP
Duke University, Durham, NC

Andrew J. Eyre, MD, MS-HPEd
Brigham and Women's Hospital/ Harvard Medical School, Boston, MA

John Kiel, DO, MPH, FACEP, CAQSM
University of Florida College of Medicine, Jacksonville, FL

Frank LoVecchio, DO, MPH, FACEP
Valleywise, Arizona State University, University of Arizona, and Creighton Colleges of Medicine, Phoenix, AZ

Sharon E. Mace, MD, FACEP
Cleveland Clinic Lerner College of Medicine/ Case Western Reserve University, Cleveland, OH

Amal Mattu, MD, FACEP
University of Maryland, Baltimore, MD

Christian A. Tomaszewski, MD, MS, MBA, FACEP
University of California Health Sciences, San Diego, CA

Steven J. Warrington, MD, MEd, MS
MercyOne Siouxland, Sioux City, IA

ASSOCIATE EDITORS
Tareq Al-Salamah, MBBS, MPH, FACEP
King Saud University, Riyadh, Saudi Arabia/ University of Maryland, Baltimore, MD

Wan-Tsu Chang, MD
University of Maryland, Baltimore, MD

Ann M. Dietrich, MD, FAAP, FACEP
University of South Carolina School of Medicine, Greenville, SC

Kelsey Drake, MD, MPH, FACEP
St. Anthony Hospital, Lakewood, CO

Walter L. Green, MD, FACEP
UT Southwestern Medical Center, Dallas, TX

John C. Greenwood, MD
University of Pennsylvania, Philadelphia, PA

Danya Khoujah, MBBS, MEHP, FACEP
University of Maryland, Baltimore, MD

Nathaniel Mann, MD
University of South Carolina School of Medicine, Greenville, SC

George Sternbach, MD, FACEP
Stanford University Medical Center, Stanford, CA

EDITORIAL STAFF
Suzannah Alexander, Editorial Director
salexander@acep.org

Joy Carrico, JD
Managing Editor

Alex Bass
Assistant Editor

Kel Morris
Assistant Editor

ISSN2325-0186 (Print)

ISSN2325-8365 (Online)

Contents

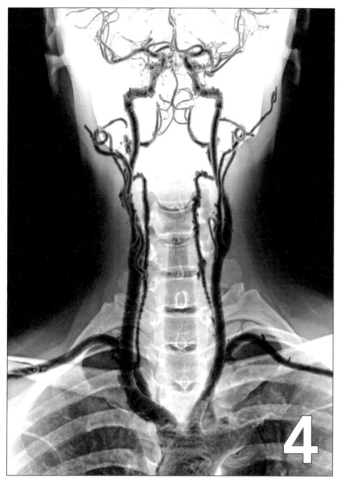

Lesson 15 4
Neck Deep
Cervical Artery Dissection
By Bushra Hussein, MD; and Erin R. Leiman, MD
Reviewed by Danya Khoujah, MBBS, MEHP, FACEP

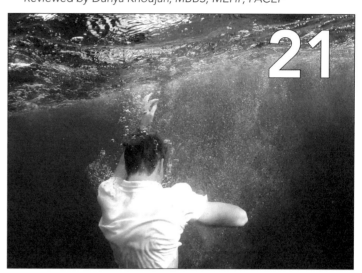

Lesson 16 21
Going Under
Drowning and Submersion Injury
By Savannah Chavez, MD; and Bethany Johnston, MD
Reviewed by Nathaniel Mann, MD

FEATURES

Clinical Pediatrics — Takayasu Arteritis 10
By Hannah Mezan, MD
Reviewed by Sharon E. Mace, MD, FACEP

The Critical ECG — Acute Pericarditis 13
By Amal Mattu, MD, FACEP

The LLSA Literature Review — 2019 AHA Update for Pediatric Advanced Life Support 14
By Christopher Fahlsing, MD, LT, MC, USN; and Daphne Morrison Ponce, MD, CDR, MC, USN
Reviewed by Andrew J. Eyre, MD, MS-HPEd

Critical Cases in Orthopedics and Trauma — Lisfranc Amputation After Crush Injury 16
By Parker Young, DO
Reviewed by John Kiel, DO, MPH

The Critical Image — Crying Infant 18
By Joshua S. Broder, MD, FACEP

The Critical Procedure — Clogged Feeding Tube Management 20
By Steven J. Warrington, MD, MEd, MS

CME Questions 30
Reviewed by Danya Khoujah, MBBS, MEHP, FACEP; and Nathaniel Mann, MD

Drug Box — Dexmedetomidine Sublingual Film 32
By Frank LoVecchio, DO, MPH, FACEP

Tox Box — Acute Triptan Overdose 32
By Christian Tomaszewski, MD, MS, MBA, FACEP

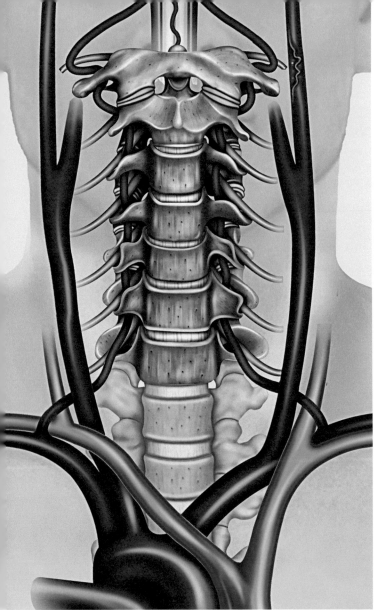

Neck Deep

Cervical Artery Dissection

LESSON **15**

Bushra Hussein, MD; and Erin R. Leiman, MD
Dr. Hussein is a resident and Dr. Leiman is an assistant professor in the Department of Emergency Medicine at Duke University Hospital in Durham, North Carolina.
Reviewed by Danya Khoujah, MBBS, MEHP, FACEP

Objectives

On completion of this lesson, you should be able to:

1. Recognize the common clinical presentations of patients with CAD.
2. Describe the most frequent complications of CAD.
3. Select the best imaging modalities to diagnose CAD.
4. Manage ischemic thromboembolic events in CAD.
5. Explain the role of thrombolysis and endovascular therapy in patients with CAD.

From the EM Model

18.0 Traumatic Disorders
   18.1 Trauma
      18.1.9 Neck Trauma
         18.1.9.3 Vascular Injuries

▬ CRITICAL DECISIONS ▬

- What are the clinical presentations of CAD?

- What are the complications of CAD?

- Which imaging modalities are used to diagnose CAD?

- What is the goal of treatment for CAD without signs of a current stroke?

- How should ischemic stroke be managed in patients with CAD?

Although the overall incidence is low, cervical artery dissection (CAD) can cause up to 20% of acute strokes in patients younger than 45 years. CAD can occur spontaneously or with trauma. Early diagnosis and treatment are important to prevent thromboembolic events and other complications.

CASE PRESENTATIONS

■ CASE ONE

A 35-year-old man with a history of migraines presents to a level I trauma center as a restrained driver in a head-on motor vehicle collision. EMS noted significant front-end damage to the patient's car with airbag deployment. The patient was able to self-extricate and was ambulatory on scene. The patient now complains of chest pain, posterior neck pain, and a migraine.

His vital signs are BP 135/69, P 101, R 20, and T 37.7°C (99.9°F); SpO$_2$ is 97% on room air. On examination, he has a seat belt abrasion to the left lateral neck as well as posterior midline cervical spine tenderness. His neurologic examination is normal, except for the reported headache and nausea. He has not vomited.

■ CASE TWO

A 41-year-old woman with a history of hypertension presents via EMS with a stroke alert. Approximately 2 hours ago, her husband noted that she had new-onset difficulty speaking, right-sided facial droop, and right-sided upper- and lower-extremity weakness. Supplemental history from her husband reveals that the patient has had a 6-day history of vertigo that was initially intermittent but has been constant during the last day. She missed several days of work due to this vertigo.

On examination, the patient is alert and tearful. She can understand commands but has dysarthria. Her neurologic deficits include a right-sided facial droop, a mild decrease in sensation on the right side, 2/5 strength in the right upper and lower extremities, and 5/5 strength in the left upper and lower extremities. Her vital signs are BP 205/103, P 72, R 18, and T 37.0°C (98.6°F); SpO$_2$ is 99% on room air.

Introduction

The incidence of CAD has increased over the last decade, likely due to improvements in imaging. CAD often occurs in the setting of trauma, including both high-mechanism and minor injuries. When overt trauma is absent, it is often called spontaneous CAD, although there may have been some triggering event or predisposing condition that can be elicited from the patient's history. CAD most commonly involves the carotid arteries, followed by the vertebral arteries (*Figure 1*). Early diagnosis and treatment of CAD significantly reduce morbidity and mortality, and one of the main roles of treatment is to prevent further thromboembolic events.

CRITICAL DECISION

What are the clinical presentations of CAD?

CAD describes the pathological tearing of the intimal layer of either the carotid or vertebral arteries, collectively known as the cervical arteries. Common symptoms of both carotid and vertebral artery dissections include unilateral headache (68%), neck pain (39%), and face pain (10%).[1] CAD can occur spontaneously, but underlying conditions such as connective tissue disorders (eg, Ehlers-Danlos syndrome, Marfan syndrome, and type I osteogenesis imperfecta), hypertension, and atherosclerosis are predisposing risk factors.[2] CAD can

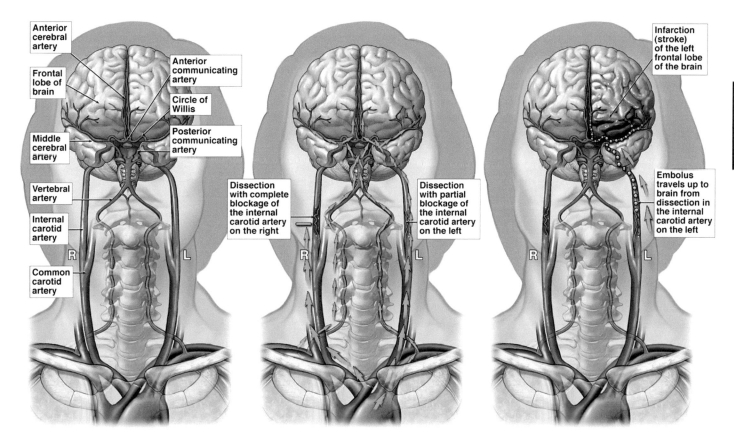

Normal Condition

Initial Condition

Condition with Stroke

FIGURE 1. Cervical artery dissection. Credit: Nucleus Medical Media Inc/Alamy Stock Photo.

also occur in the setting of trauma, including high-mechanism accidents as well as seemingly trivial events (eg, chiropractic manipulation or amusement park rides).

The average age of patients with spontaneously occurring CAD is 44 years (+/– 13), and the age of patients who sustain CAD in the setting of trauma is significantly younger at 36 years (+/– 15).[3] Trauma such as motor vehicle crashes, sporting injuries, and cervical spine manipulation can cause cervical spine injuries by direct impact, flexion or extension, hyperextension, and rotational mechanisms, which make patients vulnerable to CAD.[4-5] The clinical presentation of CAD is typically nonspecific and can be difficult to diagnose, especially if there are distracting injuries. The diagnosis of CAD requires a careful history, thorough examination, and a high clinical suspicion leading to further diagnostic testing.

Carotid Dissection

Carotid dissection commonly occurs 2 cm above the bifurcation of the common carotid artery, where the extracranial portion of the internal carotid artery travels over C2-C3. An important triad that is concerning for carotid artery dissection begins with ipsilateral neck pain; a headache that is sudden in onset, unilateral, and constant; and occasionally, partial Horner syndrome (miosis and ptosis without anhidrosis). Additionally, carotid dissections can lead to retinal or cerebral ischemia. Signs and symptoms can also include focal neurologic deficits, carotid bruits, expanding hematomas, and arterial hemorrhage.[6] Neurologic deficits may be insidious in nature because symptoms may present days or weeks after an initial injury.

Vertebral Artery Dissection

Vertebral artery dissection commonly occurs at C1-C2 due to compression at the cervical foramen and at C5-C6 at the transverse foramen. A systematic review of clinical characteristics in patients shows the most common symptoms for vertebral artery dissections are dizziness or vertigo, headache, and neck pain.[5] Some patients may have signs and symptoms that are consistent with lateral medullary ischemia (also known as Wallenberg syndrome), which is characterized by dysmetria, ataxia, and ipsilateral hemiplegia; they may also have other cerebellar signs.

CRITICAL DECISION

What are the complications of CAD?

Stroke

CAD is a common cause of stroke in young adults, with a prevalence of 20% in this population and an annual incidence rate of 2.6 to 2.9 per 100,000 in the general population. CAD patients also present with transient ischemic attacks.[7] Stroke is commonly reported in patients with vertebral artery dissections and is more prevalent in patients with extracranial vertebral artery dissections.[8]

The first mechanism of stroke is related to the endothelial injury of the affected vessel driving the coagulation cascade and thrombus formation, making a thromboembolic process more likely. In a retrospective study, 100 of 172 patients with CAD had acute strokes on diffusion-weighted image MRI; 85% of the strokes were attributed to thromboembolic events.[8] The second mechanism of stroke is by stenosis of the vessel involved, causing hypoperfusion and watershed infarction.

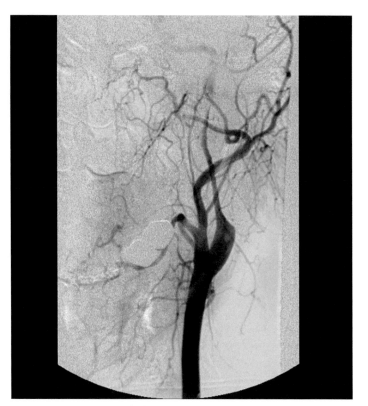

FIGURE 2. Carotid dissection with watershed infarct.
Copyright 2022 Dr. Frank Gaillard. Image courtesy of Dr. Frank Gaillard and Radiopaedia.org, rID: 5182. Used under license.

Pseudoaneurysms

Cervical artery dissections, spontaneous or otherwise, can develop pseudoaneurysms at the dissection site, which can enlarge and advance until they become symptomatic. With standard medical management of dissecting pseudoaneurysms with antiplatelet or anticoagulation therapy, the clinical course is typically benign. Most commonly, 14% of patients with dissecting pseudoaneurysms have a recurrence of nonischemic symptoms (ie, headache, neck pain, Horner syndrome, or cranial nerve palsy). Only 3% of patients have a recurrent transient ischemic attack, and typically, recurrent strokes do not occur. To mitigate the risk of rupture in patients with larger aneurysms (>10 mm in diameter), patients may undergo more aggressive treatment, endovascular stent placement, or surgical management with aneurysmal clipping. About 13% of patient have aneurysms that increase in size,

✔ Pearls

- Take a careful history in patients with neck pain or headache to evaluate for CAD, especially in the setting of trauma.
- Although the gold-standard imaging modality for CAD is conventional DSA, CTA has a high sensitivity and is more readily available in emergency departments.
- Treating extracranial CAD with either antiplatelet or anticoagulation therapy has similar efficacies; utilization of either is appropriate.
- In patients with ischemic stroke in the setting of CAD, intravenous thrombolysis should be carefully considered according to established guidelines.

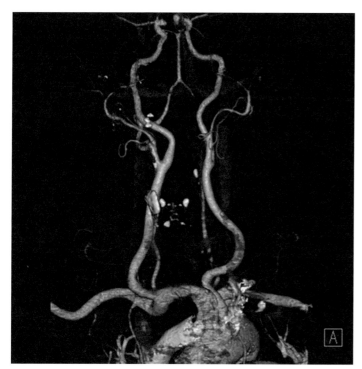

FIGURE 3. Vertebral artery dissection due to trauma. Copyright 2022 Dr. Henry Knipe. Image courtesy of Dr. Henry Knipe and Radiopaedia.org, rID: 48493. Used under license.

whereas the rest either completely resolve (30%) or remain stable (56%).[9]

CRITICAL DECISION

Which imaging modalities are used to diagnose CAD?

Patients with an acute or a subacute history of high-impact trauma, signs of cervical neck injury (eg, seat belt sign extending to the neck), symptoms of a posterior circulation injury, or focal neurologic deficits should be evaluated for CAD. Multiple imaging modalities can aid in the screening and diagnosis. The gold-standard imaging modality for CAD is digital subtraction angiography (DSA), otherwise known as invasive catheter angiography (*Figure 2*). DSA uses fluoroscopy to evaluate cerebral and cervical vessels. Although DSA detects up to 34% of asymptomatic patients with CAD, it is also more invasive than other more readily available imaging modalities for patients who acutely present to emergency departments across institutions.[5]

✖ Pitfalls

- Failing to carefully examine patients with a subacute history of any trauma, as symptoms can be subtle or insidious in nature.

- Assuming CAD patients are only at risk for thromboembolic events. CAD complications also include pseudoaneurysms. Depending on the size, they may require endovascular or surgical intervention.

- Starting endovascular therapy without expert collaboration.

A prospective study showed that CT angiography (CTA) is comparable to DSA. Both CTA and DSA were obtained in 146 patients at risk for blunt cerebrovascular injury, and CTA was found to have a high sensitivity (97.7%), specificity (100%), positive-predictive value (100%), negative-predictive value (99.3%), and accuracy (99.3%) (*Figure 3*). Unlike DSA, CTA is widely available with minimal risks when compared to the gold standard, so it is the more favorable imaging modality in emergency departments across the United States.[10]

CRITICAL DECISION

What is the goal of treatment for CAD without signs of a current stroke?

Patients with CAD are at an increased risk of having a thromboembolic event; thus, the goal of treatment is preventing an ischemic thromboembolic event. Treatment for CAD is achieved in one of two ways: antiplatelet therapy or anticoagulation. For patients with CAD, the American Heart Association recommends 3 to 6 months of treatment with either of these two therapies.

The Cervical Artery Dissection in Stroke Study (CADISS) is a randomized trial that compared these two treatment modalities in 250 patients with extracranial carotid artery dissection or vertebral artery dissection to determine their relative efficacies. Antiplatelet therapy in this trial included the use of either aspirin, dipyridamole, or clopidogrel alone or in combination. Anticoagulation therapy in this trial included the use of heparin — either low-molecular-weight or unfractionated heparin — followed by warfarin with a goal international normalized ratio of 2 to 3.[11] Overall, this study showed stroke to a be a rare complication, occurring in only 2% of patients who received treatment of any kind. The study concludes that there is no difference in efficacy when using one treatment modality versus the other. Therefore, there is no clear consensus regarding which treatment modality should be used; treatment is ultimately at the discretion of the physician or individual institutional guidelines.

CRITICAL DECISION

How should ischemic stroke be managed in patients with CAD?

Patients who present with symptoms of an acute stroke in the presence of CAD should be treated accordingly. Patients presenting within the window of intravenous thrombolytic therapy who lack absolute contraindications to thrombolysis (eg, CAD due to extension of aortic dissection) should be considered for intravenous thrombolytic therapy. Notably, thrombolysis is as effective for stroke in the setting of CAD as compared to other causes of stroke.[12] Similar to management of ischemic stroke not caused by CAD, mechanical thrombectomy should be considered when a patient has a persistent, disabling neurologic deficit, usually with a National Institute of Health Stroke Scale (NIHSS) score of ≥6.

Data are limited regarding endovascular therapy for treating CAD. The method that has been primarily used

CASE RESOLUTIONS

CASE ONE

Unfortunately, the 35-year-old man suffered a high-mechanism injury. His injuries included a C2 fracture and nondisplaced, stable sternal fractures. The patient continued to complain of neck pain and a left-sided migraine with associated nausea and vomiting. Given his injuries, there was concern for cervical artery dissection. A CTA of his neck showed left-sided vertebral artery dissection with an intimal flap. The patient was admitted to the hospital and started on heparin. His symptoms ultimately resolved, and he was transitioned to warfarin during admission.

CASE TWO

On assessment, the 41-year-old woman had a blood glucose of 103, NIHSS score of 16, and last known normal time of 2 hours ago. She had a rapid noncontract head CT scan, which was negative for intracerebral hemorrhage. CTA of the head and neck revealed an extracranial dissection of the left internal carotid artery, with a resulting left middle cerebral artery occlusion.

The patient was determined to be within the thrombolysis window and had no contraindications. After an appropriate risks and benefits discussion with her and her husband, she was treated with intravenous thrombolytics. Prior to thrombolytics, she

was started on a nicardipine drip for blood pressure management.

She was subsequently admitted to the ICU. During admission, she was also started on aspirin. Upon further history, the patient reported that she received cervical manipulation at her chiropractic office approximately 2 weeks ago. She initially had left-sided neck pain after the cervical manipulation that self-resolved. The patient reported that the vertigo she experienced started several days after the manipulation. She denied any other source of overt trauma. She recovered well, with only minor right upper-extremity weakness noted upon discharge.

---

is stent placement. The use of endovascular treatment has been employed in patients who fail antithrombotic treatment, particularly when a patient has both an embolism and hypoperfusion. Unfortunately, there are high-risk complications of stent placement, including iatrogenic arterial dissection, stent thrombosis, arterial rupture, and death.[13] Given these risks and a lack of randomized control trials, the decision for endovascular therapy is typically made with a comprehensive team, including a neurointerventionalist.

Summary

It is imperative that emergency physicians obtain a thorough history and physical examination in patients with face pain, neck pain, or headache to evaluate for CAD, especially in the setting of trauma, because symptoms are often subtle or deceptive. Risk factors for CAD that should be noted in the medical history include connective tissue disorders, hypertension, and atherosclerosis. Although the gold standard imaging modality for CAD is DSA, CTA has a high sensitivity and is more readily available in the emergency department to confirm the diagnosis.

Treating extracranial CAD with either antiplatelet or anticoagulation therapy has similar efficacies, so using either treatment can be appropriate, depending on institutional guidelines. Emergency physicians must also be aware that CAD complications not only include the risk of thromboembolic events, but also pseudoaneurysms. Depending on the size, pseudoaneurysms may require endovascular or surgical intervention. For patients with ischemic stroke in the setting of CAD, intravenous thrombolysis, mechanical thrombectomy, or endovascular therapy should be carefully considered with the appropriate expert collaboration.

REFERENCES

1. Debette S, Grond-Ginsbach C, Bodenant M, et al; Cervical Artery Dissection Ischemic Stroke Patients (CADISP) Group. Differential features of carotid and vertebral artery dissections: the CADISP study. *Neurology*. 2011;77(12):1174-1181.
2. Debette S, Leys D. Cervical-artery dissections: predisposing factors, diagnosis, and outcome. *Lancet Neurol*. 2009;8(7):668-678.
3. Xu D, Wu Y, Li J, et al. Retrospective comparative analysis of clinical and imaging features of craniocervical artery dissection: spontaneous CAD vs minor traumatic CAD. *Front Neurol*. 2022;13:836997.
4. Giacobetti FB, Vaccaro AR, Bos-Giacobetti MA, et al. Vertebral artery occlusion associated with cervical spine trauma. *Spine (Phila Pa 1976)*. 1997;22(2):188-192.
5. Shafafy R, Suresh S, Afolayan JO, Vaccaro AR, Panchmatia JR. Blunt vertebral vascular injury in trauma patients: ATLS recommendations and review of current evidence. *J Spine Surg*. 2017;3(20):217-225.
6. Cothren CC, Moore EE, Ray CE Jr, et al. Screening for blunt cerebrovascular injuries is cost effective. *Am J Surg*. 2005;190(6):845-849.
7. Blum CA, Yaghi S. Cervical artery dissection: a review of the epidemiology, pathophysiology, treatment, and outcome. *Arch Neurosci*. 2015;2(4):e26670.
8. Morel A, Naggara O, Touzé E, Raymond J, et al. Mechanism of ischemic infarct in spontaneous cervical artery dissection. *Stroke*. 2012;43(5):1354-1361.
9. Daou B, Hammer C, Chalouhi N, et al. Dissecting pseudoaneurysms: predictors of symptom occurrence, enlargement, clinical outcome, and treatment. *J Neurosurg*. 2016;125(4):936-942.
10. Eastman AL, Chason DP, Perez C, McAnulty A, Minei J. Computed tomography angiography for the diagnosis of blunt cervical vascular injury: is it ready for primetime? *J Trauma*. 2006;60(5):925-929.
11. Markus HS, Hayter E, Levi C, Feldman A, Venables G, Norris J; CADISS Trial Investigators. Antiplatelet treatment compared with anticoagulation treatment for cervical artery dissection (CADISS): a randomized trial. *Lancet Neurol*. 2015;14(4):361-367.
12. Lin J, Sun Y, Zhao S, Xu J, Zhao C. Safety and efficacy of thrombolysis in cervical artery dissection—related ischemic stroke: a meta-analysis of observational studies. *Cebrovasc Dis*. 2016;42(3-4):272-279.
13. Peng J, Liu X, Luo C, Chen L, et al. Treatment of cervical artery dissection: antithrombotics, thrombolysis, and endovascular therapy. *Biomed Res Int*. 2017;2017:3072098.

ADDITIONAL READING

Demaerschalk BM, Kleindorfer DO, Adeoye OM, et al; American Heart Association Stroke Council and Council on Epidemiology and Prevention. scientific rationale for the inclusion and exclusion criteria for intravenous alteplase in acute ischemic stroke. *Stroke*. 2016;47(2):581-641.

Jauch EC, Saver JL, Adams HP, et al; American Heart Association Stroke Council; Council on Cardiovascular Nursing; Council on Peripheral Vascular Disease; Council on Clinical Cardiology. Guidelines for the early management of patients with acute ischemic stroke: a guideline for healthcare professionals from the American Heart Association/American Stroke Association. *Stroke*. 2013;44(3):870-947.

Takayasu Arteritis

By Hannah Mezan, MD
LSU's Spirit of Charity Emergency Medicine
Residency Program, Children's Hospital,
New Orleans, Louisiana
Reviewed by Sharen E. Mace, MD, FACEP

Objective

On completion of this article, you should be able to:
- Discuss the diagnosis and management of Takayasu arteritis.

CASE PRESENTATION

A 17-year-old girl with no past medical history presents with 3 weeks of claudication. She describes significant pain in her legs with walking, which is relieved at rest. The pain progressively worsened over the past 3 weeks; she has difficulty walking across a room without severe pain. The pain began in her calves and extended up to her thighs and abdomen. She also reports numbness and tingling in her lower extremities, stating her legs feel "cold." The patient describes a brief illness that occurred 1 week prior to her symptom onset and involved abdominal pain, nausea, vomiting, fever, headaches, and fatigue. Urgent care prescribed azithromycin, and her symptoms resolved. She recalls being told her blood pressure was elevated at the time, but she was also told it was likely due to anxiety.

The patient initially presented to her primary care office with the claudication complaint; they advised her to go to the emergency department due to an elevated blood pressure of 180/100 mm Hg. Subsequent blood pressures in the emergency department were 195/99 mm Hg, 199/95 mm Hg, and 222/100 mm Hg. Blood pressures were then taken in all four extremities, which revealed a right arm pressure of 191/101 mm Hg and a left arm pressure of 189/95 mm Hg. Her right leg pressure was 139/70 mm Hg, and her left leg pressure was 131/90 mm Hg — significantly lower. Her physical examination revealed bounding radial pulses and faint dorsalis pedis pulses.

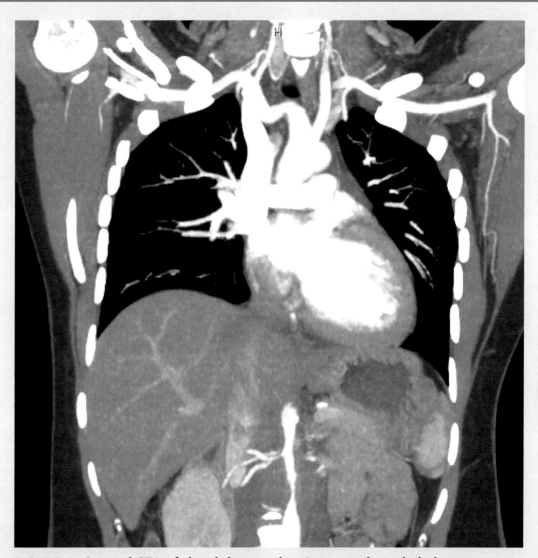

FIGURE 1. Coronal CTA of the abdomen, showing a nearly occluded aorta

The patient underwent emergent CT angiogram of the chest and abdomen (*Figures 1* and *2*), and the findings were suspicious for "periaortitis in association with midaortic syndrome with severe stenosis/near occlusion of the infrarenal aorta, bilateral renal arteries, celiac trunk, and spinal muscular atrophy. Findings may represent a vasculitis versus neoplastic process."

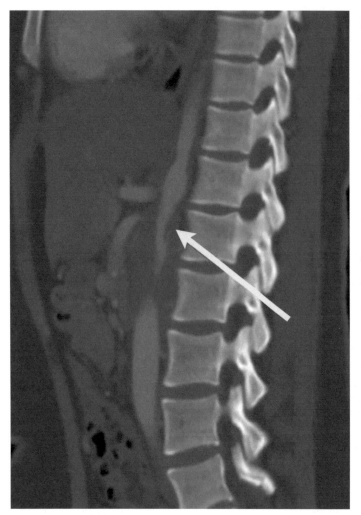

FIGURE 2. Sagittal CTA of the abdomen, emphasizing the severe narrowing of the aorta (*arrow*)

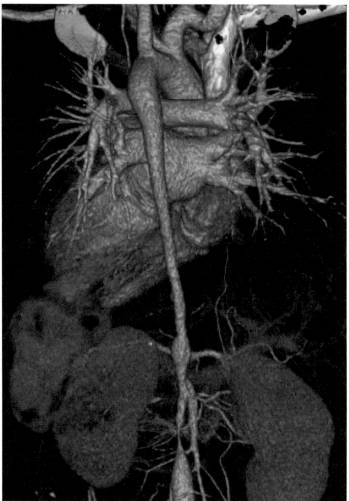

FIGURE 3. 3D reconstruction of the aorta, depicting severe narrowing of the aorta

Discussion

Takayasu arteritis is a rare form of large vessel vasculitis. It predominantly affects the aorta and its main branches. Manifestations can range from an asymptomatic disease found because of impalpable pulses to significant neurologic impairment. A two-phase process has been suggested for the disease: The first phase is marked by nonspecific inflammatory features, and the second phase involves the development of vascular insufficiency. Nonspecific inflammatory features may include fever, night sweats, malaise, weight loss, and myalgias. As the inflammation progresses to the next phase, more characteristic features become apparent — diminished or absent pulses, limb claudication or blood pressure discrepancies, vascular bruits, and hypertension. Takayasu disease incidence is highest in women (by a factor of 9 to 1), with most disease occurrence in the second or third decades of life.

Diagnosis

CT angiography (CTA) remains the gold standard for diagnosis. CTA allows for visualization of vessel wall thickening and luminal narrowing (*Figures 3* and *4*). Doppler ultrasound may also be useful for the assessment of vessel wall inflammation and has the advantage of being a noninvasive procedure. MR angiography has also been widely used.

The American College of Rheumatology defined six criteria for diagnosing Takayasu arteritis. Three of the six criteria must be met for a diagnosis to be established:

1. Age of disease onset younger than 40 years
2. Claudication of extremities
3. Decreased brachial artery pulse
4. Blood pressure difference greater than 10 mm Hg
5. Bruit over subclavian arteries or aorta
6. Arteriogram abnormality

The Ishikawa criteria later defined classification groups based on the complications and severity of the disease.

Management

Steroids are the mainstay of treatment for Takayasu arteritis; however, it is widely accepted that only about half of patients treated with steroids will respond. Immunosuppressive agents including cyclophosphamide, azathioprine, and methotrexate are often administered in combination with steroids. The other important medical issue to address is the management of hypertension.

Surgical therapy has traditionally been reserved for patients who are refractory to medical management or for those who have critical manifestations. Surgery is indicated

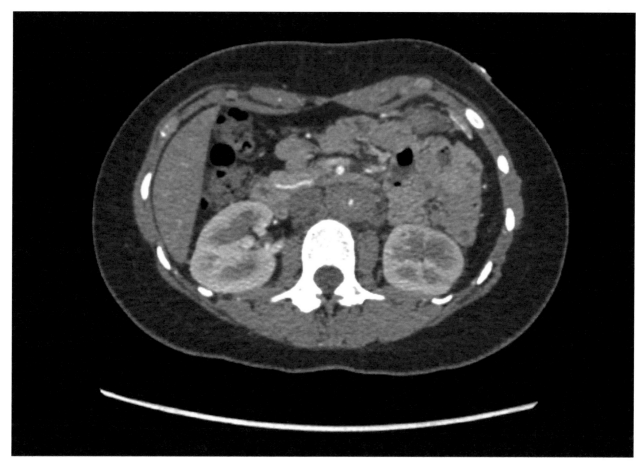

FIGURE 4. Axial CTA of the abdomen, showing the thickened walls of the aorta

when patients have hypertension with critical renal artery stenosis, extremity claudication limiting activities of daily living, cerebrovascular ischemia or critical stenoses of three or more cerebral vessels, moderate aortic regurgitation, or cardiac ischemia with confirmed coronary artery involvement.

Complications

Organ-specific manifestations of the disease may lead to disabling complications. Systemic hypertension may be associated with a higher risk of arterial vessel wall aneurysm and dissection, which is rare but life-threatening. Dilated cardiomyopathy, aortic valve insufficiency, and congestive heart failure have all been reported as cardiovascular complications. Neurologic complications include strokes, seizures, intracranial aneurysms, and encephalitis. If there is gastrointestinal involvement, there may be mesenteric ischemia caused by vasospasm of the damaged intestinal vasculature. Ocular manifestations of Takayasu arteritis can occur from occlusion or severe stenosis of the carotid arteries, such as retinal ischemia, detachment, or optic atrophy.

CASE RESOLUTION

The patient was placed on a nicardipine drip for blood pressure management and admitted to the pediatric ICU. Consults from vascular surgery, general surgery, rheumatology, nephrology, cardiology, and hematology and oncology were obtained. She was diagnosed with Takayasu arteritis and started on steroids, hydroxychloroquine, and methotrexate. She was also initiated on antihypertensive medications. The patient was discharged after a week-long hospital stay.

REFERENCES

1. Johnston SL, Lock RJ, Gompels MM. Takayasu arteritis: a review. *J Clin Path.* 2002;55(7):481-486.
2. Trinidad B, Surmachevska N, Lala V. *Takayasu Arteritis.* StatPearls Publishing. Updated 2021. Accessed July 27, 2022. https://www.ncbi.nlm.nih.gov/books/NBK459127/
3. Russo RAG, Katsicas MM. Takayasu arteritis. *Front Pediatr.* 2018;6:265.
4. Szugye HS, Zeft AS, Spalding SJ. Takayasu arteritis in the pediatric population: a contemporary United States-based single center cohort. *Pediatr Rheumatol Online J.* 2014;12:21
5. Natraj Setty HS, Vijaykumar JR, Nagesh CM, et al. Takayasu's arteritis–a comprehensive review. *J Rare Dis Res Treat.* 2017;2(2):63-68.
6. Singh H, Tanwar V, Kalra A, Ruchi. Takayasu arteritis: a rare clinical entity. *J Case Reports.* 2015;5(2):454-457.

Acute Pericarditis

By Amal Mattu, MD, FACEP

Dr. Mattu is a professor, vice chair, and director of the Emergency Cardiology Fellowship in the Department of Emergency Medicine at the University of Maryland School of Medicine in Baltimore.

Objective

On completion of this article, you should be able to:
- Recognize signs of acute pericarditis on ECG.

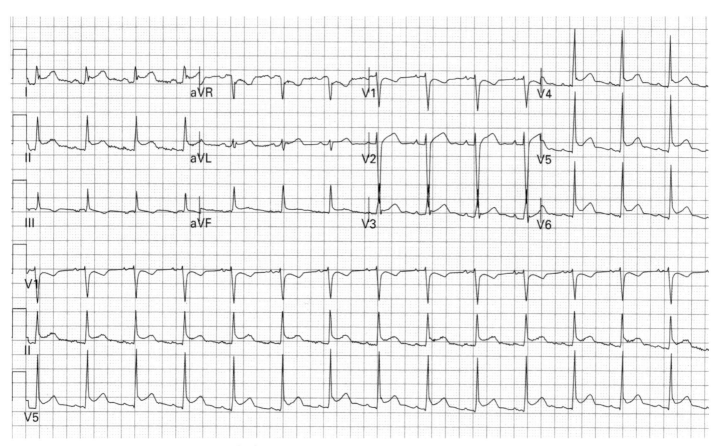

FIGURE 1. A 32-year-old woman with dyspnea

Sinus rhythm, rate 84, acute pericarditis. Diffuse ST-segment elevation (STE) is present on this ECG (*Figure 1*). Although there are many conditions that can induce STE on ECG, the major diagnostic considerations in patients with diffuse STE are large acute myocardial infarction, acute pericarditis, benign early repolarization, and left ventricular hypertrophy (LVH). LVH can be excluded by lack of voltage criteria. Of the remaining three considerations, acute pericarditis is the only one that causes PR-segment depression and downsloping, which is found in lead I and in the anterior and lateral precordial leads.

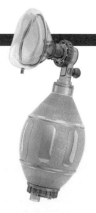

The LLSA Literature Review

2019 AHA Update for Pediatric Advanced Life Support

By Christopher Fahlsing, MD, LT, MC, USN; and
Daphne Morrison Ponce, MD, CDR, MC, USN
United States Navy
Reviewed by Andrew J. Eyre, MD, MS-HPEd

Objective
On completion of this article, you should be able to:
- Discuss the updated American Heart Association pediatric advanced life support guidelines.

Duff JP, Topjian AA, Berg MD, et al. 2019 American Heart Association focused update on pediatric advanced life support: an update to the American Heart Association guidelines for cardiopulmonary resuscitation and emergency cardiovascular care. *Pediatrics.* 2020;145(1):140(24):e20191361.

KEY POINTS

- For airway management, it is reasonable to continue BVM versus attempting an advanced airway in patients with OHCA.

- When ECMO protocols and teams are readily available, ECPR should be considered for patients with cardiac diagnoses and IHCA.

- It is reasonable to use TTM of 32°C (89.6°F) to 34°C (93.2°F) followed by 36°C (96.8°F) to 37.5°C (99.5°F) or to use TTM of 36°C (96.8°F) to 37.5°C (99.5°F) for pediatric patients who remain comatose after resuscitation.

Introduction

The 2019 focused update to the American Heart Association (AHA) pediatric advanced life support (PALS) guidelines for cardiopulmonary resuscitation (CPR) and emergency cardiovascular care (ECC) is based on three systematic reviews and the resulting "2019 International Consensus on Cardiopulmonary Resuscitation and Emergency Cardiovascular Care Science with Treatment Recommendations" (CoSTR) from the International Liaison Committee on Resuscitation (ILCOR) Pediatric Life Support Task Force. AHA guidelines for CPR and ECC are developed in concert with ILCOR's systematic review process.

The update provides recommendations for advanced airway management in pediatric cardiac arrest, extracorporeal cardiopulmonary resuscitation (ECPR) in pediatric cardiac arrest, and pediatric targeted temperature management (TTM) during postcardiac arrest care.

Airway Intervention in Pediatric Cardiac Arrest

Most pediatric cardiac arrests are triggered by respiratory deterioration. Thus, airway management and ventilation are the core components of PALS. Bag-valve-mask ventilation (BVM), endotracheal intubation, and supraglottic airway (SGA) placement are the primary airway interventions, each with its own risks and benefits. The 2019 ILCOR Pediatric Life Support Task Force and the AHA pediatric writing group reviewed 14 studies of advanced airway interventions in pediatric patients with cardiac arrest. The review included evidence for the use of an advanced airway (ie, endotracheal intubation or SGA) versus BVM only. When comparing each intervention against one another, there were no significant differences between groups in favorable neurologic outcomes or survival to hospital discharge. There is insufficient evidence to make a recommendation for BVM compared to an advanced airway for in-hospital cardiac arrests (IHCA). Additionally, no recommendation can be made for endotracheal intubation compared to SGA.

The updated 2019 recommendation is: BVM is reasonable compared to advanced airway interventions in the management of children during cardiac arrest in the out-of-hospital setting. This recommendation is classified under the American College of Cardiology and the AHA Clinical Practice Guideline Recommendation Classification System (Class) as class IIa (ie, reasonable), with a level of evidence rating of C-LD (ie, limited data). The use of advanced airways in pediatric cardiac arrest was last reviewed in 2010, and there were no significant changes to the recommendations with this most recent review. During out-of-hospital cardiac arrest (OHCA), transport time, provider skill level and experience, and equipment availability should be considered. If BVM is ineffective despite appropriate optimization, more advanced airway interventions should be considered.

ECPR for IHCA

The use of extracorporeal membrane oxygenation (ECMO) as a form of mechanical circulatory rescue for failed conventional CPR (ie, ECPR) has gained increasing popularity. ECPR is defined as the rapid deployment of ECMO during active CPR or for patients with intermittent return of spontaneous circulation (ROSC). ECPR is a resource-intense, complex multidisciplinary therapy that should be used for specialized patient populations within dedicated and highly practiced environments. The ILCOR Pediatric Life Support Task Force and the AHA pediatric writing group reviewed three studies on the use of ECPR in pediatric cardiac arrest. Two retrospective studies of pediatric IHCA, after cardiac surgery, found that the use of ECPR was associated with favorable neurologic outcomes and an increased rate of survival to hospital discharge. The third retrospective study of congenital heart disease patients with IHCA during cardiac catheterization found that the use of ECPR was associated with worse survival to hospital discharge compared to conventional CPR.

The updated 2019 recommendation is: ECPR may be considered for pediatric patients with cardiac diagnoses who have IHCA in settings with existing ECMO protocols, expertise, and equipment (Class IIb with a level of evidence of C-LD). In comparison to the 2015 AHA PALS guidelines, there were no significant changes to the recommendations within the 2019 update. Given the ethical and logistical considerations, there have been no prospective comparative analyses between CPR and ECPR. There is insufficient evidence to recommend for or against the use of ECPR for pediatric patients experiencing OHCA or for pediatric patients with noncardiac disease experiencing IHCA refractory to conventional CPR.

Postcardiac Arrest TTM

TTM refers to continuous maintenance of patient temperature within a narrowly prescribed range. Therapeutic hypothermia treats reperfusion syndrome after cardiac arrest by decreasing metabolic demand, reducing free radical production, and decreasing apoptosis. The 2019 ILCOR pediatric CoSTR summarized the evidence supporting the use of TTM (32°C [89.6°F] - 34°C [93.2°F]) after pediatric IHCA or OHCA. This pediatric review was triggered by the publication of the THAPCA-IH trial (Therapeutic Hypothermia After Pediatric Cardiac Arrest In-Hospital), a prospective randomized control trial of TTM 32°C (89.6°F) to 34°C (93.2°F)

versus TTM 36°C (96.8°F) to 37.5°C (99.5°F) for IHCA. The trial was halted for futility because the primary outcome (favorable neurobehavioral outcome at 1 year) did not differ significantly between groups (36% and 39%, respectively).

The updated 2019 recommendations are: Continuous measurement of core temperature during TTM is recommended (Class I with a level of evidence of B-NR [signifying data derived from one or more nonrandomized trials or a meta-analysis]). For infants and children who remain comatose after ROSC, it is reasonable to use either TTM 32°C (89.6°F) to 34°C (93.2°F) followed by TTM 36°C (96.8°F) to 37.5°C (99.5°F) or to use TTM 36°C (96.8°F) to 37.5°C (99.5°F) (Class IIa with a level of evidence of B-NR). Since the publication of the 2015 PALS guidelines, the second THAPCA trial and several observational studies of TTM on comatose children after cardiac arrest were published. The ILCOR Pediatric Life Support Task Force and the AHA writing group placed a higher value on pediatric data because the adult studies include patients with arrest causes, disease states, and outcomes that differ from infants and children. Regardless of strategy, providers should strive to prevent fever greater than 37.5°C (99.5°F).

Critical Decisions in Emergency Medicine's series of LLSA reviews features articles from ABEM's 2022 Lifelong Learning and Self-Assessment Reading List. Available online at acep.org/moc/llsa and on the ABEM website.

Disclosure

We are military service members. This work was prepared as part of our official duties. Title 17 USC §105 (2019) provides that "copyright protection under this title is not available for any work of the United States government." Title 17 USC §101 (2010) defines a United States government work as a work prepared by a military service member or employee of the United States government as part of that person's official duties.

The views expressed in this review article are those of the authors and do not necessarily reflect the official policy or position of the Department of the Navy, Department of Defense, or the United States government.

Lisfranc Amputation After Crush Injury

By Parker Young, DO
University of Florida College of Medicine, Jacksonville

Reviewed by John Kiel DO, MPH

Objective

On completion of this article, you should be able to:

■ Identify the complexity of a Lisfranc injury and manage it accordingly.

CASE PRESENTATION

A 44-year-old man presents with a work-related foot injury. The patient had his left foot crushed between two pallet jacks while at his warehouse job just prior to arrival. His examination is notable for a markedly swollen left foot with multiple lacerations to the dorsal and plantar surfaces. Dorsalis pedis and posterior tibial pulses are normal. Capillary refill is intact. No further trauma is identified on primary or secondary surveys. X-rays reveal open first and second displaced metatarsal fractures, third and fourth metatarsal base fractures, and fracture dislocations of all five digits. The patient is started on antibiotics, and podiatry is emergently consulted. Podiatry attempts a closed reduction at the bedside without satisfactory results, and the patient is admitted to the trauma service with a plan for urgent surgical fixation.

Discussion

The Lisfranc joint is composed proximally of three cuneiform bones and a cuboid bone linked distally with the five metatarsal bases.[1] Injuries to the Lisfranc, or tarsometatarsal, joint comprise 0.1% to 0.4% of all fractures or dislocations.[2] The joint is composed of a complex of bones and ligaments that help form the arch of the midfoot and allows supination and pronation of the forefoot.

Injuries can present a particular challenge for both diagnosis and management. Even small injuries can cause serious disability and are often missed on initial presentation. It is recommended that patients are referred to a specialist even in mild cases; surgical fixation is often required due to the high rate of atrophy and subsequent degenerative arthritis.[3-4] Only cases of ligament sprains or partial tears without static or dynamic instability are recommended for a trial of nonoperative treatment. Unstable or displaced injuries benefit from operative intervention.[5]

Initial imaging is usually plain non–weight-bearing x-rays (*Figures 1* and *2*). This imaging modality, however, is only 84.4% sensitive in revealing injury due to the complexity of the joint.[6] In subtle cases, bilateral weight-bearing films can be considered to compare the injury to the unaffected limb. If the patient has pain with weight-bearing, or concern for greater injury, CT is shown to reveal 60% more metatarsal fractures and twice as many tarsal fractures and

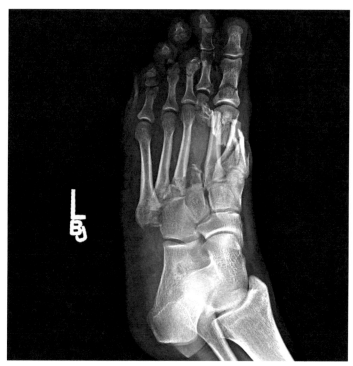

FIGURE 1. Foot x-ray (oblique), mid- and forefoot fracture dislocation

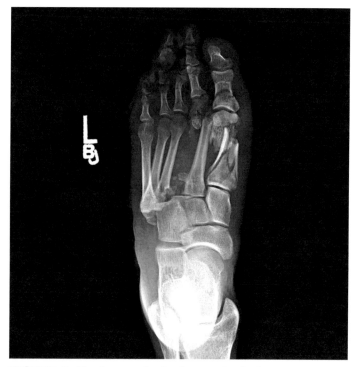

FIGURE 2. Foot x-ray (anterior-posterior), mid- and forefoot fracture dislocation

joint malalignments.[7] If x-rays and CT are inconclusive, MRI remains the gold standard specifically for ligamentous abnormalities.

Injuries are typically classified as direct and indirect trauma.[1] Indirect trauma is typically low energy and described as an axial loading placed on a plantar-flexed foot that undergoes rotation or compression. This type of injury is typically seen in athletes from football players to dancers and includes most injuries to the joint. Direct trauma is typically the result of a high-energy event such as a motor vehicle collision.[4] A crush injury, as in this case, can cause catastrophic fracture and dislocation patterns. There is often significant soft tissue swelling, which may cause compartment syndrome, and subsequent vascular and nerve complications.[4] In this case, the patient initially had intact capillary refill to all toes and an intact dorsalis pedis flow by doppler. CT angiography performed shortly after the surgery demonstrated adequate flow in the proximal dorsalis pedis artery. However, the course was complicated by swelling and ischemia to the distal foot resulting in amputation.

Lisfranc injuries, although uncommon, are a serious injury with high risk for disability. Close attention should be given to patients that present with midfoot pain, and physicians should have a low threshold for referral to a specialist.

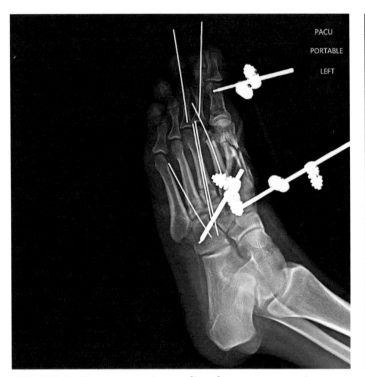

FIGURE 3. Foot x-ray, immediately post operation with external fixation

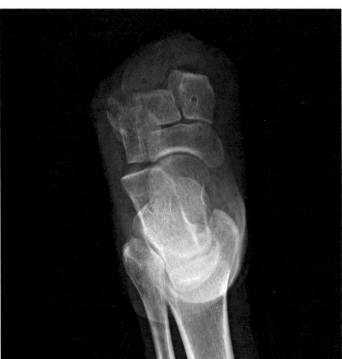

FIGURE 4. Foot x-ray, interval amputation at the Lisfranc joint

CASE RESOLUTION

The patient underwent initial external fixation of his open fracture dislocation (*Figure 3*). He had a prolonged course complicated by ischemia and necrosis of his distal foot due to compromised blood flow, which was not felt to be compartment syndrome but rather vascular compromise. The patient was seen regularly at the podiatry clinic, where wound care was performed; necrosis was found to be worsening. Roughly 5 weeks after the initial external fixation was performed, the patient underwent a left midfoot amputation (*Figure 4*). By 11 weeks post amputation, the patient was working with physical therapy and ambulating with assistance of a controlled-ankle-motion boot and crutch. The patient was also fitted with a shoe-filler device and was working on independent ambulation.

REFERENCES
1. Grewal US, Onubogu K, Southgate C, Dhinsa BS. Lisfranc injury: a review and simplified treatment algorithm. *Foot (Edinb)*. 2020;45:101719.
2. Court-Brown CM, Caesar B. Epidemiology of adult fractures: a review. *Injury*. 2006;37(8):691-697.
3. Komenda GA, Myerson MS, Biddinger KR. Results of arthrodesis of the tarsometatarsal joints after traumatic injury. *J Bone Joint Surg Am*. 1996;78(11):1665-1676.
4. Goossens M, De Stoop N. Lisfranc's fracture-dislocations: etiology, radiology, and results of treatment. A review of 20 cases. *Clin Orthop Relat Res*. 1983;176:154-162.
5. Sethi MK, Jahangir AA, Obremskey WT, eds. *Orthopedic Traumatology: An Evidence-Based Approach*. Springer; 2013.
6. Rankine JJ, Nicholas CM, Wells G, Barron DA. The diagnostic accuracy of radiographs in Lisfranc injury and the potential value of a craniocaudal projection. *AJR Am J Roentgenol*. 2012;198(4):W365-W369.
7. Sripanich Y, Weinberg MW, Krähenbühl N, et al. Imaging in Lisfranc injury: a systematic literature review. *Skeltal Radiol*. 2020;49(1):31-53.

Crying Infant

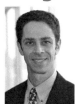

By Joshua S. Broder, MD, FACEP
Dr. Broder is a professor and the residency program director in the Department of Emergency Medicine at Duke University Medical Center in Durham, North Carolina.

Objectives

On completion of this article, you should be able to:

- Identify healing rib fractures on frontal projection and oblique chest x-rays.
- Describe the clinical importance of femur and rib fractures as indicators of nonaccidental trauma.

CASE PRESENTATION

A 3-week-old girl presents with crying. The parents report that the patient had been fussy and they moved her into their bed in an attempt to comfort her. Now, they worry they might have rolled onto the patient, causing injury while they slept.

Her vital signs are BP 114/51, P 173, R 16, and T 36.8°C (98.2°F); SpO_2 is 100% on room air. She weighs 3.4 kg (7 lb 7.9 oz). The patient is sleeping and appears to be in no distress. The examination is normal, with the exception of the left lower extremity. A clicking sensation is palpable with movement of the leg, and the infant cries with this manipulation. Pulses are normal, and there is no visible bruising on thorough examination. Femur x-rays and a skeletal survey are performed (*Figures 1, 2*, and *3*).

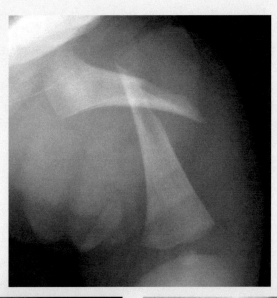

FIGURE 1. A mid-shaft, displaced, and angulated femur fracture. Femur fractures in patients younger than 12 months are rare and should be recognized as a high-risk finding for nonaccidental trauma.

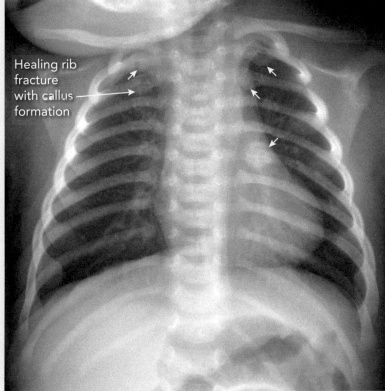

Healing rib fracture with callus formation

FIGURE 2. Frontal chest x-ray

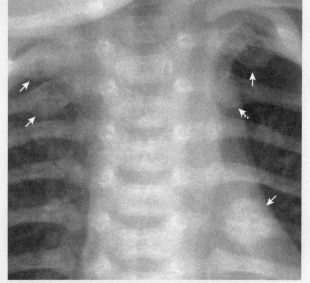

FIGURE 3. Magnified view from *Figure 2*. Chest x-ray with multiple healing posterior rib fractures, marked by callus formation. Any rib fracture in a patient younger than 12 months should raise suspicion for nonaccidental trauma. Posterior location, multiple injuries, and delayed presentation marked by healing should heighten concern.

Nonaccidental trauma (NAT) causing fractures in patients younger than 3 years may be under-recognized. In a single-center study, only 1% of patients with long bone fractures in this age group were referred for further evaluation of potential abuse, despite multiple risk factors for NAT identified on chart review.[1]

Fractures in infants younger than 12 months should particularly arouse suspicion for NAT. In this age group, 39% of fractures were attributed to abuse, compared to 8% of all fractures in children 24 to 36 months old.[2] Femur fractures in children younger than 12 months are rare and are a high-risk injury predictive of NAT.[2] Rib fractures are another high-risk indicator, with 82% of rib fractures in infants younger than 12 months resulting from NAT.[3] In children younger than 3 years, rib fracture had a positive predictive value of 95% for NAT and were the sole skeletal injury in 29%.[4] Posterior rib fractures are more common in NAT patients than in patients without NAT (43% of rib fractures versus 6% in one study).[4]

Diagnostic imaging should focus first on areas of suspected injury and those clinically relevant to the immediate care of the patient (eg, abdominal CT for patients with suspected abdominal injury or head CT for those with abnormal neurologic examinations). Once the patient has been clinically stabilized, skeletal survey x-rays are indicated to detect occult injuries in infants younger than 24 months with suspicion of NAT.[5] Oblique chest x-rays, in addition to standard frontal and lateral views, increase the sensitivity and specificity for rib fractures because they project a view of ribs without overlying heart and rib curvature (*Figures 4* and *5*).[6] Bone callus formation is a delayed x-ray finding, with estimates between 4 and 14 days after injury;[7] it is not possible to exactly determine the age of a fracture by x-ray.[5] Consequently, callus formation visible on x-ray provides additional evidence of multiple episodes of injury over time or injuries not fitting the clinical history (see *Figures 2–5*).

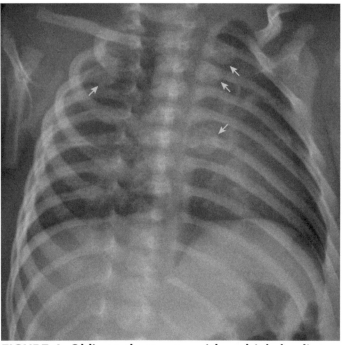

FIGURE 4. **Oblique chest x-ray with multiple healing posterior rib fractures**

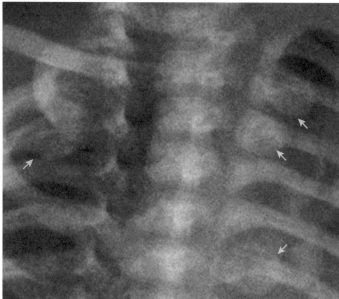

FIGURE 5. **Magnified view from *Figure 4*.** When obtained in addition to standard frontal and lateral views, oblique views may improve sensitivity and specificity for rib fracture.

CASE RESOLUTION

The patient was admitted for further evaluation of suspected NAT.

Feature Editor: Joshua S. Broder, MD, FACEP. See also *Diagnostic Imaging for the Emergency Physician* (Winner of the 2011 Prose Award in Clinical Medicine, the American Publishers Award for Professional and Scholarly Excellence) and *Critical Images in Emergency Medicine* by Dr. Broder.

REFERENCES

1. Taitz J, Moran K, O'Meara M. Long bone fractures in children under 3 years of age: is abuse being missed in emergency department presentations? *J Paediatr Child Health.* 2004;40(4):170-174.
2. Leventhal JM, Thomas SA, Rosenfield NS, Markowitz RI. Fractures in young children. Distinguishing child abuse from unintentional injuries. *Am J Dis Child.* 1993;147(1):87-92.
3. Bulloch B, Schubert CJ, Brophy PD, Johnson N, Reed MH, Shapiro RA. Cause and clinical characteristics of rib fractures in infants. *Pediatrics.* 2000;105(4):E48.
4. Barsness KA, Cha ES, Bensard DD, et al. The positive predictive value of rib fractures as an indicator of nonaccidental trauma in children. *J Trauma.* 2003;54(6):1107-1110.
5. Expert Panel on Pediatric Imaging; Wootton-Gorges SL, Soares BP, Alazraki AL, et al. ACR Appropriateness Criteria® suspected physical abuse-child. *J Am Coll Radiol.* 2017;14(suppl 5):S338-S349.
6. Ingram JD, Connell J, Hay TC, Mackenzie T. Oblique radiographs of the chest in nonaccidental trauma. *Emerg Radiol.* 2000;7:42-46.
7. McKinley DW, Chambliss ML. Follow-up radiographs to detect callus formation after fractures. *Arch Fam Med.* 2000;9:373-374.

The Critical Procedure

Clogged Feeding Tube Management

By Steven J. Warrington, MD, MEd, MS
MercyOne Siouxland, Sioux City, Iowa

Objective

On completion of this article, you should be able to:

■ Demonstrate how to use a Fogarty catheter to unclog a feeding tube.

Introduction

Patients may present with a variety of feeding tube issues, ranging from displacement to clogs. While replacement with a new feeding tube may be ideal, it is not always possible, such as in the case of a newly placed feeding tube. When nothing is passing and there is concern for an obstruction, attempting to unclog the tube may solve the issue.

Contraindications

■ None

Benefits and Risks

The primary benefit of attempting to clear a feeding tube is to allow the existing tube to remain in place. Depending on the instrument used, a theoretical risk of perforation of the feeding tube and bowel or stomach exists if it is advanced past the portion of tube able to be visualized. There is also a risk of damaging the tube, which can cause immediate or delayed failure. Otherwise, there are no significant risks aside from the potential for displacement or failure to resolve the situation.

Alternatives

There are multiple methods for unclogging a feeding tube. The one described below uses a Fogarty catheter; however, there are some commercially available devices. Additionally, the literature suggests other methods, such as using carbonated beverages, milking the tube, or using increased pressure.

Aside from unclogging the feeding tube, a replacement tube is the primary alternative. Replacing the tube may be done in the emergency department but is dependent on how newly placed the site is, the type and location of the feeding tube, and the availability of supplies (ie, tubes).

Reducing Side Effects

If a hard or rigid instrument is used to attempt unclogging, maintaining visualization throughout the entire process theoretically reduces the risk associated with puncture and perforation. Measuring and marking distances on the instrument being used to unblock the tube (eg, a Fogarty catheter) also reduces risks associated with mucosal injury or perforation by ensuring the instrument does not extend beyond the feeding tube.

Special Considerations

Because unclogging could increase pressure on the feeding tube and cause a perforation, leak, or tube aneurysm, it is beneficial to assess tube integrity after the procedure using contrast and plain x-rays. This is similar to the method used to assess for placement, except with a focus on maintaining contrast within the feeding tube.

TECHNIQUE

1. **Obtain** consent of the patient, gather materials, and bring them to the bedside. A No. 4 catheter for 10Fr or 12Fr tubes and a No. 5 catheter for 14Fr tubes are recommended.
2. **Identify** the length of the indwelling feeding tube.
3. **Measure** and mark the Fogarty catheter, so it is not extended beyond the expected tip of the feeding tube.
4. **Insert** the tip of the Fogarty catheter and advance to the end of the measured distance (ie, expected end of feeding tube). In the event some resistance is met, inflate and then deflate the balloon and attempt to advance it farther. Repeat as necessary to reach the distal end of the feeding tube.
5. **Inflate** and then deflate the balloon once the end of the feeding tube is reached.
6. **Withdraw** the catheter while intermittently stopping to inflate and deflate the balloon. Be aware that attempting to withdraw the catheter with the balloon inflated can cause movement of the feeding tube itself rather than the intended clearing of the obstruction.

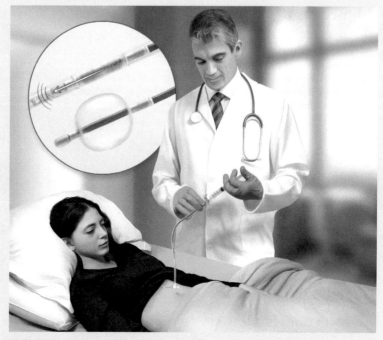

FIGURE 1.
Clearance of obstruction using a Fogarty catheter

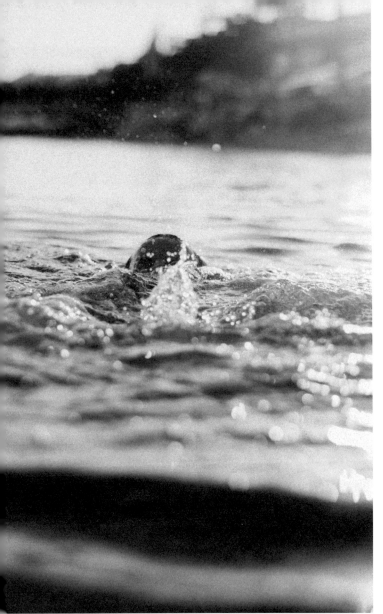

Going Under

Drowning and Submersion Injury

LESSON 16

By Savannah Chavez, MD; and Bethany Johnston, MD
Dr. Chavez is chief resident and Dr. Johnston is an associate EMS medical director and associate director of the Virtual Care Simulation Lab at Summa Health Emergency Medicine in Akron, Ohio.
Reviewed by Nathaniel Mann, MD

Objectives

On completion of this lesson, you should be able to:

1. Define drowning and emphasize the importance of standardized terminology.
2. Recognize drowning as a pathophysiologic process characterized by an initial pulmonary insult followed by delayed clinical deterioration, rather than as an event.
3. Identify the most critical elements of the patient history for treatment and prognosis.
4. Assess and stabilize a drowning victim and triage for admission or observation.
5. Diagnose and treat concomitant conditions associated with submersion injuries.

From the EM Model

6.0 Environmental Disorders
   6.5 Submersion Incidents

CRITICAL DECISIONS

- How is drowning defined?

- What is the pathophysiology of drowning?

- What important prehospital information should be obtained?

- How should drowning patients be assessed and managed?

- What tests are predictors of outcome?

- How long should asymptomatic patients be observed, and which patients are safe to discharge?

Summertime is the time to break out the floaties, sunscreen, and lounge rafts, but with fun in the sun comes the risk of serious tragedies from drowning events. Thus, emergency physicians must understand the appropriate definitions, management, and disposition of drowning patients.

CASE PRESENTATIONS

■ CASE 1

A 10-year-old boy arrives via EMS after he was found at the bottom of his cousin's in-ground swimming pool. Family pulled him from the water, attempted rescue breaths, and started chest compressions. EMS placed a supraglottic airway device and performed bag-valve-mask ventilation, with ROSC just before arrival. The patient's father states that the patient was seen diving headfirst into the shallow end of the pool. He was last seen outside of the pool about 12 minutes before EMS was called.

■ CASE 2

A 39-year-old woman is brought in by her friends after "drifting off" in the jacuzzi while drinking. She slipped beneath the surface of the water and was underneath only briefly before her friends pulled her out. She occasionally coughs, and she is still intoxicated. Otherwise, she is acting as expected, according to her friends. She has no past medical history, but she occasionally smokes cigarettes.

Introduction

Drowning is one of the most preventable causes of morbidity and mortality in adults and children, yet it is a routine cause of death globally. Classic risk factors for drowning include age younger than 4 years or adolescence, non-Caucasian, drug and alcohol use, and male sex, the latter accounting for 80% of deaths by drowning. Many pediatric drowning deaths occur in the presence of at least one adult and can occur with even momentary lapses in supervision.[1]

Despite ongoing public health initiatives to prevent these incidents, there are about 8,000 emergency department visits annually for drownings, approximately 3,900 of which are ultimately fatal. Many statistics exclude traumatic or disaster-related drownings.[2] There are innumerable circumstances in which drowning can occur; however, emergency physicians typically see community incidents from freshwater bodies, swimming pools, bathtubs, or buckets.[2] Most of these drownings are pediatric or young adult patients, but all age groups are susceptible. Other unique scenarios may include scuba diving incidents with concomitant barotrauma, drownings complicated by marine envenomation, swimming-induced pulmonary edema, commercial boating or fishing accidents, and motor vehicle collisions that result in drowning.

CRITICAL DECISION

How is drowning defined?

Historically, terminology to classify "types" of drowning has included water salinity, mechanism, and a multitude of other features that were thought to be important distinctions for clinical management. For example, there were once concerns that the tonicity of aspirated water significantly altered serum electrolytes and would continue to do so throughout hospitalization.[3] Much of the data supporting these ideas were based on artificially drowned animals. Understanding of the effects of drowning has improved over time: It is now accepted that hypoxemia and its sequelae are the main factors for drowning morbidity and mortality, and the adjectives used to characterize these events do not alter this final pathway.

Additional terminology appearing in the literature includes phrases such as "dry drowning," "wet drowning," "secondary drowning," or "near-drowning," among others. As of 2002, Utstein-Style guidelines and expert consensus defined drowning or submersion injury as "a process resulting in primary respiratory impairment from submersion/immersion in a liquid medium," with or without morbidity, mortality, or even aspiration.[4] The guidelines elaborate: "implicit in this definition is that a liquid/air interface is present at the entrance of the victim's airway, preventing the victim from breathing air. The victim may live or die after this process, but whatever the outcome, he or she has been involved in a drowning incident." This definition covers a multitude of scenarios and a spectrum of clinical presentations, each of which has the potential for alveolar disruption, acute lung injury (ALI), and hypoxemia. It is critical to standardize the language for present inter-physician communication and future data collection and analysis. In 2015, the Second International Utstein-Style Consensus Conference on Drowning developed updated guidelines for collecting and reporting data. A series of reporting tables are available to guide investigators in drowning research.[5]

Limitations of data interpretation due to poorly standardized terminology, the retrospective and observational nature of most data, and heavy use of animal models to extrapolate human drowning physiology make providing evidence-based guidelines for drowning management difficult. Additionally, most drowning data comes from pediatric populations, which raises potential issues with treatment algorithms for adults. Therefore, adjunct treatments for associated conditions largely fall to existing guidelines for those conditions as if they occurred in isolation.

CRITICAL DECISION

What is the pathophysiology of drowning?

Complex pathophysiologic mechanisms contribute both to the drowning event itself as well as downstream complications such as ALI or cardiac arrest (*Figure 1*). Reflexes that occur during drowning are responses both to immersion of the body itself and submersion of the airway beneath an air-liquid interface. Ultimately, involuntary laryngospasm and voluntary breath-holding are overcome either by unconsciousness or the hypercapnic drive to ventilate. Additionally, in cases of rapid exposure to cold water, two seemingly conflicting reflexes can occur: the cold shock reflex and mammalian dive reflex (*Figure 2*).

The *cold shock reflex* results from a rapid drop in skin temperature. Receptors within the skin induce gasping, hyperventilation, and increased sympathetic outflow and cardiac output, and, therefore, oxygen demand.[6] This is a two-fold problem in drowning because victims can no longer voluntarily protect their airway and can aspirate when they are already at an oxygen deficit. This reflex occurs at approximately 25°C (77°F), and its intensity is inversely proportional to the temperature.

Alternatively, the *mammalian dive reflex* results from afferent trigeminal nerve receptors in the nares reacting to rapid immersion in cold water. Three autonomic responses result: apnea, bradycardia, and increased peripheral vascular resistance. This reflex should theoretically offer some protection by decreasing the risk of aspiration, decreasing cardiac oxygen demand, and increasing oxygen delivery to the brain and other vital organs by shunting blood away from the peripheral circulation and large muscle groups. It is thought to contribute to cases of survival after prolonged submersion times. However, the cold shock and dive reflexes seemingly have conflicting effects on heart rate, and there is ongoing discussion about whether this conflict contributes to cardiac dysrhythmia in drowning.[7]

Lastly, the role of laryngospasm in response to the first few milliliters of liquid aspirated can theoretically provide either a protective or harmful effect in drowning. While it may briefly prevent some fluid from entering the lungs, there is potential for mechanical or shearing damage to sensitive alveolar tissues when inhaling against a closed glottis. It is impossible to definitively identify the cases in which this type of damage is incurred and difficult to assess the extent to which this type of injury contributes to ALI compared to aspiration.

Most drowning cases likely result in the aspiration of at least some liquid. Both saltwater and freshwater aspiration can disturb normal lung surfactant, which contributes to the development of ALI. The actual volume required to trigger acute respiratory distress syndrome (ARDS) has been extensively studied but remains inconclusive. However, it is generally believed that amounts as small as 1 to 3 mL/kg are enough to disrupt lung surfactant.[6] Compromised surfactant results in alveolar collapse, shearing injury, and alterations in membrane permeability, triggering the release of pro-inflammatory cytokines. Cytokines recruit neutrophils into lung tissue, where they release cytotoxic mediators

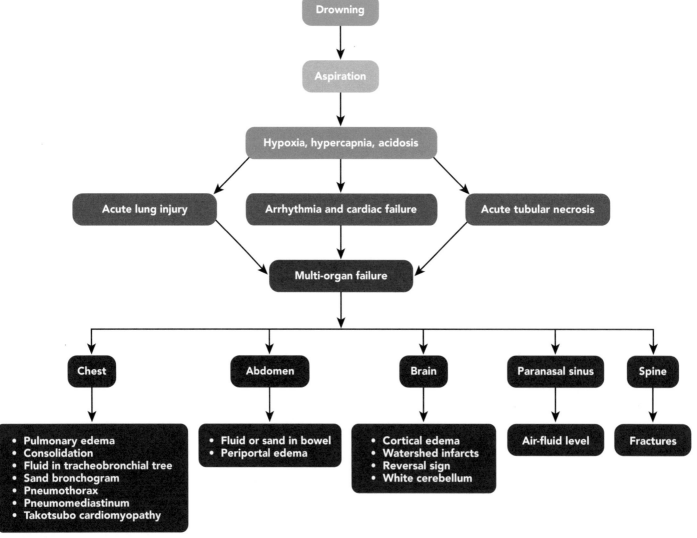

FIGURE 1. Pathophysiology and imaging findings of drowning. Adapted from Restrepo CS, Ortiz C, Singh AK, Sannananja B. Near-drowning: epidemiology, pathophysiology and imaging findings. *J Trauma Care.* 2017;3(3)1026.

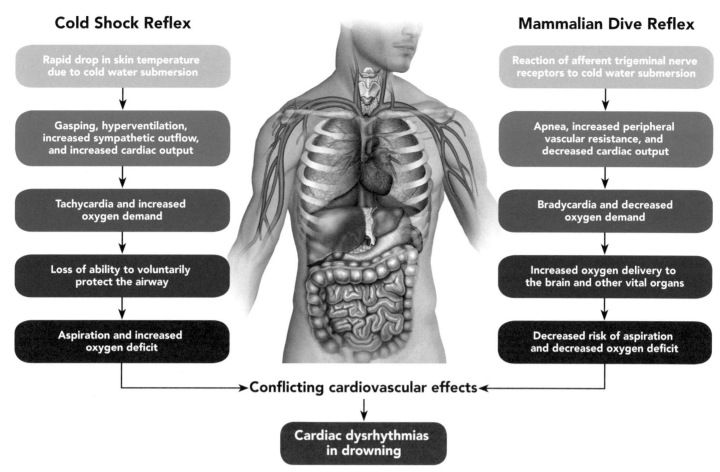

Cold Shock Reflex

Rapid drop in skin temperature due to cold water submersion

↓

Gasping, hyperventilation, increased sympathetic outflow, and increased cardiac output

↓

Tachycardia and increased oxygen demand

↓

Loss of ability to voluntarily protect the airway

↓

Aspiration and increased oxygen deficit

Mammalian Dive Reflex

Reaction of afferent trigeminal nerve receptors to cold water submersion

↓

Apnea, increased peripheral vascular resistance, and decreased cardiac output

↓

Bradycardia and decreased oxygen demand

↓

Increased oxygen delivery to the brain and other vital organs

↓

Decreased risk of aspiration and decreased oxygen deficit

→ Conflicting cardiovascular effects ←

↓

Cardiac dysrhythmias in drowning

FIGURE 2. Comparison of the cold shock reflex and mammalian dive reflex.
Credit: ACEP and ilusmedical/Shutterstock.com.

that further damage sensitive alveolar tissue; this self-perpetuating inflammatory cascade leads to ARDS and severe hypoxemia.

Ultimately, systemic hypoxia is the driving force behind morbidity and mortality in drowning. Severe hypoxemia drives cardiac dysrhythmias and arrest, neurologic injury, multisystem organ failure, and shock in drowning patients. Clinically significant intravascular shifts depending on the tonicity of aspirated fluid have largely been debunked.[8] Hypotension is more likely related to hypoxic or acidemic cardiovascular dysfunction, rather than hypovolemia.[9]

CRITICAL DECISION

What important prehospital information should be obtained?

The full history of the environment, preceding and surrounding events, and on-scene resuscitation dictate priorities in management beyond the initial airway and breathing assessments.

Submersion Time and On-scene Bystander or EMS CPR

The duration of submersion has the most robust evidence supporting its use as a predictor of outcomes, including survival and neurologic recovery.[10] Due to the compensatory mechanisms discussed, it is difficult to differentiate actual anoxic time from submersion time. However, mortality quickly increases beyond 5 minutes of total submersion, with near 100% mortality at submersion greater than 25 minutes.

Morbidity between 5 and 25 minutes of submersion is most often related to neurologic injury. Neurologically, isolated hypoxic events without ischemia are understood to be more survivable due to continued delivery of other nutrients compared to those that occur with cardiac arrest. As a result, if the submersion time is short and cardiopulmonary resuscitation rapidly follows, there is still a chance for some neurologic recovery. Submersion time reported by bystanders is often, at best, an estimate and, at worst, inaccurate. Still, this information can be useful for prognosis. Time from first possible submersion to first resuscitation attempt should be obtained if possible.

Location, Type, or Temperature of Water

Distinctions between fresh water and salt water are no longer clinically relevant to the management of most drownings. Both water types can cause surfactant washout, disrupt alveolar integrity, and lead to noncardiogenic pulmonary edema, or ARDS.[11] However, it is still important to note the body of water where the drowning occurred to maintain suspicion for downstream infectious complications. While all water should be presumed to be contaminated, water containing sewage or foreign bodies such as sand or feces can raise the likelihood of later infection, including pneumonia, pulmonary or extrapulmonary abscess formation, or even bacteremia.[12] By the same token, some bacteria are specific to water types, such as *Legionella* in fresh water. Although there is a high likelihood of polymicrobial infection, the type of water can promote the correct empiric coverage if infection develops. However, in awake patients who can be discharged, there is currently no evidence to promote prophylactic antibiotics. In patients who require intubation, monitoring for nosocomial pneumonia and subsequent treatment should be pursued, as in any other intubated patient.

The temperature of the water and surrounding environment should inform physicians about possible concomitant thermal injuries that resulted in or from the drowning or the possibility of survival despite a prolonged submersion time. There have been case reports suggesting that rapid-onset hypothermia resulting from icy water drowning can modulate the effect of submersion duration, resulting in better outcomes with longer submersion times.[13-16] Some drowning victims have survived more than 60 minutes in extremely cold water, demonstrating the neuroprotective effect cold exposure can have. In one famous case, Dr. Anna Bågenholm, who found an air pocket that enabled her to breathe, survived with neurologic recovery after a reported 80 minutes of submersion in freezing water and a core temperature of 13.7°C (56.6°F). Such reports have lent support to the adage, "no one is dead until warm and dead." Generally, water must be 6°C (42.8°F) or colder to rapidly cool the body and offer the neuroprotective effect against hypoxia. The observed neuroprotective features of hypothermia may be attributable to hypothermia itself and its dampening effects on cellular metabolism and oxygen demand or due to the mammalian dive reflex.

While this specific circumstance is rarer in the United States and does not guarantee survival, it is a useful consideration for physicians providing online medical control to any prehospital personnel who may be evaluating a prolonged submersion. Additionally, these temperatures are more extreme than those used in targeted temperature management (TTM) and occur *prior* to rescue and in parallel with the drowning event as opposed to being initiated after rescue. Currently, there is insufficient evidence to support the use of extreme hypothermia or even traditional TTM after rescue in unconscious drowning patients who did not suffer cardiac arrest. There may still be a role for TTM in drowning patients who require CPR as a part of routine post–cardiac arrest care.

Circumstances Leading to Drowning

Understanding the events preceding drowning may provide information regarding possible trauma, abuse, or other medical emergencies that may have led to drowning. This information is particularly important in pediatric populations, such as infant and toddler drownings. While it is important to maintain suspicion for possible child abuse, drowning can occur quickly, quietly, and with very brief lapses in adult supervision.

Patient State Prior to Submersion

In teenage and adult patients, drugs and alcohol are large contributors to drowning events and may alter their circulatory response both during and after resuscitation. While the context may be known, it is also important to consider suicidality or intentional overdoses in unwitnessed or nonrecreational drowning events.

Known Comorbidities and Medications

A complete past medical history, as available, is useful in determining possible medical causes of drowning (eg, acute coronary syndromes, dysrhythmias, seizures) as well as the potential for recovery or decompensation.

Layperson Rescue Attempts

Most bystanders are not specifically trained in water rescue. Whether the initial victim is an adult or child, there are numerous reports of secondary victims who drown while attempting rescue.[17] A systemic, delayed response can occur even in seemingly minimal cases of aspiration, such as that of rescuers. While evaluating drowning patients, consideration should be given to any potential bystanders who attempted water rescue in case they also incurred a submersion injury. Even when apparently stable, these individuals may benefit from formal evaluation and emergency department observation. If accompanying drowning patients to the hospital, this information can be crucial if the rescuers decompensate in the emergency department as visitors. This circumstance is also an important consideration for prehospital clinicians, who should consider counseling rescuers to undergo an evaluation.

CRITICAL DECISION

How should drowning patients be assessed and managed?

Airway and Breathing

There are several considerations to maintain while caring for drowning patients, but as with all medical resuscitations, assessment begins with airway and breathing. Because hypoxemia is the driving pathologic mechanism in these patients, optimizing oxygenation and ventilation is paramount. Assessment of the airway begins with evaluating the rate, depth, and quality of respirations as well as any supplemental oxygen needs.

Asymptomatic Patients

For all drowning patients, with or without symptoms or respiratory distress, supplemental oxygen should be provided when SpO_2 is less than 94%. Because of the alveolar damage caused by aspiration, even initially asymptomatic drowning victims may progress to ARDS (*Figure 3*). Repeat pulmonary assessment and SpO_2 monitoring should be routine for all patients.

Symptomatic Patients

A spectrum of symptoms can result from drowning and may be as mild as an isolated cough or as severe as cardiac arrest. In awake patients, important physical examination findings have been associated with increasing mortality. A mild cough alone has not been correlated with significant morbidity or decompensation. Abnormal lung sounds on auscultation, severe cough, frothy sputum, foamy material in the airway, and hypotension are ominous predictors of a poor outcome in drowning. Hypoxemia, increased work of breathing, or dyspnea are all indications for inpatient admission.

Establishing an airway in obtunded or coding patients is intuitive; deciding to secure the airway in awake patients who suffered an aspiration event is more nebulous. The assessment of these patients relies primarily on their clinical presentation. In patients who are in respiratory distress but able to follow commands, a trial of noninvasive positive-pressure ventilation (NIPPV) is reasonable. In cases where patients are unable to follow commands or there is persistent respiratory distress and hypoxia despite optimization on NIPPV, intubation is likely required. Vomitus may be present in drowning victims' airways from the gag reflex during aspiration, rescue breaths, or chest compressions; this scenario should be anticipated and managed accordingly during intubation.

Drowning victims who require intubation have likely progressed to severe ARDS, so ventilatory management should rely on the principles of a lung-protective strategy. An extensive discussion of ARDS ventilatory management is outside the scope of this lesson; however, the primary principles in ARDS management and a lung-protective strategy include optimization of positive end-expiratory pressure, avoiding excessive volutrauma and barotrauma (use tidal volumes 6-8 mL/kg of ideal body weight, target plateau pressures <30 mm Hg) and minimizing damage from oxygen free radicals (use minimum FiO_2 to achieve SpO_2 88%-95% or PaO_2 55-80 mm Hg) per the ARDSnet protocol (ardsnet.org). Persistent, severe hypoxemia and poor lung compliance on the ventilator despite optimal settings, or cases involving extreme refractory hypothermia, likely indicate a need for extracorporeal membrane oxygenation (ECMO).

Additional Airway Considerations

A definitive airway should be prioritized in arresting patients. Although supraglottic airways (SGAs) are generally favored in the prehospital setting, pulmonary edema, massive aspiration, and significant vomitus caused by drowning can hinder their effectiveness. In the standard resuscitation of out-of-hospital cardiac arrest patients, prehospital supraglottic airways avoid interruptions in chest compressions for definitive airway placement. Physicians often (appropriately) elect to leave the SGA in place during the duration of resuscitation for certain cases of cardiac arrest. However, alterations to lung function, including low compliance and higher resistance, necessitate higher positive pressures to achieve adequate oxygenation.[18] While patients with other causes of out-of-hospital cardiac arrest may be oxygenated or ventilated adequately with an SGA, these devices may not be effective enough to reverse drowning pathology caused by massive aspiration or pulmonary edema and could impede the return of spontaneous circulation (ROSC). While still an appropriate prehospital measure, establishing a definitive airway in drowning patients after hospital arrival or even switching to bag-valve-mask ventilation may be the most reasonable choice to counter such lung dysfunction if adequate chest rise is not visible.[19]

There is no evidence to support mechanically removing aspirated water from the lungs or trachea other than what is typical with routine airway suction. Attempts to estimate the volume of water aspirated to aid in determining the prognosis are unlikely to work because small volumes of water can cause drastic and long-standing changes in pulmonary physiology. It is likewise impossible to estimate the potential alveolar shearing injury incurred when a drowning victim inhales and exerts significant negative inspiratory pressure against a closed glottis.[20]

Circulation

There is a predictable progression of cardiac dysrhythmia from the hypoxia and acidosis that occurs in drowning. Patients typically progress from sinus tachycardia to bradycardia to pulseless electrical activity, and, ultimately, to asystole.[21] Ventricular tachycardia or fibrillation is less common in drowning or as a result of hypoxia.[22] Thus, cardiac arrest in this setting should be presumed to be from hypoxia and hypercapnia unless a preceding event raises suspicion for an arrest prior to or causing the drowning. This re-emphasizes the need for aggressive, early airway management.

Correction of hypoxia should be the mainstay of treatment, and hypotension should be managed with vasopressors or careful fluid resuscitation given the complex interplay of noncardiogenic pulmonary edema and myocardial depression from hypoxia in these patients.

The selection of fluid does not need to be made based on the type of water aspirated. In cases of severe hypothermia, patients should be rewarmed to obtain ROSC, prevent cardiac arrhythmias, or reverse hypotension. Regarding the duration of cardiac resuscitative measures, pediatric studies suggest that ROSC beyond 30 minutes after drowning and resuscitation suggests a poor outcome.[9] Access to ECMO capabilities is an evolving therapy strategy with new ventures into portable ECMO devices and field cannulation.

Disability

Significant morbidity and mortality result from global hypoxic-ischemic injury to the brain in drowning, which is the most common cause of death in patients surviving initial resuscitation efforts.[23] Managing anoxic brain injury requires maintaining adequate cerebral perfusion, euglycemia, seizure prophylaxis, electrolyte management, and TTM in cases of cardiac arrest. CT imaging of the head in obtunded or unconscious drowning patients may have significant bearing on prognosis and further treatment.

✔ Pearls

- Submersion duration and time to CPR after rescue are useful for prognosis.
- Airway and breathing are a priority in all drowning victims. Supraglottic airways may not be sufficient in cases of aspiration and should be exchanged for definitive airway early in the treatment process.
- Clinical observation and pulmonary reassessment are more useful than initial laboratory tests and imaging for determining disposition.
- Mechanical ventilation should follow lung-protective principles.

Exposure

During the initial assessment, patients should be immediately exposed for a thorough physical examination. Removal of wet clothing is crucial to begin addressing environmental hypothermia. The question of induced hypothermia in drowning victims has largely been a subject of conflicting theory, data, and clinical outcomes. The temperature observed to achieve neuroprotection in cases of prolonged submersion must have occurred rapidly and, importantly, during submersion, not after rescue. In postarrest patients, therapeutic hypothermia may be considered based on standard therapy for post–cardiac arrest care and neurologic recovery; it is not specific to drowning alone. There are no evidence-based guidelines recommending therapeutic hypothermia as an intervention for unconscious drowning patients with a pulse. Likewise, in awake patients, management of hypothermia should follow standard guidelines.

Additional Considerations

Trauma

Trauma may occur both as a cause and result of drowning. After the primary survey, patients should be assessed for traumatic injury as indicated clinically and based on history and physical examination findings. Cervical spine stabilization has largely been a reflexive recommendation in drowning victims regardless of context. Generally, there is a low incidence of cervical spine injury unless a specific history of diving, multiple traumatic injuries, or obvious evidence of head and neck injury exists.[24] Outside of a history suggesting obvious traumatic injury, reflexive C-spine precautions are likely unnecessary. For example, a toddler who presents from a suburban pool party is less likely to have trauma than an adult who fell from a raft into rocky rapids or a teenager who failed to emerge immediately after jumping head-first from a diving board. It is important to weigh the low incidence of injury against the inhibitory nature of C-spine protection when trying to establish a definitive airway, which may likely have greater benefit.[25]

Medical and Social Background

More broadly, depending on the available history, etiologies that contributed to the drowning should be considered, such as seizure, cardiac arrhythmia or ischemia, and stroke. As able, a detailed physical and neurologic examination should be performed after initial resuscitation to evaluate for additional medical conditions occurring in parallel. Depending on the clinical context and availability of information, patients may need to be worked up as altered or syncopal patients. Additionally, social considerations such as suicidal or homicidal intent should be evaluated if the circumstances raise suspicion for them, although these drownings are less common than other methods. A toxicology evaluation corroborated by available history findings is warranted in this setting and may help in determining disposition in awake patients. Patients acutely intoxicated with ethanol, benzodiazepines, or other drugs may merit longer observation due to added respiratory insult. In pediatric patients, the potential for child abuse should be considered and elucidated from the history, particularly in infants.

CRITICAL DECISION

What tests are predictors of outcome?

The routine use of laboratory tests in evaluating and determining disposition for drowning victims has no value in predicting subsequent decompensation or outcome. While there was long believed to be fluid and electrolyte shifts resulting in hemodilution and metabolic derangements, these ideas largely came from studies where animal models were intentionally drowned with volumes likely much larger than those typically aspirated in human drownings. Significant volume shifts or electrolyte derangements are less likely in real human drownings. A complete blood count and basic metabolic panel cannot guide management in the context of drowning but are better suited to identify other processes that may have contributed to the drowning event, if applicable.

Chest x-rays are part of the routine workup of any patient with breathing difficulties. Initial x-ray findings in drowning may include edema, pneumothorax, or pneumomediastinum, but most commonly, initial chest x-rays are unremarkable. There are cases, however, of patients with initially normal chest x-rays who progressed to severe disease requiring ventilatory support (*Figures 3* and *4*).[26] Thus, normal chest imaging should not be used as an anchor for a disposition without an adequate period of observation.

In the largest study evaluating CT head findings in pediatric drownings, abnormal initial head CTs on arrival were predictive of poor outcomes.[27] Conversely, most initial head CTs were normal but did not necessarily predict a favorable outcome. Many patients with normal head CTs went on to develop brain abnormalities, including cerebral edema and hypoxic sequelae either on subsequent CTs or MRI. Of note, CT imaging in drowned patients who received CPR did not demonstrate evidence of hemorrhage. In pediatric populations where abuse is a consideration, head CT may serve to distinguish or elevate this suspicion if hemorrhagic findings are noted. Additionally, mental status as measured by the Glasgow Coma Scale (GCS) in these patients was severely depressed (<4) when compared to patients presenting with nonaccidental trauma, who generally have a GCS score higher than 4. General recommendations do not promote routine head CTs as

---

✖ Pitfalls

- Failing to prioritize and reassess airway and breathing.
- Discharging patients too early based on an initial negative chest x-ray or before 6 to 8 hours of observation.
- Ignoring possible emergencies that may have contributed to the drowning incident, including traumatic, cardiac, neurologic, metabolic, or abusive events.

part of a drowning evaluation if the patient is awake. Evidence of trauma, severely depressed GCS, or any observed neurologic change should dictate CT imaging as it would in isolation.

MRI may be more useful in predicting outcomes, but its use is unlikely during an emergent resuscitation. It is more useful several days after the event.[28] Since the incidence of cervical spine injury is low in drowning victims unless there is a history of trauma or other suspicious mechanism, CT imaging of the cervical spine should not be part of routine evaluation unless clinically indicated.[25]

Arterial blood gases should be used as an adjunct to guide management of any patient with ARDS who requires NIPPV or mechanical ventilation. However, initial airway management decisions in the emergency department should be primarily driven by clinical presentation. Of note, an initial pH of less than 7.10 is associated with poorer outcomes in drowning.[29]

CRITICAL DECISION

How long should asymptomatic patients be observed, and which patients are safe to discharge?

Emergency physicians should view drowning as a process rather than a single event and expect potential decompensation regardless of initial presentation. Patients arriving asymptomatic or with minimal symptoms have been shown to decompensate up to 7 hours after immersion.[30] While classification tools and algorithms have been proposed to predict outcomes and even the level of inpatient care required, overall disposition from the emergency department is straightforward. Healthy, asymptomatic patients with a normal chest x-ray, physical examination, and vital signs are candidates for discharge after an observation period of at least 6 to 8 hours with no clinical change. Mild cough alone may be an exception, depending on clinical judgment. In a review of 1,831 drowning cases, Spzilman found 0% mortality when cough is the *only* clinical abnormality; x-rays closer to the end of the observation period are preferred as radiographic findings can evolve (see *Figures 3* and *4*).[31,32] All others should be admitted to a monitored setting. Cardiopulmonary comorbidities should be taken into consideration when deciding on a period of emergency department observation versus immediate admission.

With all populations, discharge counseling is imperative. Providing instructions regarding delayed respiratory distress and infectious complications is integral to ensuring adequate follow-up care and return visits. Additionally, it is important to counsel parents on the various preventative strategies for child drownings, including physical barriers, approved personal flotation devices, and constant supervision. While the ability to swim is important, it does not fully protect against drowning, and parents should be advised that swimming ability does not preclude active adult supervision.

Summary

Drowning is a complex process of respiratory impairment that does not cease with rescue. Immediate complications revolve around hypoxemia, acidosis, and structural insult to the lungs, both because of liquid aspiration and the circulatory response to submersion. Hypoxic cardiac arrest, hypoxic brain injury,

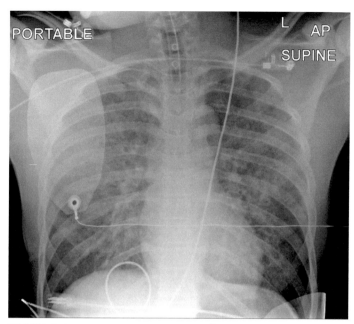

FIGURE 3. Resuscitation room chest x-ray. Copyright 2022 Dr. Jan Frank Gerstenmaier. Image courtesy of Dr. Jan Frank Gerstenmaier and Radiopaedia.org, rID: 24685. Used under license.

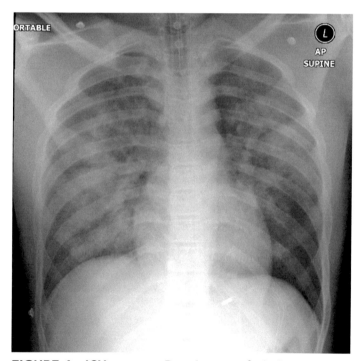

FIGURE 4. ICU x-ray on Day 1 post admission. Copyright 2022 Dr. Jan Frank Gerstenmaier. Image courtesy of Dr. Jan Frank Gerstenmaier and Radiopaedia.org, rID: 24685. Used under license.

and respiratory complications are the predominant sources of morbidity and mortality in drowning. Initial management should be aimed at optimizing respiratory status, and emergency department evaluation and management are primarily driven by clinical presentation. Asymptomatic patients with a normal examination, vitals, and chest x-ray may be discharged after an observation period of 6 to 8 hours.

CASE RESOLUTIONS

■ CASE 1

With the history of a possible diving injury and drowning, the patient had a definitive endotracheal tube placed with cervical spine stabilization. He received a CT scan of the head and cervical spine without evidence of global anoxic brain injury or cervical fracture. He was admitted to the pediatric ICU and went on to develop cerebral edema, with repeat head CT imaging demonstrating diffuse edematous changes and loss of gray-white matter differentiation. With an unknown submersion time of up to 12 minutes, his potential for neurologic recovery was low. Care was ultimately withdrawn by the family.

■ CASE 2

This patient was observed for 6 hours and did not develop any new symptoms beyond the minimal cough, which significantly improved. Her lung sounds remained clear, and her chest x-ray was normal. She was re-evaluated when clinically sober and did not feel subjectively short of breath. She was discharged home with precautions to be re-evaluated if she developed any new symptoms.

REFERENCES

1. Peden A, Franklin R. Causes of distraction leading to supervision lapses in cases of fatal drowning of children 0-4 years in Australia: a 15-year review. *J Paediatr Child Health*. 2019;56(3):450-456.

2. CDC WONDER. Centers for Disease Control and Prevention. Accessed April 16, 2022. https://wonder.cdc.gov/

3. Noble CS, Sharpe N. Drowning: its mechanism and treatment. *Can Med Assoc J*. 1963;89(9):402-404.

4. Idris AH, Berg RA, Bierens J, et al. Recommended guidelines for uniform reporting of data from drowning: the "Utstein Style." *Circulation*. 2003;108(20):2565-2574.

5. Idris AH, Bierens JJLM, Perkins GD, et al. 2015 revised Utstein-Style recommended guidelines for uniform reporting of data from drowning-related resuscitation: an ILCOR advisory statement. *Circ Cardiovasc Qual Outcomes*. 2017;10(7):e000024.

6. Bierens J, Lunetta P, Tipton M, Warner DS. Physiology of drowning: a review. *Physiology (Bethesda)*. 2016;31(2):147-166.

7. Shattock MJ, Tipton MJ. "Autonomic conflict": a different way to die during cold water immersion? *J Physiol*. 2012;590(14):3219-3230.

8. Orlowski JP, Abulleil MM, Phillips JM. The hemodynamic and cardiovascular effects of near-drowning in hypotonic, isotonic, or hypertonic solutions. *Ann Emerg Med*. 1989;18(10):1044-1049.

9. Szpilman D. Near-drowning and drowning classification: a proposal to stratify mortality based on the analysis of 1,831 cases. *Chest*. 1997;112(3):660-665.

10. Quan L, Bierens JJLM, Lis R, Rowhani-Rahbar A, Morley P, Perkins GD. Predicting outcome of drowning at the scene: a systematic review and meta-analyses. *Resuscitation*. 2016;104:63-75.

11. Layon AJ, Modell JH. Drowning: update 2009. *Anesthesiology*. 2009;110(6):1390-1401.

12. Ender P, Dolan MJ. Pneumonia associated with near-drowning. *Clin Infect Dis*. 1997;25(4):896-907.

13. Huckabee HC, Craig PL, Williams JM. Near drowning in frigid water: a case study of a 31-year-old woman. *J Int Neuropsychol Soc*. 1996;2(3):256-260.

14. Samuelson H, Nekludov M, Levander M. Neuropsychological outcome following near-drowning in ice water: two adult case studies. *J Int Neuropsychol Soc*. 2008;14(4):660-666.

15. Golden FS, Tipton MJ, Scott RC. Immersion, near-drowning and drowning. *Br J Anaesth*. 1997;79(2):214-225.

16. Eich C, Bräuer A, Kettler D. Recovery of a hypothermic drowned child after resuscitation with cardiopulmonary bypass followed by prolonged extracorporeal membrane oxygenation. *Resuscitation*. 2005;67(1):145-148.

17. Turgut A, Turgut T. A study on rescuer drowning and multiple drowning incidents. *J Safety Res*. 2012;43(2):129-132.

18. Baker PA, Webber JB. Failure to ventilate with supraglottic airways after drowning. *Anaesth Intensive Care*. 2011;39(4):675-677.

19. Schmidt A, Sempsrott JR, Hawkins SC, Arastu AS, Cushing TA, Auerbach PS. Wilderness Medical Society clinical practice guidelines for the treatment and prevention of drowning: 2019 update. *Wilderness Environ Med*. 2019;30(4S):S70-S86.

20. Layon AJ, Modell JH. Drowning: update 2009. *Anesthesiology*. 2009;110(6):1390-1401.

21. Eich C, Bräuer A, Timmermann A, et al. Outcome of 12 drowned children with attempted resuscitation on cardiopulmonary bypass: an analysis of variables based on the "Utstein Style for drowning." *Resuscitation*. 2007;75(1):42-52.

22. Grmec S, Strnad M, Podgorsek D. Comparison of the characteristics and outcome among patients suffering from out-of-hospital primary cardiac arrest and drowning victims in cardiac arrest. *Int J Emerg Med*. 2009;2(1):7-12.

23. Centers for Disease Control and Prevention. Nonfatal and fatal drownings in recreational water settings — United States, 2001-2002. *MMWR Morb Mortal Wkly Rep*. 2004;53(21):447-452.

24. Hwang V, Shofer FS, Durbin DR, Baren JM. Prevalence of traumatic injuries in drowning and near drowning in children and adolescents. *Arch Pediatr Adolesc Med*. 2003;157(1):50-53.

25. Watson, R. Scott, et al. "Cervical spine injuries among submersion victims." *J Trauma* 2001;51(4):658-662.

26. Gregorakos L, Markou N, Psalida V, et al. Near-drowning: clinical course of lung injury in adults. *Lung*. 2009;187(2):93-97.

27. Rafaat K, Spear RM, Kuelbs C, Parsapour K, Peterson B. Cranial computed tomographic findings in a large group of children with drowning: diagnostic, prognostic, and forensic implications. *Pediatr Crit Care Med*. 2008;9(6):567-572.

28. Dubowitz DJ, Bluml S, Arcinue E, Dietrich RB. MR of hypoxic encephalopathy in children after near drowning: correlation with quantitative proton MR spectroscopy and clinical outcome. *AJNR Am J Neuroradiol*. 1998;19(9):1617-1627.

29. Hooper AJ, Hockings, LE. Drowning and immersion injury. *Anaesth Intensive Care Med*. 2011;12(9):399-402.

30. Causey AL, Tilelli JA, Swanson ME. Predicting discharge in uncomplicated near-drowning. *Am J Emerg Med*. 2000;18(1):9-11.

31. Spzilman D. Near-drowning and drowning classification: a proposal to stratify mortality based on the analysis of 1,831 cases. *Chest*. 1997;112(3):660-665.

32. Szpilman D, Bierens JJLM, Handley AJ, Orlowski JP. Drowning. *N Eng J Med*. 2012;366(22):2102-2110.

CME Questions

Reviewed by **Danya Khoujah, MBBS, MEHP, FACEP; and Nathanial Mann, MD**

Qualified, paid subscribers to *Critical Decisions in Emergency Medicine* may receive CME certificates for up to 5 ACEP Category I credits, 5 *AMA PRA Category 1 Credits*™, and 5 AOA Category 2-B credits for completing this activity in its entirety. Submit your answers online at acep.org/cdem; a score of 75% or better is required. You may receive credit for completing the CME activity any time within 3 years of its publication date. Answers to this month's questions will be published in next month's issue.

1 Although it is a relatively rare cause of stroke overall, cervical artery dissection is a common cause of ischemic stroke in what age group?
   - A. <18 years
   - B. 18-45 years
   - C. 45-60 years
   - D. >60 years

2 What is the most common presenting symptom of cervical artery dissection?
   - A. Arm weakness
   - B. Headache or neck pain
   - C. Miosis or ptosis
   - D. Vomiting

3 Cervical artery dissection is caused by a tear in which layer of the vessel?
   - A. Adventitia
   - B. Intima
   - C. Media
   - D. Vasa vasorum

4 Carotid artery dissection most commonly occurs at what location?
   - A. 2 cm above the bifurcation of the common carotid artery
   - B. At the C2 cervical foramen
   - C. At the C5-C6 transverse foramen
   - D. Below the bifurcation of the common carotid artery

5 A patient presents with headache and neck pain after a visit to the chiropractor but has an unrevealing cranial nerve examination. The emergency physician is concerned for cervical artery dissection. What study is considered most readily accessible with minimal risks in the emergency department to aid in diagnosis?
   - A. Cerebral angiography
   - B. CT angiography
   - C. Lumbar puncture
   - D. MRI

6 What is a stroke caused by cervical artery dissection most commonly attributed to?
   - A. Pseudoaneurysm formation
   - B. Subarachnoid hemorrhage
   - C. Thromboembolic events
   - D. Vessel stenosis

7 What is the goal of treatment of cervical artery dissection?
   - A. To help heal and recanalize vessels
   - B. To prevent a subarachnoid hemorrhage
   - C. To prevent dissection extension
   - D. To prevent thromboembolic complications

8 What did the CADISS trial determine?
   - A. Anticoagulants have a higher 30-day mortality rate when treating cervical artery dissection
   - B. Antiplatelet medications are a more efficacious treatment than anticoagulants in treating cervical artery dissection
   - C. At 12-months' follow-up, a cervical artery dissection patient's risk of recurrent stroke is 10%
   - D. There was no significant difference in developing stroke between patients treated with antiplatelets or anticoagulants

9 Which finding can be considered as an absolute contraindication to intravenous thrombolysis?
   - A. Aortic arch dissection
   - B. Cervical artery dissection
   - C. Intracranial dissection
   - D. Persistent BP of 180/100 mm Hg

10 A patient presents 12 hours after the onset of unilateral weakness and is found to have cervical artery dissection on initial imaging. Mechanical thrombectomy should be considered in all but which scenario?
   - A. Patient has already received intravenous thrombolytics
   - B. Patient has an acute ischemic stroke caused by a proximal intracranial arterial occlusion
   - C. Patient has an NIH stroke scale score of 5
   - D. Patient is at a stroke center with appropriate expertise

11 **What is acceptable terminology to describe a drowning victim?**

A. Dry drowning
B. Near drowning
C. Submersion injury
D. Wet drowning

12 **Which patient did not drown?**

A. Infant who fell under the bathwater surface, was apneic, and requires CPR
B. 5-year-old who fell into a swimming pool, was rescued within 1 minute, and is awake and coughing
C. 23-year-old intoxicated man who got his swimming shoes stuck in a submerged tree at the lake for 5 seconds, resurfaced on his own, and has a mild cough
D. 30-year-old woman wearing a life vest who fell off a river raft and onto a rock where she clung to it yelling for help, suffering no cough or symptoms of respiratory impairment the rest of the day

13 **What is an acceptable amount of time to observe a patient who suffered a drowning event?**

A. 30 minutes if asymptomatic on arrival and with a normal initial chest x-ray
B. 2 hours after a negative chest x-ray
C. 6 hours on 2 L/min O_2 nasal cannula supplementation or less
D. 9 hours and when clinically sober

14 **Which drowning victim can likely be safely discharged?**

A. 8-year-old girl with faint right lower lobe lung opacity on emergency department chest x-ray
B. 27-year-old man who is intoxicated and has a productive cough after an unwitnessed submersion
C. 48-year-old man with an occasional cough but with no symptoms and a negative chest x-ray
D. 60-year-old woman normally on 3 L/min O_2 via nasal cannula at home, now requiring 5 L/min O_2 with a severe cough

15 **What information is most useful in determining the potential for recovery from a drowning event?**

A. Initial arterial blood gas pH 7.19
B. Required trial of noninvasive positive-pressure ventilation on arrival
C. Time beneath the surface
D. Water temperature

16 **Which risk factor is not classically associated with drowning?**

A. Age younger than 4 years
B. History of chronic obstructive pulmonary disease
C. History of seizure
D. Intoxication

17 **For which patient is the temperature of the water theoretically beneficial in drowning?**

A. 45-year-old intoxicated tourist submerged in 35°C (95°F) hot springs
B. Ice climber who fell into 4°C (39.2°F) water
C. Toddler who fell into a cooler of ice water at a summer birthday party
D. Triathlete who lost consciousness during training in 15°C (59°F) lake water

18 **Which drowning victim should have a CT of the cervical spine?**

A. 15-year-old who fell off a boat in the middle of a lake
B. 25-year-old man who did not resurface while cliff diving
C. Fully clothed toddler who was rescued from the bottom of the deep end of the pool
D. Infant left unattended in a bathtub

19 **Which pulmonary complication is possible with drowning?**

A. Acute respiratory distress syndrome
B. Extrapulmonary abscess
C. Pneumothorax
D. All of these

20 **Which physiologic response is unassociated with immersion or submersion?**

A. Bradycardia
B. Laryngospasm
C. Myoclonus
D. Tachycardia

ANSWER KEY FOR JULY 2022, VOLUME 36, NUMBER 7

1	2	3	4	5	6	7	8	9	10	11	12	13	14	15	16	17	18	19	20
C	C	B	D	D	C	B	D	D	A	C	D	B	D	D	C	A	A	B	D

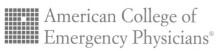
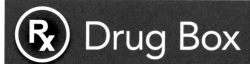

Drug Box

DEXMEDETOMIDINE SUBLINGUAL FILM

By Frank LoVecchio, DO, MPH, FACEP
Valleywise Health and ASU, Phoenix, Arizona

Objective
On completion of this column, you should be able to:
- Describe the use of dexmedetomidine sublingual film to subdue symptoms of acute agitation associated with schizophrenia and bipolar disorder.

Acute agitation in patients with bipolar disorder often requires urgent chemical de-escalation. In April 2022, the FDA approved dexmedetomidine sublingual film for the treatment of adults with agitation associated with schizophrenia and bipolar I and bipolar II disorders.

Mechanism of Action
Selective α-2 adrenergic receptor agonist that is orally absorbed quickly; α-2 receptor affinity, binding, and upregulation occur after prolonged use.

Research
Two double-blinded, placebo-controlled, randomized trials evaluated the use of the drug for the acute treatment of agitation associated with schizophrenia or bipolar I or II disorder. In adults with bipolar disorder and mild to moderate agitation, treatment with sublingual dexmedetomidine 180 µg, 120 µg, or placebo resulted in a mean reduction in the total score of the Positive and Negative Syndrome Scale, Excited Component at 2 hours after treatment. Patients were not eligible for the drug if their systolic blood pressure was less than 110 mm Hg, their diastolic blood pressure was less than 70 mm Hg, their heart rate was less than 55 bpm, or they had evidence of hypovolemia or orthostatic hypotension. Maximal reductions of blood pressure and heart rate were observed 2 hours post dose. Further study is welcome to clarify the appropriate use for emergency department patients.

Dosing for Film, Sublingual, as Hydrochloride
Mild or moderate agitation: Administered either sublingually or buccally. Initial dose of 120 µg. If agitation persists, up to 2 additional doses of 60 µg may be administered at least 2 hours apart. Maximum dose of 240 µg/day.
Severe agitation: Administered sublingually or buccally. Initial dose of 180 µg. If agitation persists, up to 2 additional doses of 90 µg may be administered at least 2 hours apart. Maximum dose of 360 µg/day.

Adverse Effects
Most common: Somnolence, paresthesia or oral hypoesthesia, light-headedness, dry mucous membranes and mouth, hypotension, and orthostatic hypotension (incidence ≥5% and at least twice the rate of placebo)
Cardiovascular: Can cause a biphasic blood pressure response (a short hypertensive phase with hypotension thereafter) related to α-2 adrenergic receptor subtypes α-2B (responsible for hypertensive effects) and α-2A (responsible for hypotension).
Pediatrics and pregnancy: Decreases sinus and atrioventricular nodal function in pediatric patients. Safety of the sublingual formulation for pregnant patients and children has not been studied.

REFERENCE
Preskorn SH, Zeller S, Citrome L, et al. Effect of sublingual dexmedetomidine vs placebo on acute agitation associated with bipolar disorder: a randomized clinical trial. *JAMA.* 2022;327(8):727-736.

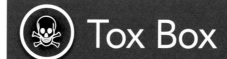

Tox Box

ACUTE TRIPTAN OVERDOSE

By Christian Tomaszewski, MD, MS, MBA, FACEP
University of California San Diego Health

Objective
On completion of this column, you should be able to:
- Recognize the signs of an overdose of triptans and commence treatment.

Triptans are a family of drugs used for migraine and cluster headaches. They are not associated with death after oral overdose except in combination with other drugs, which may lead to serotonergic syndrome.

Mechanism of Action
- Serotoninergic 5-HT1 receptor agonist
- Vasoconstriction of intracranial extracerebral arteries by direct effect on cerebral vascular smooth muscle
- Inhibition of neuropeptide release by sensory dural nerve fibers

Pharmacokinetics
- Moderate bioavailability
- A single dose of up to 400 mg sumatriptan is tolerated well.

Clinical Manifestations
- *Gastrointestinal:* Nausea, vomiting, and diarrhea
- *Cardiac:* Chest pain, hypertension, tachycardia, coronary ischemia, and dysrhythmia
- *Neurologic:* Drowsiness, dizziness, vertigo, paresthesias, and possible CVA
- *Skin:* Diaphoresis
- *Serotonin syndrome:* Agitation, autonomic hyperactivity, tremor, and clonus

Diagnostics
- Basic metabolic panel if indicated
- ECG if symptomatic
- Acetaminophen concentration screening in intentional overdoses

Treatment
- Activated charcoal if early and significant overdose (multiple doses are ineffective)
- Benzodiazepines for agitation
- IV nitroprusside, phentolamine, clevidipine, or labetalol for refractory symptomatic hypertension
- Nitroglycerin for coronary vasospasm
- Lidocaine or amiodarone for ventricular dysrhythmias

Disposition
- Symptomatic exposures require observation and treatment.
- If asymptomatic at 6 hours after ingestion, the patient can be medically cleared.

Critical decisions
in emergency medicine

Volume 36 Number 9: **September 2022**

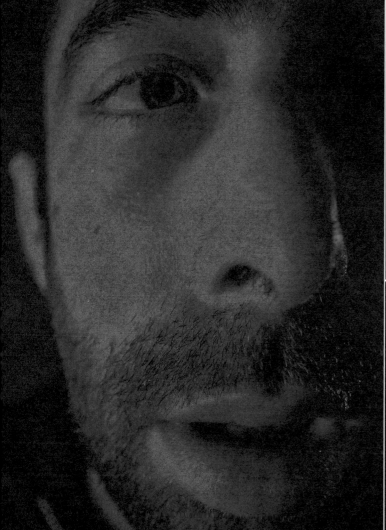

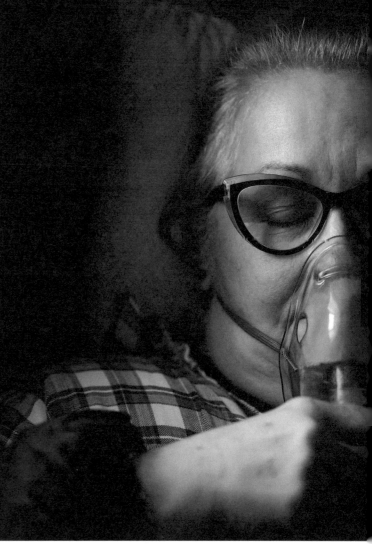

Off the Hook

The opioid crisis continues to rage, with overdose now the leading cause of death in adults younger than 50 years. For patients in moderate to severe withdrawal, initiating buprenorphine for opioid use disorder in the emergency department is safe, effective, and easy to deliver. Emergency physicians must, therefore, be prepared to treat these vulnerable patients.

Old School

The recent pandemic has highlighted important differences in caring for older adults. Geriatric patients are more likely to require critical interventions and often use more resources than younger patients. As such, emergency department personnel must learn how to best care for these patients to improve morbidity and mortality and decrease unnecessary hospitalizations.

THE OFFICIAL CME PUBLICATION OF THE AMERICAN COLLEGE OF EMERGENCY PHYSICIANS

Contributor Disclosures. In accordance with the ACCME Standards for Commercial Support and policy of the American College of Emergency Physicians, all individuals with control over CME content (including but not limited to staff, planners, reviewers, and authors) must disclose whether they have any relevant financial relationship(s) to learners prior to the start of the activity. These individuals have indicated that they have a relationship, which, in the context of their involvement in the CME activity, could be perceived by some as a real or apparent conflict of interest (eg, ownership of stock, grants, honoraria, or consulting fees), but these individuals do not consider that it will influence the CME activity. Joshua S. Broder, MD, FACEP, is a founder and president of OmniSono Inc, an ultrasound technology company and a consultant on the Bayer USA Cardiac Imaging Advisory Board. Sharon E. Mace, MD, FACEP, performs contracted research funded by Biofire Corporation, Genetesis, Quidel, and IBSA Pharma. All remaining individuals with control over CME content have no significant financial interests or relationships to disclose.

This educational activity consists of two lessons, eight feature articles, a post-test, and evaluation questions; as designed, the activity should take approximately 5 hours to complete. The participant should, in order, review the learning objectives for the lesson or article, read the lesson or article as published in the print or online version until all have been reviewed, and then complete the online post-test (a minimum score of 75% is required) and evaluation questions. Release date September 1, 2022. Expiration date August 31, 2025.

Accreditation Statement. The American College of Emergency Physicians is accredited by the Accreditation Council for Continuing Medical Education to provide continuing medical education for physicians.

The American College of Emergency Physicians designates this enduring material for a maximum of 5 *AMA PRA Category 1 Credits™*. Physicians should claim only the credit commensurate with the extent of their participation in the activity.

Each issue of *Critical Decisions in Emergency Medicine* is approved by ACEP for 5 ACEP Category I credits. Approved by the AOA for 5 Category 2-B credits.

Commercial Support. There was no commercial support for this CME activity.

Target Audience. This educational activity has been developed for emergency physicians.

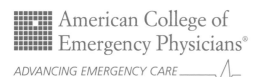

ADVANCING EMERGENCY CARE

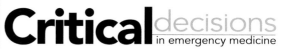

Critical Decisions in Emergency Medicine is the official CME publication of the American College of Emergency Physicians. Additional volumes are available.

EDITOR-IN-CHIEF
Michael S. Beeson, MD, MBA, FACEP
Northeastern Ohio Universities,
Rootstown, OH

SECTION EDITORS
Joshua S. Broder, MD, FACEP
Duke University, Durham, NC

Andrew J. Eyre, MD, MS-HPEd
Brigham and Women's Hospital/
Harvard Medical School, Boston, MA

John Kiel, DO, MPH, FACEP, CAQSM
University of Florida College of Medicine,
Jacksonville, FL

Frank LoVecchio, DO, MPH, FACEP
Valleywise, Arizona State University, University of Arizona,
and Creighton Colleges of Medicine, Phoenix, AZ

Sharon E. Mace, MD, FACEP
Cleveland Clinic Lerner College of Medicine/
Case Western Reserve University, Cleveland, OH

Amal Mattu, MD, FACEP
University of Maryland, Baltimore, MD

Christian A. Tomaszewski, MD, MS, MBA, FACEP
University of California Health Sciences,
San Diego, CA

Steven J. Warrington, MD, MEd, MS
MercyOne Siouxland, Sioux City, IA

ASSOCIATE EDITORS
Tareq Al-Salamah, MBBS, MPH, FACEP
King Saud University, Riyadh, Saudi Arabia/
University of Maryland, Baltimore, MD

Wan-Tsu Chang, MD
University of Maryland, Baltimore, MD

Ann M. Dietrich, MD, FAAP, FACEP
University of South Carolina School of Medicine,
Greenville, SC

Kelsey Drake, MD, MPH, FACEP
St. Anthony Hospital, Lakewood, CO

Walter L. Green, MD, FACEP
UT Southwestern Medical Center, Dallas, TX

John C. Greenwood, MD
University of Pennsylvania, Philadelphia, PA

Danya Khoujah, MBBS, MEHP, FACEP
University of Maryland, Baltimore, MD

Nathaniel Mann, MD
University of South Carolina School of Medicine,
Greenville, SC

George Sternbach, MD, FACEP
Stanford University Medical Center, Stanford, CA

EDITORIAL STAFF
Suzannah Alexander, Editorial Director
salexander@acep.org

Joy Carrico, JD
Managing Editor

Alex Bass
Assistant Editor

Kel Morris
Assistant Editor

ISSN2325-0186 (Print)   ISSN2325-8365 (Online)

Contents

Lesson 17 4
Off the Hook
Management of Opioid Use Disorder
By Sharon Long, MD; Mitchell Katona, MD, MPH;
Jason Kolb, MD; and Amanda dos Santos, MD
Reviewed by Wan-Tsu Chang, MD

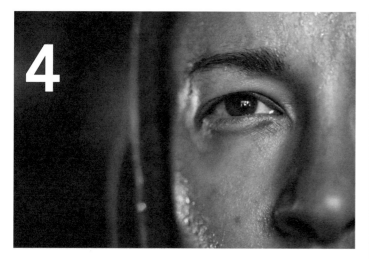

Lesson 18 22
Old School
New Approaches to Geriatric Care
By Nicole E. Cimino-Fiallos, MD, FACEP;
and Danya Khoujah MBBS, MEHP, FACEP
Reviewed by Nathaniel Mann, MD

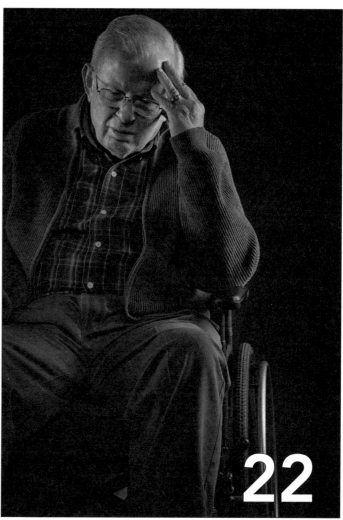

FEATURES

Clinical Pediatrics — Ectopic Pregnancy 12
    By Eric Reed, MD; and Courtney Smalley, MD
    Reviewed by Sharon E. Mace, MD, FACEP

The Literature Review — Community-Acquired Pneumonia.............................14
    By Jason Morris, MD; and Andrew J. Eyre, MD, MS-HPEd

The Critical Procedure — Irrigation of the Eyes.......................................16
    By Steven J. Warrington, MD, MEd, MS

The Critical ECG — Accelerated Junctional Tachycardia 17
    By Amal Mattu, MD, FACEP

Critical Cases in Orthopedics and Trauma — Occult Talus Fracture....................18
    By John Kiel, DO, MPH

The Critical Image — The Importance of Incidental Findings...........................20
    By Joshua S. Broder, MD, FACEP

CME Questions 30
    Reviewed by Wan-Tsu Chang, MD; and Nathaniel Mann, MD

Drug Box — Fidaxomicin 32
    By Frank LoVecchio, DO, MPH, FACEP

Tox Box — Carbamazepine Poisoning...32
    By Christian A. Tomaszewski, MD, MS, MBA, FACEP

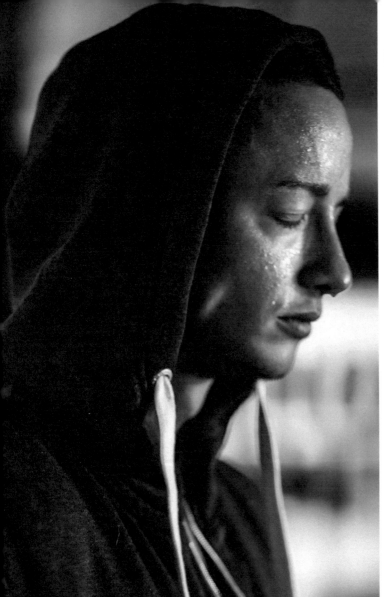

Off the Hook

Management of Opioid Use Disorder

LESSON 17

By Sharon Long, MD; Mitchell Katona, MD, MPH;
Jason Kolb, MD; and Amanda dos Santos, MD

Dr. Long is the assistant program director of the emergency medicine residency program and an affiliate faculty member in the Division of Emergency Medicine, Department of Surgery and Perioperative Care, and Dr. Katona is an emergency medicine resident at The University of Texas at Austin Dell Medical School. Dr. Kolb is an emergency physician and medical director of the emergency department–based MOUD program, and Dr. dos Santos is an emergency medicine resident at Summa Health System in Akron, Ohio.

Reviewed by Wan-Tsu Chang, MD

Objectives

On completion of this lesson, you should be able to:

1. Screen and identify patients with OUD and opioid withdrawal symptoms.
2. State the indications and contraindications for using buprenorphine and naloxone.
3. Explain the pharmacology, dosing, and administration of buprenorphine in the treatment of OUD and opioid withdrawal.
4. Identify steps for linking patients to outpatient care after buprenorphine is initiated.
5. Describe the impact of stigma and harm reduction on the health care outcomes of people with OUD.

From the EM Model

14.0 Psychobehavioral Disorders
    14.1 Substance Use Disorders
        14.1.6 Opioid Use Disorder

■ CRITICAL DECISIONS ■

- How do physicians identify OUD in patients?
- What is buprenorphine, and how does it work?
- What are the indications for using buprenorphine for OUD, and how is it initiated?
- What are the best next steps after patients are given or prescribed buprenorphine?
- Do physicians need special training or certification to prescribe buprenorphine?
- What role does stigma play in the health outcomes of patients who use drugs?
- What harm reduction strategies should be considered when treating patients with OUD?

The opioid crisis continues to rage, with overdose now the leading cause of death in adults younger than 50 years. For patients in moderate to severe withdrawal, initiating buprenorphine for opioid use disorder (OUD) in the emergency department is safe, effective, and easy to deliver to this vulnerable population at high risk of death.

CASE PRESENTATIONS

◼ CASE ONE

A 22-year-old man with no known past medical history presents via ambulance. The paramedics state that a bystander called 911 after noticing the patient slumped over in his parked car. The paramedics found him unresponsive with slow, shallow respirations but normal pulses. His initial vital signs included BP 102/56, P 62, R 5, and T 37°C (98.6°F). They administered two sequential 4-mg doses of intranasal naloxone, and the patient's mental status and respirations improved significantly. On arrival at the emergency department, the patient is alert but appears uncomfortable. He is vomiting and has difficulty sitting still while being placed on the monitor. Vital signs include BP 122/66, P 94, R 16, and T 37°C (98.6°F). On physical examination, his face is flushed, and his pupils are dilated. The remainder of the examination is unremarkable, including normal peripheral perfusion, clear lung sounds, and a nontender abdomen.

◼ CASE TWO

A 38-year-old man experiencing homelessness with a history of chronic back pain after a motor vehicle collision presents with a chief complaint of myalgias. Over the last several months, he has had increasing full-body aches that are worse over the lumbar spine, but he denies any recent trauma, fever, weakness, numbness, or bowel or bladder symptoms. He discloses that since the collision, he has developed a "problem with pain pills" and has recently begun purchasing "street oxy" tablets that he crushes and snorts. He denies any use of hypodermic needles but reveals that he took pain pills 30 minutes prior to arrival. He previously tried "quitting cold turkey" but began feeling ill and having intense cravings. He states that he wants to quit but is unsure whether he can do it by himself and asks for help. His vital signs include BP 118/68, P 72, R 18, and T 37°C (98.6°F). Physical examination is reassuring with normal peripheral perfusion, clear respirations bilaterally, and no spinal tenderness or neurologic deficits.

◼ CASE THREE

A 23-year-old woman presents for evaluation of a skin infection on her left arm. She notes one large and several small areas of redness, swelling, and pain that have been present for several days. Due to the increased association of soft tissue infections with OUD, the physician asks about intravenous drug use, and the patient acknowledges ongoing intravenous use of fentanyl. She says she last used fentanyl 36 hours ago. The patient also reports a positive home pregnancy test last week. In addition to the skin complaints, she reports sweating, muscle aches, restlessness, nausea, vomiting, and diarrhea. She has had no fever, no abdominal or pelvic pain, and no vaginal bleeding. On examination, vital signs include BP 110/70, P 105, R 18, and T 36.7°C (98.1°F). She has beads of sweat on her forehead and widely dilated pupils despite a bright room. Her left arm shows acute and chronic needle tracks as well as a 4-cm fluctuant mass and several small areas of cellulitis. The rest of the skin shows gooseflesh, and there is mild tremor with extension of the upper extremities.

Introduction

Despite increased attention from health care organizations, government agencies, and physician groups, the opioid epidemic remains one of the most serious health problems in the United States. From April 2020 to April 2021, the CDC reported over 100,000 drug overdose deaths, with over 75,000 of these deaths attributed to opioids — a marked increase from the 56,000 opioid-related deaths in the year prior.[1] The 1-year mortality rate following a nonfatal opioid overdose is up to 5.5% (similar to acute myocardial infarction), with 4.6% of these deaths occurring within 2 days and 20.5% occurring within 1 month of the overdose.[2] Additionally, nonfatal opioid overdoses carry a high risk of death due to complications. For many patients with OUD, the emergency department is their entry point to health care; therefore, emergency physicians must be skilled in the recognition, evaluation, and treatment of OUD. Treating these patients aligns with the core mission of emergency medicine — to improve the outcomes of patients who present with conditions of high mortality and morbidity with evidence-based treatments. Emergency physicians can have a great impact on outcomes in these cases by providing appropriate and timely intervention.

Initiation of buprenorphine in the emergency department lowers both overdose and all-cause mortality in patients with OUD.[3] It can be ordered in the emergency department, hospital, or clinic setting by any physician, without the need for any special waivers. For patients in moderate to severe opioid withdrawal, buprenorphine controls symptoms within 1 hour, requires no testing, and uses minimal emergency department resources. The improvement in symptoms can be dramatic and gratifying for the patient as well as the physician.

CRITICAL DECISION

How do physicians identify OUD in patients?

The emergency department is a primary point of engagement with health care for many patients with OUD. Patients who present with opioid overdose or who are specifically seeking OUD treatment are easily identified. However, when OUD is indeterminate or the patient does not self-identify as using opioids, the opportunity for OUD treatment may be missed. Physician awareness of subtle or associated presentations of OUD and effective screening are essential to identifying these patients early in their course. Educating staff on the effectiveness of medication for OUD (MOUD) in reducing mortality can change traditionally biased attitudes toward patients and improve screening and identification.

Screening for OUD

Many substance use screening tools are available to emergency physicians to identify patients with OUD. It is especially important to screen for OUD in pregnant women because of the effects of OUD on newborns. Departments with more tailored resources for this patient population, such as social workers or substance use navigators, may have access to lengthier substance use screening tools. Emergency

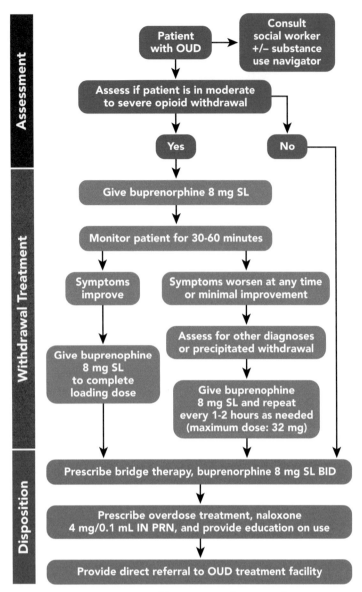

FIGURE 1. Initiation of buprenorphine in the emergency department

departments with fewer resources may have to rely on a more simplified screening process.

One emergency department used a simple, single-question suicide screen as a model to screen for OUD in all patients.[4] Triage nurses asked, "In the last week, have you struggled with painkillers or used heroin or fentanyl?"[4] This screen was found to be more sensitive than other methods, such as reviewing prior health records.[4] Staff reported it was streamlined, empowering, and nondisruptive, adding an average of only 12 seconds to triage time.[4] Patients with a positive screen were assessed early in their medical care for opioid withdrawal, allowing for timely treatment when indicated.[4]

Patients may be reluctant to reveal their substance use to medical staff due to prior health care experiences and the stigma associated with drug use.[5,6] Emergency departments can improve patients' level of comfort in seeking care for OUD by encouraging a culture of compassion. This strategy includes empathic interviewing when screening patients and displaying educational resources about the availability of OUD treatments in departments' public spaces.

Nonobvious OUD Presentations

Because OUD often has significant associated comorbidities, patients with OUD may present with a variety of complaints that are less obviously linked to OUD and affect multiple body systems.

OUD frequently coexists with psychiatric disorders. All patients with complaints of anxiety, depression, mania, psychosis, or suicidal ideation should be asked about substance use, including opioids. Skin and soft tissue infections are common, especially among patients with OUD who use drugs intravenously. Patients experiencing opioid withdrawal may also have gastrointestinal complaints. Spinal epidural abscess, spine osteomyelitis, and discitis can also be associated with OUD. Back pain with fever and neurologic deficits are symptoms highly concerning for these conditions, and patients who present with these symptoms should be screened for OUD. Signs and symptoms of endocarditis, including fever, chest pain, dyspnea, heart murmur, Osler nodes, and Janeway lesions, should also prompt an OUD screening.

Patients may want to leave before completing medical treatment because they suffer from OUD and are experiencing opioid withdrawal or fear its onset. Thus, emergency physicians who recognize the presence of OUD should provide MOUD treatment, so these patients can continue appropriate medical care for other conditions.

CRITICAL DECISION

What is buprenorphine, and how does it work?

Buprenorphine is an opioid with *low activity* (partial agonist) but *high affinity* at the μ-opioid receptor.[7,8] As a *partial* agonist, buprenorphine only partially stimulates the μ-opioid receptor, allowing for some release of endorphins and other neurotransmitters.[7] This process mitigates withdrawal symptoms and controls cravings without the euphoria and abuse potential of *full*-agonist opioids. These unique properties result in buprenorphine's high safety profile and ceiling effect for respiratory depression and sedation, which are absent in other opioids such as methadone, a full agonist used to treat OUD and chronic pain. In fact, no overdose deaths have been related to buprenorphine without coexisting ingestions (such as benzodiazepines).[7,9] Buprenorphine's high-affinity binding to the μ-opioid receptor prevents other opioids from binding to and activating the receptor and can displace other opioids already bound to these receptors. Replacing full agonists like fentanyl with partial agonists like buprenorphine can precipitate withdrawal.[7,9]

Formulations of Buprenorphine

Buprenorphine for the treatment of OUD is typically delivered in sublingual preparations, either as a film or tablet.[7] Absorption is rapid, and first-pass metabolism by the liver is avoided. Some formulations combine naloxone with buprenorphine to decrease misuse (eg, snorting or injection). Naloxone is not active when taken sublingually but is active if injected or snorted.[7] Plain buprenorphine is sometimes referred to as monotherapy, and buprenorphine-naloxone preparations are called dual therapy. Given its rapid absorption and onset

HEART RATE

0	HR <81
1	HR 81-100
2	HR 101-120
4	HR >120

GASTROINTESTINAL UPSET

0	None
1	Stomach cramps
2	Nausea or loose stool
3	Vomiting or diarrhea
5	Multiple episodes of vomiting or diarrhea

SWEATING

0	None
1	Reports chills or flushing
2	Observable flushed or moist face
3	Beads of sweat on face
4	Sweat streaming off face

TREMOR

0	None
1	Felt but not observed
2	Observable
4	Gross tremor or twitching

RESTLESSNESS

0	None
1	Subjective only
3	Frequent shifting or extremity movements
5	Cannot sit still for more than a few minutes

YAWNING

0	None
1	Once or twice
2	3+ times
4	Several times per minute

PUPILS

0	Normal or constricted
1	Mildly dilated for room light
2	Moderately dilated for room light
5	Very dilated with only rim of iris visible

ANXIETY/IRRITABILITY

0	None
1	Subjective
2	Obviously anxious or irritable
4	Assessment difficult due to severity

BONE/JOINT PAIN

0	None
1	Mild, diffuse discomfort
2	Subjectively severe
4	Observable discomfort (eg, rubs joints)

SKIN

0	Normal
3	Observable piloerection
5	Prominent piloerection

RHINORRHEA/TEARING

0	None
1	Nasal congestion or unusually moist eyes
2	Rhinorrhea or tearing
4	Constant rhinorrhea or tears streaming down face

TOTAL

0-7	Unlikely to require immediate buprenorphine
8-36	Give stat buprenorphine

FIGURE 2. COWS scoring

of action, dosing buprenorphine in patients in moderate to severe opioid withdrawal provides rapid relief of withdrawal symptoms. As a partial opioid agonist, symptom control is superior to nonopioid adjunct medications such as clonidine, antiemetics, and NSAIDs, although all of these can be considered for patients with opioid withdrawal.[9] Buprenorphine is also available as a once-monthly depot injection and a subcutaneous implant lasting for 6 months.

CRITICAL DECISION

What are the indications for using buprenorphine for OUD, and how is it initiated?

Opioid withdrawal may result from abstinence or following the administration of naloxone or buprenorphine.[7,9,10] Buprenorphine has two primary indications in the emergency department: It may be used immediately for the treatment of opioid withdrawal or as an outpatient prescription for treatment of OUD as bridge therapy to primary care (*Figure 1*).[9-11]

Home induction of buprenorphine is appropriate when a patient is not yet in withdrawal. It may also be prescribed for patients weeks after they have completely "detoxed."[1,7,8] No testing is required prior to buprenorphine initiation.[9,12]

Diagnosis of Opioid Withdrawal

Accurate diagnosis is important since untreated opioid withdrawal portends a high mortality risk at discharge.[12] Symptoms may be severe and include anxiety, irritability, gastrointestinal distress, and diffuse pain, while clinical signs may include restlessness, tachycardia, diaphoresis, mydriasis, yawning, and piloerection.[7,9,10] The Clinical Opiate Withdrawal Scale (COWS) score uses such signs and symptoms to quantify withdrawal severity, with a score of 8 or higher indicating a low likelihood of precipitated withdrawal (*Figure 2*).[9] Alternatively, patients may be assessed subjectively by asking if they are experiencing withdrawal and objectively by identifying a clinical sign (eg, moist forehead, tachycardia, or restlessness).

Immediate Buprenorphine Administration for Opioid Withdrawal

As soon as a patient is determined to be in moderate or severe withdrawal with no contraindication, buprenorphine should be given.[12] Clinical presentation is a more reliable assessment of withdrawal than timing of last use. The onset of withdrawal can vary from 6 to 72 hours after last use, depending on the half-life of the opioid used.[7,9,10,12]

The recommended initial dose of buprenorphine is 8 mg SL.[9-12] The sublingual film should completely dissolve under the tongue and should not be swallowed. Patients should have nothing else by mouth for 15 minutes, should be monitored for 30 to 60 minutes, and then should be assessed for response. If symptoms improve, they should receive a second dose of 8 mg SL to complete the loading dose.[9-12] The recommended total dose on the first day of treatment is between 16 and 32 mg to maximize relief from withdrawal symptoms and minimize the risk of cravings.[7,9,10,12] Lower initial doses are not recommended because they are inferior for preventing cravings and may, paradoxically, precipitate withdrawal.[8-12] If symptoms are unchanged or worsen, consider precipitated withdrawal or an alternative diagnosis.

Buprenorphine- or naloxone-precipitated withdrawal is treated with a higher dose of buprenorphine, up to 8 to 16 mg every 1 to 2 hours to a maximum of 32 mg.[9-12] Both opioid withdrawal and buprenorphine can cause nausea. Antiemetic agents such as ondansetron may be used.[9]

Home Initiation of Buprenorphine

Patients with OUD who do not meet criteria for immediate buprenorphine administration in the emergency department should be offered a prescription for buprenorphine for home initiation.[7-12] Although there is a paucity of literature supporting a specific regimen for buprenorphine, particularly in the case of home initiation, a reasonable approach to home initiation is 4 mg SL every 2 hours as needed for withdrawal symptoms up to a recommended total dose of 24 mg on the first day.[9,10] Patients should be given careful guidance to wait until they experience moderate withdrawal symptoms before initiating MOUD and to return to the emergency department if their symptoms worsen after taking buprenorphine.[9] After this first day of MOUD treatment, patients should begin taking a bridge therapy regimen.

MOUD Bridge Therapy

All patients with OUD who are not already receiving treatment should be offered MOUD, regardless of whether they are currently in withdrawal. Initiation of buprenorphine in the emergency department lowers the risk of overdose and all-cause mortality.[1,3,5,8-12] Patients started on MOUD are twice as likely to remain in treatment and less likely to require hospitalization, return to the emergency department, transmit infectious diseases, or engage in criminal activities.[2,3,9] Most patients ultimately reach a stable long-term dose between 8 to 24 mg per day, and thus, a reasonable approach to bridge therapy (prescription at discharge) is 8 mg SL twice daily.[9] Patients should be discharged with a sufficient bridge prescription to last at least until their expected referral appointment.[11]

Buprenorphine in Pregnancy

Buprenorphine is safe and effective for use in pregnant patients for both withdrawal and outpatient treatment of OUD.[9,13] In addition to buprenorphine's other advantages, it reduces the severity of neonatal abstinence syndrome in newborns of pregnant patients treated with buprenorphine through delivery with no increased risk of maternal-fetal adverse events.[13-15] Previously, formulations that combine buprenorphine with naloxone were not recommended due to concerns of teratogenicity or precipitated withdrawal from fetal exposure to naloxone; however, buprenorphine-naloxone has been shown to be safe and effective in multiple studies.[9,13] Because buprenorphine is minimally transferred in breast milk, mothers should continue taking buprenorphine while breast feeding.[13]

CRITICAL DECISION

What are the best next steps after patients are given or prescribed buprenorphine?

First, all patients with OUD should receive linkage to outpatient-based opioid treatment (OBOT) and receive a prescription for and education about nasal naloxone. Additionally, the Drug Addiction Treatment Act of 2000 (DATA 2000) requires that patients prescribed buprenorphine be counseled and receive a phone number for OBOT follow-up. Providing an appointment or a direct referral is useful in linking patients to OBOT through primary care clinics, hospital-based addiction clinics, office-based opioid treatment programs, and telehealth opioid treatment programs.[12] A comprehensive treatment approach includes MOUD, counseling services, and social support or peer recovery coaches. Substance use navigators and social workers can be particularly helpful with the referral process for treatment clinics in the community.[11]

CRITICAL DECISION

Do physicians need special training or certification to prescribe buprenorphine?

Legislation passed in the early 20th century outlawed prescribing opioids to treat patients with OUD. In the 1960s, an exception was made when methadone maintenance therapy emerged and was shown to be successful for multiple outcomes in OUD. However, methadone maintenance therapy can only be administered in heavily regulated, certified opioid treatment programs ("methadone clinics") where patients must present almost daily for dosing. In 2002, when buprenorphine was introduced as a safe and effective outpatient treatment and received FDA approval for treating

✔ Pearls

- Buprenorphine is a partial-agonist opioid that is safe, effective, and easy to use to treat patients with OUD. Its rapid absorption sublingually provides quick relief for opioid withdrawal symptoms.

- Buprenorphine has been proven to decrease all-cause mortality in patients with OUD.

- Emergency physicians should use language and behaviors that reduce the stigma of OUD and should provide proven harm reduction strategies, such as dispensing naloxone to OUD patients.

- Any physician with a standard DEA registration can prescribe buprenorphine.

OUD, a waiver became necessary to further circumvent existing regulations on using opioids to treat OUD. DATA 2000 provided a means to obtain that waiver, the X-waiver, where physicians could prescribe buprenorphine for patients with OUD.[8]

However, on December 29, 2022, Congress eliminated the "DATA-Waiver Program" with the signing of the Consolidated Appropriations Act of 2023. As a result, an X-waiver is no longer required to prescribe buprenorphine for the treatment of OUD. Only a standard DEA registration number is required, and there is no limit on the number of patients a prescriber may treat for opioid use disorder. The This bill also requires health care providers, as a condition of receiving or renewing a DEA registration, to complete a one-time training on managing patients with substance use disorders. The DEA and SAMHSA will provide detailed guidance prior to June 2023, when the training requirement will take effect.

CRITICAL DECISION

What role does stigma play in the health outcomes of patients who use drugs?

Only a minority of people suffering from OUD receive treatment each year. In addition to concerns surrounding treatment readiness, availability, and affordability, frequently reported reasons for not seeking treatment include stigma and fear of social repercussions.[3,5,16]

Stigma is particularly dangerous in health care because it hinders quality of care and health outcomes.[16] Emergency physicians are responsible for recognizing and addressing stigma and discrimination in the workplace. Physicians can start by debunking misguided beliefs, concentrating on scientific information about addiction and treatment in their communications with staff, and advocating for change in discriminatory policies that hurt patients. One potential source of stigma in the emergency department is routine drug screens, which are inherently flawed, can lead to legal and societal repercussions, and can perpetuate harmful biases and discrimination.

The stigma toward people with substance use disorder (SUD) is rooted in the antiquated belief that addiction is a moral failing. A stigma involves labeling someone (eg, an addict) and using it to stereotype everyone with that label (eg, dirty addicts).[16] When physicians believe the stereotype, they may unintentionally react negatively toward an individual or promote harmful discriminatory practices or policies. Public stigma contributes to self-stigma, which can keep patients from seeking treatment, harm reduction services, and even care for illnesses unrelated to SUD.[16]

It is important to interact kindly and compassionately with patients who have SUD and to be respectful when talking with colleagues about them. Evidence suggests that certain words evoke automatic negative thoughts in clinicians, leading to inferior quality of care and less standardized treatments.[16] Terms such as "substance abuser," "addict," and "clean" tend to elicit implicit biases and negative explicit behaviors from treatment professionals. Alternatively, person-first language, such as "a person with substance use disorder," tends to elicit more empathetic behaviors toward these patients.[16] In 2017, the White House Office of National Drug Control Policy published "Change the Language of Addiction" that urges health care professionals to replace common stigmatizing terms with clinical and scientific language.[17]

CRITICAL DECISION

What harm reduction strategies should be considered when treating patients with OUD?

As with any other chronic illness, prevention is key. However, once a disease has developed, lifelong treatment and secondary prevention may be required. Since the emergency department is the entry point to health care for many patients with SUD, harm reduction strategies should be employed to reduce complications from drug use. Emergency physicians can create a safe and therapeutic space for every patient they serve.

Not every patient encountered, however, will be ready and willing to start treatment. In these cases, physicians should "meet them where they are." The emergency department should be a place where patients can discuss safe drug injection practices, such as not using drugs alone; always carrying naloxone; using drug testing strips; using clean needles, syringes, cookers, and filters; using sharps container disposal; washing hands and prepping the skin with alcohol swabs; and inserting the needle bevel up to prevent vessel injury.[18] This not only prevents community spread of communicable diseases, infections, injury, and death, but also shows patients that physicians have their best interests at heart. It seeds trust between patients and emergency physicians should these patients return for OUD treatment in the future.

In addition to candid discussions, patients with SUD should be offered HIV and hepatitis C screening. Physicians should dispense naloxone to all patients with OUD, regardless of the reason for their visit or treatment stage, and refer patients to local services in their community, such as state-sponsored, free naloxone programs (https://www.naloxoneforall.org) and needle exchange programs that provide new, sterile needles to drug users along with other services and resources (https://nasen.org/map).

It is important to avoid creating needless barriers to MOUD treatment for people with concomitant poly-SUDs.

✖ Pitfalls

- Neglecting to adequately screen patients for OUD.

- Overlooking the important role emergency departments play in treating patients with OUD.

- Failing to assess patients for opioid withdrawal when they screen positive and to promptly initiate buprenorphine when indicated.

- Neglecting to dispense nasal naloxone and link all patients with OUD to definitive follow-up care.

Although MOUD is intended specifically for opioids, studies have shown that MOUD treatment correlates with significant decreases in other drug use, including alcohol, sedatives, cocaine, and amphetamines.[6] Additionally, after 6 months of treatment, patients report improved overall health, decreased disability, and less pain, anxiety, and depression.[6]

Emergency physicians should be mindful that OUD is a chronic disease often characterized by relapses, similar to other chronic diseases. Treatment retention rates at 12 months past MOUD initiation are roughly 35%.[19] Emergency physicians should have an open-door policy and reassure patients that they can again receive MOUD treatment after relapse of opioid use.

Treatment of Acute Pain

Treating patients in acute pain who are already on MOUD can be challenging for both patients and physicians. Patients may fear untreated pain and OUD relapse. Experts strongly recommend that buprenorphine be continued at the patient's usual dosage in the emergency department, during hospitalization, and in the perioperative period to prevent a return to opioid use.[20] Buprenorphine is a potent analgesic, and given its high affinity for μ-opioid receptors, it may prevent full agonists from binding unless used at very high doses. The mainstay of pain management is multimodal analgesia with local adjuvants combining pharmacologically different drugs, such as acetaminophen, NSAIDs, ketamine, α-2 agonists (eg, clonidine, dexmedetomidine, tizanidine), gabapentinoids, and intravenous lidocaine. Alternatively, physicians can direct patients to continue their home dose of buprenorphine but divided into more frequent intervals, with additional doses of intravenous or sublingual buprenorphine as needed for pain control.[20] Patients' baseline daily dose may be increased up to 32 mg a day, divided into doses given every 6 or 8 hours. If pain is still refractory to these measures, full opioid agonists may be administered *after* discussing the risks and benefits with patients. Refractory pain will require exceedingly higher doses.[20] In this situation, emergency physicians may want to consider consulting a pain specialist at their institution, if available.

Summary

OUD carries high morbidity and mortality and is commonly encountered in the emergency department. Emergency physicians have the opportunity to help this vulnerable population with evidence-based treatment that lowers morbidity and mortality. Emergency physicians must be skilled in the recognition of OUD, especially less obvious cases, and in treatment options, including use of buprenorphine. With compassionate words, attitudes, and actions, physicians can reduce OUD-associated stigma and encourage more patients to get treatment. Physicians should use proven harm reduction modalities for every patient, which includes dispensing or prescribing naloxone. Although the trend in drug overdose is discouraging, it highlights why it is important for emergency physicians to do their part in addressing this ongoing public health emergency.

REFERENCES

1. Ahmad FB, Rossen LM, Sutton P. Provisional drug overdose death counts. National Center for Health Statistics. 2022. Accessed on July 20, 2022. https://www.cdc.gov/nchs/nvss/vsrr/drug-overdose-data.htm

2. Weiner SG, Baker O, Bernson D, Schuur JD. One-year mortality of opioid overdose victims who received naloxone by emergency medical services. *Ann Emerg Med*. 2017;70(4 suppl):S158.

3. Santo T Jr, Clark B, Hickman M, et al. Association of opioid agonist treatment with all-cause mortality and specific causes of death among people with opioid dependence: a systematic review and meta-analysis. *JAMA Psychiatry*. 2021;78(9):979-993.

4. Lowenstein M, McFadden R, Abdel-Rahman D, et al. Redesign of opioid use disorder screening and treatment in the ED. *NEJM Catal Innov Care Deliv*. 2022;3(1).

5. Substance Abuse and Mental Health Services Administration. Key substance use and mental health indicators in the United States: results from the 2020 national survey on drug use and health. Center for Behavioral Health Statistics and Quality, Substance Abuse and Mental Health Services Administration. 2021. https://www.samhsa.gov/data/sites/default/files/reports/rpt35325/NSDUHFFRPDFWHTMLFiles2020/2020NSDUHFFR1PDFW102121.pdf

6. Duber HC, Barata IA, Cioè-Peña E, et al. Identification, management, and transition of care for patients with opioid use disorder in the emergency department. *Ann Emerg Med*. 2018;72(4):420-431.

7. Coe MA, Lofwall MR, Walsh SL. Buprenorphine pharmacology review: update on transmucosal and long-acting formulations. *J Addict Med*. 2019;13(2):93-103.

8. Substance abuse and mental health services administration. SAMHSA. Accessed May 13, 2022. https://www.samhsa.gov/

9. Strayer RJ, Hawk K, Hayes BD, et al. Management of opioid use disorder in the emergency department: a white paper prepared for the American Academy of Emergency Medicine. *J Emerg Med*. 2020;58(3):522-546.

10. Herring AA, Perrone J, Nelson LS. Managing opioid withdrawal in the emergency department with buprenorphine. *Ann of Emerg Med*. 2019;73(5):481-487.

11. Treat patients with opioid use disorder on-shift. CA Bridge. Published March 2022. Accessed May 13, 2022. https://cabridge.org/tools/on-shift

12. Snyder H, Kalmin MM, Moulin A, et al. Rapid adoption of low-threshold buprenorphine treatment at California emergency departments participating in the CA Bridge program. *Ann Emerg Med*. 2021;78(6):759-772.

13. Committee on Obstetric Practice American Society of Addiction Medicine. Committee opinion no. 711: opioid use and opioid use disorder in pregnancy. *Obstet Gynecol*. 2017;130(2):e81-e94.

14. Jumah NA, Edwards C, Balfour-Boehm J, et al. Observational study of the safety of buprenorphine+naloxone in pregnancy in a rural and remote population. *BMJ Open*. 2016;6(10):e011774.

15. Jones HE, Kaltenbach K, Heil SH, et al. Neonatal abstinence syndrome after methadone or buprenorphine exposure. *N Engl J Med*. 2010;363(24):2320-2331.

16. Ashford RD, Brown AM, Curtis B. Substance use, recovery, and linguistics: the impact of word choice on explicit and implicit bias. *Drug Alcohol Depend*. 2018;189:131-138.

17. Botticelli MP, Koh HK. Changing the language of addiction. *JAMA*. 2016;316(13):1361-1362.

CASE RESOLUTIONS

■ CASE ONE

Based on the history given by EMS and the physical examination, a diagnosis of naloxone-induced opioid withdrawal was made. A COWS score was obtained and found to be 15, indicating moderate withdrawal. The patient was treated initially with 8 mg SL buprenorphine, and a social worker was consulted to refer the patient to a local opioid treatment clinic after discharge. After 45 minutes, the patient was reassessed and reported resolution of his symptoms. A second dose of 8 mg SL buprenorphine was given to complete a loading-induction dose, and the patient was further observed for a minimum of 2 hours following the last dose of naloxone. He had no recurrent symptoms or sedation. The patient was counseled on the use of naloxone and buprenorphine, and outpatient follow-up was discussed in detail. He was discharged with prescriptions for naloxone 4 mg/0.1 mL intranasal and buprenorphine-naloxone sublingual film 8 mg/2 mg twice daily, with ample supply to last until his clinic appointment.

■ CASE TWO

Along with compassionate interviewing, the physician thanked the patient for asking for help and discussed treatment options with him, including offering MOUD. The patient was assessed for withdrawal with a COWS score of 1, indicating no active withdrawal. Based on this score, he was advised and agreed to undergo home initiation of buprenorphine. Social work was then consulted and connected him to a local opioid treatment program and coordinated a primary care appointment. The patient was counseled specifically on home initiation, including waiting for moderate withdrawal symptoms, and advised to return immediately if he experienced symptoms of precipitated withdrawal. He was further counseled on the use of naloxone, and outpatient follow-up was discussed in detail. He was discharged with a prescription for naloxone 4 mg/0.1 mL intranasal as well as buprenorphine-naloxone sublingual film 4 mg/1 mg, with instructions to take 1 film (4 mg) every 2 hours for withdrawal symptoms up to 6 films (24 mg) on the first day, followed by 2 films (8 mg) twice daily.

■ CASE THREE

Complete blood count and lactic acid results were normal. A pelvic ultrasound showed a single, live intrauterine pregnancy measuring 8 weeks and 5 days. The left arm abscess was successfully drained. The patient's tachycardia was correctly attributed to opioid withdrawal, and assessment of her COWS score was 12, indicating moderate withdrawal. After a discussion of MOUD, the patient was given an 8-mg dose of buprenorphine with significant but not complete improvement of her symptoms. A second 8-mg dose was administered 1 hour later with near total relief of withdrawal symptoms. The hospital's high-risk obstetrics service had experience treating pregnant patients with buprenorphine, and the social worker made the patient a follow-up appointment for 5 days later. A 5-day bridge prescription was written for buprenorphine 8 mg twice daily.

18. Getting off right: a safety manual for injection drug users. National Harm Reduction Coalition. Accessed March 7, 2022. https://harmreduction.org/issues/safer-drug-use/injection-safety-manual/

19. Reuter QR, Santos AD, McKinnon J, Gothard D, Jouriles N, Seaberg D. Long-term treatment retention of an emergency department initiated medication for opioid use disorder program. *Am J Emerg Med.* 2022;55:98-102.

20. Buresh M, Ratner J, Zgierska A, Gordin V, Alvanzo A. Treating perioperative and acute pain in patients on buprenorphine: narrative literature review and practice recommendations. *J Gen Intern Med.* 2020;35(12):3635-3643.

ADDITIONAL READING

Quinones S. *Dreamland: The True Tale of America's Opiate Epidemic.* Bloomsbury Publishing; 2019.

PHYSICIAN RESOURCES

The Consolidated Appropriations Act, 2023 — how it benefits integrated behavioral health. Agency for Healthcare Research and Quality. Published January 31, 2023. https://integrationacademy.ahrq.gov/news-and-events/news/consolidated-appropriations-act-2023-how-it-benefits-integrated-behavioral

National Clinician Consultation line: (855)300-3595 (M-F 6 AM-5 PM PST)

PATIENT RESOURCES

https://www.naloxoneforall.org/
https://dancesafe.org/shop/
https://nasen.org/map/
https://cabridge.org/

Ectopic Pregnancy

By Eric Reed, MD; and Courtney Smalley, MD
Case Western Reserve University Medical School,
Cleveland, Ohio

Reviewed by Sharon E. Mace, MD, FACEP

Objective

On completion of this article, you should be able to:

- Evaluate information about ectopic pregnancy to manage pregnant patients.

CASE PRESENTATION

A 16-year-old girl presents with her mother. She is experiencing sudden-onset abdominal pain that started 6 hours ago; within that time, she has had 3 episodes of syncope. She reports that she is 8 weeks' pregnant, determined by her last menstrual period and a positive home pregnancy test. She has had vaginal bleeding for the past week. Triage staff are unable to obtain her blood pressure; her other vital signs include P 107, R 47, and T 36.7°C (98.1°F). The examination is remarkable only for skin pallor and diffuse lower abdominal tenderness with rebound and guarding.

The patient is rushed back to a resuscitation bay and placed in the Trendelenburg position. Manual blood pressure records a systolic pressure of 80 mm Hg, and fluid resuscitation is initiated. A focused assessment with sonography in trauma examination is performed and is positive for free fluid in all abdominal views. Subsequent pelvic views fail to demonstrate a gestational or yolk sac in the endometrial cavity.

The gynecology resident is paged and evaluates the patient, whereupon the resident requests a formal ultrasound. Given the patient's hemodynamic instability, the ultrasound technician performs the study at the bedside and confirms complex free fluid in the pelvis with the left adnexa concerning for a possible ectopic pregnancy (*Figures 1-3*). Quantitative human chorionic gonadotropin (hCG) returns in the 700s. In the meantime, the mother of the patient verbally consents to blood products, and a transfusion of the first two units of uncrossmatched blood is initiated.

Discussion

Ectopic pregnancy may be as common as 0.6% to 2% of all pregnancies. It is more common with increased maternal age, estimated at 4% to 5% of all pregnancies in those older than 40 years.[1-3] The prevalence is higher in patients who present with first-trimester bleeding or pain, estimated between 6% and 16%. In up to half of patients who present with ectopic pregnancy, the ectopic pregnancy is not identified.[4]

Pathophysiology

Ectopic pregnancy is the implantation of a fertilized ovum outside of the endometrial cavity, which can occur in the cervix, uterine interstitium, fallopian tube (most common), ovary, or the peritoneal or abdominal cavities. The suspected mechanisms behind ectopic implantation include anatomical tubal obstruction, impaired ciliary function, and abnormal chemotactic factors.[5]

Risk Factors

The risk factors associated with the highest odds of ectopic pregnancy are prior tubal surgery or prior ectopic pregnancy.[3,4] Approximately 30% of pregnancies following tubal ligation are ectopic. A history of pelvic inflammatory disease (PID) is also associated with increased odds of ectopic pregnancy; interestingly, the rate of ectopic pregnancy has increased fivefold since 1970,

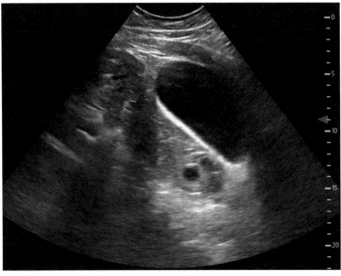

FIGURE 1. Right adnexal view demonstrating an ovoid-shaped hypoechoic mass concerning for ectopic pregnancy

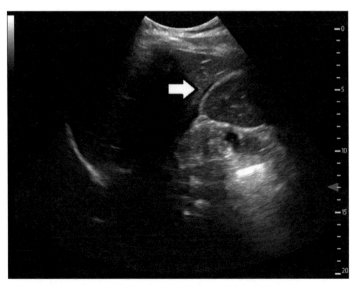

FIGURE 2. Coronal midaxillary view of the right upper quadrant demonstrating free fluid in Morison pouch

attributed in part to the increasing incidence of PID.[2] While intrauterine device (IUD) use confers a lower risk of ectopic pregnancy overall, those who become pregnant with an IUD in place have a 50% rate of ectopic pregnancy.[5] Up to half of patients with ectopic pregnancy have no recognized risk factors for it.[5]

Complications

Development of the embryo outside of the endometrial cavity can lead to rupture of the associated structure and massive intraperitoneal hemorrhage. This complication accounts for an estimated 4% to 9% of pregnancy-related deaths.[1,4] If the ectopic pregnancy is treated and resolves, subsequent pregnancies carry an increased risk of recurrent ectopy, with an odds ratio of 8.3.[4]

Diagnosis

Abdominal or pelvic pain and vaginal bleeding are the most common presenting complaints of ectopic pregnancy.[1] If ruptured, the patient is more likely to present with abdominal tenderness and guarding. Even in the absence of rupture, vaginal bleeding may be present. No combination of examination findings and risk factors has been identified to sufficiently rule out ectopic pregnancy.[4]

Pregnancy may be confirmed with urine hCG testing. Ultrasonography should be the initial imaging modality in the setting of a known pregnancy. If imaging is indeterminate, quantitative hCG should be pursued. However, no single measurable quantitative hCG level can rule out an ectopic pregnancy or predict a benign clinical course, and an ectopic pregnancy may present with rising, stable, or falling hCG levels. Falling levels confirm nonviability but do not rule out ectopic pregnancy.[4]

On ultrasound, a gestational sac and yolk sac should be visible via the transabdominal approach when the hCG surpasses 6,500 IU/L or via the transvaginal approach at 1,000 to 2,000 IU/L. These values with each ultrasound approach are termed the discriminatory threshold. An intrauterine fluid collection (ie, pseudogestational sac) may also be seen in ectopic pregnancies; therefore, a gestational sac alone is insufficient to confirm an intrauterine pregnancy (IUP).[4] Outside of the uterus, up to 75% of tubal ectopic pregnancies are visible on transvaginal ultrasound.[5]

Failure to identify an IUP on ultrasound is associated with an ectopic pregnancy risk of approximately 36%, and simultaneous identification of free pelvic fluid increases that risk. The presence of an IUP effectively rules out ectopic pregnancy, except for those patients who have undergone ovulation induction or assisted conception. These patients are at greater risk of a heterotopic pregnancy, which is reported to be as common as 1 in 100 pregnancies in this population.[4]

Management

In the past, ectopic pregnancy was considered a surgical emergency requiring laparotomy, but early diagnosis with

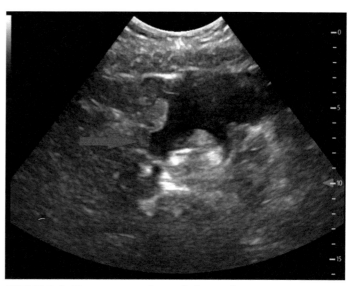

FIGURE 3. Transverse view of the pelvis demonstrating hypoechoic free fluid

hCG testing and ultrasonography allows for increased use of laparoscopy and medical management with methotrexate. The most common treatment remains surgical, including salpingectomy or organ-preserving methods of salpingotomy or transampullary expression in the case of tubal pregnancies. Surgical treatment has been associated with infection and an increased rate of subsequent ectopic pregnancy.[2]

An estimated 20% to 35% of ectopic pregnancies are now managed nonsurgically, the majority with methotrexate.[2] Expectant management is possible because some ectopic pregnancies resolve spontaneously, although the patient must be asymptomatic and willing to accept the potential risks of hemorrhage. Scant evidence makes expectant management an uncommon option.[5,6] Up to 15% of patients managed with methotrexate require subsequent surgical management. In emergent cases of rupture and hemorrhage, surgical management remains the only option.[2,6]

REFERENCES

1. Seeber BE, Barnhart KT. Suspected ectopic pregnancy. *Obstet Gynecol.* 2006;107(2)(part 1):339-413.
2. Van Den Eeden SK, Shan J, Bruce C, Glasser M. Ectopic pregnancy rate and treatment utilization in a large managed care organization. *Obstet Gynecol.* 2005;105(5)(part 1):1052-1057.
3. Bouyer J, Coste J, Shojaei T, et al. Risk factors for ectopic pregnancy: a comprehensive analysis based on a large case-control, population-based study in France. *Am J Epidemiol.* 2003;157(3):185-194.
4. Murray H, Baakdah H, Bardell T, Tulandi T. Diagnosis and treatment of ectopic pregnancy. *CMAJ.* 2005;173(8):905-912.
5. Taran FA, Kagan KO, Hübner M, Hoopmann M, Wallwiener D, Brucker S. The diagnosis and treatment of ectopic pregnancy. *Dtsch Arztebl Int.* 2015;112(41):693-703.
6. Hoover KW, Tao G, Kent CK. Trends in the diagnosis and treatment of ectopic pregnancy in the United States. *Obstet Gynecol.* 2010;115(3):495-502.

CASE RESOLUTION

Upon receiving the results of the formal ultrasound and quantitative hCG testing, the gynecology team immediately admitted the patient for diagnostic laparoscopy and postoperative monitoring. A ruptured left fallopian tube ectopic pregnancy with active bleeding was confirmed. Approximately 3.3 L of hemoperitoneum was evacuated. Her postoperative course was notable for acute blood loss anemia, requiring one additional unit of packed red blood cells. She was discharged from the hospital after 3 days.

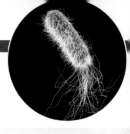

The Literature Review

Community-Acquired Pneumonia

By Jason Morris, MD; and Andrew J. Eyre, MD, MS-HPEd
Harvard Affiliated Emergency Medicine Residency; and
Brigham & Women's Hospital in Boston, Massachusetts

Objective

On completion of this article, you should be able to:

■ Recall the major elements of the ATS and IDSA clinical guidelines on CAP.

Metlay JP, Waterer GW, Long AC, et al. Diagnosis and treatment of adults with community-acquired pneumonia. an official clinical practice guideline of the American Thoracic Society and Infectious Diseases Society of America. *Am J Respir Crit Care Med.* 2019;200(7):e45-e67.

KEY POINTS

■ Sputum and blood cultures should be obtained in patients with severe CAP and in all patients empirically covered for MRSA or *P. aeruginosa* infections.

■ An initial procalcitonin level should not determine the need for antibacterial therapy.

■ Steroids should not routinely be used in the treatment of CAP.

■ The HCAP categorization should be abandoned and replaced by evaluating local MRSA and *P. aeruginosa* risk factors when selecting antibiotic regimens.

■ The routine use of follow-up chest imaging is not recommended.

Introduction

In 2019, the American Thoracic Society (ATS) and Infectious Diseases Society of America (IDSA) released an update on their guidelines for community-acquired pneumonia (CAP) framed as a series of questions and answers.

QUESTION 1: In adults with CAP, should an initial sputum Gram stain and culture be obtained?
ANSWER: Do not obtain an initial sputum Gram stain and culture in the outpatient setting. In the inpatient setting, only obtain an initial sputum Gram stain and culture if treating patients with severe CAP or if they are at high risk for methicillin-resistant *Staphylococcus aureus* (MRSA) or a *Pseudomonas aeruginosa* infection.

QUESTION 2: In adults with CAP, should initial blood cultures be obtained?
ANSWER: Do not obtain initial blood cultures in the outpatient setting. In the inpatient setting, only obtain initial blood cultures if treating patients with severe CAP or patients at high risk for MRSA or a *P. aeruginosa* infection.

QUESTION 3: In adults with CAP, should initial *Legionella* and pneumococcal urinary antigen testing be performed?
ANSWER: Not unless patients have severe CAP or are at high risk for a *Legionella* infection.

QUESTION 4: In adults with CAP, should initial testing for the influenza virus be performed?
ANSWER: Yes, if influenza is present in the community at that time. A rapid molecular assay (eg, influenza nucleic acid amplification test) is recommended over a rapid antigen test.

QUESTION 5: In adults with CAP, should initial procalcitonin be used to withhold initiation of antibiotic treatment?
ANSWER: An initial serum procalcitonin level should not hinder the initiation of empiric antibiotic therapy.

QUESTION 6: Should a clinical prediction rule for prognosis plus clinical judgment versus clinical judgment alone be used to determine the disposition for adults with CAP?
ANSWER: Use validated tools — the Pneumonia Severity Index is preferred over the CURB-65 (a tool based on confusion, urea level, respiratory rate, blood pressure, and age ≥65 years) — to determine the need for hospitalization.

QUESTION 7: Should a clinical prediction rule for prognosis plus clinical judgment versus clinical judgment alone be used to determine floor versus ICU admission for adults with CAP?
ANSWER: All patients with hypotension who require pressors or need mechanical ventilation should be admitted to the ICU. Patients with severe CAP, as defined by the IDSA/ATS criteria and by clinical judgment, may qualify for a higher level of care (*Table 1*).

Critical Decisions in Emergency Medicine's literature review features articles from various reading lists, including the Academic Affairs Committee. Available online at acep.org/moc/llsa.

QUESTION 8: In the outpatient setting, which antibiotics are recommended for empiric treatment of CAP in adults?

ANSWER: In patients with no comorbidities, amoxicillin, doxycycline, *or* a macrolide (in areas with low pneumococcal macrolide resistance) may be used. In patients with comorbidities, a combination therapy of amoxicillin *and* clavulanate or a cephalosporin *and* a macrolide or doxycycline may be used. Additionally, monotherapy with a respiratory fluoroquinolone may be used.

QUESTION 9: In the inpatient setting, which antibiotic regimens are recommended for empiric treatment of CAP in adults without risk factors for MRSA and *P. aeruginosa*?

ANSWER: In nonsevere CAP, a combination therapy of a beta-lactam *and* a macrolide or a monotherapy with a respiratory fluoroquinolone may be used. Alternatively, a beta-lactam *and* doxycycline can be used. In severe CAP, a combination therapy of a beta-lactam *and* a macrolide or respiratory fluoroquinolone may be used.

QUESTION 10: In the inpatient setting, should patients with suspected aspiration pneumonia receive additional anaerobic coverage beyond standard empiric treatment for CAP?

ANSWER: Not unless empyema or a lung abscess is suspected.

QUESTION 11: In the inpatient setting, should adults with CAP and risk factors for MRSA or *P. aeruginosa* be treated with extended-spectrum antibiotic therapy instead of standard CAP regimens?

ANSWER: Use of the prior categorization of health care–associated pneumonia (HCAP) should no longer be used in the selection of extended antibiotic coverage. Empiric coverage should be based on locally validated risk factors. For MRSA coverage, vancomycin or linezolid is recommended. For *P. aeruginosa*, piperacillin-tazobactam, cefepime, ceftazidime, aztreonam, meropenem, or imipenem can be used.

QUESTION 12: In the inpatient setting, should adults with CAP be treated with corticosteroids?

ANSWER: Not typically. However, if patients have refractory septic shock, then steroids may be considered.

QUESTION 13: In adults with CAP who test positive for influenza, should the treatment regimen include antiviral therapy?
ANSWER: Yes.

Validated Definition Includes Either One Major Criterion or Three or More Minor Criteria
Minor criteria
Respiratory rate ≥30 breaths/min
PaO$_2$/FiO$_2$ ratio ≤250
Multilobar infiltrates
Confusion/disorientation
Uremia (blood urea nitrogen level ≥ 20 mg/dL)
Leukopenia* (white blood cell count < 4,000 cells/μL)
Thrombocytopenia (platelet count < 100,000/μL)
Hypothermia (core temperature < 36°C [96.8°F])
Hypotension requiring aggressive fluid resuscitation
Major criteria
Septic shock with need for vasopressors
Respiratory failure requiring mechanical ventilation
* Due to infection alone (ie, not chemotherapy induced)

TABLE 1. 2007 IDSA/ATS Criteria for Defining Severe CAP. Reprinted with permission of the American Thoracic Society. Copyright 2022 American Thoracic Society. All rights reserved. *Cite:* Metlay JP, Waterer GW, Long AC, et al. Diagnosis and treatment of adults with community-acquired pneumonia. an official clinical practice guideline of the American Thoracic Society and Infectious Diseases Society of America. *Am J Respir Crit Care Med.* 2019;200(7):e45-e67. The *American Journal of Respiratory and Critical Care Medicine* is an official journal of the American Thoracic Society.

QUESTION 14: In adults with CAP who test positive for influenza, should the treatment regimen include antibacterial therapy?

ANSWER: Yes.

QUESTION 15: In adults with CAP who are improving, what is the appropriate duration of antibiotic treatment?
ANSWER: Five days or until clinical stability is achieved, whichever is later.

QUESTION 16: In adults with CAP who are improving, should follow-up chest imaging be obtained?
ANSWER: If symptoms improve as expected, repeat imaging is usually unnecessary.

The Critical Procedure
Irrigation of the Eyes

By Steven J. Warrington, MD, MEd, MS
MercyOne Siouxland, Sioux City, Iowa

Objective

On completion of this article, you should be able to:
■ Use nasal cannulas to irrigate patients' eyes.

Introduction

Eye injuries and contaminations that require irrigation can occur with a variety of substances, and emergency physicians must consider multiple aspects of the procedure to help patients better tolerate eye irrigation.

Contraindications

■ Suspected globe perforation should prompt caution and a discussion with a specialist prior to irrigation.

Benefits and Risks

The benefit of eye irrigation depends on the situation, but the aim is often to prevent further damage and remove any foreign material. Aside from potentially causing corneal abrasions and discomfort, the procedure has relatively little risk associated with it.

Alternatives

The technique described in this article uses material and equipment readily available in most emergency departments. Emergency physicians should also keep in mind that commercial products are available, such as decontamination solutions for initial irrigation or balanced salt solutions for ongoing irrigation. Additionally, commercially available instruments may be used during irrigation.

Reducing Side Effects

Eye irrigation should not be delayed to await transport to the emergency department or to await setting up for formal irrigation. If patients are in a room in the emergency department, it may be wise to have them irrigate with tap water until a more formal irrigation setup is ready.

The following irrigation technique uses a nasal cannula over the bridge of the nose. Emergency physicians must ensure that the entire area, including under the eyelids, is irrigated and evaluated to prevent retained foreign bodies. Use gauze to lift and retract the lids to expose fornices and allow for focal irrigation and removal of any contaminants or foreign bodies.

Special Considerations

Irrigation of the eyes can cause anxiety and discomfort in patients. Aside from systemic therapies, multiple strategies can be employed to help patients better tolerate the procedure. Initial anesthetic drops can be placed in the eyes; anesthetic can also be mixed with a bag of normal saline. One recommendation is to use 10 mL of 1% lidocaine in a 1 L bag of saline that is being used for irrigation. Moreover, warmed fluids may be easier for patients to tolerate than room-temperature fluids. Using lactated ringers or adding bicarbonate to normal saline has also been done; however, results are inconclusive as to which approach is better at alleviating patient discomfort. Additionally, pH should be tested in cases of chemical exposure.

TECHNIQUE

1. **Obtain** materials and supplies and deliver them to the bedside.
2. **Evaluate** the eyes to rule out globe perforation.
3. **Anesthetize** the eyes (eg, with a drop of topical proparacaine).
4. **Consider** adding 10 mL of 1% lidocaine to a 1 L bag of warmed, normal saline.
5. **Spike** the saline bag with IV tubing and hook up the end of the IV tubing to the nasal cannula, which should allow the saline to flow out through the nasal prongs.
6. **Place** the nasal cannula over the bridge of the nose, allowing saline to flow out over both eyes.
7. **Retract** the upper and lower eyelids using gauze and ensure irrigation of the fornices. Consider sweeping the fornices with a cotton swab.
8. **Determine** if testing the pH after irrigation is warranted.
9. **Complete** the rest of the eye evaluation as indicated.

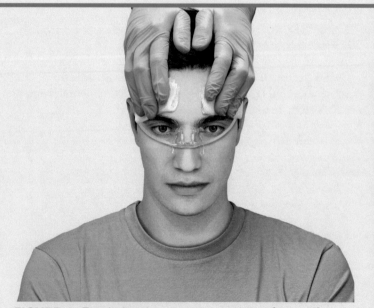

FIGURE 1. Eye irrigation setup using nasal cannula over the bridge of the nose

The Critical ECG

Accelerated Junctional Tachycardia

By Amal Mattu, MD, FACEP

Dr. Mattu is a professor, vice chair, and director of the Emergency Cardiology Fellowship in the Department of Emergency Medicine at the University of Maryland School of Medicine in Baltimore.

Objective

On completion of this article, you should be able to:

■ Recognize the ECG characteristics of accelerated junctional tachycardia.

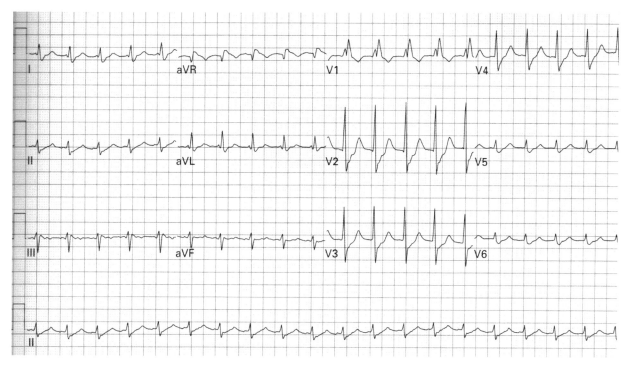

FIGURE 1. A 67-year-old man with palpitations

Accelerated junctional tachycardia, rate 115, bifascicular block (right bundle branch block [RBBB] and left anterior fascicular block [LAFB]), prolonged QT-interval (*Figure 1*). Subtle P waves are noted on the rhythm strip. However, the PR interval is too short (<120 msec) for normal sinus rhythm, unless an accessory pathway was present. (There is no evidence of an accessory pathway.) The most likely alternative cause of such a short PR interval is a junctional rhythm. A normal atrioventricular junctional rate is 40 to 60 beats/min; thus, this is referred to as an accelerated junctional tachycardia. An RBBB (QRS duration >120 msec, rSR′ pattern in lead V_1, wide S waves in the lateral leads) and LAFB (leftward axis, rS pattern in lead III and qR in I and aVL) are also present.

This patient was initially misdiagnosed as having sinus tachycardia. He was treated for several hours with intravenous fluids with the assumption that the tachycardia was due to hypovolemia. When his rate showed no evidence of improvement, the proper diagnosis was finally made. He then received a small dose of a beta-blocker medication and immediately converted to sinus rhythm with a rate of 75.

From Mattu A, Brady W. *ECGs for the Emergency Physician 2*. BMJ Publishing. Reprinted with permission.

Occult Talus Fracture

By John Kiel DO, MPH

Dr. Kiel is an assistant professor of emergency medicine and sports medicine at the University of Florida College of Medicine – Jacksonville

Objective

On completion of this article, you should be able to:

■ Recognize the need for advanced imaging in patients with traumatic ankle pain.

CASE PRESENTATION

A 44-year-old woman with a history of anxiety, depression, and tobacco use presents following a motor vehicle collision. She was restrained during the collision and denies loss of consciousness. Although she was initially ambulatory at the scene, pain in her ankle has progressively worsened despite oral narcotics. On examination, her right ankle is noted to be grossly edematous without any focal findings. She is neurovascularly intact. Initial x-rays do not identify any traumatic pathology (*Figures 1* and *2*). Because of her persistent and worsening pain, a CT of the ankle is obtained and shows a nondisplaced fracture through the neck and body of the talus with intra-articular extension (*Figure 3*).

Discussion

Talus fractures are relatively rare, representing around 3% to 5% of all foot and ankle fractures.[1] This injury typically occurs due to high-energy mechanisms such as falls from height or motor vehicle collisions. Occasionally, diagnosis is delayed when the talus fracture is due to a lower-energy mechanism and x-rays are normal. Associated injuries include other ipsilateral limb fractures and subtalar dislocations. Patients with talus fractures report ankle pain and an inability to bear weight. On physical examination, these patients often have bruising, swelling, reduced range of motion, and tenderness; they are frequently unable to perform a gait examination. Deformity may or may not be present.

Diagnostic evaluation can be tricky. X-rays of the ankle remain the imaging modality of choice and should be obtained prior to advanced imaging in virtually all cases. However, sensitivity is low at 74% but increases as displacement increases.[2] The Canale view can be used to optimize talus visualization, which involves the foot in maximal equinus and at 15° pronation and an x-ray beam that is at a 75° angle cranial from horizontal.

Once a talus fracture is known or suspected, CT remains the imaging modality of choice. When talus fractures are identified on x-rays, CT is useful for surgical planning and for assessing the degree of comminution and articular involvement. If x-rays do not reveal a talus fracture but suspicion still exists, CT should be obtained to confirm the diagnosis.

Unfortunately, patients with talus fractures are at high risk of complications, especially avascular necrosis (AVN). The risk of AVN correlates with the severity of the displacement of fragments or dislocation of joints. Both tibiotalar and subtalar dislocations greatly increase the risk of AVN. Other talus fracture complications include

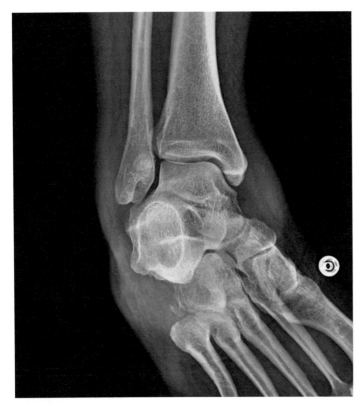

FIGURE 1. Mortise view of the ankle identifying no traumatic pathology

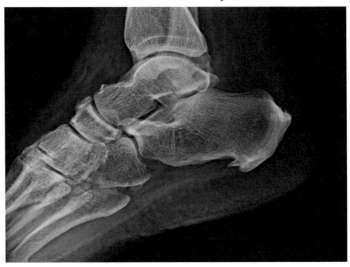

FIGURE 2. Lateral view of the ankle identifying no traumatic pathology

osteoarthritis (50%), infection (20%), and nonunion (5%-10%).[3] Nonoperative management can be considered in patients with nondisplaced body, head, or process fractures. However, because of the high morbidity associated with talus fractures, an orthopedic and podiatric specialist should be consulted before deciding to manage the fracture nonoperatively. In the emergency department, patients should be reduced and fitted with a posterior short-leg splint with or without a stirrup. If closed reduction cannot be achieved, emergent surgical intervention is indicated.

REFERENCES

1. Fournier A, Barba N, Steiger V, et al. Total talar fracture — long-term results of internal fixation of talar fractures. a multicentric study of 114 cases. *Orthop Traumatol Surg Res.* 2012;98(4)(suppl 1):S48-S55.

2. Dale JD, Ha AS, Chew FS. Update on talar fracture patterns: a large level I trauma center study. *AJR Am J Roentgenol.* 2013;201(5):1087-1092.

3. Dodd A, Lefaivre KA. Outcomes of talar neck fractures: a systematic review and meta-analysis. *J Orthop Trauma.* 2015;29(5):210-215.

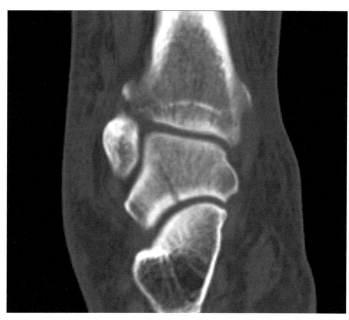

FIGURE 3. CT demonstrating a nondisplaced fracture through the body of the talus

CASE RESOLUTION

The patient was found to have a nondisplaced, intra-articular talus fracture. She was seen by podiatry who recommended a trial of nonoperative management and outpatient follow-up. She was placed in a well-padded posterior splint and made non–weight-bearing to that limb. Following discharge, the patient was subsequently lost to follow-up.

The Importance of Incidental Findings

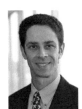

By Joshua S. Broder, MD, FACEP
Dr. Broder is a professor and the
residency program director in
the Department of Emergency
Medicine at Duke University
Medical Center in Durham,
North Carolina.

Objectives

On completion of this article, you should be able to:

■ Describe the importance of incidental findings on CT.

■ Recognize CT and chest x-ray findings of possible tuberculosis.

■ Outline next steps for patients with potential tuberculosis.

CASE PRESENTATION

A 50-year-old man presents by EMS after losing consciousness at a bus station. Bystanders reported that he had been drinking alcohol and fell, striking his head. His vital signs are BP 102/83, P 93, R 16, and T 36°C (96.8°F); SpO_2 is 96% on room air. The patient is awake and alert but appears intoxicated. A cervical collar is in place, and the patient has no obvious spinal step-offs or tenderness. His head examination shows no signs of trauma. He has normal cardiopulmonary and abdominal examinations and no focal neurologic deficits. The patient undergoes an evaluation including cervical spine CT, and the images are reviewed (*Figure 1*).

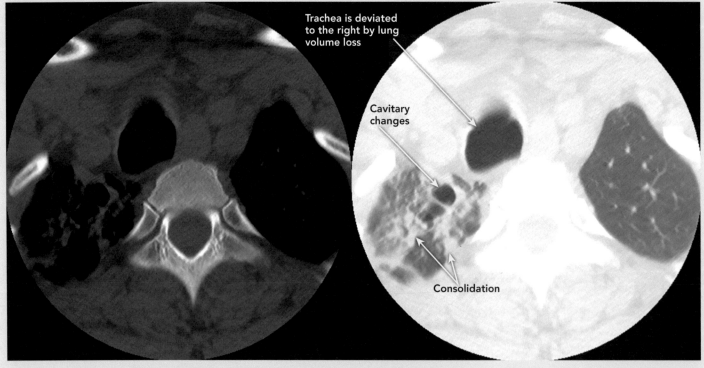

FIGURE 1. CT cervical spine (*left*, bone window; *right*, lung window). While no fractures are visible, incidental findings suggest tuberculosis. Normally a midline structure, the trachea deviates to the patient's right due to volume loss in the right lung. The right lung apex shows cavitary and consolidative changes. Findings are more obvious when the image is viewed using a lung window rather than the default bone window used when assessing the cervical spine for trauma.

Discussion

Incidental findings on cervical spine CT for trauma assessment are common, occurring in up to 28.3% of patients, but are included in radiology reports at low rates (2.9% in one study).[1,2] In a retrospective study, 33.4% of trauma CTs of the head, chest, and abdomen and pelvis had documented incidental findings, of which only 9.8% were reported to patients in written discharge materials.[3] The clinical significance of incidental findings varies widely from unimportant to highly relevant. Physicians can be held accountable for informing patients of incidental findings and referring them for appropriate follow-up care. The ACEP

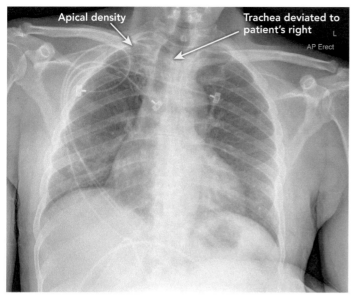

FIGURE 2. **Posterior-anterior chest x-ray.** Chest x-ray findings include tracheal deviation (indicating volume loss) and subtle increased density with cavitary abnormalities in the right lung apex, more clearly seen on the patient's CT.

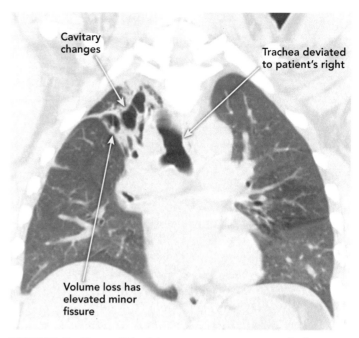

FIGURE 3. **Chest CT without contrast, coronal view, lung window.** Chest CT confirms findings seen on cervical spine CT and chest x-ray.

clinical policy on interpretation of diagnostic imaging tests calls for communication of incidental findings to patients.[4]

In 2021, 7,860 new tuberculosis (TB) cases were reported in the United States, with an incidence of 2.4 per 100,000.[5] Patients with suspected active TB should undergo chest x-ray as the initial imaging test, with CT generally reserved for patients with equivocal chest x-ray findings (*Figures 2* and *3*).[6]

While reporting requirements may vary by locality, the CDC recommends that all suspected or confirmed cases of TB be reported within 24 hours; penalties may apply for failure to report.[7] Even latent TB must be reported in some jurisdictions.[7]

The American College of Radiology Appropriateness Criteria Imaging of Possible Tuberculosis notes that apical cavitary disease is a high-risk feature that, when active tuberculosis is clinically suspected, warrants respiratory isolation pending sputum testing.[6] Patients should be assessed for signs and symptoms of active tuberculosis and risk factors for latent disease.

High-risk CT features that suggest active disease, which is confirmed by positive acid-fast bacilli (AFB) smears or a positive TB culture, include cavitation, apical or superior lobe consolidation, clustered tree-in-bud or miliary nodules, lymphadenopathy, and pleural effusion.[8] Scarring, which can cause lung volume loss and traction on adjacent structures, may be seen in previously treated inactive tuberculosis.[9]

REFERENCES

1. Beheshtian E, Sahraian S, Yousem DM, Khan MK. Incidental findings on cervical spine computed tomography scans: overlooked and unimportant? *Neuroradiology.* 2018;60(11):1175-1180.
2. Barboza R, Fox JH, Shaffer LE, Opalek JM, Farooki S. Incidental findings in the cervical spine at CT for trauma evaluation. *AJR Am J Roentgenol.* 2009;192(3):725-729.
3. Thompson RJ, Wojcik SM, Grant WD, Ko PY. Incidental findings on CT scans in the emergency department. *Emerg Med Int.* 2011;2011:624847.
4. American College of Emergency Physicians. Interpretation of diagnostic imaging tests. *Ann Emerg Med.* 2018;72(4):e51-e52.
5. Filardo TD, Feng PJ, Pratt RH, Price SF, Self JL. Tuberculosis — United States, 2021. *MMWR Morb Mortal Wkly Rep.* 2022;71(12):441-446.
6. Ravenel JG, Chung JH, Ackman JB, et al; Expert Panel on Thoracic Imaging. ACR Appropriateness Criteria® imaging of possible tuberculosis. *J Am Coll Radiol.* 2017;14(5)(suppl 1):S160-S165.
7. Menu of suggested provisions for state tuberculosis prevention and control laws. Centers for Disease Control and Prevention. 2012. Accessed August 25, 2022. https://www.cdc.gov/tb/programs/laws/menu/caseid.htm
8. Yeh JJ, Yu JKL, Teng WB, et al. High-resolution CT for identify patients with smear-positive, active pulmonary tuberculosis. *Eur J Radiol.* 2012;81(1):195-201.
9. Nachiappan AC, Rahbar K, Shi X, et al. Pulmonary tuberculosis: role of radiology in diagnosis and management. *Radiographics.* 2017;37(1):52-72.

CASE RESOLUTION

The patient was found to have undergone therapy for AFB-confirmed TB more than 15 years earlier but denied current signs or symptoms, although his ongoing alcohol use is a risk factor for reactivation. A report was filed with the local health department, and the patient was discharged with instructions for follow-up.

Feature Editor: Joshua S. Broder, MD, FACEP. See also *Diagnostic Imaging for the Emergency Physician* (Winner of the 2011 Prose Award in Clinical Medicine, the American Publishers Award for Professional and Scholarly Excellence) and *Critical Images in Emergency Medicine* by Dr. Broder.

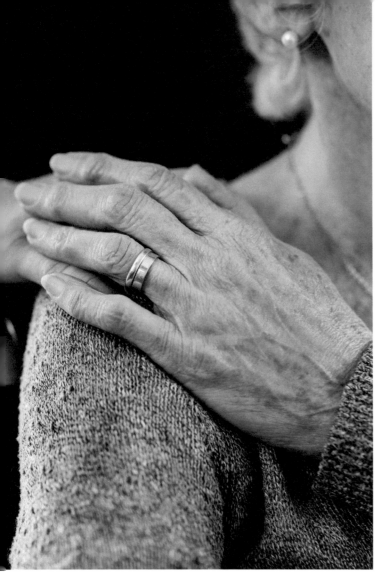

Old School

New Approaches to Geriatric Care

LESSON 18

By Nicole E. Cimino-Fiallos, MD, FACEP; and Danya Khoujah MBBS, MEHP, FACEP

Dr. Cimino-Fiallos is the assistant medical director of the Department of Emergency Medicine at Meritus Medical Center in Hagerstown, Maryland. Dr. Khoujah is an attending physician in the Department of Emergency Medicine at AdventHealth in Tampa, Florida. She is also a volunteer adjunct assistant professor in the Department of Emergency Medicine at the University of Maryland School of Medicine.

Reviewed by Nathaniel Mann, MD

Objectives

On completion of this lesson, you should be able to:

1. Discuss the vulnerability of older adults diagnosed with COVID-19 and prescribe effective prevention methods and treatments to decrease the likelihood of hospitalization and death.
2. List the unique challenges facing geriatric patients in the emergency department.
3. Recognize the shortcomings of current triage systems regarding geriatric patients.
4. Initiate simple emergency department improvements to enhance the care of older patients.
5. Identify strategies and resources to improve knowledge of best practices in geriatric emergency care.
6. Use evidence-based strategies for discharge planning for geriatric patients.

From the EM Model

20.0 Other Core Competencies of the Practice of Emergency Medicine
    20.4 Systems-Based Practice

CRITICAL DECISIONS

- What are the main differences between treating older adults and their younger counterparts for COVID-19?

- What are geriatric emergency departments, and are they needed?

- Are geriatric patients being triaged correctly?

- What interventions can make an emergency department more geriatric friendly, and do these interventions improve outcomes?

- How can safe discharge be used to minimize the likelihood that patients return or require hospitalization in the near future?

- How can physicians who are not specially trained in geriatrics boost their knowledge?

The recent pandemic has highlighted important differences in caring for older adults. This vulnerable patient population is more likely to require critical interventions and often uses more resources than younger patients. Learning more about how to care for geriatric patients can lead to improved morbidity and mortality and fewer unnecessary hospitalizations. Thus, all emergency department personnel should employ techniques to improve the quality of care delivered to aging patients.

CASE PRESENTATIONS

■ CASE ONE

A 76-year-old man presents with chest pain. He has had the pain for 3 days but was trying to avoid the emergency department because he feared COVID-19 exposure. His ECG shows new Q waves in the anterior leads and diffuse T-wave inversions. His case is discussed with the on-call cardiologist who reports that the patient's ECG does not meet the criteria for an emergent catheterization and that he should be managed medically. His troponin level is elevated. The patient is treated with nitroglycerin and aspirin. His chest pain improves, and he is admitted.

■ CASE TWO

A 75-year-old woman presents after a fall. She lost her balance on an escalator, falling approximately eight steps. She is taken to the local emergency department and reports neck and hip pain. She does not think she hit her head or lost consciousness. On arrival, her vital signs include BP 110/70, P 98, and R 20; SpO_2 is 98% on room air. She is afebrile. She appears uncomfortable, grimaces with range of motion of her left hip, and has some tenderness to her cervical spine. The rest of her examination is normal. She is evaluated, and x-rays of her neck and hip are ordered. The x-rays are unremarkable, the patient is discharged home with a prescription for acetaminophen, and she is wheeled to her son's car in the parking lot.

■ CASE THREE

A 67-year-old woman presents with shortness of breath. She requires 2 L of O_2 via nasal cannula to maintain an oxygen saturation above 90%. Her vital signs include BP 150/70, P 98, and R 24. X-ray shows bilateral patchy infiltrates suspicious for viral pneumonia. Her COVID-19 rapid antigen test is positive. The hospital is full, and the patient is healthy with a medical history of only hypertension. She is not vaccinated against COVID-19. She is discharged home with steroids, home oxygen, and a pulse oximeter to monitor her oxygen saturations.

Introduction

Patients older than 65 years are the fastest growing segment of the population, and accordingly, their visits to the emergency department and hospital admissions are on the rise.[1,2] Knowing how to care for older patients is critical to optimizing care, avoiding iatrogenic harm, decreasing morbidity and mortality, and avoiding unnecessary hospitalizations. Fellowships in geriatric emergency care and specially designated geriatric emergency departments are two approaches to enhancing the delivery of age-appropriate care to older patients; however, neither is common nor cheap. Reality mandates that all emergency physicians be cognizant of the differences in the care required for older patients. As generations age and the geriatric population expands, emergency departments must be able to accommodate the special needs of these unique patients. Simple changes to emergency department design, modification of the triage protocol, proper discharge planning, medication reconciliation, and targeted educational initiatives for emergency physicians and nurses can pay dividends to improve the quality of care delivered to older patients. New data also suggest that these investments improve outcomes and save the health care system money.[3]

CRITICAL DECISION

What are the main differences between treating older adults and their younger counterparts for COVID-19?

The global COVID-19 pandemic assaulted the world but ravaged the geriatric population. In 2022, older adults in the United States are still 5 to 10 times more likely to require hospitalization and 65 to 330 times more likely to die from COVID-19 than an 18-year-old patient.[4] The frailty syndrome that plagues older adults in other disease processes also increases their risks of morbidity and mortality from COVID-19.[5] Diagnosing this infection remains challenging, as some emergency departments and hospital systems are unable to perform universal testing of patients due to limitations on testing supplies.

Older adults may present atypically. Instead of the traditional symptoms of fever and cough, they may come to the emergency department with altered mental status or generalized weakness. Certain risk factors, in addition to age, seem to predict disease severity. A history of congestive heart failure or chronic obstructive pulmonary disease, the presence of delirium, a chest x-ray that shows more than two lobes of disease involvement, tachypnea, tachycardia, hypoxia, and a lack of vaccination for COVID-19 all increase the risk of worse outcomes in COVID-19 cases.

Thankfully, vaccinations against COVID-19 improve outcomes in geriatric patients. Older adults who receive both doses of a COVID-19 vaccine have a 94% reduced risk of COVID-19–related hospitalization.[6] Emergency physicians should consider offering COVID-19 vaccinations to older adults who may be unable to access them through more traditional avenues.[7]

Several medications are now in use for the treatment of COVID-19. Dexamethasone is used for the treatment of patients with hypoxia. The risks associated with steroid use in older adults include hyperglycemia, psychiatric effects, and susceptibility to other infections.[8] Remdesivir, an antiviral medication, reduces the time to clinical improvement for hospitalized patients but has shown no mortality benefit. It should be avoided in patients with advanced kidney disease (ie, a glomerular filtration rate <30). A combination of nirmatrelvir and ritonavir is a newer option for the treatment of COVID-19 in high-risk patients. It reduces the need for hospitalization but has numerous drug-drug interactions and requires renal dosing in patients with kidney dysfunction. Molnupiravir is another option for outpatient treatment and may prevent hospitalization in high-risk patients. The mortality benefit is, as yet, unclear.[9] By using these medications and appropriately risk stratifying patients, emergency physicians can reduce COVID-19 hospitalizations in older adults, improve outcomes, and decrease the strain on an overburdened health care system.

The effects of the pandemic are not strictly limited to those who are infected with the virus. According to one

Volume 36 Number 9: **September 2022** 23

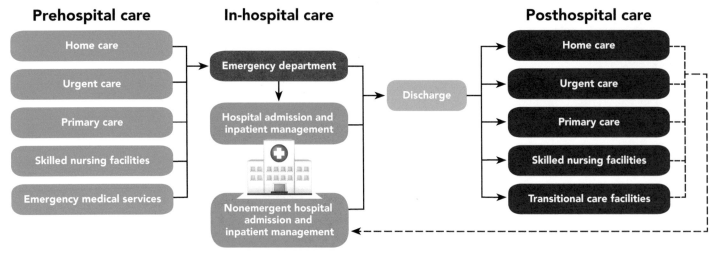

FIGURE 1. Emergency department management in the geriatric health care continuum

study, one-third of older US individuals delayed health care during the COVID-19 pandemic.[10] Rates of emergency department presentations for stroke, myocardial infarction, and traumatic injuries in older adults all decreased in the beginning of the pandemic.[11] Patients were also forced to defer preventative and elective care. It will take years to study the effects of these delays.

The physical and mental health effects of the restrictions of the COVID-19 pandemic on older adults are yet to be fully quantified. In the emergency department alone, the consequences of stringent visitor exclusion policies have been substantial. By classifying all visitors under one umbrella, hospital systems minimize the roles of family and caregivers who provide important medical information, orientation cues, and emotional support to geriatric patients and their health care teams. Family members and caregivers advocate on behalf of these patients and often act as surrogate decision makers. Family members and caregivers would have been especially valuable to have with patients in the emergency department during the pandemic because face masks potentially worsen patients' disorientation and miscommunication between patients and staff. Additionally, constrained staff limit the hospital's ability to attend to the needs of older and disabled patients. Preliminary data also suggest that these visitor restrictions had only a modest impact on transmission of the COVID-19 virus in emergency departments and that hospitals should be hesitant to reinstate these restrictions in future waves.[12]

CRITICAL DECISION

What are geriatric emergency departments, and are they needed?

In 2010, 15% of the 130 million people who visited emergency departments in the United States were older than 65 years.[1] Caring for older patients requires special attention because of the high rates of cognitive impairment, falls, functional impairment, depression, and long lists of home medications.[13] These patients have more emergent problems, need more diagnostic tests, and are more likely to be admitted to the hospital or ICU than any other age group.[14] Compared to the general population, visits to the emergency department are high-risk events that put geriatric patients at increased risk of medical errors, adverse drug interactions, and falls.[15]

Older patient visits to emergency departments have steadily increased, and the number of those admitted to the hospital has increased more than those who are discharged, with the use of ICU services almost doubling between 2001 and 2009.[2] These changes may indicate a more critically ill population or could be due to overutilization of services. There are dangers to hospitalization, including delirium, hospital-acquired infections, falls, iatrogenic complications, and loss of functional status. With Medicare deducting reimbursements for iatrogenic complications such as catheter and wound infections, the incentive to take better care of admitted older patients now has a financial aspect.[16]

Geriatric patients also require more services after discharge to prevent medical recidivism (*Figure 1*). Even if the services they require are provided, they are still at higher risk of bouncing back to the emergency department and requiring readmission than their younger counterparts.[17]

Functional problems and geriatric syndromes affect most patients older than 75 years. Approximately half are dependent on others in one or more aspects of personal activities of daily living. Up to two-thirds of emergent patients in this age group require assistive care. About a quarter of older patients seen in the emergency department exhibit one form of cognitive impairment, and half cannot walk unsupervised.[18]

The unique challenges facing this population and the success of prior initiatives that focused on disease entities, such as stroke care, or patient populations, such as pediatrics, have contributed to the birth of the concept of geriatric emergency departments. These facilities are designed with the older patient in mind. A safer layout, specially trained staff, case managers, and applicable protocols are in place to improve safety, decrease admissions, optimize discharges, and decrease moribund outcomes.[16,19] They are focused not only on chief complaints, but also on approaching the older patient as a whole and addressing comorbidities such as depression, cognitive impairment, and medication interactions. Geriatric-focused emergency departments have been associated with a decreased rate of hospital admission and a reduction in costs to the health care system.[3,15,19]

CRITICAL DECISION

Are geriatric patients being triaged correctly?

The most common triage system used in the United States is based on the Emergency Severity Index (ESI), which risk stratifies patients according to the severity of their presentation and how quickly they should be seen.[20] In a study by Baumann et al that specifically looked at the older patient population, the third iteration of the ESI algorithm (ESI-3) demonstrated validity because it correlates with hospitalization, length of stay, resource utilization, and survival.[21] This is important from a patient safety standpoint because it ensures that sicker patients are seen first; however, when addressing individual outcomes in older patients, the ESI has many shortcomings. Its dependence on vital signs makes it less sensitive; vital signs can be deceptively normal in older patients.[22] Specifically, a trigger for the "danger zone" in the ESI is a heart rate of 100 beats/min, but tachycardia is not easily mounted by older patients. In addition, altered mental status or "disorientation" warrants a higher acuity triage level, yet delirium is frequently missed on evaluation of older patients.[23] Older adults without grossly abnormal vital signs, nonfocal complaints, or atypical presentations, or those with dementia or other cognitive disorders, can easily be assigned to lower triage acuities.[24] Under-triage leads to increased wait times and worsened outcomes, a more negative patient experience, "discomfort, nervousness, mistrust, and confusion," and feelings of abandonment and anxiety.[25,26]

These challenges have led many experts to propose geriatric-specific modifications to the ESI by increasing the sensitivity of vital signs and level of consciousness, which follows the logic of pediatric-specific parameters (*Table 1*). Research is still required to test this approach. Another important intervention is to encourage the involvement of a family member or caretaker in the process, especially for patients who are cognitively impaired.[16]

Even when geriatric patients are triaged appropriately, they are less likely to be seen within the appropriate time frame for their assigned urgency.[27] It is unclear why older patients wait longer for care, even though they are likely to be sicker and to require admission and critical care.

An area of robust interest is triage for trauma patients. As injuries to older people increase, so do their morbidity and mortality. These increases are not limited to major traumatic injuries; they also occur among people with seemingly minor injuries, such as after falls. One obvious reason for the twofold to fivefold increase in mortality in this population is their abundance of comorbidities. Under-triage becomes an additional complicating factor.[28] An estimated one-third of older trauma patients are under-triaged, with the rate climbing to almost 60% of patients aged 90 years and older, negatively affecting mortality rates and costs.[28, 29] A unique initiative in Ohio started in 2009 used an evidence-based triage protocol in the field for injured patients older than 70 years to determine destination, using lower thresholds for transfer to a trauma center. This protocol improved the sensitivity of identifying the severity of injury and increased the proportion of individuals discharged home, but it failed to change the mortality rate.[29,30]

CRITICAL DECISION

What interventions can make an emergency department more geriatric friendly, and do these interventions improve outcomes?

Triage

In addition to traditional triage and emergent care, emergency department visits are used as opportunities to screen patients for a variety of conditions (eg, depression, suicide, abuse, and substance abuse) and direct them toward appropriate resources. When assessing older patients, consideration should be given to identifying those at high risk of an adverse event after discharge, such as readmission, a repeat emergency visit, institutionalization, functional decline, or death. This awareness focuses the use of time, personnel, and resources, which are hot commodities in this era of decreased federal funding for health care.[16]

A meta-analysis by Carpenter et al evaluated a variety of screening tools for their ability to identify at-risk patients during triage and thereby improve care through targeted management (*Table 2*).[31] By definition, screening tools should be sensitive, have a good negative predictive value, and be simple and reproducible. Unfortunately, none of the screening tools evaluated in this review yielded "compelling evidence" to justify recommendation of their use.[31,32] A review article by Graf et al evaluated a targeted screening process, where geriatric patients underwent a brief evaluation to identify high-risk patients.[32] These patients then underwent a comprehensive geriatric assessment. In this review, there was evidence to support this two-step screening process to identify at-risk patients in need of further intervention and to decrease emergency department readmissions.[32] Given the lack of statistical evidence, the authors of the Carpenter review could not advocate for any specific screening test; however, they did emphasize the need for a focused, evidence-based screening tool that can identify high-risk populations at the time of triage and influence management decisions, consistent with the Geriatric Emergency Department Guidelines.[16,31]

Physical Environment

Building a geriatric emergency department with amenities specifically designed to accommodate older patients may seem like a fantasy for many physicians. Not all changes, however, require a large amount of money or a contractor (*Table 3*). When asked

Screening Tools
• Identification of Seniors at Risk (ISAR)
• Triage Risk Screening Tool (TRST)
• Silver Code
• Variables Indicative of Placement (VIP) risk
• Mortality Risk Index
• Rowland questionnaire
• Runciman questionnaire
• Score Hospitalier d'Evaluation du Risque de Perte d'Autonomie (SHERPA)

TABLE 2. Tools used in emergency departments to risk stratify older patients according to risk of short-term adverse outcomes

Vital Sign	Current Abnormal Threshold	Proposed Threshold
Heart Rate	>100 bpm	>90 bpm
Blood Pressure	<90 mm Hg	<110 mm Hg
Temperature	>38°C (100.4°F) oral	>37.4°C (99.3°F) oral

TABLE 1. Suggested thresholds for vital signs in older patients

what they would like to see in an emergency department, older patients reported that they wanted to see their independence, mobility, and safety prioritized.[32] Ideally, the hallways should be clear from clutter and easily accessible by someone using a walker or wheelchair. Handrails should be installed, and signage with easy-to-read graphics should be clearly visible to direct patients to amenities like the bathroom, waiting room, and exit to parking. Orientation aids in each patient's room should include an easy-to-read clock and a sign denoting the date and day of the week, especially for patients at high risk of delirium.[33]

Improved lighting is a simple way to decrease the risk of adverse events such as falls and delirium; older adults require three times as much light as younger adults for visual clarity. Patients should be able to control the light in their room, including turning off the lights at night, which lessens disruption to their circadian rhythm and subsequently the risk of delirium. Indirect light is preferred to spot lighting, which increases glare and makes it more difficult for older people to see.[16]

Older patients are at significant risk of falls. Some interventions such as fall-risk bracelets have failed to improve outcomes; others may decrease this risk and should be implemented. Beds should be kept at low levels to allow patients to stand more easily. Bed rails should not be used because they do not reduce fall risk and actually increase the risk of injury if the patient does fall.[16] Elevated doorway thresholds should be removed. Uneven walking surfaces, textured tiles, rugs, and carpets should be avoided. Reducing the number of patient transfers during the emergency department visit also decreases the risk of falls.[16] Bedside radiologic studies and portable laboratory equipment for bedside blood draws limits the number of transports and decreases the risk of disorientation by keeping the patients in one treatment space for their entire stay.[16]

Geriatric patients are at high risk of skin breakdown while in the hospital. Some simple changes in practice can reduce this risk. The use of medical tape and adhesive should be limited because they can injure frail skin.[15] Extra-thick, soft mattresses are usually available in the hospital and should be requested for geriatric patients expected to have extended stays. Patients should be given the option of using a soft reclining chair instead of a stretcher if it does not interfere with their treatment. Other furniture choices should consider ease of cleaning and softness to protect fragile skin.

Geriatric delirium in the emergency department is common and may have an iatrogenic component. Interventions that can decrease the risk of delirium include frequently orienting patients to the time and place using signs or sitters, avoiding unnecessary tethering in the form of monitor leads or urinary catheters, and turning the lights off in patients' rooms at night.[16] Patients should be encouraged to use their glasses and hearing aids to help them remain oriented and engaged.

Staffing

Polypharmacy is prevalent in older patients, making them prone to medication errors, adverse events, and drug interactions. In addition, given the physiologic changes and comorbidities typical among older patients, some medications have been deemed inappropriate for this age group and have been identified in several initiatives (eg, Beers Criteria, the Screening Tool of Older Persons' Prescriptions [STOPP]).[34,35] Subsequently, emergency department pharmacists may play a significant role

in addressing this population and improving outcomes. Shaw et al reported that an emergency department–based pharmacist or clinical pharmacy specialist often identified at least one medication-related problem in almost half of older patients.[36] However, the presence of a pharmacist was not associated with improved clinical outcomes in previous studies.[36]

Many emergency departments have limited budgets and staff but may have access to a plethora of hospital volunteers. Engaging this supplemental workforce to improve geriatric outcomes can pay off with improved patient experiences. On patient satisfaction surveys, many older adults report not receiving enough attention and reassurance in the emergency department. They describe the emergency department as busy and chaotic and that their basic needs, such as being hungry or needing to use the toilet, are not addressed sufficiently. A robust volunteer service could fill many of these gaps and support a strained emergency department staff.[33]

Patient Care Initiatives

Several aspects of geriatric patient care should be addressed specifically during the care of every older patient in the emergency department. For example, delirium screening can be effective in decreasing in-hospital morbidity and can detect patients at heightened risk of death, thereby prompting appropriate interventions. When physicians do not use a dedicated screening tool, they miss the diagnosis of delirium more than 50% of the time.[37] Although the Mini-Mental Status Exam (MMSE) is cumbersome and unsuitable for the emergency department, alternatives include the Quick Confusion Scale, Brief Confusion Assessment Method (bCAM), and Modified Richmond Agitation and Sedation Scale (mRASS). These tests are more feasible for use in the emergency department because each should take less than 1 minute to administer. The Quick Confusion Scale is a shorter version of the MMSE and is the test with the best performance to time.[32] The bCAM is derived from the Confusion

Physical Environment
Handrails
Clutter-free hallways
Large clocks
Signage indicating date
Ambient light
Lower-level beds
Even walking surfaces
Bedside interventions
Avoidance of medical tape
Thick, soft mattresses

Staffing
Pharmacists
Volunteers
Social workers or case managers
Physical therapists

Patient Care Initiatives
Frailty assessment
Delirium detection
Pain management
Palliative care

TABLE 3. Interventions that improve outcomes for geriatric patients in emergency departments

Assessment Method (CAM), which is used in ICUs for detection of delirium.

Undertreatment of pain is also a common problem for geriatric patients. In fact, a study by Platts-Mills et al showed that older patients are 20% less likely than younger patients to receive any pain medications.[38] This difference probably stems from concerns about the use of narcotics in older patients. Alternatives to narcotics for pain management, such as acetaminophen, topical treatments (such as lidocaine patches), and nerve blocks, should be considered. The use of low-dose narcotics, with titration, is safe in older patients; however, increased bioavailability and medication interactions in this population must be factored into dosing decisions. Finally, uncontrolled pain, especially after an injury, increases the risk of delirium in susceptible patients and is frequently associated with functional decline, disability, and an increased risk of falls.

Introducing the concept of palliative care early and correctly is essential in the care of all patients, but especially in those with multiple comorbidities. Palliative care and hospice care are not the same. Palliative care is interdisciplinary care focused on improving the quality of life for patients of any age (and their families) who are living with significant pain or serious illness. By contrast, hospice care provides palliative care to dying patients in their final months of life. Clarifying this distinction is important because it enables patients and their families to accept a referral to palliative care if appropriate, improving the quality of life for the patient, reducing hospital stays, and decreasing costs.[39]

CRITICAL DECISION

How can safe discharge be used to minimize the likelihood that patients return or require hospitalization in the near future?

Before discharging geriatric patients from the emergency department, consider this: "Up to 80% of older people discharged from an [emergency department] have at least one unrecognized geriatric problem such as delirium, dementia, depression, undernutrition, or unmet social service needs."[40] Remembering to look for insidious diagnoses prior to discharging an older patient is an important part of designing a safe discharge plan.

A multidisciplinary approach is necessary for a safe discharge and can improve outcomes: An emergency department pharmacist should review the medication list; a geriatric life specialist should conduct screenings for depression, neglect, abuse, and other geriatric-specific topics; a social worker should create a safety plan; and a physical therapist should assess the patient's needs.[15] Kelley et al noted that one barrier to the safe discharge of older patients from the emergency department is the limited availability of ancillary staff, such as social workers, who typically work during usual business hours. Expanding the resources that are already in place can improve the discharge process.

Prior to discharge, a few things must be addressed. One is the patient's mobility, which affects safety and fall risk at home.[16] Interestingly, older adults overestimate their ability to perform simple tasks — specifically, getting out of bed, walking 10 feet, and then returning to bed — up to 20% of the time, and even more so if they are dependent on a walking device. Therefore, a member of the emergency care team should directly observe the patient's mobility prior to discharge. The timed Get Up and Go Test is used in inpatient settings and emergency departments as a predictor of return visits and hospitalizations.[41]

The importance of discharge protocols that enhance communication between the emergency team and outpatient care has been acknowledged by various specialty societies.[16] However, McCusker et al found that communication between community physicians and emergency physicians is infrequent and that telephone follow-up after discharge is rare.[42] As expressed in the Geriatric Emergency Department Guidelines, personnel should contact patients' outpatient care teams to solidify a follow-up plan and to relay information about the complaints that brought them to the emergency department, available test results, treatments administered, patients' responses to treatment, consultations obtained, discharge diagnoses, and new prescriptions.[16] The discharge instructions handed to geriatric patients should be in a large font; as applicable, they can be shared with family members in accordance with the parameters of HIPAA.

Emergency department personnel can improve the discharge experience by providing additional information about geriatric topics to patients and their families. Topics that were popular in a geriatric patient survey included information about advance care directives, elder services in the community, and how to create a list of medications.[33] If written in layman's terms in an easy-to-read style, patients often appreciate this relevant information.

The most appropriate disposition for a patient may not be to the place they left to come to the emergency department. For example, a patient coming from home might be better served by entering hospice or an assisted living facility. Other placement considerations should include the need for rehabilitation or observation.[15]

If a patient is discharged home, follow-up phone calls can play a significant role in reducing the likelihood of bounce backs and improving outcomes. In a study by Aldeen and associates, nurses with training in geriatric emergency medicine made follow-up calls 1 to 3 days after discharge and again at 10 to 14 days after discharge.[43] The calls aimed to assess pain, answer medication questions, confirm the scheduling of outpatient follow-up appointments, and inquire about home health care status. Rates of return visits within 3 days and hospital admissions were lower in the group that received the follow-up consultation. Follow-up

✔ Pearls

- "Bounce back" visits can be reduced by making follow-up phone calls to high-risk older patients.
- Therapies to treat COVID-19 exist to improve outcomes in older adults.
- Patients want more information about advance care directives, elder services in the community, and the compilation of medication lists; therefore, this material should be included in standard discharge paperwork.
- Making small physical changes to the emergency department (eg, placing a clock with large numerals in each room) can help prevent complications like delirium.
- Educational resources for staff about caring for geriatric patients are readily available.

phone calls are a cheap and easy way to reduce expensive admissions and returns to the emergency department.

CRITICAL DECISION

How can physicians who are not specially trained in geriatrics boost their knowledge?

In a perfect geriatric emergency department, the physicians would be fellowship-trained geriatric emergency physicians with a support staff that includes geriatric life specialists and nurses with special training in elder care.[15] These expectations are unrealistic for most emergency departments, but physicians and nurses can pursue education in geriatric topics with minimal extra effort. In surveys about the care given to geriatric patients, physicians reported moral angst about the quality of care and cited lack of education as a main reason for their discomfort.[33]

When surveyed about their comfort level in caring for geriatric patients in the emergency department, staff cited a need for education and training on geriatric-specific issues such as health problems that come with aging, communication with older patients, elder abuse, and cultural sensitivity.[33] They also wanted to learn more about managing patients with dementia and about responding to confusion, aggression, and agitation appropriately.[33] Some other topics that might benefit an emergency department staff with an interest in improving geriatric care include living wills and available community services.

The Geriatric Emergency Department Guidelines are presented as a consensus document of the American College of Emergency Physicians, American Geriatrics Society, Emergency Nurses Association, and Society for Academic Emergency Medicine. They are not a mandate or requirement, but they provide evidence-based material that is relevant to the daily care of geriatric patients in the emergency department. Topics include atypical presentations of disease, pain management and palliative care, effects of comorbid conditions on current presentation, common complaints that prompt older patients to seek care, and the logistics of making an emergency department more geriatric friendly. These high-yield topics can help physicians target areas where geriatric patients suffer delays in diagnosis or worse outcomes than their younger counterparts.

✖ Pitfalls

- Failing to recognize that even when appropriately triaged, older patients are still more likely to wait longer than is appropriate given their acuity level.
- Failing to recognize that 80% of older patients have delirium, dementia, depression, under-nutrition, or unmet social service needs at the time of discharge.
- Neglecting to sufficiently treat geriatric patients' pain or to educate them on quality-of-life services, such as palliative care.
- Overlooking the need to beware of medication interaction or the need for renal dosing when prescribing medications for COVID-19.

Summary

Older patients require careful consideration. They are at high risk of complications and have increased morbidity and mortality compared to other patient groups. While not all hospitals can afford to create dedicated geriatric emergency departments, physicians can make small changes to their existing departments and focus on continuing medical education in this field to improve the experience and outcomes of vulnerable geriatric patients.

REFERENCES

1. National Center for Health Statistics. Health, United States, 2014: with special features on adults aged 55-64. U.S. Department of Health and Human Services. 2014. http://www.cdc.gov/nchs/data/hus/hus14.pdf#086
2. Pines JM, Mullins PM, Cooper JK, Feng LB, Roth KE. National trends in emergency department use, care patterns, and quality of care of older adults in the United States. J Am Geriatr Soc. 2013;61(1):12-17.
3. Hwang U, Dresden SM, Vargas-Torres C, et al. Association of a geriatric emergency department innovation program with cost outcomes among Medicare beneficiaries. JAMA Netw Open. 2021;4(3):e2037334.
4. Risk for COVID-19 infection, hospitalization, and death by age group. Centers for Disease Control and Prevention. Accessed July 6, 2022. https://www.cdc.gov/coronavirus/2019-ncov/covid-data/investigations-discovery/hospitalization-death-by-age.html
5. Prendki V, Tiseo G, Falcone M; ESCMID Study Group for Infections in the Elderly. Caring for older adults during the COVID-19 pandemic. Clin Microbiol Infect. 2022;28(6):785-791.
6. COVID-19 risks and vaccine information for older adults. Centers for Disease Control and Prevention. Accessed August 5, 2022. https://www.cdc.gov/aging/covid19/covid19-older-adults.html
7. Waxman MJ, Moschella P, Duber HC, et al. Emergency department-based COVID-19 vaccination: where do we stand? Acad Emerg Med. 2021;28(6):707-709.
8. Jung C, Wernly B, Fjölner J, et al. Steroid use in elderly critically ill COVID-19 patients. Eur Respir J. 2021;58(4):2100979.
9. Wen W, Chen C, Tang J, et al. Efficacy and safety of three new oral antiviral treatment (molnupiravir, fluvoxamine and Paxlovid) for COVID-19: a meta-analysis. Ann Med. 2022;54(1):516-523.
10. Na L. Characteristics of community-dwelling older individuals who delayed care during the COVID-19 pandemic. Arch of Gerontol Geriatr. 2022;101:104710.
11. Mitra B, Mitchell RD, Cloud GC, et al. Presentations of stroke and acute myocardial infarction in the first 28 days following the introduction of state of emergency restrictions for COVID-19. Emerg Med Australas. 2020;32(6):1040-1045.
12. Lo AX, Wedel LK, Liu SW, et al. COVID-19 hospital and emergency department visitor policies in the United States: impact on persons with cognitive or physical impairment or receiving end-of-life care. J Am Coll Emerg Physicians Open. 2022;3(1):e12622.
13. Hwang U, Shah MN, Han JH, Carpenter CR, Siu AL, Adams JG. Transforming emergency care for older adults. Health Aff (Millwood). 2013;32(12):2116-2121.
14. Platts-Mills TF, Glickman SW. Measuring the value of a senior emergency department: making sense of health outcomes and health costs. Ann Emerg Med. 2014;63(5):525-527.
15. Burton J, Young J, Bernier C. The geriatric ED: structure, patient care, and considerations for the emergency department geriatric unit. Int J Gerontol. 2014;8(2):56-59.
16. American College of Emergency Physicians; American Geriatric Society; Emergency Nurses Association; Society of Academic Emergency Medicine; Geriatric Emergency Department Guidelines Task Force. Geriatric emergency department guidelines. Ann Emerg Med. 2014;63(5):e7-e25. https://www.acep.org/globalassets/uploads/uploaded-files/acep/clinical-and-practice-management/resources/geriatrics/geri_ed_guidelines_final.pdf
17. Di Bari M, Salvi F, Roberts AT, et al. Prognostic stratification of elderly patients in the emergency department: a comparison between the "Identification of Seniors at Risk" and the "Silver Code." J Gerontol A Biol Sci Med Sci. 2011;67(5):544-550.
18. Gray LC, Peel NM, Costa AP, et al. Profiles of older patients in the emergency department: findings from the interRAI Multinational Emergency Department Study. Ann Emerg Med. 2013;62(5):467-474.

CASE RESOLUTIONS

CASE ONE

The patient's care was delayed because of his fear of a COVID-19 exposure in the emergency department. He was started on a heparin drip, and his serial troponin measurements trended up. He was taken for a nonemergent catheterization and was found to have a proximal left anterior descending artery occlusion. After stenting, his ECG showed anterior wall hypokinesis and an ejection fraction of 25%.

CASE TWO

This patient should have met the criteria for transfer to a trauma center. CT is the test of choice for an evaluation of the cervical spine in older adults, and the patient was at risk of a missed diagnosis. Older adults are also at higher risk of ligamentous injuries and need a thorough examination, including gait, reflex, and sensory testing to rule out spinal cord pathologies. The patient did not ambulate prior to discharge. She returned 2 days later with a report of persistent hip pain and an inability to bear weight on her leg. MRI revealed an occult hip fracture, and she ultimately required surgical repair.

CASE THREE

When the patient returned home, her shortness of breath worsened, but she could not find her glasses. Thus, she could not read her discharge instructions and was unsure about when to return to the hospital. She called her primary care physician who recommended she return to the emergency department. She was admitted to the hospital with hypoxia and treated with a high-flow nasal cannula and intravenous dexamethasone and remdesivir. She was discharged to a rehabilitation and skilled nursing facility 5 days later.

19. Keyes DC, Singal B, Kropf C, Fisk A. Impact of a new senior emergency department on emergency department recidivism, rate of hospital admission, and hospital length of stay. *Ann Emerg Med.* 2014;63(5):517-524.

20. Gilboy N, Tananbe P, Travers D, Rosenau AM. Emergency Severity Index (ESI): a triage tool for emergency department care, version 4. EMSC Innovation and Improvement Center. 2012. Accessed August 11, 2022. https://media.emscimprovement.center/documents/ESI_Handbook2125.pdf

21. Baumann MR, Strout TD. Triage of geriatric patients in the emergency department: validity and survival with the Emergency Severity Index. *Ann Emerg Med.* 2007;49(2):234-240.

22. Platts-Mills TF, Travers D, Biese K, et al. Accuracy of the Emergency Severity Index triage instrument for identifying elder emergency department patients receiving an immediate life-saving intervention. *Acad Emerg Med.* 2010;17(3):238-243.

23. Han JH, Zimmerman EE, Cutler N, et al. Delirium in older emergency department patients: recognition, risk factors, and psychomotor subtypes. *Acad Emerg Med.* 2009;16(3):193-200.

24. Tucker G, Clark NK, Abraham I. Enhancing ED triage to accommodate the special needs of geriatric patients. *J Emerg Nurs.* 2013;39(3):309-314.

25. Guttmann A, Schull MJ, Vermeulen MJ, Stukel TA. Association between waiting times and short term mortality and hospital admission after departure from emergency department: population based cohort study from Ontario, Canada. *BMJ.* 2011;342:d2983.

26. Shankar KN, Bhatia BK, Schuur JD. Toward patient-centered care: a systematic review of older adults' views of quality emergency care. *Ann Emerg Med.* 2014;63(5):529-550.e1.

27. Freund Y, Vincent-Cassy C, Bloom B, Riou B, Ray P; APHP Emergency Database Study Group. Association between age older than 75 years and exceeded target waiting times in the emergency department: a multicenter cross-sectional survey in the Paris metropolitan area, France. *Ann Emerg Med.* 2013;62(5):449-456.

28. Staudenmayer KL, Hsia RY, Mann NC, Spain DA, Newgard CD. Triage of elderly trauma patients: a population-based perspective. *J Am Coll Surg.* 2013;217(4):569-576.

29. Ichwan B, Darbha S, Shah MN, et al. Geriatric-specific triage criteria are more sensitive than standard adult criteria in identifying need for trauma center care in injured older adults. *Ann Emerg Med.* 2015;65(1):92-100.e3.

30. Caterino JM, Brown NV, Hamilton MW, et al. Effect of geriatric-specific trauma triage criteria on outcomes in injured older adults: a statewide retrospective cohort study. *J Am Geriatr Soc.* 2016;64(10):1944-1951.

31. Carpenter CR, Shelton E, Fowler S, et al. Risk factors and screening instruments to predict adverse outcomes for undifferentiated older emergency department patients: a systematic review and meta-analysis. *Acad Emerg Med.* 2015;22(1):1-21.

32. Graf CE, Zekry D, Giannelli S, Michel JP, Chevalley T. Efficiency and applicability of comprehensive geriatric assessment in the emergency department: a systematic review. *Aging Clin Exp Res.* 2011;23(4):244-254.

33. Kelley ML, Parke B, Jokinen N, Stones M, Renaud D. Senior-friendly emergency department care: an environmental assessment. *J Health Serv Res Policy.* 2011;16(1):6-12.

34. American Geriatrics Society 2015 Beers Criteria Update Expert Panel. American Geriatrics Society 2015 updated Beers criteria for potentially inappropriate medication use in older adults. *J Am Geriatr Soc.* 2015;63(11):2227-2246.

35. O'Mahony D, O'Sullivan D, Byrne S, O'Connor MN, Ryan C, Gallagher P. STOPP/START criteria for potentially inappropriate prescribing in older people: version 2. *Age Ageing* 2015;44(2):213-218.

36. Shaw PB, Delate T, Lyman A Jr, et al. Impact of a clinical pharmacy specialist in an emergency department for seniors. *Ann Emerg Med.* 2016;67(2):177-188.

37. Han JH, Wilson A, Vasilevskis EE, et al. Diagnosing delirium in older emergency department patients: validity and reliability of the delirium triage screen and the brief confusion assessment method. *Ann Emerg Med.* 2013;62(5):457-465.

38. Platts-Mills TF, Esserman DA, Brown DL, Bortsov AV, Sloane PD, McLean SA. Older US emergency department patients are less likely to receive pain medication than younger patients: results from a national survey. *Ann Emerg Med.* 2012;60(2):199-206.

39. Kahn JH, Magauran BG Jr, Olshaker JS, Shankar KN. Current trends in geriatric emergency medicine. *Emerg Med Clin North Am.* 2016;34(3):435-452.

40. Rosted E, Wagner L, Hendriksen C, Poulsen I. Geriatric nursing assessment and intervention in an emergency department: a pilot study. *Int J Older People Nurs.* 2012;7(2):141-151.

41. Roedersheimer KM, Pereira GF, Jones CW, Braz VA, Mangipudi SA, Platts-Mills, TM. Self-reported versus performance-based assessments of a simple mobility task among older adults in the emergency department. *Ann Emerg Med.* 2016;67(2):151-156.

42. McCusker J, Verdon J, Vadeboncoeur A, et al. The elder-friendly emergency department assessment tool: development of a quality assessment tool for emergency department-based geriatric care. *J Am Geriatr Soc.* 2012;60(8):1534-1539.

43. Aldeen AZ, Courtney DM, Lindquist LA, Dresden SM, Gravenor SJ. Geriatric emergency department innovations: preliminary data for the geriatric nurse liaison model. *J Am Geriatr Soc.* 2014;62(9):1781-1785.

ADDITIONAL READING

Caplan GA, Williams AJ, Daly B, Abraham K. A randomized, controlled trial of comprehensive geriatric assessment and multidisciplinary intervention after discharge of elderly from the emergency department — The DEED II study. *J Am Geriatr Soc.* 2004;52(9):1417-1423.

Carpenter C, Bromley M, Caterino JM, et al. Optimal older adult emergency care: introducing multidisciplinary geriatric emergency department guidelines from the American College of Emergency Physicians, American Geriatrics Society, Emergency Nurses Association, and Society for Academic Emergency Medicine. *J Am Geriatr Soc.* 2014;62(7):1360-1363.

Carpenter CR, Dresden SM, Shah MN, Hwang U. Adapting emergency care for persons living with dementia. GEAR Network. Accessed August 22, 2022. https://gearnetwork.org/2022/08/10/adapting-emergency-care-for-persons-living-with-dementia/

Rosenberg M, Rosenberg L. The geriatric emergency department. *Emerg Med Clin North Am.* 2016;34(3):629-648.

Samaras N, Chevalley T, Samaras D, Gold G. Older patients in the emergency department: a review. *Ann Emerg Med.* 2010;56(3):261-269.

CME Questions

Reviewed by Wan-Tsu Chang, MD; and Nathaniel Mann, MD

Qualified, paid subscribers to *Critical Decisions in Emergency Medicine* may receive CME certificates for up to 5 ACEP Category I credits, 5 *AMA PRA Category 1 Credits*™, and 5 AOA Category 2-B credits for completing this activity in its entirety. Submit your answers online at acep.org/cdem; a score of 75% or better is required. You may receive credit for completing the CME activity any time within 3 years of its publication date. Answers to this month's questions will be published in next month's issue.

1   A patient with a history of opioid use disorder presents with restlessness, vomiting, piloerection, and tachycardia. **What is the best next step?**
A.   Administer ondansetron 4 mg IV
B.   Complete a urine drug screen
C.   Complete Clinical Opiate Withdrawal Scale scoring and discuss buprenorphine with the patient
D.   Notify a social worker to link the patient to follow-up care

2   A patient with a history of opioid use disorder presents with chronic back pain. Physical examination and vital signs are normal. The patient reports regular heroin use and requests help addressing his addiction. He denies current symptoms of opioid withdrawal. **What is the best next step?**
A.   Administer buprenorphine 8 mg SL and discharge with buprenorphine 8 mg SL twice daily and naloxone 4 mg/0.1 mL nasal spray
B.   Administer naloxone 0.2 mg IV
C.   Complete Clinical Opiate Withdrawal Scale scoring
D.   Discharge with education on home-initiation dosing of buprenorphine and a bridge prescription for 8 mg SL twice daily and naloxone 4 mg/0.1 mL nasal spray

3   **Which patient is most likely to benefit from immediate administration of buprenorphine?**
A.   A patient, brought in by a friend, stuporous and with a low respiratory rate but an otherwise normal physical examination
B.   A patient with a history of opioid use disorder who presents with anxiety, a temperature of 40°C (104°F), a pulse of 125, and erythema and induration surrounding a wound on the forearm but who is otherwise asymptomatic with a normal physical examination
C.   A patient with a history of opioid use disorder who presents with chills, difficulty sitting still, stomach cramps, and anxiety but who is otherwise asymptomatic with a normal physical examination
D.   A pregnant patient with a history of opioid use disorder who presents with anxiety and vomiting, a pulse of 105, diaphoresis, and obvious tremulousness but who is otherwise asymptomatic with a normal physical examination

4   A patient who presents in moderate opioid withdrawal, characterized primarily by agitation and vomiting, is given buprenorphine 8 mg SL. One hour later, the patient is reassessed, and their symptoms are unchanged. **What is the best next step?**
A.   Administer droperidol 1.25 mg IV because the patient is not responding to buprenorphine and requires nonagonist treatment for agitation and vomiting
B.   Give a second dose of buprenorphine 8 mg SL and continue monitoring for clinical improvement
C.   Give a second dose of buprenorphine 8 mg SL and discharge with naloxone 4 mg/0.1 mL nasal spray PRN and appropriate follow-up
D.   Monitor for an additional 30 minutes because the patient may need more time for onset of symptom relief

5   A patient presents in moderate opioid withdrawal. Per chart review, the patient was treated for naloxone-induced withdrawal at their last visit 1 month ago and was discharged with prescriptions for buprenorphine and naloxone with outpatient follow-up. The patient reports relapsing on heroin. **What is the best next step?**
A.   Administer buprenorphine 2 mg SL and monitor symptoms for 30 to 60 minutes
B.   Administer buprenorphine 8 mg SL and monitor symptoms for 30 to 60 minutes
C.   Discharge after counseling the patient on continuing treatment with buprenorphine and outpatient follow-up
D.   Notify hospital administration about the patient's misuse of emergency department resources and create a plan to prevent future malingering

6   EMS reports that they are 5 minutes away transporting Ana Smith, a 35-year-old woman, well known to the team for being verbally and physically aggressive during frequent visits for substance-related complaints. EMS found her apneic in cardiac arrest after a suspected opioid overdose. They have administered naloxone six times, and she is still in pulseless electrical activity. The staff asks, "What is coming in?" **What is an appropriate response?**
A.   "Ana Smith, one of our frequent fliers. She is an alcoholic with a history of substance abuse and has overdosed again. Get ready for advanced cardiovascular life support."
B.   "High-acuity case of a young female in pulseless electrical activity arrest. She has history of substance use disorder, and EMS suspect accidental opioid overdose. Please get multiple doses of naloxone ready alongside advanced cardiovascular life support drugs and ensure we have reliable access."
C.   "Remember that junkie who is always aggressive, requiring restraints when she comes in drunk and high? EMS is bringing her in. They gave her tons of naloxone and are doing chest compressions. Get ready for intraosseous line and short advanced cardiovascular life support."
D.   "There is an addict coming in after an overdose. Double up on our gloves and personal protective equipment and get ready for advanced cardiovascular life support."

7   **What are the unique pharmacologic mechanisms that contribute to buprenorphine's safety profile?**
A.   Full μ-opioid agonist with high receptor affinity
B.   Full μ-opioid agonist with low receptor affinity
C.   Full μ-opioid antagonist with high receptor affinity
D.   Partial μ-opioid agonist with high receptor affinity

8   A 55-year-old man presents with recurrent abscesses. He has a history of polysubstance use disorder and uses methamphetamine and fentanyl via smoking and injecting. He is vomiting, has clammy skin and dilated pupils, and anxiously states "I just need an antibiotic prescription and need to be somewhere in 30 minutes. I'm not staying in the hospital." He refuses an offer to speak to him about treatment with buprenorphine. **What is the best response?**
A.   Because the patient is clearly withdrawing, administer intravenous antibiotics along with injectable long-acting buprenorphine and give him a prescription for buprenorphine so that he can continue it when he feels ready. Recommend primary care follow-up for his abscess.
B.   Compassionately try to convince him to stay in the hospital and tell him that he must stop using drugs. If he refuses, obtain testing for HIV and hepatitis C but do not provide antibiotics, as he will likely not take them and clearly wants to leave to go use drugs.
C.   Convince him that he needs to stay in the hospital but do not offer buprenorphine because he is clearly not ready and does not qualify for medication for opioid use disorder since he is using multiple drugs. Review inpatient detox options until you find one that the patient likes.
D.   Perform a complete medical screening and examination and then reassure him that he is welcome to return any time he is ready for treatment. Counsel him on clean drug injection practices, provide him with naloxone and resources for needle exchange programs, and prescribe appropriate antibiotics with return precautions.

9 A 16-year-old girl with opioid use disorder presents after a mechanical fall. X-rays confirm a left fibula Maisonneuve nondisplaced fracture. After consulting orthopedic surgery and ensuring there are no other injuries, the plan is to splint her leg and discharge her with analgesia and outpatient orthopedics follow-up. She reports that her pain is 9/10 and that she recently started buprenorphine. She is using 16 mg each morning for maintenance therapy. Her mother is at the bedside and is concerned that this injury could lead to a relapse. What medications should be chosen?

A. Give her 0.1 mg/kg of IV morphine because one dose will not jeopardize her sobriety, discharge her with continuation of her maintenance dose of buprenorphine, and prescribe a short 5-day course of oral oxycodone for breakthrough pain

B. Give her IV ketorolac and acetaminophen and discharge with oral NSAIDs and acetaminophen because she worked hard on her sobriety and it should not be jeopardized

C. Offer her either a dose of IV ketamine or IV buprenorphine now for breakthrough pain, recommend outpatient multimodal analgesia including acetaminophen and NSAIDs, and prescribe a short course of 8 mg SL buprenorphine for breakthrough pain

D. She is already on a high dose of buprenorphine and does not need additional analgesia, so recommend that she should divide the dose and take 8 mg in the morning and 8 mg at night

10 In which patient group should physicians be particularly concerned with the potential for opioid use disorder and more keenly screen and interview?

A. Patients who experience frequent respiratory infections
B. Patients with difficulty adhering to prescribed medications
C. Patients with multiple cardiovascular comorbidities
D. Pregnant patients

11 Which intervention decreases the risk of falls for older patients?

A. Bed rails
B. Elevated beds
C. Fall-risk bracelets
D. Flat, even floors

12 Which statement regarding pain management in older patients is true?

A. Fentanyl patches are safer in older adults than oral opiates for the treatment of pain.
B. Ibuprofen is typically all that is needed for older patients with severe injuries.
C. Selecting a medication from the Beers Criteria is the safest way to prescribe medications to geriatric patients.
D. Uncontrolled pain is an independent risk factor for delirium.

13 Which initiative is unlikely to make the discharge process safer for older patients?

A. Compressing all discharge instructions to fit on one piece of paper
B. Including family members in the discharge process if the patient agrees
C. Providing a hand-off to the patient's primary care physician, detailing the plan of care, and requesting a close follow-up appointment for the patient
D. Typing all instructions in simple language and personally reviewing them with the patient

14 A prolonged emergency department stay can result in all of the following except which scenario?

A. Bed sores
B. Delirium
C. Improved patient satisfaction
D. Increased mortality

15 What should be a first step in the treatment of agitated geriatric patients?

A. Administration of haloperidol
B. Application of restraints
C. Removal of family or caregivers from the room to decrease stimulation
D. Reorientation and verbal de-escalation with the assistance of family or caregivers at the bedside

16 An 86-year-old woman presents after a fall. During the review of systems, she reports that she has had burning while urinating. Her urinalysis is positive for leukocytes, >50 WBCs/μL, large bacteria, and nitrites. What should the emergency physician do prior to discharging this patient?

A. Arrange to have the patient taken to her car in a wheelchair after discharge so that she does not have to walk and risk falling in the emergency department
B. Discuss the planned antibiotic therapy with the emergency department pharmacist or consult Beers Criteria for Potentially Inappropriate Medication Use in Older Adults for guidance
C. Explain to the patient why adding another medicine to her medication regimen is dangerous and then do not give her a prescription for antibiotics
D. Since an antibiotic is warranted, prescribe one without checking the patient's home medication list

17 Triaging older patients appropriately can be challenging. Which statement about triage is false?

A. Even when triaged appropriately, geriatric patients wait longer to be seen than expected, given their assigned triage level.
B. Heart rate is the most sensitive vital sign for the appropriate triage of elderly patients.
C. Inappropriate field triage can direct elderly trauma patients away from level I trauma centers and put them at greater risk of delays in appropriate care.
D. The ESI triage system is not always accurate when triaging elderly adults.

18 Which statement regarding pain management in older adults is true?

A. Acetaminophen, non-narcotic medications, and topical anesthetics are not useful in the geriatric population and should not be used in lieu of more effective opiates.
B. Palliative care can help to create safe and effective pain management plans for elderly patients and should not be limited to hospice patients.
C. Palliative care is most appropriate for patients with terminal illnesses and is not useful for patients with complex pain.
D. Regional nerve blocks have not been shown to reduce pain in older patients and should not be used for pain control.

19 A 70-year-old woman presents at 10 PM with gout, for which she is given 8 mg of morphine. After receiving it, she becomes delirious, falls trying to get up, and sustains a femoral neck fracture. Which intervention could have prevented this adverse series of events?

A. Application of a fall-risk bracelet
B. Consideration of low-dose or non-narcotic analgesics to treat the patient's pain initially
C. Hourly vital signs and re-evaluation by the nurse
D. Placement of a Foley catheter

20 A 76-year-old woman presents and is diagnosed with COVID-19. Which factor is not a risk for clinical decompensation?

A. History of ACE-inhibitor use
B. History of congestive heart failure and chronic obstructive pulmonary disease
C. Lack of vaccination against COVID-19
D. Presence of delirium

ANSWER KEY FOR AUGUST 2022, VOLUME 36, NUMBER 8

1	2	3	4	5	6	7	8	9	10	11	12	13	14	15	16	17	18	19	20
B	B	B	A	B	C	D	D	A	C	C	D	D	C	C	B	B	B	D	C

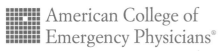

American College of
Emergency Physicians®

ADVANCING EMERGENCY CARE

Post Office Box 619911
Dallas, Texas 75261-9911

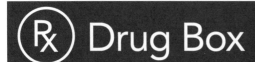

Fidaxomicin

By Frank LoVecchio, DO, MPH, FACEP
Valleywise Health and ASU, Phoenix, Arizona

Objective
On completion of this column, you should be able to:
- Discuss the current recommendations for the treatment of CDI.

Fidaxomicin is the suggested first-line drug to treat diarrhea caused by *Clostridioides* (formerly *Clostridium*) *difficile* infections (CDI) in adults and children older than 6 months. In 2021, the American College of Gastroenterology updated its clinical practice guidelines for CDI. The Infectious Diseases Society of America and the Society for Healthcare Epidemiology of America also published clinical practice guidelines, stating that a 10-day course of fidaxomicin is the preferred treatment for an initial episode of CDI. A 10-day course at a standard dosing of oral vancomycin is an acceptable alternative. These changes were supported by data presented at the 2022 Digestive Disease Week Annual Meeting, which evaluated real world data via a retrospective review of Medicare beneficiaries.[1] Data reveal that after the initial CDI episode sample, fidaxomicin has a 13.5% higher rate of 4-week sustained responses than vancomycin (71.7% vs 58.2%; P = 0.0058). There is also a 13.2% higher response rate detected at 8 weeks with fidaxomicin (63.2% vs 50.0%; P = 0.0114).

Mechanism of Action
Fidaxomicin inhibits the σ subunits in bacterial RNA polymerases, resulting in the inhibition of protein synthesis and cell death in susceptible organisms such as *C. difficile.*

Adult Dosing
Initial infection: 200 mg twice daily PO for 10 days. If treatment response is delayed, a longer duration (ie, up to 14 days) may be appropriate.
Recurrent infection: 200 mg twice daily PO for 10 days or 200 mg twice daily PO for 5 days, followed by 200 mg once every other day PO for 20 days.
There is no dose adjustment for hepatic or renal impairment.

Adverse Effects (>10%)
Gastrointestinal: Nausea (11% in adults)
Miscellaneous: Fever (13% in infants, children, and adolescents)
Pregnancy risk factor: Unknown, but limited systemic absorption may limit fetus drug levels

Contraindications
Hypersensitivity to fidaxomicin or any component of the formulation is possible. There is minimal absorption, but potentially, hypersensitivity can occur in patients with a macrolide allergy.

REFERENCE
1. Iapoce C. Fidaxomicin superior to vancomycin in reaching desired *C. difficile* outcomes. HCP Live. May 31, 2022. Accessed August 17, 2022. https://www.hcplive.com/view/fidaxomicin-superior-vancomycin-desired-c-diff-outcomes

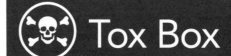

Carbamazepine Poisoning

By Christian A. Tomaszewski, MD, MS, MBA, FACEP
University of California San Diego Health

Objective
On completion of this column, you should be able to:
- Manage patients with carbamazepine poisoning.

Carbamazepine is a common antiepileptic drug also utilized for mood stabilization. Neurotoxicity predominates with prolonged use, and delayed toxicity can occur. Deaths, however, are rare. Altered mental status can occur with as little as 20 mg/kg, and cardiac toxicity can occur with ingestion of >50 mg/kg.

Mechanism of Action
- Binds to sodium channels in an inactivated state
- Inhibits neuronal depolarization and glutamate release
- May be anticholinergic in massive ingestions

Pharmacokinetics
- Peak levels after oral ingestion can be delayed 12 hours or more (>96 hours in extended release).
- Elimination half-life is >18 hours, becoming zero-order in overdose.

Clinical Manifestations
- *Neurologic:* Sedation, ataxia, myoclonus, seizures, and coma
- *Ocular:* Nystagmus and mydriasis
- *Cardiac:* Tachycardia, hypotension, and QRS prolongation
- *Anticholinergic:* Flushing and dry mucous membranes and skin

Diagnostics
- Serial serum carbamazepine levels
- Glucose and acetaminophen screenings
- ECG

Treatment
- Oral activated charcoal if <1-2 hours post ingestion and airway is protected
- Repeat activated charcoal and whole-bowel irrigation in sustained-release formulation carbamazepine
- Bolus IV fluids and/or pressors for hypotension
- Sodium bicarbonate IV for QRS widening
- Benzodiazepines or propofol for seizures
- May consider hemodialysis for refractory seizures or cardiac instability

Disposition
- Discharge home if asymptomatic at 4-6 hours post ingestion with decreasing levels.

Critical decisions
in emergency medicine

Volume 36 Number 10: **October 2022**

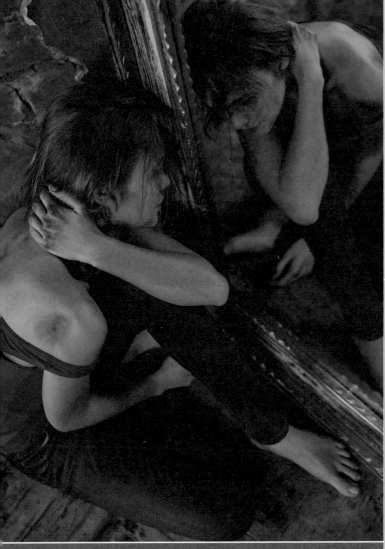

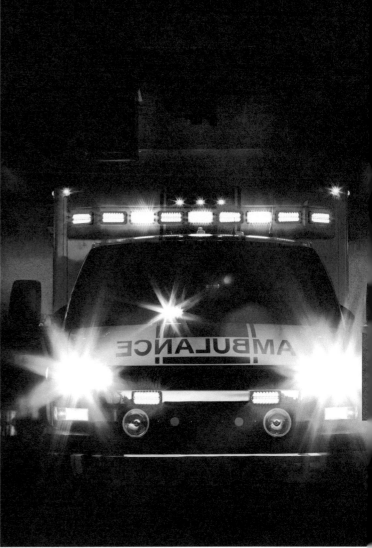

Under Attack

More than half of sexual assault victims never report the crime or seek medical care. Nevertheless, emergency physicians must understand the jurisdictional requirements and established procedures to evaluate and manage these patients to provide proper care and support, obtain high-quality evidence for law enforcement, treat injuries, and protect victims from sexually transmitted infections.

Shifting Gears

Narrowing down the myriad options for transferring critically ill patients to a higher level of care can be a complex and urgent task. Emergency physicians must know what transfer options are available and how to select the most appropriate critical care transport to decrease the risk of patients decompensating during transport and to quickly get them to a higher level of care.

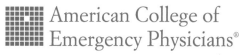

American College of Emergency Physicians®

ADVANCING EMERGENCY CARE

Critical decisions
in emergency medicine

Critical Decisions in Emergency Medicine is the official CME publication of the American College of Emergency Physicians. Additional volumes are available.

EDITOR-IN-CHIEF

Michael S. Beeson, MD, MBA, FACEP
Northeastern Ohio Universities, Rootstown, OH

SECTION EDITORS

Joshua S. Broder, MD, FACEP
Duke University, Durham, NC

Andrew J. Eyre, MD, MS-HPEd
Brigham and Women's Hospital/ Harvard Medical School, Boston, MA

John Kiel, DO, MPH, FACEP, CAQSM
University of Florida College of Medicine, Jacksonville, FL

Frank LoVecchio, DO, MPH, FACEP
Valleywise, Arizona State University, University of Arizona, and Creighton Colleges of Medicine, Phoenix, AZ

Sharon E. Mace, MD, FACEP
Cleveland Clinic Lerner College of Medicine/ Case Western Reserve University, Cleveland, OH

Amal Mattu, MD, FACEP
University of Maryland, Baltimore, MD

Christian A. Tomaszewski, MD, MS, MBA, FACEP
University of California Health Sciences, San Diego, CA

Steven J. Warrington, MD, MEd, MS
MercyOne Siouxland, Sioux City, IA

ASSOCIATE EDITORS

Tareq Al-Salamah, MBBS, MPH, FACEP
King Saud University, Riyadh, Saudi Arabia/ University of Maryland, Baltimore, MD

Wan-Tsu Chang, MD
University of Maryland, Baltimore, MD

Ann M. Dietrich, MD, FAAP, FACEP
University of South Carolina School of Medicine, Greenville, SC

Kelsey Drake, MD, MPH, FACEP
St. Anthony Hospital, Lakewood, CO

Walter L. Green, MD, FACEP
UT Southwestern Medical Center, Dallas, TX

John C. Greenwood, MD
University of Pennsylvania, Philadelphia, PA

Danya Khoujah, MBBS, MEHP, FACEP
University of Maryland, Baltimore, MD

Nathaniel Mann, MD
University of South Carolina School of Medicine, Greenville, SC

George Sternbach, MD, FACEP
Stanford University Medical Center, Stanford, CA

EDITORIAL STAFF

Suzannah Alexander, Editorial Director
salexander@acep.org

Joy Carrico, JD
Managing Editor

Alex Bass
Assistant Editor

Kel Morris
Assistant Editor

ISSN2325-0186 (Print)   ISSN2325-8365 (Online)

Contents

Lesson 19 4
Under Attack
Care for Sexual Assault Victims
By Heather V. Rozzi, MD, FACEP; and
Ralph J. Riviello, MD, MS, FACEP
Reviewed by Kelsey Drake, MD, MPH, FACEP

Lesson 20 23
Shifting Gears
Selecting Appropriate Critical Care Transport
By Ani Aydin, MD, FACEP; Christie Fritz, MD, MS;
Luke Duncan, MD; and Jason Cohen, DO, FACEP
Reviewed by Nathaniel Mann, MD

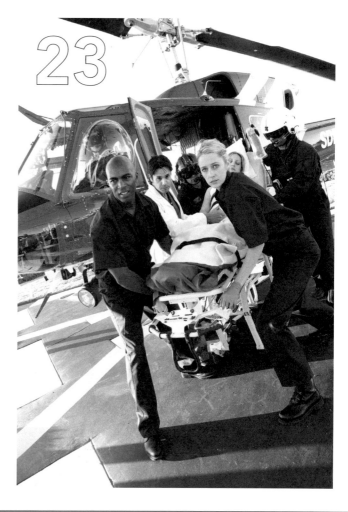

23

4

FEATURES

The Critical ECG — Acute Posterior Myocardial Infarction 11
  By Amal Mattu, MD, FACEP

The Literature Review — Moderate Temperature Management After
  Nonshockable-Rhythm Cardiac Arrest 12
  By Chinezimuzo Ihenatu, MD; and Michael E. Abboud, MD, MSEd
  Reviewed by Andrew J. Eyre, MD, MS-HPEd

The Critical Procedure — Traction Splinting a Midshaft Femur Fracture 14
  By Steven J. Warrington, MD, MEd, MS

Critical Cases in Orthopedics and Trauma — Recurrent Prosthetic Hip Dislocation 16
  By Julie Shaner, MD
  Reviewed by John Kiel, DO, MPH

The Critical Image — A Pregnant Trauma Patient 18
  By Joshua S. Broder, MD, FACEP

Clinical Pediatrics — Moyamoya Disease–Induced Stroke 20
  By Jonathan Blalock, BS; Sarah Guess, MD; and Laurie Malmstrom, MD
  Reviewed by Sharon E. Mace, MD, FACEP

CME Questions 30
  Reviewed by Kelsey Drake, MD, MPH, FACEP; and Nathaniel Mann, MD

Drug Box — Tecovirimat 32
  By Frank LoVecchio, DO, MPH, FACEP

Tox Box — Dinitrophenol Overdose 32
  By Christian A. Tomaszewski, MD, MS, MBA, FACEP

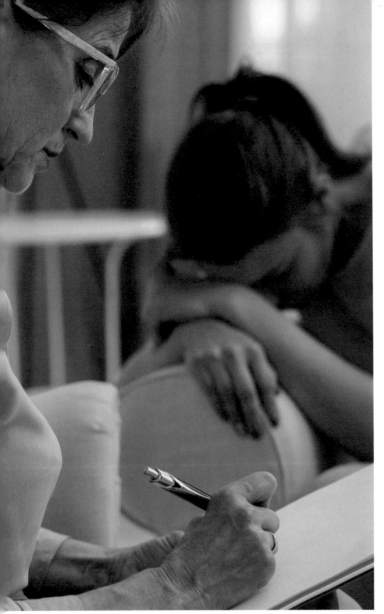

Under Attack

Care for Sexual Assault Victims

LESSON 19

By Heather V. Rozzi, MD, FACEP; and
Ralph J. Riviello, MD, MS, FACEP

Dr. Rozzi is an attending physician and a core faculty member at WellSpan York Hospital in York, Pennsylvania. She is an assistant professor of emergency medicine at Pennsylvania State University College of Medicine and an adjunct clinical assistant professor of emergency medicine at Drexel University College of Medicine. Dr. Rozzi also serves as medical director for the WellSpan York Hospital's Forensic Examiner Team, York County Children's Advocacy Center, and Adams County Children's Advocacy Center. Dr. Riviello is chair and professor of the Department of Emergency Medicine at UT Health San Antonio in Texas.

Reviewed by Kelsey Drake, MD, MPH, FACEP

Objectives

On completion of this lesson, you should be able to:

1. Perform a complete sexual assault evaluation with appropriate documentation.
2. Explain the evidence collection process for patients after sexual assault.
3. Describe the required prophylaxis for patients after sexual assault.
4. Discuss the legal requirements of caring for a patient who has been sexually assaulted.
5. Identify issues specific to the care of special populations after sexual assault.

From the EM Model

14.0 Psychobehavioral Disorders
    14.6 Patterns of Violence/Abuse/Neglect
        14.6.3 Sexual Assault

■ CRITICAL DECISIONS ■

- What are the dynamics of sexual assault?
- What is the role of SANEs, and what is a SART?
- What are key elements of the history, examination, and evidence collection in sexual assault cases?
- What are key elements of documentation for sexual assault patients?
- What prophylaxis and follow-up should be provided to patients after sexual assault?
- What are the legal requirements when caring for patients after sexual assault?
- What are some considerations when working with sexual assault victims in special populations?

Sexual assaults account for 4.4% of emergency department visits for interpersonal violence, but this percentage likely underrepresents the prevalence of sexual assault. Emergency physicians must understand the jurisdictional requirements and established procedures to evaluate and manage sexual assault victims to provide care and support, obtain high-quality evidence for law enforcement, treat injuries, and protect victims from sexually transmitted infections (STIs).

CASE PRESENTATIONS

■ CASE ONE

An 86-year-old woman with dementia presents with unusual vaginal discharge, which was noticed while she was being bathed. She is bedbound. Her only remaining family is a daughter, who is her health care power of attorney. Because of her dementia, the patient is unable to provide a history. On examination, bruising to her face and inner thighs are noted (*Figure 1*). A thick, yellow discharge is noted in her underwear.

■ CASE TWO

A 19-year-old woman is brought in by her college roommate. The patient is tearful, and her hair is disheveled. She states that she was on a second date with a male classmate. She awoke in an unfamiliar apartment and found her clothes in a pile on the floor. She denies pain and has not noted any physical injuries.

■ CASE THREE

A 12-year-old boy is brought in by his mother after disclosing that his wrestling coach has been sexually abusing him. The patient is reluctant to discuss the abuse but states that the last sexual contact was earlier that day. He reports rectal pain.

Introduction

More than 50% of women and almost 30% of men have experienced sexual violence involving physical contact. About 4% of men and 25% of women have been a victim of rape or attempted rape.[1] These numbers are likely significantly underestimated because fewer than half of sexual assault victims report the crime to law enforcement or seek medical care. In addition, the prevalence in many vulnerable populations, such as those who are homeless or institutionalized, has not been studied. Patients who have been sexually assaulted may suffer from physical injuries and significant psychological sequelae. These issues can be chronic, affecting patients' long-term health, family relationships, and employment.

CRITICAL DECISION

What are the dynamics of sexual assault?

Numerous myths about sexual assault pervade and create bias against patients who have been assaulted. For example, when asked to describe the idea of sexual assault, many would describe an unknown perpetrator using violence with, perhaps, a weapon to physically injure a young, attractive woman.[2] In reality, most sexual assaults are committed by perpetrators known to patients. According to the National Intimate Partner and Sexual Violence Survey, only 12.1% of female and 13.7% of male victims were assaulted by a stranger.[3]

The use of a weapon during sexual assault is also rare. A recent study found that of the total rapes in the United States in 2020, the vast majority (277,823) did not involve a weapon. In cases that involved weapons, 9,651 involved a knife, 1,680 involved a firearm, and 18,718 cases involved other weapons.[4] Surprisingly, 6,242 victims did not know if a weapon was used, and 5,833 victims did not know what type of weapon was used.[4]

The primary motivation for sexual assault is not sexual gratification.[5] Typically, perpetrators rape to exert power and control over their victims and derive satisfaction from taking away the right to consensual sexual activity. Male perpetrators of sexual assault often experience some form of sexual dysfunction during the assault, including erectile dysfunction or lack of ejaculation.

Men are the perpetrators of sexual assault 99.6% of the time when rape victims are women and 85.2% of the time when rape victims are men.[6] Women and girls constitute most rape victims (85.8% women versus 14.2% men).

Most sexual assaults do not involve significant physical violence, and victims rarely present with serious injuries. The reported incidence of nongenital physical injuries ranges from 23% to 85% of sexual assault patients based on published studies with varying methodologies.[7] The incidence of genital injury

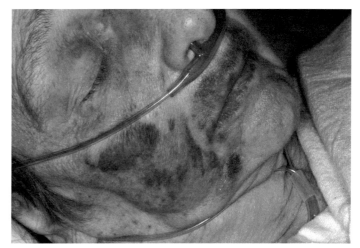

FIGURE 1. A patient with bruising after an assault.
Credit: York Hospital Forensic Examiner Team.

following sexual assault ranges from 5% by direct visualization to 87% using techniques such as colposcopy and toluidine blue staining.[8,9] Male victims of sexual assault may be at a higher risk for serious injury than female victims. The rate of nonanogenital injury in male victims appears to range between 17% and 38%. Approximately 66% of male victims suffer bodily injury.[10-12]

CRITICAL DECISION

What is the role of SANEs, and what is a SART?

Sexual assault nurse examiners (SANEs) are nurses who specialize in caring for and collecting evidence from patients who were sexually assaulted. SANEs perform time-intensive forensic examinations following clearly defined protocols that lead to more effective prosecutions of perpetrators. When available, SANEs should be consulted to perform a medical forensic examination for any patient who reports a sexual assault. In addition to their specialized training, SANEs are well versed in available community resources. When SANEs are available to perform these time-intensive examinations, emergency physicians can focus on the management of other patients. In any event, evaluations should be conducted within 7 days of the incident, although most hospitals have a cutoff of 5 days.

In addition to needing timely medical care and postexposure prophylaxis (PEP), sexual assault patients also have complex emotional and legal needs. A patient-focused multidisciplinary, multiagency approach is best for meeting these needs. Individuals and organizations involved in the initial response to these patients are known as the sexual assault response team (SART). These teams are cost-effective, allow patients to be examined sooner, are

Members of the SART	
Medical	• Hospitals • Physicians • SANE • Sexual assault forensic examiner • Medical personnel
Legal	• Police • Law enforcement personnel • Crime lab • Judicial system • Prosecutors • Corrections officers
Social services	• Rape crisis center staff • Domestic violence agencies • Protective services personnel from agencies such as the states' adult and child protective services • Patient advocates • Survivors of sexual assault • Clergy and faith community • Schools • Sex offender treatment

TABLE 1. SART members. *Source:* Adapted from data at https://www.ovcttac.gov/saneguide/multidisciplinary-response-and-the-community/collaboration-with-community-partners/

better at collecting evidence, and increase rates of reporting sexual assault. Key team members include medical personnel, patient advocates, prosecutors, protective services personnel, and law enforcement personnel (*Table 1*). The SANE Program Development and Operation Guide, published by the Office for Victims of Crime within the Department of Justice, is an outstanding resource for more information regarding SART programs.[13]

CRITICAL DECISION

What are key elements of the history, examination, and evidence collection in sexual assault cases?

Like all other patients, sexual assault patients must have a medical screening examination (MSE) upon presentation prior to the sexual assault examination. Although serious physical injury after sexual assault is rare, if a patient is seriously injured, medical care takes precedence over evidence collection.

As with any other procedure, consent must be obtained prior to performing a sexual assault examination. Emergency physicians must know the requirements of the jurisdictions they practice in when performing these examinations.[14,15] Some jurisdictions, as dictated by state and local statutes, require emergency physicians to notify law enforcement of the sexual assault. Jurisdictions also often mandate which chart forms and sexual assault kits to use during the examination.

The key elements of the history and physical examination for sexually assaulted patients depend on each emergency department's policy for its clinicians. If the department policy is for emergency clinicians to provide only an MSE before patients are managed by the SANE, then the only history needed is that information necessary to identify an emergency medical condition, questions about injuries, areas of pain or bleeding, or whether strangulation occurred. Patients should also be asked about suicidal or homicidal ideation, both of which are common after sexual assault. Information obtained while taking the medical history will guide the physical examination. If there is no SANE and the emergency clinician is also providing the forensic examination, then a complete history of the event, forensic history, physical examination, and

evidence collection should be completed. Forensic evidence collection is just one part of the total care provided in the emergency department. The decision to collect evidence depends on the areas of penetration and the time interval since the assault, with each area having different time limits. Current guidelines are:

• Vaginal penetration — 120 hours (5 days);
• Anal penetration — 72 hours (3 days);
• Oral penetration — 24 hours (1 day); and
• Bite marks or saliva on skin — 96 hours (4 days).[14]

There may be unique situations in which these timelines can be extended. For instance, in cases of sexual assault on children, pediatric evidence collection is based on jurisdictional guidance and may follow the guidelines above. However, for pediatric cases that present past these timelines, specialized outpatient examination by a child abuse pediatrician or pediatric SANE is preferred to emergency department examination and evidence collection.[16]

The forensic history details what occurred during the sexual assault. Most jurisdictions use specialized forms to document the forensic history. Some key features of the forensic history include:

• Date of last consensual sexual activity and, if recent, acts performed and with whom;
• History of the sexual assault;
• Use of any force, weapons, strangulation, or other assaultive events;
• Acts during the assault (eg, areas of penetration, type of penetration, use of condoms and lubricant, kissing, biting, sucking, ejaculation, and, if so, location of ejaculation); and
• Acts post assault (eg, wiping, douching, showering, and bathing).

After the forensic history is gathered, the physical examination is performed. The physical examination is divided into body and anogenital examinations. The body examination includes a head-to-toe assessment to identify and photograph debris, injuries, and potential evidence and palpation of areas that may indicate injuries. The body examination can be enhanced by using an alternate light source (ALS) to look for possible biological evidence.[17,18] The ALS is a device that produces light at specific wavelengths to fluoresce substances that are normally invisible to the naked eye, such as semen, vaginal secretions, and saliva. One disadvantage of using ALS, however, is that many other nonbiological agents can also fluoresce.

✔ Pearls

■ In addition to the need for timely medical care and STI PEP, sexual assault patients have complex emotional and legal needs best met by a patient-focused, multidisciplinary, and multiagency approach using a SART program.

■ Patients who have been victims of sexual violence require a comprehensive physical examination by a SANE, when possible, including evidence collection and careful and thorough documentation of injuries.

■ Although testing for STIs can be deferred in asymptomatic sexual assault patients, STI PEP should be offered per current CDC recommendations.

■ Male victims, the elderly, patients with disabilities, and members of the military face special challenges when seeking care for sexual assault.

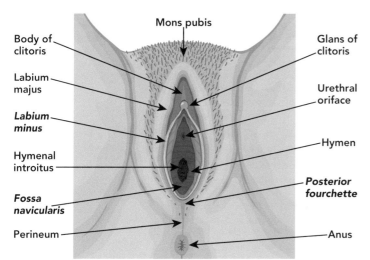

FIGURE 2. Common sites of genital injury. Genital areas injured after sexual assault most commonly include the fossa navicularis, labium minus, and posterior fourchette. *Credit:* logika600/Shutterstock.com.

Labels on figure: Mons pubis, Body of clitoris, Labium majus, *Labium minus*, Hymenal introitus, *Fossa navicularis*, Perineum, Glans of clitoris, Urethral oriface, Hymen, *Posterior fourchette*, Anus

If potential biological or debris evidence is found, it should be packaged using a two-swab technique. In this technique, two cotton-tipped applicators are lightly moistened with saline or sterile or distilled water and rolled over the area using light pressure. The swabs are allowed to air dry and then packaged according to jurisdictional protocol.[14]

If the patient reports the occurrence of strangulation during the assault, a strangulation-specific history and physical examination should also be performed. Strangulation occurs in approximately 15% of sexual assaults. When the sexual assault occurs in an intimate relationship, the incidence of strangulation increases to 25%.[19] Many patients will not disclose strangulation, but serious injury, such as carotid artery dissection, may result from strangulation, even when there are no obvious signs of trauma. To avoid missing this diagnosis, clinicians should ask specific questions such as, "Were you choked or strangled?" Most emergency departments use a dedicated history-taking and documentation tool that includes questions and body maps pertinent to strangulation, focusing on patients' head and neck region.

Next, the anogenital examination is performed. Unlike a non–sexual assault pelvic examination in women, the medical forensic examination emphasizes visual inspection of the external genitalia and vulva. The posterior fourchette, fossa navicularis, and labia minora are the most common areas of sexual assault injury in women (*Figure 2*). Visualization is aided by using a separation-and-traction technique: The labia should be gently separated with downward traction while looking for debris, biological evidence, and injury. An ALS may be used here as well. The process is:

- Visualizing, photographing as indicated, collecting debris, and swabbing the external genitalia and vulva;
- Applying and then removing toluidine blue, if being used, and revisualizing and photographing the area;
- Inserting the speculum;
- Visualizing and swabbing the vaginal vault and cervix;
- Visualizing, photographing as indicated, and swabbing the perineum and perianal area;
- Visualizing, photographing as indicated, and swabbing the anus and rectum (*Figure 3*);
- Inspecting the anal sphincter;
- Applying toluidine blue to the anus to enhance visualization of any injury found; and

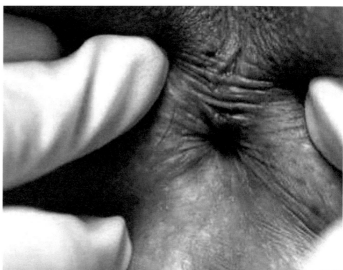

FIGURE 3. Laceration near the anus. *Credit:* Ralph J. Riviello, MD.

- Using an anoscope to aid in visualizing rectal mucosa and swabbing the anus and rectum.

Recommendations for the anogenital examination include:
- Using a labial separation-and-traction technique to visualize the posterior fourchette and fossa navicularis, where most genital injuries are seen (see *Figure 2*)[20];
- Describing the location of external genitalia injuries based on a clockface after documenting the patient's position (the clock position changes with the patient's position);
- Using toluidine blue to visually enhance injuries to the external genitalia by:
  - Applying it to the area from 3 to 6 o'clock,
  - Removing it with acetic acid solution, a baby wipe, or water-based lubricant on a cotton ball, and
  - Remembering not to confuse dye accumulation with an actual injury;
- Using colposcopy or a digital camera to enhance visualization of anogenital injury and to capture images;
- Inserting a speculum *after* dye application because an iatrogenic injury from insertion could be mistaken for an assault-related injury; and
- Using the TEARS mnemonic to describe anogenital injuries (**T**ears or lacerations, **E**cchymosis, **A**brasions, **R**edness, and **S**welling).

Dry items collected for evidence, such as clothing and sheets containing debris, may be sealed in paper bags marked with the patient's name (or number, if reporting anonymously) and stored with the evidence kit. Wet items of clothing should be dried prior to packaging. If drying at the emergency department is not possible, law enforcement should be alerted that the items need to be dried prior to storage.

Once collected, the evidence kit must remain in a clinician's direct line of sight or securely stored until collected by law enforcement. Most kits include a chain of custody form, often on the outside of the container, to document the custody, control, and transfer of evidence. Failure to maintain the chain of custody may render collected evidence inadmissible in court.

Drug-Facilitated Sexual Assault

Alcohol and drugs are involved in one- to two-thirds of all sexual assaults. Alcohol is the most common substance used to incapacitate victims.[6] Drugs that cause sedation or disinhibition, such as flunitrazepam, methylenedioxymethamphetamine (MDMA), ketamine, and gamma-hydroxybutyrate (GHB), may be used as "date rape drugs." Ketamine and GHB cause sedation. MDMA has stimulatory and hallucinogenic properties and reduces inhibitions. Flunitrazepam, a benzodiazepine legally sold in Latin America and Europe but not approved for sale in the United States, produces anterograde amnesia. In one study, these drugs were found in 5% of patients who were sexually assaulted.[21]

Alcohol- and drug-facilitated sexual assault (ADFSA) should be considered in patients who present with amnesia of events, severe nausea and vomiting, drowsiness, fatigue, dizziness, memory loss, impaired motor skills, or severe intoxication. ADFSA should also be considered in those whose level of intoxication is disproportionate to the amount of alcohol consumed.[22] If ADFSA is suspected, urine and blood samples should be obtained for testing, preferably using the first available urine specimen, per jurisdictional policy. Specimens should be sent to specialized forensic laboratories instead of to the in-hospital laboratory. Specimen collection for ADFSA can be performed up to 96 hours post assault; however, the chance of recovery is better when the evidence is collected closer to the time of the incident.

CRITICAL DECISION

What are key elements of documentation for sexual assault patients?

Comprehensive and objective documentation is crucial when caring for patients who were sexually assaulted. It can expedite the legal process and reduce the need for the clinician to testify in court. Body maps and photography should be used; these features are built into most modern electronic medical records. Physicians should consider using the "hide from patient portal" feature of the electronic medical record if patients want documentation to remain private. Using a standardized charting document ensures that important points of the history and examination are not missed. Several forms are available to assist with this process, but many jurisdictions have their own specific documentation forms.

Documentation should include the medical and forensic histories, any injuries noted on physical examination, and any forensic evidence collected. Document the patient's own words: Patient statements are powerful during legal proceedings, and they help guide physical examination and imaging decisions. If the patient was strangled, documentation should also include the method of strangulation and the assailant's position relative to the patient.

The final documented diagnosis should avoid the use of loaded terms like "alleged" and "rule out" when referring to sexual assault. Better alternatives include descriptions like "evaluation following sexual assault," "sexual assault," and "reported sexual assault." Specific injury diagnoses or physical findings should also be included in the final patient record.

CRITICAL DECISION

What prophylaxis and follow-up should be provided to patients after sexual assault?

Testing

Because testing for STIs immediately after the sexual assault does not provide evidence of infection acquired during the sexual assault, STI testing can be deferred, especially if patients are willing to undergo prophylactic treatment. If patients decline prophylactic treatment for STIs, testing should be considered.

HIV nPEP Factors
Assailant factors
• HIV status
• Characteristics and HIV risk behaviors in assailant (eg, injection drug abuse, men who have sex with men)
• Presence of mucosal lesions
Local epidemiology/prevalence of HIV/AIDS
Time elapsed since assault
Risk and benefits of treatment
Assault characteristics
• Multiple assailants
• Vaginal or anal penetration
• Condom use
• Ejaculation onto mucosal membranes
• Presence of mucosal lesions on victim
• Genital injury or trauma

TABLE 2. Considerations for HIV nPEP

Current recommendations from the CDC are nucleic acid amplification testing (NAAT) for chlamydia and gonorrhea at the site of exposure and for vaginal trichomonas. Serum testing is recommended for syphilis, HIV, and hepatitis B.[23]

Treatment

Empiric treatment for gonorrhea, chlamydia, and trichomoniasis should be given based on current CDC recommendations, which occasionally change based on patterns of resistance. Prophylaxis for hepatitis B should be tailored to patients' vaccination status. Patients who have had hepatitis B or are vaccinated against it do not require immunization after sexual assault. HPV vaccination status should also be considered; patients who have not been previously vaccinated against HPV may want to get immunized after sexual assault.

While data regarding the transmission of HIV during sexual assault is lacking, HIV seroconversion has occurred in patients whose only risk factor was sexual assault or abuse. Although the exact risk of transmission is unknown, it seems to depend on the type of exposure and may be higher in sexual assault due to genital injuries sustained through the use of force.[24] The risk of an HIV infection is zero when the assailant is known to be HIV negative, but the assailant's HIV status is often unknown. Occupational PEP use has been extrapolated to sexual assault patients. During the initial examination, the risk of HIV exposure should be assessed, and high-risk victims should be informed about the possible benefits of nonoccupational PEP (nPEP). The sooner nPEP is initiated, the more effective it is. Ideally, nPEP should be administered within 72 hours of the assault and continued for 28 days. There are several factors that influence the medical recommendation for nPEP (*Table 2*). If the treatment is offered, the victim must be informed of the necessity of early initiation, close follow-up care, and adherence to the treatment regimen as well as the potential side effects. Patients should either be given a starter pack of medications with arrangements for close follow-up or be provided with the full course of nPEP at the initial emergency department visit. Follow-up care should be arranged with a physician who has experience with nPEP and HIV.[25] Unfortunately, the number of patients who accept HIV nPEP remains low and the rate of treatment compliance even lower, even though HIV is a serious illness and the nPEP regimen is easy and has minimal complications.

For female patients of reproductive age, and when permitted by the jurisdiction's law, postcoital contraception should be offered following a negative pregnancy test. Commonly available single-dose regimens include levonorgestrel and ulipristal. Both are highly effective if given early after assault, although ulipristal may be more effective for women with a higher body mass index (>25) and if treatment is started more than 72 hours after the assault.[26]

Follow-up

Sexual assault has long-reaching physical and emotional consequences, the management of which is beyond the scope of emergency physicians. These patients should be screened for suicidal and homicidal thoughts prior to discharge. Patients who were sexually assaulted have an increased incidence of post-traumatic stress disorder, depression, and anxiety and may experience somatic symptoms such as migraines and pelvic pain. Insomnia is common, and patients may have problems with intimate relationships after sexual assault.

Clinicians should be aware of resources within their communities for victims of sexual assault. Many communities have sexual assault resource centers that provide clients with mental health services and legal advocacy. Patients should be provided with resources for medical follow-up and STI testing follow-up, including HIV. If nPEP is given, follow-up should be with an expert in HIV PEP. Referrals to rape crisis or victim advocacy centers should be included.

CRITICAL DECISION

What are the legal requirements when caring for patients after sexual assault?

Legal obligations and reporting requirements vary from state to state, and emergency physicians must understand the requirements for the jurisdictions in which they practice. Jurisdiction requirements can usually be found through the state's department of health or attorney general's website. Some states require that all cases of sexual assault be reported to law enforcement. Patients may choose to remain anonymous but should still be notified by law enforcement prior to evidence being destroyed.

Patient consent should be obtained prior to sexual assault examination and evidence collection. Most health care facilities have a written policy on caring for sexually assaulted patients who cannot give consent, such as those who are unconscious or mentally altered. In many cases, family members may be able to provide consent. Because evidence collection is time sensitive, some emergency departments collect forensic evidence as an anonymous case until consent can be obtained to transfer the evidence to law enforcement.

✖ Pitfalls

- Failing to have an organized SART response to sexual assault patients that includes multiple disciplines and agencies.
- Neglecting to perform a head-to-toe physical examination with evidence collection per jurisdictional protocols.
- Forgetting to offer STI PEP to patients who were sexually assaulted.
- Overlooking the importance of linking sexual assault patients to outpatient resources, including local rape crisis centers.

CRITICAL DECISION

What are some considerations when working with sexual assault victims in special populations?

Male Patients

Male victims are far less likely than female victims to report sexual assault for several reasons, including cultural resistance to the idea that men can be victims of these crimes. In addition, significant social and emotional barriers discourage sexual assault victims from coming forward, including shame, guilt, embarrassment, a desire to keep the incident secret from family and friends, concerns about confidentiality, and fear of not being believed.[27] Particularly for men, trepidation of being perceived as gay deters them from reporting being abused, but sexual violence is nondiscriminatory — every adult and child is a potential victim. Male victims are twice as likely as female victims to be attacked by multiple assailants.[28,29] This reality has important implications in evidence collection and analysis and in determining the need for HIV prophylaxis.

Older Patients

Sexual assault perpetrators often seek out victims who are easy to overpower and unlikely to report the incident. Older patients who rely on others for necessities of daily living are especially vulnerable to sexual assault, and their dependence on others can make reporting difficult or impossible. Many jurisdictions have legal reporting requirements for the sexual assault of older patients, even when they do not require reporting for sexual assault of other adults.

Patients With Disabilities

Patients with disabilities are sexually assaulted at a higher rate than the general population and may be unable to provide informed consent for sexual activity when they are intellectually disabled.[30] Patients with disabilities, both physical and intellectual, may be dependent on others, making reporting difficult or impossible.

Patients in the Military

The Department of Defense received 6,236 reports of sexual assault in the fiscal year 2019.[31] Because of the overwhelming volume of men in the military, men are almost twice as likely as women to be victimized but are far less likely to report the crime. Reporting sexual assault presents unique challenges for military personnel. Military members who have been sexually assaulted may live and work with their perpetrators; in some cases, perpetrators outrank them. Work is ongoing within the Department of Defense to improve the response to sexual violence in the military.

Summary

The emergency department is often the first and sometimes the only place where patients are treated for sexual assault. Thus, a multidisciplinary response that includes medical personnel, patient advocates, prosecutors, protective services personnel, and law enforcement personnel is important. Patients who were sexually assaulted should receive a head-to-toe examination, have evidence collected per jurisdictional protocols, and be started on STI PEP. Because sexual victimization can have long-term physical and emotional consequences, outpatient referrals for medical follow-up and counseling should be provided prior to discharge.

CASE RESOLUTIONS

■ CASE ONE

After receiving consent from the patient's daughter, the patient was evaluated by the emergency physician and SANE. In addition to bruising on the face and thighs, the patient had a laceration to the posterior fourchette and purulent drainage from the cervix. Evidence was collected and turned over to law enforcement. Samples were sent for chlamydia, gonorrhea, trichomonas, syphilis, HIV, and hepatitis B. Empiric treatment was given per CDC recommendations. Adult Protective Services was notified, and the patient was hospitalized pending placement in a different nursing facility.

■ CASE TWO

The patient's physical examination was normal. She was uncertain whether she wanted to press charges but agreed to anonymous evidence collection. Given the patient's amnesia of events, the physician sent serum and urine to the forensic laboratory for alcohol and drug testing. A sexual assault evidence kit was collected, the patient's clothing was placed in paper bags, and the evidence was secured per jurisdictional protocols.

■ CASE THREE

After ensuring the child's safety, the physician notified law enforcement and Child Protective Services. The on-call rape crisis advocate and SANE were called in. The SANE found swelling and redness of the anal fold and a small tear (see *Figure 3*). STI prophylaxis was initiated. The SANE collected evidence and turned it over to the police. The patient was discharged with standard sexual assault referrals.

REFERENCES

1. Fast facts: preventing sexual violence. Centers for Disease Control and Prevention. 2022. https://www.cdc.gov/violenceprevention/sexualviolence/fastfact.html
2. Lonsway KA, Archambault J. Dynamics of sexual assault: what does sexual assault really look like? End Violence Against Women International. 2020. https://evawintl.org/wp-content/uploads/Module-2_Dynamics-11.9.2020.pdf
3. Basile KC, Smith SG, Kresnow MJ, Khatiwada S, Leemis RW. The National Intimate Partner and Sexual Violence Survey: 2016/2017 report on sexual violence. Centers for Disease Control and Prevention. 2022. https://www.cdc.gov/violenceprevention/pdf/nisvs/nisvsreportonsexualviolence.pdf
4. Number of forcible rape and sexual assault victims in the United States in 2020, by weapon presence. Statista Research Department. 2021. https://www.statista.com/statistics/251931/usa--reported-forcible-rape-cases-by-weapon-presence/
5. Yonack L. Sexual assault is about power: how the #MeToo campaign is restoring power to victims. Psychology Today. 2017. https://www.psychologytoday.com/us/blog/psychoanalysis-unplugged/201711/sexual-assault-is-about-power
6. Tjaden P, Thoennes N. Extent, nature, and consequences of rape victimization: findings from the National Violence Against Women Survey. Office of Justice Programs. 2006. https://www.ojp.gov/pdffiles1/nij/210346.pdf
7. Green WM. Sexual assault. In: Riviello RJ, ed. *Manual of Forensic Emergency Medicine: A Guide for Clinicians.* Jones and Bartlett; 2010:107-121.
8. Massey JB, García CR, Emich JP Jr. Management of sexually assaulted females. *Obstet Gynecology.* 1971;38(1):29-36.
9. Slaughter L, Brown CR. Colposcopy to establish physical findings in rape victims. *Am J Obstet Gynecology.* 1992;166(1)(part 1):83-86.
10. Larsen ML, Hilden M. Male victims of sexual assault; 10 years' experience from a Danish assault center. *J Forensic Leg Med.* 2016;43:8-11.
11. Nesvold H, Worm AM, Vala U, Agnarsdóttir G. Different Nordic facilities for victims of sexual assault: a comparative study. *Acta Obstet Gynecol Scand.* 2005;84(2):177-183.
12. Riggs N, Houry D, Long G, Markovchick V, Feldhaus KM. Analysis of 1,076 cases of sexual assault. *Ann Emerg Med.* 2000;35(4):358-362.
13. SANE program development and operation guide. Office for Victims of Crime. https://www.ovcttac.gov/saneguide/introduction/
14. Sexual Assault Forensic Evidence Reporting (SAFER) Act Work Group. National best practices for sexual assault kits: a multidisciplinary approach. Office of Justice Programs. 2016. https://www.ojp.gov/pdffiles1/nij/250384.pdf
15. Office on Violence Against Women. *A National Protocol for Sexual Assault Medical Forensic Examinations.* 2nd ed. US Department of Justice; 2013. https://www.ojp.gov/pdffiles1/ovw/241903.pdf
16. Office on Violence Against Women. *A National Protocol for Sexual Abuse Medical Forensic Examinations: Pediatric.* US Department of Justice; 2016. https://www.justice.gov/ovw/file/846856/download

17. Eldredge K, Huggins E, Pugh LC. Alternate light sources in sexual assault examinations: an evidence-based practice project. *J Forensic Nurs.* 2012;8(1):39-44.
18. Mackenzie B, Jenny C. The use of alternate light sources in the clinical evaluation of child abuse and sexual assault. *Pediatr Emerg Care.* 2014;30(3):207-210.
19. Zilkens RR, Phillips MA, Kelly MC, Mukhtar SA, Semmens JB, Smith DA. Non-fatal strangulation in sexual assault: a study of clinical and assault characteristics highlighting the role of intimate partner violence. *J Forensic Leg Med.* 2016;43:1-7.
20. Slaughter L, Brown CR, Crowley S, Peck R. Patterns of genital injury in female sexual assault victims. *Am J Obstet Gynecol.* 1997;176(3):609-616.
21. Negrusz A, Juhascik M, Gaensslen RE. Estimate of the incidence of drug-facilitated sexual assault in the US: final report. Office of Justice Programs. 2005. https://www.ojp.gov/pdffiles1/nij/grants/212000.pdf
22. Examination process – alcohol and drug facilitated sexual assault. Sexual Assault Forensic Examination Technical Assistance. https://www.safeta.org/page/examprocessadfsa
23. Sexually transmitted infections treatment guidelines, 2021: sexual assault and abuse and STIs. Centers for Disease Control and Prevention. 2021. https://www.cdc.gov/std/treatment-guidelines/sexual-assault.htm
24. Association of Nurses in AIDS Care; International Association of Forensic Nurses; National Alliance to End Sexual Violence; the National Sexual Violence Resource Center. Position statement: universal access to anti-HIV medication. National Sexual Violence Resource Center. 2013. https://www.nsvrc.org/sites/default/files/2013-08/publications_nsvrc_position-universal-access-anti-hiv-medication.pdf
25. Announcement: updated guidelines for antiretroviral postexposure prophylaxis after sexual, injection-drug use, or other nonoccupational exposure to HIV — United States, 2016. *MMWR Morb Mortal Wkly Rep.* 2016;65(17):458.
26. Chao YS, Frey N. *Ulipristal Versus Levonorgestrel for Emergency Contraception: A Review of Comparative Clinical Effectiveness and Guidelines.* Canadian Agency for Drugs and Technologies in Health; 2018. https://www.ncbi.nlm.nih.gov/books/NBK538737/
27. Sable MR, Danis F, Mauzy DL, Gallagher SK. Barriers to reporting sexual assault for women and men: perspectives of college students. *J Am Coll Health.* 2006;55(3):157-162.
28. McLean IA. The male victim of sexual assault. *Best Pract Res Clin Obstet Gynaecol.* 2013;27(1):39-46.
29. Stermac L, Del Bove G, Addison M. Stranger and acquaintance sexual assault of adult males. *J Interpers Violence.* 2004;19(8):901-915.
30. Harrell E. Crime against persons with disabilities, 2009-2019 – statistical tables. Bureau of Justice Statistics. 2021. https://bjs.ojp.gov/content/pub/pdf/capd0919st.pdf
31. Sexual Assault Prevention and Response. Department of Defense annual report on sexual assault in the military: fiscal year 2019. US Department of Defense. 2020. https://media.defense.gov/2020/Apr/30/2002291660/-1/-1/1/1_DEPARTMENT_OF_DEFENSE_FISCAL_YEAR_2019_ANNUAL_REPORT_ON_SEXUAL_ASSAULT_IN_THE_MILITARY.PDF

Acute Posterior Myocardial Infarction

By Amal Mattu, MD, FACEP
Dr. Mattu is a professor, vice chair, and director of the
Emergency Cardiology Fellowship in the Department
of Emergency Medicine at the University of Maryland
School of Medicine in Baltimore.

Objective

On completion of this article, you should be able to:

- Recognize the characteristics of an acute posterior myocarial infarction on ECG.

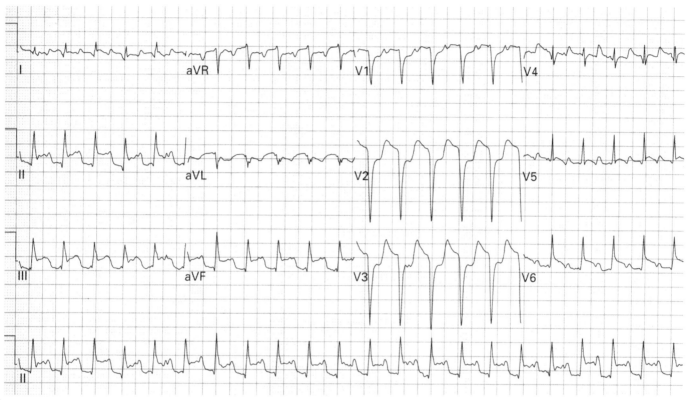

FIGURE 1. A 53-year-old man with a prior history of MI presents with chest pain and diaphoresis

ST with first-degree atrioventricular (AV) block, rate 130, acute inferior-lateral myocardial infarction (MI) with possible posterior MI, anteroseptal MI of undetermined age, and a prolonged QT interval. ST-segment elevation (STE) is present in the inferior and lateral leads consistent with acute myocardial infarction (AMI). Pronounced ST-segment depression is present in leads V_1-V_3. In the presence of an inferior AMI, ST-segment depression in the anteroseptal leads can represent either reciprocal change, or it can indicate acute posterior MI. Reciprocal ST-segment depression is usually shallow and downsloping, whereas ST-segment depression due to an acute posterior MI is usually horizontal and depressed by more than 2 mm. Therefore, the ST-segment depression in this case appears more likely to be due to an acute posterior MI.

Another expected finding in posterior MI is large R waves in leads V_1-V_3. In this case, however, large Q waves presumably from a prior anteroseptal MI prevent the development of large R waves. Confirmation of acute posterior MI could be accomplished by repeating the ECG with posterior leads and finding STE. A slightly prolonged QT interval is also present, which might be caused by acute cardiac ischemia. Other possible causes of QT-interval prolongation include hypokalemia, hypomagnesemia, hypocalcemia, elevated intracranial pressure, drugs with sodium channel–blocking effects, hypothermia, and congenital prolonged QT syndrome.

From Mattu A, Brady W. *ECGs for the Emergency Physician 2*. BMJ Publishing. Reprinted with permission.

Moderate Temperature Management After Nonshockable-Rhythm Cardiac Arrest

By Chinezimuzo Ihenatu, MD; and
Michael E. Abboud, MD, MSEd
University of Pennsylvania
Department of Emergency Medicine, Philadelphia
Reviewed by Andrew J. Eyre, MD, MS-HPed

Objective

On completion of this article, you should be able to:
- Describe the benefits of therapeutic hypothermia in nonshockable-rhythm cardiac arrest patients.

Lascarrou JB, Merdji H, Le Gouge A, et al; CRICS-TRIGGERSEP Group. Targeted temperature management for cardiac arrest with nonshockable rhythm. *N Engl J Med.* 2019;381(24):2327-2337.

KEY POINTS

- Prior data on the benefits of moderate therapeutic hypothermia for patients with nonshockable-rhythm cardiac arrest are inconclusive.

- In patients with nonshockable rhythms, moderate therapeutic hypothermia at 33°C (91.4°F) significantly improves favorable neurologic outcomes at 90 days after cardiac arrest compared to normothermia at 37°C (98.6°F); moderate hypothermia has an NNT of 22.

- Therapeutic hypothermia at 33°C (91.4°F) compared to normothermia at 37°C (98.6°F) in patients with nonshockable-rhythm cardiac arrest does not demonstrate any differences in outcomes secondary to neurologic function (eg, mortality, ICU length of stay, adverse events, or mechanical ventilation duration).

- Due to findings from this study, the AHA now recommends therapeutic hypothermia for patients in cardiac arrest with an initial nonshockable rhythm.

Introduction

Therapeutic hypothermia has been a topic of interest in cardiac arrest literature for decades and gained broad acceptance in the early 2000s. Since then, targeted hypothermia has become a mainstay of practice. Large national and international organizations such as the American Heart Association (AHA) and the International Liaison Committee on Resuscitation endorse therapeutic hypothermia for patients after out-of-hospital, shockable-rhythm cardiac arrest who have achieved return of spontaneous circulation (ROSC) but remain comatose. Data from prior important cardiac arrest studies on targeted temperature management (TTM) are not robust for patients with nonshockable rhythms. Because nonshockable rhythms have a poor prognosis and an increasing prevalence in cardiac arrests, postarrest hypothermia for nonshockable rhythms requires further investigation. A 2019 study by Lascarrou et al, dubbed the HYPERION trial, attempted to address this gap in knowledge.

This study was a randomized controlled trial (RCT), the first of its kind to investigate the effects of moderate hypothermia on the neurologic outcomes of patients 90 days after a cardiac arrest with nonshockable rhythms. The study was an open-label, blinded-outcome-assessor, multicenter trial conducted in 25 ICUs in France. The study was composed of adult patients who achieved ROSC after a nonshockable-rhythm cardiac arrest. Patients with a "no-flow time" longer than 10 minutes, those who received CPR for longer than 60 minutes, certain cirrhosis patients, and pregnant patients were excluded from the study. The two main arms of the study were patients who underwent therapeutic hypothermia (33°C [91.4°F] for the first 24 hours) and those kept at normothermia (37°C [98.6°F]). Patients at each center were randomly assigned in a 1:1 ratio. Blinded psychologists then used the Cerebral Performance Category scale to estimate the postarrest neurologic status for each patient 90 days after cardiac arrest.

The findings show that there is a significant difference in neurologic outcomes at 90 days between the 33°C (91.4°F) group and the 37°C (98.6°F) group. Favorable neurologic outcomes at 90 days occurred in 10.2% of the patients in the hypothermia group compared to 5.7% in the normothermia group (*P* = 0.04). There were no significant differences between the two treatment arms in secondary outcomes (eg, mortality, ICU length of stay, mechanical ventilation

Critical Decisions in Emergency Medicine's literature review features articles recommended by the Academic Affairs Committee. Available online at acep.org/moc/llsa.

12   *Critical Decisions in Emergency Medicine*

days, and prespecified adverse events). Furthermore, this study's number needed to treat (NNT) for hypothermia to produce a favorable outcome in 1 patient at 90 days was 22. Comparatively, the NNT for epinephrine in cardiac arrest is 112 and for bystander CPR is 15. These results highlight the potential importance of cooling patients regardless of initial rhythm. About 75% of the cardiac arrests experienced by these patients were out-of-hospital, underscoring the study's applicability to the emergency department patient population.

There are several limitations to this study. One main limitation encompasses a statistical component: This trial has a low fragility index, which means that changes in outcomes to only a couple of patients would be enough to change the outcome of the study. A bigger sample size would have improved the internal validity of the study. Additional limitations include varying the rewarming times, including the data from febrile patients (those with a temperature of 38°C [100.4°F] after the TTM period), using telephone interviews to assess neurologic function, and counting patients with missing data as deceased. Further studies that replicate findings in this RCT and address these limitations are warranted.

Despite these limitations, this study prompted the AHA to change its guidelines; it now recommends moderate hypothermia after cardiac arrest for all rhythms. Importantly, this study focused on neurologic outcomes as an end result rather than focusing on survivability. Although there was no survival benefit demonstrated in this study, the findings presented promising data on the relationship between cooling body temperatures and higher functional status for people who survive. Functional status, arguably, has a greater impact on population health and is more in line with patient preferences than survivability alone. From an emergency medicine perspective, this study demonstrated that moderate hypothermia has the potential to help shockable- *and* nonshockable-rhythm cardiac arrest patients experience a higher neurologic function post arrest.

Traction Splinting a Midshaft Femur Fracture

By Steven J. Warrington, MD, MEd, MS
MercyOne Siouxland, Sioux City, Iowa

Objective

On completion of this article, you should be able to:

- Set a traction splint for a midshaft femur fracture.

Introduction

Traction splinting of femur fractures has been used for the past century in military, prehospital, and hospital settings. There are currently multiple commercially available traction splints with similar principles and methods of use.

Contraindications

- Additional fracture of the same leg, aside from midfoot or distal to midfoot

Benefits and Risks

Traction splints are a noninvasive method; they immobilize femur fractures and decrease associated pain more than simple splinting. Traction splinting may also reduce hemorrhage, although there is debate in the literature and no definitive evidence. Interestingly, there is limited evidence on the benefit of traction splinting, aside from a recent study on decreased pain and a distant study on mortality, which may have been rendered moot by more recent advances.

Risks of traction splints include skin complications, such as skin sloughing and pressure sores; neurovascular injuries; compartment syndrome; distraction of associated fractures; perineal injuries; and urethral injuries.

Alternatives

One basic alternative to traction splints is simple splints that only immobilize the extremity. These splints can be anything from pneumatic and prefabricated splints to a much simpler stabilization with rigid supports. Another alternative that provides traction and requires no additional

TECHNIQUE

1. **Discuss** the traction splinting procedure with the patient and consider if written consent is necessary or appropriate for the situation.

2. **Gather** equipment and staff for the procedure. Fully expose the affected extremity from the pelvis down, evaluate the extremity for other possible fractures or injuries, and assess distal neurovascular status.

3. **Prepare** the traction splint:

   a. For traction splints with adjustable length, measure to the appropriate length, which includes approximately 6 inches past the ankle.

   b. For traction splints with a heel stand, unfold and lock the stand.

   c. Open and prepare the straps on the traction splint, so they are ready to be fastened to the patient.

4. **Apply** manual traction to reduce the fracture and improve alignment. For traction splints with a heel stand or upward angulation, ensure manual traction is at a similar upward angle.

5. **Slide** the traction splint into place.

6. **Apply** the ankle strap or harness.

7. **Ensure** there is appropriate tension to the ankle strap or harness.

8. **Apply** the other supportive straps of the traction splint.

9. **Assess** distal neurovascular status.

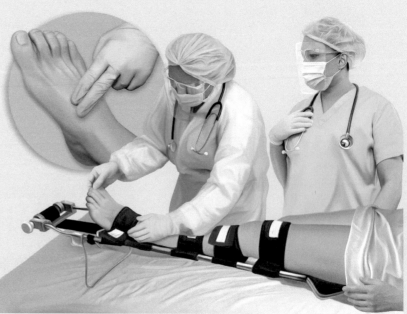

FIGURE 1. Application of a traction splint

skill is Buck or Hamilton-Russell traction. These types of traction are also skin traction (ie, noninvasive); they require equipment commonly available in a hospital setting. A final traction option is skeletal traction, which is an invasive method using pins or wires.

Reducing Side Effects

Assessing patients for concomitant injuries can reduce complications during splint application and traction. Even though traction splints reduce pain, patients may need adjunctive therapy, such as regional or intravenous analgesic agents.

Another key factor in reducing side effects is the re-evaluation of patients' neurovascular and skin status after splint application.

Recognizing that a traction splint, after placement, can lead to neurovascular compromise or pressure ulcers (in cases of prolonged splinting) can help prevent long-term complications.

Special Considerations

With multiple traction splint models available, physicians must consider which traction splint to use. Although the differences between the models may not matter in most cases, there is a model for splinting bilateral femur shaft fractures that may be useful depending on the patient's injuries. Another consideration is that some traction splints extend farther than others; this can cause issues depending on the space available, bed size, and height of the patient.

Recurrent Prosthetic Hip Dislocation

By Julie Shaner, MD
University of Florida College of Medicine – Jacksonville

Reviewed by John Kiel, DO, MPH

Objective

On completion of this article, you should be able to:

■ Describe how to manage prosthetic hip dislocations.

CASE PRESENTATION

A 69-year-old woman with a medical history of bilateral hip replacements presents after falling at home. She reports having bent over to put groceries in the refrigerator when her leg gave out, causing her to fall and become unable to walk. On arrival, she complains of sharp and severe pain in her left hip. The examination reveals an externally rotated hip with gross tenderness, intact motor function, and a dorsalis pedis pulse. She is also noted to have hyperesthesia of the peroneal and tibial nerves. Initial x-rays diagnose an anterosuperior dislocation of the left femoral prosthesis (*Figures 1* and *2*).

Discussion

Native hip dislocations are relatively uncommon when compared with other joints such as shoulders, ankles, and fingers. Prosthetic hip dislocations, however, are slightly more common, with an average incidence of 0.14% (95% CI, 0.08%-0.21%). The national estimate of prosthetic hip dislocations presenting to US emergency departments rose significantly between 2000 (n = 2,395; 95% CI, 1,264-3,526) and 2017 (n = 8,094; 95% CI, 4,276-11,912) (*P* <0.001). The rate of total hip arthroplasty (THA) dislocation is projected to increase because the number of THAs is increasing annually. Dislocation is the most frequent complication of THAs, occurring in up to 10% of all primary replacements and 28% of revisions; it is also a common indication for a revision surgery of a primary THA.[1,2]

Multiple factors are calculated in determining the risk of prosthetic dislocation. The vast majority of prosthetic dislocations occur within 6 weeks of surgery, and of those, about one-third become recurrent dislocations.[3] Patient factors associated with increased risk of dislocation include an age older than

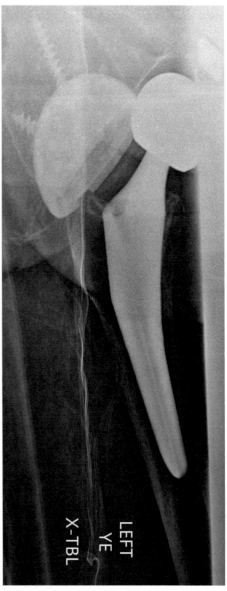

FIGURE 2. Lateral view confirming anteriorsuperior positioning of the prosthetic femoral head

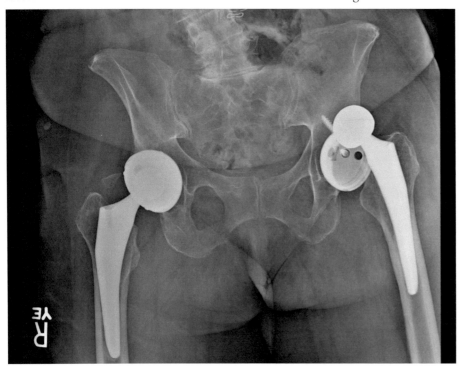

FIGURE 1. Anteriorposterior view of the pelvis showing left prosthetic hip dislocation

70 years, female sex, musculoligamentous laxity, a history of revision surgery, weakness of the abductor muscles, and altered spinopelvic mechanics. Implant factors such as improper cup placement or failure to recreate appropriate limb length and offset increase the risk of dislocation. The surgical approach also contributes to the prediction of prosthetic stability. In general, the posterolateral approach has a higher incidence of dislocation than the anterior and lateral approaches.

Patients with prosthetic hip dislocations frequently present to the emergency department after a low-energy mechanism causes injury. Initial x-rays should be obtained to determine the type of dislocation. Similar to native hips, most prosthetic hip dislocations occur posteriorly, causing the hip to be shortened and internally rotated. Managing prosthetic hip dislocations, similar to managing native ones, should include adequate procedural sedation, muscle relaxation, and reduction techniques (eg, the Allis maneuver and Captain Morgan technique). If a hip is dislocated anteriorly, an alternative reduction technique involving straight traction and forward hip flexion followed by internal rotation can be used. Internal rotation is done because anterior dislocations typically result in an externally rotated limb.

There may be some questions about who is best suited to reduce a prosthetic hip. Emergency physicians are adequately trained to reduce them, and a study by Lawerey et al demonstrated that there is no difference between emergency and orthopedic physicians in the proportion of successful hip reductions or associated complications.[4] However, patients treated by emergency physicians are discharged much sooner than those treated by orthopedic physicians.

The following are some indications that an orthopedic surgery consultation or a transfer to an emergency department with orthopedic surgical services is necessary.

- Patients within the first 6 weeks post surgery require special consideration because they may still have unhealed surgical incisions and wound-related issues.
- Any hip replacement that has a reconstructed acetabulum warrants expert evaluation. On imaging, a reconstructed acetabulum appears more complicated than a simple cup. It may have augments or phalanges extending from the cup,

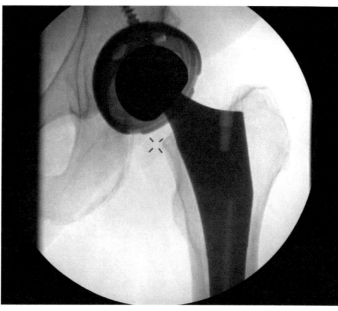

FIGURE 3. Confirmation of closed reduction in the operating room with fluoroscopy

or it may have extraneous periacetabular hardware.
- Hip replacements with a concomitant periprosthetic fracture, signs of a grossly loose femoral implant, a grossly loose cup, or a broken implant all indicate orthopedic consultation.
- Patients with poor proximal femoral bone stock are likely to need care beyond the scope of the emergency department.
- Patients with implant-specific designs including constrained liners or dual-mobility femoral-head implants warrant specialized attention.

If emergency physicians reduce a hip dislocation, the patient's orthopedic surgeon must be notified for proper follow-up. If hospital admission is not required, discharge instructions should include no bending of the hip past 90°, no crossing of the midline, no inward rotation, and use of an abduction pillow. If there are further concerns, the patient can also be restricted to toe-touch weight-bearing.

CASE RESOLUTION

The patient had spontaneously dislocated her left hip several times and previously presented for the same issue. The emergency physician made several attempts at a closed reduction, but the patient became hypoxic and apneic during procedural sedation. She was then admitted to the hospital for manipulation under general anesthesia. In the operating room, with the patient paralyzed, her left hip was reduced using a combination of axial traction, flexion, and external rotation (*Figure 3*). After a brief period in the recovery room, the patient insisted on discharge. She is currently waiting to follow up with the hip reconstruction specialist for revision of her left hip arthroplasty.

REFERENCES

1. Parvizi J, Picinic E, Sharkey PF. Revision total hip arthroplasty for instability: surgical techniques and principles. *J Bone Joint Surg Am.* 2008;90(5):1134-1142.
2. Bozic KJ, Kurtz SM, Lau E, Ong K, Vail TP, Berry DJ. The epidemiology of revision total hip arthroplasty in the United States. *J Bone Joint Surg Am.* 2009;91(1):128-133.
3. Sikes CV, Lai LP, Schreiber M, Mont MA, Jinnah RH, Seyler TM. Instability after total hip arthroplasty: treatment with large femoral heads vs constrained liners. *J Arthroplasty.* 2008;23(7)(suppl):59-63.
4. Lawrey E, Jones P, Mitchell R. Prosthetic hip dislocations: Is relocation in the emergency department by emergency medicine staff better? *Emerg Med Australas.* 2012;24(2):166-174.

A Pregnant Trauma Patient

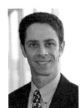

By Joshua S. Broder, MD, FACEP
Dr. Broder is a professor and the residency program director in the Department of Emergency Medicine at Duke University Medical Center in Durham, North Carolina.

Objectives

On completion of this article, you should be able to:

- Describe the safety of CT in pregnancy.
- Identify CT findings of placental abruption.
- Recognize limits of imaging for placental abruption and describe alternative monitoring for fetal distress.

CASE PRESENTATION

An 18-year-old woman at 36 weeks 6 days' gestation presents after a head-on motor vehicle collision. The patient is awake and alert but does not recall the events; EMS reports significant vehicle damage and airbag deployment. The patient complains of low back pain but denies other symptoms such as abdominal pain, vaginal bleeding, and vaginal fluid leak. She is uncertain whether she feels fetal movement. Her vital signs are BP 131/90, P 115, R 16, and T 36.6°C (97.9°F); SpO$_2$ is 99% on room air.

The patient has blood in her nares and a cervical collar in place. She is tachycardic with clear and equal breath sounds. Her abdomen is gravid and rigid, and her lumbar spine is tender. No blood or fluid is noted at the vaginal introitus. The focused assessment with sonography in trauma examination is negative. Fetal ultrasound shows a heart rate of 158 bpm without clear signs of placental abruption. Given the concern for multisystem trauma, CT is performed (*Figure 1*).

Discussion

Although fetal exposure to ionizing radiation should be limited in keeping with the ALARA principle (ie, "As Low As Reasonably Achievable"), the American College of Obstetrics and Gynecology notes that CT scans expose fetuses to a level of radiation well below the threshold associated with fetal harm. "If…[the technique is] necessary … or… *more readily available for the diagnosis in question*, [it] should not be withheld from a pregnant patient [italics added]."[1] The American College of Radiology states CT of the abdomen and pelvis with an intravenous contrast agent is "usually appropriate" in hemodynamically stable pregnant patients with major blunt trauma.[2] CT of the abdomen and pelvis provides an estimated fetal dose of 25 mGy; fetal radiation doses below 50 mGy are not associated with an increased risk of fetal loss or anomaly.[3] Despite these recommendations, one study found that only 34.4% of pregnant trauma patients with high-risk mechanisms had undergone guideline-recommended CT imaging, perhaps because of radiation concerns.[4]

When performed, CT is used primarily for assessment of maternal injuries. Fetal injuries may be noted, and the placenta is also visible on intravenous contrast-enhanced CT. Placental abruption is a critical diagnosis because of the risk of fetal morbidity and mortality (20%-60%) and maternal risks (eg, hemorrhage, disseminated intravascular coagulation [DIC], and death).[5] Ultrasound is routinely used for assessing the fetus, but it has a sensitivity for placental abruption as low as 24%, although specificity is high (92%-96%).[6] A retrospective study found that clinical abdominal CT reports for pregnant trauma patients were only 42.9% sensitive but 89.7% specific for placental abruption. This result may reflect a relative lack of familiarity with normal and abnormal CT placental appearance because of intentional CT avoidance during pregnancy. When a radiologist was cued to look for placental abruption in the study's images, sensitivity

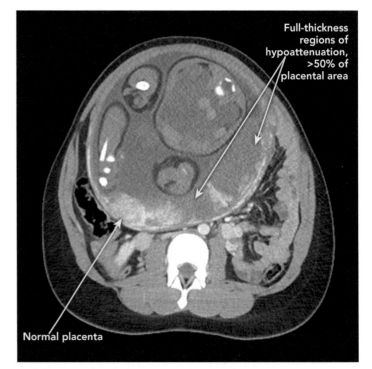

FIGURE 1. CT abdomen with intravenous contrast (soft-tissue window), axial image. Hypoattenuated regions span the full thickness of the placenta and encompass more than 50% of its cross-sectional area, strongly suggesting placental injury.

rose to 100%, while specificity fell to 79.5% (ie, a false positive rate of 20.5%). When trained on normal and abnormal placental images first, radiologists achieved a sensitivity of 100% and a specificity of 82.1%.[5] The study authors noted that false negative results may have occurred because radiologists were not evaluating the placenta during CT interpretation. Once radiologists were specifically instructed to examine the placenta, they were able to readily identify placental abnormalities that had been overlooked in routine clinical reports. Although a CT's sensitivity for placental abruption may increase when a radiologist specifically examines the placenta, this study's findings suggest overall that emergency physicians should be cautious about relying on CT for this crucial diagnosis.

False positive interpretations of placental abruption on CT can occur because the normal CT appearance of the placenta evolves over the course of pregnancy, and these changes can be mistaken for injury and abruption. The placenta is divided into a fetal section (closest to the fetus and amniotic cavity), a middle section, and a maternal section (closest to the uterine myometrium). In the second and third trimesters, the placenta commonly has a heterogeneous contrast-enhancement pattern, which can be misidentified as areas of injury or hypoperfusion associated with abruption.[5] Small subchorionic hemorrhages within the fetal section of the placenta are common and usually do not threaten the fetus. Normal placental cotyledons (arborizing placental vascular structures that facilitate oxygen and nutrient exchange between fetal and maternal blood) that occur by 24 weeks' gestation have a rounded, hypoattenuating appearance. In the third trimester, normal chorionic plate indentations within the fetal section and venous lakes within the maternal section of the placenta have a low-attenuation appearance. Physiologic myometrial contraction causes thickening and bulging of the myometrium, which can be misinterpreted as a region of underperfused placenta. Myometrial contraction usually displays an obtuse angle between regions of high- and low-enhancement on the fetal surface of the placenta, whereas placental abruption is typically associated with acute angles. Small wedge-shaped placental infarcts are sometimes seen in later pregnancy without apparent clinical significance.

False negative interpretations of placental abruption can also occur. For instance, large retroplacental hematomas can be mistaken for normal findings because they have a low-enhancement pattern similar to the myometrium.

Highly specific findings for placental abruption are areas of hypoenhancement approaching or exceeding 50% of the cross-sectional area of the placenta in a CT image (see *Figure 1*).

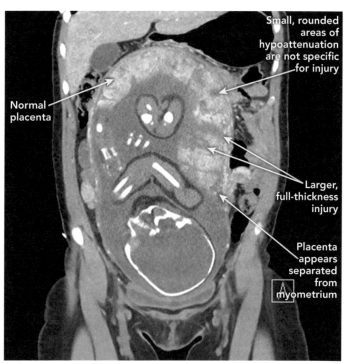

FIGURE 2. CT abdomen with intravenous contrast (soft-tissue window), coronal image. While small, rounded areas of hypoattenuation can be normal features of the placenta, larger, full-thickness regions are suspicious for injury. An acute-angle hypodensity at the margin of the placenta suggests abruption.

Full-thickness areas of placental hypoattenuation should be strongly considered as signs of abruption, in contrast to normal findings that typically cause only partial-thickness areas of hypoattenuation (*Figure 2*). Undermining of the placenta by a hypoenhancing region of hematoma with a "beaked" or acute-angle leading edge is also suspicious for abruption.

If initial fetal and placental assessment is reassuring, continuous fetal heart rate monitoring remains the clinical standard for diagnosis of fetal distress, given the limits of ultrasound and CT. Fetal distress can occur in the absence of placental abruption (eg, as a consequence of other maternal injuries such as hemorrhage from other common traumatic sources).

CASE RESOLUTION

The patient's CT was negative for other injuries. Immediately following CT, fetal monitoring became nonreassuring, so the patient underwent rapid cesarean section. The newborn had Apgar scores of 1 and 5 but subsequently improved. The patient developed DIC and had 3 L of operative blood loss, requiring ICU admission. Later, the patient and baby were discharged home in good condition.

Feature Editor: Joshua S. Broder, MD, FACEP. See also *Diagnostic Imaging for the Emergency Physician* (Winner of the 2011 Prose Award in Clinical Medicine, the American Publishers Award for Professional and Scholarly Excellence) and *Critical Images in Emergency Medicine* by Dr. Broder.

REFERENCES

1. Committee opinion no. 723: guidelines for diagnostic imaging during pregnancy and lactation. *Obstet Gynecol.* 2017;130(4):e210-e216.
2. Shyu JY, Khurana B, Soto JA, et al; Expert Panel on Major Trauma Imaging. ACR Appropriateness Criteria® Major Blunt Trauma. *J Am Coll Radiol.* 2020;17(5)(suppl):S160-S174.
3. Raptis CA, Mellnick VM, Raptis DA, et al. Imaging of trauma in the pregnant patient. *Radiographics.* 2014;34(3):748-763.
4. Shakerian R, Thomson BN, Judson R, Skandarajah AR. Radiation fear: impact on compliance with trauma imaging guidelines in the pregnant patient. *J Trauma Acute Care Surg.* 2015;78(1):88-93.
5. Wei SH, Helmy M, Cohen AJ. CT evaluation of placental abruption in pregnant trauma patients. *Emerg Radiol.* 2009;16(5):365-373.
6. Fadl SA, Linnau KF, Dighe MK. Placental abruption and hemorrhage-review of imaging appearance. *Emerg Radiol.* 2019;26(1):87-97.

Moyamoya Disease–Induced Stroke

By Jonathan Blalock, BS; Sarah Guess, MD; and Laurie Malmstrom, MD

University of South Carolina School of Medicine Greenville and Prisma Health, Department of Emergency Medicine, Greenville, South Carolina

Reviewed by Sharon E. Mace, MD, FACEP

Objective

On completion of this article, you should be able to:

■ Discuss how to diagnose and manage moyamoya disease in pediatric patients.

CASE PRESENTATION

A previously healthy 5-year-old African-American boy presents with seizure-like activity that started upon awakening. He was in his usual state of health the previous evening but woke up around 4 AM complaining of nausea. When he reawoke at 7 AM, he had developed rhythmic jerking of the left arm, left-sided weakness, and aphasia. On initial examination, he seems hypervigilant and is unable to focus or make eye contact. His upper body is braced in a defensive posture. The examination is also significant for tachycardia (126 to 160 bpm); hypotonia of the left upper and lower extremities; tonic-clonic contractions of the left upper extremity, manifesting as left shoulder shrugging; and left hemineglect. His Glasgow Coma Scale score is 14 due to confusion. His aphasia affects both expressive and receptive language. These findings are concerning for ongoing seizure, a postictal state, or ongoing stroke. He is given a total of 3 mg of intravenous lorazepam and loaded with 20 mg/kg of levetiracetam, which resolve his convulsions. Laboratory evaluation is significant for a normal glucose level, normal renal function, and a normal leukocyte count with a mildly elevated platelet count. Emergent head CT reveals a large area of hypoattenuation in the right middle cerebral artery distribution concerning for an acute infarction, with involvement of the frontal, parietal, and temporal lobes (*Figure 1*). CT angiogram of the head and neck demonstrates multifocal stenoses and occlusions of the bilateral internal carotid arteries along with enlarged lenticulostriate and thalamoperforating arteries. These findings suggest moyamoya vasculopathy; pediatric neurology is consulted. The patient is admitted to the pediatric ICU in stable condition.

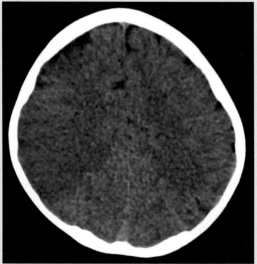

FIGURE 1. CT demonstrating wedge-shaped hypoattenuation in the right middle cerebral artery distribution consistent with ischemic infarction

Pathophysiology

Moyamoya disease (MMD) refers to a noninflammatory, progressive arteriopathy characterized by stenosis of the internal carotid arteries. The disease often progresses to involve the anterior and middle cerebral arteries (*Figure 2*). Severe stenosis of the intracranial vasculature causes compensatory collateral circulation to form through the lenticulostriate, leptomeningeal, thalamoperforating, and dural arteries, giving rise to the classic "puff of smoke" appearance (*Figure 3*).[1] This vessel network consists of abnormally fragile vessels, and changes in flow dynamics can lead to secondary aneurysms.

Moyamoya is divided into two main categories, MMD and moyamoya syndrome (MMS). MMS refers to the association of this vasculopathy with other conditions such as neurofibromatosis type 1, trisomy 21, thyroid disease, sickle cell anemia, and prior radiation therapy. When this vasculopathy is idiopathic, it is referred to as MMD. Multiple genetic mutations associated with the development of moyamoya have been discovered. In these cases, moyamoya is considered MMD rather than MMS.

Presentation

Patients with MMD typically present with signs and symptoms of cerebral ischemia or hemorrhage and their associated sequelae. In more than 80% of pediatric cases of MMD, clinical presentation is related to ischemia and includes transient ischemic attacks (TIAs) and infarcts.[2] Provocative maneuvers that cause hypocapnia, such as straining or hyperventilation, cause vasoconstriction and can induce neurologic symptoms. Adults with MMD, by contrast, are more likely to suffer from hemorrhagic events.[3,4] As patients with MMD become adults, their brains develop collateral vessels to augment circulation in areas of diminished blood flow. Even though collateral vessels dilate to increase blood flow during periods of ischemia, they are fragile and prone to rupture. Hemorrhage most often occurs in the basal ganglia and thalamus but can also occur from associated aneurysmal ruptures. Yamamoto et al described the development of lenticulostriate and choroidal channels in patients with childhood-onset MMD and noted that these channels tend to be more developed than in patients with adult-onset MMD, even though there are no significant differences in the Suzuki staging of collaterals (*Table 1*, see also *Figure 2*).[5] Rupture of collateral channels is an etiology for hemorrhagic stroke, primarily seen in patients with longer-standing disease. Incidence is close to 1 in 300,000 in Japan with variable incidence reported among sources.[6,7]

In the United States, incidence is documented at 0.086 in 100,000.[7] There are a few studies that examine the prevalence of disease in the African American populations in the US, and there is limited mixed data on the incidence in African Americans, with some reports indicating increased frequency in Caucasian Americans, while others report increased frequency in African Americans.[6,7]

Diagnosis and Differential Diagnosis

The diagnosis of MMD should be considered in patients with symptoms of cerebral ischemia or hemorrhage without an obvious cause. Most patients first undergo CT, which may demonstrate findings of ischemic stroke or hemorrhage. If TIA is causing symptoms, the CT scan may be unremarkable. CT angiography can demonstrate stenosis and occlusions typical of MMD. However, the use of MRI is favorable because, with diffusion-weighted imaging, it has higher sensitivity for acute infarct and can detect change in normal flow–related signal loss (ie, flow voids). MRI combined with MR angiography has a 92% sensitivity and 100% specificity for diagnosis.[8] MR modalities are preferred for diagnosing MMD in children because of the higher accuracy and avoidance of radiation exposure.

The gold standard and most reliable method for diagnosis is conventional cerebral digital subtraction angiography (DSA), which allows for excellent visualization of the intracranial vasculature and is the most accurate technique for cerebro-vascular investigation. Overall, DSA is a safe and reliable method for MMD diagnosis, but it requires significant radiation exposure and large amounts of contrast medium, making it a better option for patients without a definite diagnosis or for those who are undergoing evaluation before or after intervention.[9]

Regardless of angiographic technique, the characteristic MMD pattern is stenosis and occlusion of the internal carotid arteries, a network of collateral vessels in the basal ganglia, and possibly, transdural anastomoses and collaterals from the external carotid artery system.

Disease Staging

The landmark paper from Suzuki and Takaku in 1969 described the characterization of MMD using DSA.[1] This paper was published shortly after the discovery of the disease in children of Japanese descent in 1960. The study looked at 1,400 patients with MMD and characterized vascular findings on cerebral angiography to develop a staging system (see *Table 1*).

Management

The management of MMD in the acute setting generally parallels the management of ischemic stroke, intracerebral hemorrhage (ICH), and seizures. For those with ischemic-type symptoms, antiplatelet therapy is typically recommended for both children and adults. Antiplatelet therapy with agents such as aspirin or cilostazol is associated with improved survival in patients with MMD.[10] However, because MMD also increases the risk of both ischemia and hemorrhage, the decision to continue antiplatelet agents is complex. There is no medical treatment that reverses or prevents the progression of MMD. For ICH due to MMD, surgical intervention may be warranted if the ICH meets the criteria for evacuation.

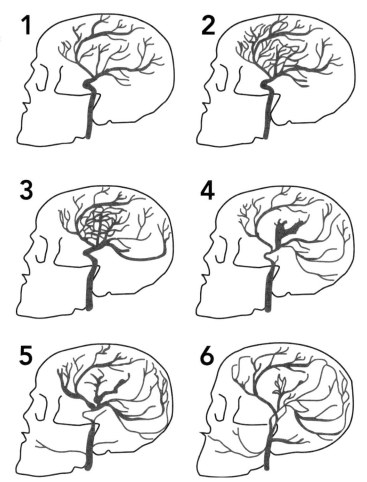

FIGURE 2. Graphic illustration of MMD progression by Suzuki staging as seen on DSA. *Credit:*Sarah Guess, MD.

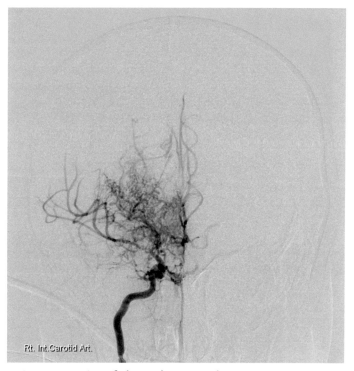

FIGURE 3. DSA of the right carotid artery demonstrating the classic "puff-of-smoke" appearance in MMD. *Credit:* Copyright 2022 Dr. Andrew Dixon. Image courtesy of Dr. Andrew Dixon and Radiopaedia.org, rID: 10586. Used under license.

Intraventricular hemorrhage that results in acute obstructive hydrocephalus may require placement of an external ventricular drain.

Chronic management of MMD consists of surgical revascularization to improve cerebral perfusion and prevent future complications. All patients with symptomatic or asymptomatic MMD should be referred for neurosurgical evaluation. Surgical treatment is performed on a nonemergent basis when patients are deemed stable. Direct, indirect, and combined revascularization techniques are shown to improve outcomes in patients with MMD.[11,12] Direct revascularization is performed through external carotid–internal carotid bypass, which typically involves direct anastomosis of the superficial temporal artery (STA) to a branch of the middle cerebral artery, allowing for immediate increases in cerebral blood flow. However, direct bypass requires highly skilled microsurgical techniques and favorable donor and recipient vessels. Because children's blood vessels have a smaller caliber and are less durable, indirect bypass remains the preferred method for surgical revascularization in pediatric MMD.

The two main indirect bypass techniques are encephaloduroarteriosynangiosis (EDAS) and encephalomyosynangiosis (EMS). EDAS involves carefully dissecting and freeing the superficial temporal artery before creating a small craniotomy and attaching the STA to the dura mater. In EMS, a flap of the temporalis muscle is placed directly over the cerebral cortex. The goal of both techniques is to provide a stimulus and source for neovascularization to augment cerebral perfusion. The development of pial collaterals allows for increased perfusion, with revascularization occurring over a period of 6 to 12 months.

Stage	Name	Description
1	Narrowing of the carotid fork	No other abnormalities are noted.
2	Initiation of moyamoya	The carotid fork is "large and obscure," main arterial vessels are enlarged, and no collaterals are noted.
3	Intensification of moyamoya	Changes develop in the main intracerebellar arteries, and some main vessels are replaced by moyamoya.
4	Minimization of moyamoya	Occlusion is noted in the internal carotid artery up to the junction of the posterior communicating artery (this vessel may not be seen on angiogram). Moyamoya is noted to be rough with a poor network of vessels.
5	Reduction of moyamoya	Branches from the internal carotid artery begin to disappear, and moyamoya continues to minimize other vessels. Collateral flow continues to increase.
6	Disappearance of moyamoya	Vessels originally seen with moyamoya at the base of the brain have disappeared. Primarily only collaterals remain, and only the vertebral or external carotid artery maintains flow.

TABLE 1. Stages of MMD as described by Suzuki and Takaku in 1969 based on angiographic findings. Names of the stages are taken directly from the publication. Suzuki J, Takaku A. Cerebrovascular "moyamoya" disease: disease showing abnormal net-like vessels in base of brain. *Arch Neurol.* 1969;20(3):288-299.

CASE RESOLUTION

The patient was admitted to the pediatric ICU for 1 day and was discharged from the hospital on day 4 following an uneventful admission. Additional studies included ECG and DNA microarray testing, neither of which detected any abnormalities. Consultants included pediatric neurosurgery, neuroendovascular surgery, and pediatric neurology. At discharge, the patient had residual left-sided paresis and no further seizures. Medications at discharge included aspirin (40.5 mg daily) and levetiracetam (350 mg twice daily).

Two weeks after discharge, the patient presented for a possible TIA but was discharged home. He is currently attending physical and occupational therapies and is followed by outpatient neurology and neurosurgery. Because there has been no further seizure activity, pediatric neurosurgery plans to proceed with a nonemergent indirect revascularization procedure.

REFERENCES

1. Suzuki J, Takaku A. Cerebrovascular "moyamoya" disease: disease showing abnormal net-like vessels in base of brain. *Arch Neurol.* 1969;20(3):288-299.
2. Lee S, Rivkin MJ, Kirton A, deVeber G, Elbers J; International Pediatric Stroke Study. Moyamoya disease in children: results from the International Pediatric Stroke Study. *J Child Neurol.* 2017;32(11):924-929.
3. Okada Y, Shima T, Nishida M, Yamane K, Yamada T, Yamanaka C. Effectiveness of superficial temporal artery-middle cerebral artery anastomosis in adult moyamoya disease: cerebral hemodynamics and clinical course in ischemic and hemorrhagic varieties. *Stroke.* 1998;29(3):625-630.
4. Chiu D, Shedden P, Bratina P, Grotta JC. Clinical features of moyamoya disease in the United States. *Stroke.* 1998;29(7):1347-1351.
5. Yamamoto S, Kashiwazaki D, Uchino H, et al. Clinical and radiological features of childhood onset adult moyamoya disease: implication for hemorrhagic stroke. *Neurol Med Chir (Tokyo).* 2020;60(7):360-367.
6. Guey S, Tournier-Lasserve E, Herve D, Kossorotoff M. Moyamoya disease and syndromes: from genetics to clinical management. Dovepress. 2015 Feb. 16;2015:49-68. https://www.dovepress.com/moyamoya-disease-and-syndromes-from-genetics-to-clinical-management-peer-reviewed-fulltext-article-TACG
7. Moyamoya Disease. NORD. 2018. https://rarediseases.org/rare-diseases/moyamoya-disease
8. Yamada I, Suzuki S, Matsushima Y. Moyamoya disease: comparison of assessment with MR angiography and MR imaging versus conventional angiography. *Radiology.* 1995;196(1):211-218.
9. Hasuo K, Tamura S, Kudo S, et al. Moya moya disease: use of digital subtraction angiography in its diagnosis. *Radiology.* 1985;157(1):107-111.
10. Seo WK, Kim JY, Choi EH, et al. Association of antiplatelet therapy, including cilostazol, with improved survival in patients with moyamoya disease in a nationwide study. *J Am Heart Assoc.* 2021;10(5):e017701.
11. Golby AJ, Marks MP, Thompson RC, Steinberg GK. Direct and combined revascularization in pediatric moyamoya disease. *Neurosurgery.* 1999;45(1):50-60.
12. Miyamoto S, Yoshimoto T, Hashimoto N, et al; JAM Trial Investigators. Effects of extracranial-intracranial bypass for patients with hemorrhagic moyamoya disease: results of the Japan Adult Moyamoya Trial. *Stroke.* 2014;45(5):1415-1421.

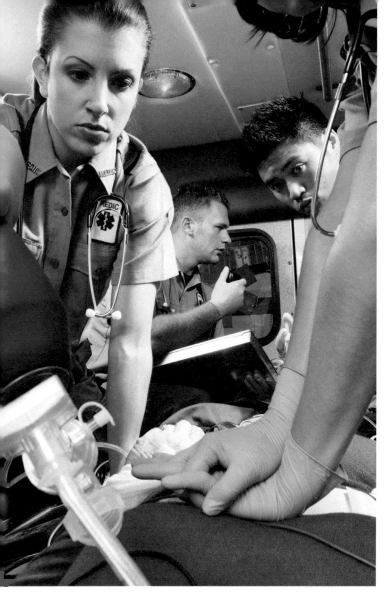

Shifting Gears
Selecting Appropriate Critical Care Transport
LESSON 20

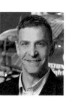

By Ani Aydin, MD, FACEP; Christie Fritz, MD, MS; Luke Duncan, MD; and Jason Cohen, DO, FACEP

Dr. Aydin is an assistant professor in the Department of Emergency Medicine, medical director of SkyHealth and Adult Ground Critical Care Transport, and associate medical director of EMS and critical care at Yale University School of Medicine in New Haven, Connecticut. Dr. Fritz is an emergency physician and medical director of Beth Israel Deaconess Medical Center Ambulance Service, clinical instructor at Harvard Medical School, and assistant program director for the Harvard-Affiliated Emergency Medicine Residency at Beth Israel in Boston, Massachusetts. Dr. Duncan is an associate professor, chief of the Division of Critical Care, and medical director of the ECLS program at Albany Medical Center in Albany, New York. Dr. Duncan is also medical director of LifeNet New York. Dr. Cohen is a physician in the Division of Trauma, Burns, Surgical Critical Care, and Emergency General Surgery in the Department of Surgery at Brigham and Women's Hospital in Boston, Massachusetts, and chief medical officer of Boston MedFlight.

Reviewed by Nathaniel Mann, MD

Objectives

On completion of this lesson, you should be able to:

1. Recall important factors used for selecting interfacility transport for critically ill patients.
2. Describe the training and experience of transport personnel.
3. Identify staffing models and their capabilities.
4. Define the levels of care provided during transport.
5. Recognize potential limitations of care during transport.
6. Discuss the responsibilities of sending and receiving physicians and the CCT medical director.
7. State how to access local and regional interfacility transport resources.

From the EM Model

20.0 Other Core Competencies of the Practice of Emergency Medicine
      20.4 Systems-Based Practice
           20.4.4 Health Care Coordination
           20.4.5 Regulatory/Legal
                20.4.5.5 Emergency Medical Treatment and Active Labor Act (EMTALA)

▬ CRITICAL DECISIONS ▬

- What factors should be considered when selecting interfacility transport for critically ill patients?
- What are the training and experience levels of transport personnel?
- What ad hoc transport staffing models are available to transport critically ill patients?
- Who makes up CCT and specialty teams?
- What are the limitations of clinical care during transport?
- What are the responsibilities of sending and receiving physicians and CCT medical directors?
- How can physicians identify and contact local and regional transport resources?
- What are the accrediting bodies for services involved in interfacility CCT?

Narrowing down the myriad options for transferring critically ill patients to a higher level of care can be a complex and urgent task. Emergency physicians must know what transfer options are available and how to select the most appropriate critical care transport (CCT) to decrease the risk of patients decompensating during transport and to quickly get them to a higher level of care.

■ CASE ONE

A 38-year-old man with no significant medical history presents after 3 days of dyspnea on exertion, lower-extremity edema, dizziness, and near syncope following a mild viral illness. His initial workup is notable for bilateral perihilar edema with an enlarged cardiac silhouette, elevated troponin and B-type natriuretic peptide levels, and a negative D-dimer test. A bedside ECG shows decreased left ventricular function and a dilated inferior vena cava. During the evaluation, the patient clinically decompensates, with worsening hypotension and hypoxemia. His work of breathing improves on moderate BiPAP settings, and his blood pressure improves with diuresis and an epinephrine infusion. The patient is accepted to the ICU at the closest cardiac center. The transfer center asks if they should send their CCT team to retrieve the patient, which may take several hours, or if the local ALS transportation agency is adequate. The receiving physician also asks whether the patient should be intubated for the transport.

■ CASE TWO

A previously healthy 8-year-old girl presents via EMS from the local urgent care clinic with dyspnea and lethargy.

She was seen at urgent care the day prior, diagnosed with bilateral otitis media, and discharged home with a prescription for amoxicillin. On return to urgent care, she was tachypneic with an increased work of breathing, given dexamethasone, and transferred to the emergency department. On arrival, the patient is ill appearing, tachypneic to 36 breaths/min with an SpO$_2$ of 93% on room air, and tachycardic to 140 bpm with a blood pressure of 123/72 mm Hg. Her laboratory results are notable for a blood glucose of 508 mg/dL, a pH of 6.9 with a PaCO$_2$ of 7 mm Hg, and a serum bicarbonate level of less than 5 mEq/L. She is treated with 20 mL/kg of normal saline, started on an insulin infusion, and given potassium repletion. The patient remains ill appearing but is stable as the physician calls regional referral hospitals for an available pediatric ICU bed. She is eventually accepted to a center approximately 70 miles away. The receiving hospital offers to send their ground specialty CCT team to retrieve the patient; however, their estimated time of arrival is approximately 3 hours from now. The sending hospital has a contract with the local ALS service that can be available for transport in about 1 hour. Finally, there are two helicopter EMS services in the region, but the first service contacted declines due to poor weather conditions.

■ CASE THREE

A 75-year-old man with a history of hypertension presents with scalp bleeding after falling down five stairs and striking his head. He is not on antiplatelet agents or anticoagulants and has an initial Glasgow Coma Scale (GCS) score of 14. He is complaining of left hip pain and left-sided chest pain worsened by breathing. A bedside extended focused assessment with sonography in trauma ultrasound examination shows a left-sided pneumothorax, so a chest tube is placed. There are no signs of hemoperitoneum on ultrasound. CT imaging shows a 2-cm right-sided subdural hematoma without midline shift and left-sided rib 6 through 10 fractures with a minimal residual pneumothorax after proper chest tube placement. X-ray shows a left midshaft femur fracture. The patient is accepted for transfer to a level I trauma center. The closest CCT team is 1.5 hours away, and the closest ALS transfer resource is parked in the ambulance bay. While the physician tries to secure an accepting transfer facility, the patient's GCS score declines to 12, and he has increasing left thigh swelling with a systolic blood pressure drop to 80 mm Hg.

Introduction

Emergency physicians often stabilize critically ill and injured patients, but to provide definitive care, physicians must keep in mind hospital and community resources and their limitations. When interfacility transfer is necessary for a higher level of care or expert consultation, emergency physicians must be aware of available transport resources (ie, the various modes of transport and the capabilities and scope of practice of transport personnel) as well as how to facilitate transport safely and effectively.[1] Emergency physicians must consider the limitations of the transport service, which can range from the basic life support (BLS) of EMS services to the advanced care of CCT and specialty teams, and plan accordingly to mitigate the risks associated with interfacility transfers.[2-5]

CRITICAL DECISION

What factors should be considered when selecting interfacility transport for critically ill patients?

Many factors should be considered during the interfacility transport of critically ill patients (*Table 1*). For example, with time-sensitive conditions, such as ST-elevation myocardial

Condition	Factors to Consider
Is the condition time sensitive?	• STEMI • Stroke • Trauma
How much active management is needed en route?	• Hemodynamic stability • CCT access to online medical control • Transport personnel's training and scope of practice
What special devices, equipment, or therapies are needed?	• Mechanical ventilators • Infusion pumps • Blood products • Isolettes for neonates
Is a specialty transport team needed?	• Neonatal • Pediatric • ECMO • HiROB • Mobile stroke units
What are the unmodifiable factors that influence available options?	• Availability of EMS and CCT teams • Weather • Distance to receiving facility • Traffic patterns • Landing zones for rotor wing transport

TABLE 1. Factors to consider for selecting the mode and level of transport

Personnel Type	Approximate Hours of Training	Typical Scope of Care
EMR	50 hours	**Basic lifesaving interventions** • Tourniquet application • First aid • CPR, automated external defibrillator, bag-valve-mask use • Autoinjectors
EMT	150 hours	**BLS and transportation** • Assisting patients with prescribed medications • Placing oral and nasal airways • Supplemental oxygen use • Splinting and immobilization • Uncomplicated vaginal deliveries • Naloxone atomizer
A-EMT	200 hours	**BLS and limited ALS and transport** • Limited pharmacological interventions • Intravenous or intraosseous placement • Cardiac monitoring • Supraglottic airway placement • Nebulized medications
Paramedic	1,100 hours	**ALS and transport** • ECG interpretation • Pacing, cardioversion, defibrillation • Advanced cardiovascular life support medications • Noninvasive positive-pressure ventilation • Endotracheal intubation • Percutaneous cricothyroidotomy • Medication delivery via pump • Needle decompression • Maintenance of blood product transfusion
CCT	Dictated by medical director	**ALS with additional specialty training** • Advanced noninvasive and invasive mechanical ventilation • Advanced airway techniques, video laryngoscopy • Cardiac assist devices • Intracranial pressure monitoring • Blood product administration • Invasive-line monitoring • Advanced medication administration and titrations

TABLE 2. Training and scope of practice of EMS and CCT personnel

infarctions (STEMIs), acute ischemic strokes, and traumatic injuries, patients should be transported expeditiously while also considering their needs for advanced monitoring and ongoing treatment during transport.

Some critically ill patients may require active management during transport, such as the independent initiation or titration of vasopressor agents, airway management, active manipulation of mechanical ventilation parameters, or blood product administration. They may also need specialty equipment, such as mechanical ventilators, transfusion pumps, cardiac assist devices, or invasive monitoring equipment (eg, an arterial line or intracranial pressure monitor).[2] In these cases, the transport team's training and comfort level with this type of equipment must be considered.[2] In some instances, specialty teams may be deployed to care for critically ill patients during transport and may include mobile extracorporeal membrane oxygenation (ECMO) teams, neonatal or pediatric transport teams, or those capable of caring for high-risk obstetric (HiROB) patient emergencies.[6,7]

Several nonmodifiable and environmental factors should also be considered, such as weather conditions, travel distance, and the availability of on-site versus remote landing zones for air transport at individual hospitals. The various

modes of transport range from ground to helicopter to fixed-wing services. Importantly, the vehicle type does not necessarily equate with the level of care. Many specialty and CCT-level services operate via ground ambulances. Likewise, several air (helicopter and fixed-wing) services operate primarily at an advanced life support (ALS) level of care.[8]

CRITICAL DECISION

What are the training and experience levels of transport personnel?

Traditionally, EMS personnel respond to local 911 emergencies, patient transport requests, and calls to transport patients between health care facilities. The EMS system is composed of multitiered responders who have competency-based requirements and varied scopes of practice based on their training (*Table 2*). EMS personnel include emergency medical responders (EMRs), emergency medical technicians (EMTs), advanced emergency medical technicians (A-EMTs), and paramedics.[9]

EMRs undergo between 45 and 60 hours of training and can provide some immediate lifesaving treatments while awaiting the arrival of advanced EMS personnel.[9] EMTs receive between 150 and 180 hours of training and perform basic life support (BLS) techniques.[9] In addition to the skills of EMRs, EMTs can assist patients in administering some of their own medications, provide a limited spectrum of oral medications, insert oropharyngeal or nasopharyngeal airways, provide supplemental oxygen, splint and immobilize extremities, and perform emergency vaginal deliveries.[9] They are unable to initiate, monitor, or maintain intravenous infusions. They are skilled in facilitating safe and efficient transport of patients via ambulance, without providing invasive care.[9] A-EMTs require approximately 200 hours of training and, in addition to the lifesaving maneuvers of basic EMTs, can insert supraglottic airways, treat patients with nebulized medications, insert intravenous and intraosseous lines, monitor cardiac functions, and monitor and maintain simple intravenous fluid infusions (nonmedications), such as crystalloid solutions.[9]

Paramedics are the highest level of EMS personnel, often requiring more than 1,200 hours of training.[9] In addition to having the skills required of A-EMTs, paramedics can perform ALS, including ECG interpretation and advanced cardiac life support, medication-facilitated intubations and cricothyroidotomies, mechanical and noninvasive ventilation, decompressive thoracostomies, infusions of medications, and maintenance of blood product transfusions.[9]

CRITICAL DECISION

What ad hoc transport staffing models are available to transport critically ill patients?

Occasionally, patients' conditions may exceed the level of care that can be provided in the available transport ambulance, even when staffed at the paramedic level.[1,9] In such cases, the ideal solution is to include a dedicated CCT team from the sending or receiving facility or a third-party organization as part of the transfer team.

If a CCT team is unavailable for an appropriate time frame, sending physicians must weigh the risks against the benefits of waiting for CCT availability, sending patients via a lower level of care, or forming an ad hoc transport team by sending their hospital staff with an existing transport team to augment its capabilities and scope of practice.[10] For example, some EMS agencies cannot initiate a transfusion of blood products due to local regulations or agency protocols. This scenario may require hospital staff, such as a registered nurse, to travel with the team to initiate a transfusion during transport. The sending physician must decide if the benefits of transfusing a patient during transport are worth the loss of a nurse in the emergency department and the challenges to the transport team of an additional caregiver. The decision may be contingent on several factors, including local resources, transport times to the nearest receiving facility, and background and training of ad hoc transport team members.

Respiratory therapists (RTs), specialty-care nurses from various ICUs, perfusionists, nurse practitioners (NPs), physician assistants (PAs), and physicians may also be called into service to help transport critically ill patients. However, most of these ad hoc team members are unfamiliar with the challenges, limitations, and safe operations of an out-of-hospital transfer or do not grasp the importance of cohesion in a team that has trained together. All of these

factors must go into the deliberation of sending physicians when they decide which transport service to use.

CRITICAL DECISION

Who makes up CCT and specialty teams?

BLS teams are usually made up of two EMTs; ALS teams are typically an EMT and a paramedic, although ALS teams can also be two paramedics.[1] CCT teams can include physicians, NPs, PAs, RTs, and critical care–trained nurses and paramedics.[9] Paramedic and nurse teams are the most common patient care teams, although this varies based on available resources and the sponsoring health care organization.[10,11] The medical director of each CCT team, in conjunction with the sponsoring body, establishes the crew configuration, training, and treatment protocols during prehospital and interfacility transports while keeping in mind each clinician's scope of practice.[10]

Specialty transport teams are often used for special high-risk populations, such as pediatric, neonatal, and HiROB patients.[6,12,13] Special procedural teams may also exist in the community, including mobile ECMO teams, which may include intensivists, cardiac surgeons, perfusionists, and RTs.[7]

CRITICAL DECISION

What are the limitations of clinical care during transport?

Ideally, interfacility transport brings additional resources and training to critically ill patients before transfer and provides expedient and safe transport while maintaining a high level of care en route.[3,9] However, these benefits do not routinely occur in the United States, given the constraints of EMS systems, scarcity of specialty resources, and limitations of financial reimbursement for transport. Nevertheless, the *minimum* goal of interfacility transport should be to continue the level of care initiated at the sending facility while being capable of employing mitigation tools and strategies

---

✔ Pearls

- Emergency physicians must be aware of their local and regional interfacility transport capabilities and the scope and training of crew members.
- For safe, patient-centered transports, emergency physicians should stabilize patients as much as possible prior to transfer and consider the risks and limitations of available care during transport.
- The mode and level of transport used for interfacility transfers depends on the time-sensitive need for expert consultation; risk of patient deterioration during transfer; and training, scope, and capability of transport personnel.
- Air and ground CCT teams have additional training, as dictated by their medical director, to provide ongoing specialty care and treat the causes of patient deterioration if it occurs during transfer to the destination facility.

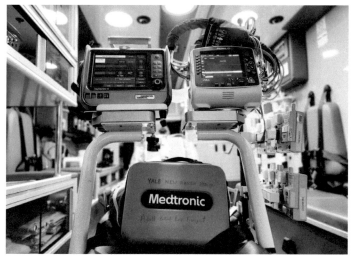
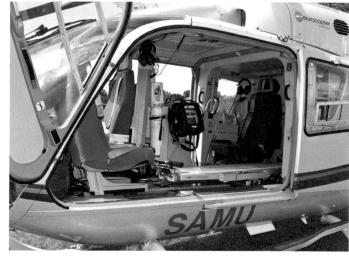

FIGURE 1. CCT ground and air transport vehicles with equipment. *Credit:* (*left*) Dr. Ani Aydin; (*right*) Ed Buziak/Alamy Stock Photo

to prevent and treat potential decompensation.[9] Sending physicians must be aware of the limitations that exist during interfacility transport, so they choose the appropriate mode and level of care.[9,10]

The composition of the transport team determines the clinical care provided during transport.[9,10] Although the scope and certification of health care professionals who make up CCT teams vary by state, and sometimes by service, most critical care patients transported between facilities in the United States are cared for by specially trained paramedics and nurses.[11] Most staff on CCT-designated teams are required to complete additional training to maintain readiness and provide a higher level of care.[9] Several national courses and certification programs provide this extra training, including the International Association of Flight and Critical Care Paramedics certifications (FP-C or CCP-C) and the Air and Surface Transport Nurses Association (ASTNA) certifications (CFRN or CTRN).[12] The specialized training of CCT teams prepares them to care for critically ill patients in transit and teaches mitigation strategies if patients decompensate during transport.[9,10]

Sometimes, ALS-level personnel without education beyond their initial certification must care for critically ill patients. Lack of specialized training may significantly limit the care team's ability to effectively manage changes in patients' status.[2-5] For example, although many patients can be continued on the same mechanical ventilation strategy or vasopressor support during transport, a specifically trained and experienced team has the skills and online medical control support to address clinical decompensation if it occurs during transport. Endotracheal intubation and advanced airway management are within the scope of traditional paramedics, but medication-facilitated or rapid sequence intubation may not be.

Physicians must consider how limitations of space and resources in ground and air transport vehicles can affect complex, patient-centered care and safety. Access to patients may be limited by the vehicle's cabin configuration (*Figure 1*). For instance, some helicopters limit access to the lower extremities, and some ambulances limit access to one side of the patient. Patient access during transport may also be impacted by the requirement that team members use seat restraints during transport.

The eventuality of a prolonged transport is a major planning consideration for CCT teams. Should CCT teams need to initiate new medications or blood products to patients en route, their choices are limited to those on the transport vehicle. More importantly, limitations in personnel quantity can have a significant impact on patient care. For example, one busy resuscitation in an emergency department may require 6 to 10 people, including physicians, nurses, NPs, PAs, RTs, and pharmacists. During transport, only one or two responders may be available.

CRITICAL DECISION

What are the responsibilities of sending and receiving physicians and CCT medical directors?

When emergency physicians recognize that the needs of a critically ill patient exceed their capabilities, they may need to facilitate a transfer to a hospital capable of providing such care. In the United States, emergency physicians are obligated to complete a screening medical examination per the Emergency Medical Treatment and Labor Act (EMTALA) and must do their best to stabilize patients.[10,12] When the need for transfer to a higher level of care is identified, EMTALA designates the sending physician as the one responsible for choosing the most appropriate level of care and mode of transport based on the patient's clinical condition, likelihood of decompensation, and clinical needs during transport, including any specialty devices.[10,12]

Medical directors of transport services are responsible for dictating the basic crew configurations and their training and scope of practice, understanding that specialty teams have differing scopes of practice depending on the available personnel.[8-10] Medical directors can also provide additional support during transit by establishing criteria for online medical direction assistance in cases of patient deterioration.[10]

Accepting physicians must ensure that the receiving hospital has the capacity, expertise, and personnel to care for transferred patients.[12] Accepting physicians may also provide expert consultation, including advising sending physicians or transport teams on how to stabilize patients during transit.[10] Receiving hospitals cannot make their acceptance of patients contingent on their own CCT team undertaking the transfer.

CRITICAL DECISION

How can physicians identify and contact local and regional transport resources?

Similar to learning about resource and resuscitation equipment availability in the emergency department, emergency physicians must learn how to locate resources in their communities. Local EMS medical directors can discuss the capabilities and availability of the various services in the area.[10] Additionally, state offices or bureaus of EMS, usually within public health departments, frequently provide regulatory oversight and strategic planning for EMS.

Air medical transport, particularly helicopter transport, is susceptible to weather limitations.[8] Calling multiple air medical transport operators after a declined transport mission due to dangerous weather conditions, also known as "weather shopping," is discouraged because it may prompt flying in detrimental conditions and has been linked to adverse events.[13,14] The prohibitive weather conditions for one air transport service likely apply to others, unless an agency operates under instrument flight rules (IFR), which increase weather minimums. Agencies that operate under IFR, however, are uncommon in the United States helicopter EMS industry. In general, a single weather decline should prompt physicians to consider opting for ground transport or delaying patient transfer unless the physician knows a service that operates under IFR.

CRITICAL DECISION

What are the accrediting bodies for services involved in interfacility CCT?

In the civilian medical community in the United States, outside of state and regional licensure for ground and air ambulance services, voluntary, independent industry bodies set the national operational and clinical standards for safe patient transports. The Commission on Accreditation of Medical Transport Systems (CAMTS) is the primary accrediting body for air and ground CCT organizations in the United States.[14] As with other credentialing bodies,

CAMTS offers transport organizations the chance to complete a voluntary evaluation to ensure compliance with accreditation standards and demonstrate the ability to provide quality service. CAMTS is comprised of 21 nonprofit organizations, including the American College of Emergency Physicians (ACEP), National Association of EMS Physicians (NAEMSP), Emergency Nurses Association (ENA), Association of Critical Care Transport (ACCT), and American Academy of Pediatrics, and is a member of the American National Standards Institute.[14] Although CAMTS does not mandate accreditation, many states have adopted mandatory CAMTS accreditation to be licensed at the CCT level.

Some areas of the country may not have access to any of the more than 160 agencies that have invested the resources and organizational commitment toward CAMTS accreditation. For ground ambulance organizations, the Commission on Accreditation of Ambulance Services (CAAS) independently accredits organizations and reviews if they are adhering to "nationally accepted standards," irrespective of the level of care provided. The CAAS is led by a board that has representation from the American Ambulance Association, NAEMSP, ENA, and ACEP.[15]

Beyond the CAMTS and CAAS, differentiating and validating standards of care in CCT services in the United States can be challenging. Physicians in these circumstances may be forced to rely on their personal knowledge of organizations and their leadership when determining the best option for transporting critically ill patients to a higher level of care.

The ACCT offers a set of additional operational and clinical standards for CCT organizations to increase their quality of care.[9] Similarly, the ASTNA has published its second edition of *Standards for Critical Care and Specialty Transport*. These standards attempt to provide a framework for expectations of CCT programs. NAEMSP, in conjunction with ACEP and the Air Medical Physicians Association, also offers various position statements on air medical utilization and the necessity for strong quality assurance programs.

Summary

CCT teams include personnel specifically trained to care for critically ill patients during interfacility transfers, including continuing care initiated at the sending hospital and treating clinical deteriorations that may occur during transport.[3,9] Additionally, CCT teams, based on their training and scope as dictated by a medical director, can care for patients requiring specialty devices and titrate medications during transport, comparable to mobile ICUs.[9,10] Specialty teams are trained to care for medically vulnerable patients (eg, pediatric or neonatal) who require additional expertise for safe and effective care during interfacility transports.[6,10] When emergency physicians need to transfer critically ill patients to a higher level of care or specialty hospital, they must be aware of their roles and responsibilities, the transport resources in their communities, the training and scope of the transport personnel, and the limitations and risks of transport.

✖ Pitfalls

- Neglecting to arrange additional resources for more emergent transfers and delaying transport of critically ill patients with time-sensitive conditions.
- Failing to understand how transport mode and level of care available in the community can lead to unsafe conditions during transport.
- Overlooking the importance of the training, scope, and capabilities of transport personnel in providing the appropriate level of care and increasing patient safety during transfer to a higher level of care.

CASE RESOLUTION

CASE ONE

The emergency physician elected to avoid intubation prior to transport because the patient was alert and much improved with BiPAP. Additionally, the physician was concerned about hemodynamic collapse with rapid sequence intubation. The local EMS agency could not transport patients on BiPAP without taking the hospital RT, a vital hospital resource. It was decided to wait for the CCT team that could stabilize the patient's airway and hemodynamic status should he need it during transport. When the patient was transitioned to the transport BiPAP, he decompensated, but the CCT team appropriately responded by titrating the BiPAP settings and vasopressor support. The rest of the transport was uneventful, and the patient was diagnosed with viral myocarditis and ultimately required a percutaneous mechanical circulatory support device. An eventual full recovery is expected.

CASE TWO

The emergency physician decided to wait for the ground CCT team because they were specially trained to care for critically ill pediatric patients. Approximately 3 hours later, the CCT team arrived and assessed the patient. Following protocol, the CCT team contacted their pediatric intensivist for online medical direction, who instructed them to initiate an infusion of hypertonic saline due to the patient's declining mental status and readminister a second dose during transport if her mental status did not improve.

The patient's mental status initially improved but then deteriorated en route. An additional bolus of hypertonic saline was administered, and with concerns about her ability to compensate for her acidemia, she underwent rapid sequence intubation. The patient was ventilated using a strategy driven by the CCT team's bedside blood gas analyzer, and she was given a sodium bicarbonate infusion and electrolyte replacement. On arrival at the receiving hospital's pediatric ICU, a CT head scan revealed diffuse cerebral edema. The patient received aggressive osmotic therapy and a decompressive craniotomy, improving her cerebral edema and neurologic status with minimal residual deficits.

CASE THREE

With the patient's declining mental status and time-sensitive condition, the emergency physician elected to intubate the patient while awaiting ALS transfer. His blood pressure improved after receiving a unit of packed RBCs. The ALS crew arrived and expressed concern about the patient's clinical instability. The sending physician and transport service's medical director discussed the case and its risks and agreed that the patient's condition was time sensitive and required immediate transport. To augment the ALS crew's capabilities, the sending physician arranged for an emergency department nurse and an RT to accompany the transport team. A transfusion of fresh frozen plasma was initiated before transfer, and one unit of packed RBCs was sent in a cooler with the team. The patient arrived at the level I trauma center in stable but critical condition and was emergently transferred to the operating room for a subdural hematoma evacuation by neurosurgery.

REFERENCES

1. National Highway Traffic Safety Administration. National EMS scope of practice model. EMS. 2007. https://www.ems.gov/education/EMSScope.pdf

2. Droogh JM, Smit M, Hut J, de Vos R, Ligtenberg JJ, Zijlstra JG. Inter-hospital transport of critically ill patients: expect surprises. Crit Care. 2012;16(1):R26.

3. Warren J, Fromm RE Jr, Orr RA, Rotello LC, Horst HM; American College of Critical Care Medicine. Guidelines for the inter- and intrahospital transport of critically ill patients. Crit Care Med. 2004;32(1):256-262.

4. Murata M, Nakagawa N, Kawasaki T, et al. Adverse events during intrahospital transport of critically ill patients: a systematic review and meta-analysis. Am J Emerg Med. 2022;52:13-19.

5. Nonami S, Kawakami D, Ito J, et al. Incidence of adverse events associated with the in-hospital transport of critically ill patients. Crit Care Explor. 2022;4(3):e0657.

6. Patel SC, Murphy S, Penfil S, Romeo D, Hertzog JH. Impact of interfacility transport method and specialty teams on outcomes of pediatric trauma patients. Pediatr Emerg Care. 2018;34(7):467-472.

7. Bonadonna D, Barac YD, Ranney DN, et al. Interhospital ECMO transport: regional focus. Semin Thorac Cardiovasc Surg. 2019;31(3):327-334.

8. Araiza A, Duran M, Surani S, Varon J. Aeromedical transport of critically ill patients: a literature review. Cureus. 2021;13(5):e14889.

9. Association of Critical Care Transport. Critical care transport standards. National Association of State EMS Officials. 2016. https://nasemso.org/wp-content/uploads/ACCT-Standards-Version1-Oct2016.pdf

10. Shelton SL, Swor RA, Domeier RM, Lucas R. Medical direction of interfacility transports: National Association of EMS Physicians standards and clinical practice committee. Prehosp Emerg Care. 2000;4(4):361-364.

11. Greene MJ. 2012 critical care transport workplace and salary survey. Air Med J. 2012;31(6):276-280.

12. Examination and treatment for emergency medical conditions and women in labor. Social Security Administration. 1986. https://www.ssa.gov/OP_Home/ssact/title18/1867.htm

13. Aircraft accident report: helicopter air ambulance collision with terrain Survival Flight Inc. Bell 407 helicopter, N191SF near Zaleski, Ohio January 29, 2019. National Transportation Safety Board. 2020. https://www.ntsb.gov/investigations/AccidentReports/Reports/AAR2001.pdf

14. Commission on Accreditation of Medical Transport Systems. Eleventh edition accreditation standards of the Commission on Accreditation of Medical Transport Systems. 2018. https://www.camts.org/wp-content/uploads/2017/05/CAMTS-11th-Standards-DIGITAL-FREE.pdf

15. About CAAS. Commission on Accreditation of Ambulance Services. 2022. https://caas.org/about

ADDITIONAL READING

National Highway Traffic Safety Administration. National Emergency Medical Service Education Standards. 2021. https://www.ems.gov/pdf/EMS_Education_Standards_2021_v22.pdf

Reviewed by Kelsey Drake, MD, MPH, FACEP; and Nathaniel Mann, MD

Qualified, paid subscribers to *Critical Decisions in Emergency Medicine* may receive CME certificates for up to 5 ACEP Category I credits, 5 *AMA PRA Category 1 Credits*™, and 5 AOA Category 2-B credits for completing this activity in its entirety. Submit your answers online at acep.org/cdem; a score of 75% or better is required. You may receive credit for completing the CME activity any time within 3 years of its publication date. Answers to this month's questions will be published in next month's issue.

1 Which statement is a characteristic of sexual assault against male victims?

A. Male victims are more likely than female victims to be assaulted by multiple assailants.

B. Male victims are three times more likely than female victims to report the assault.

C. Male victims of sexual assault do not require postexposure prophylaxis for sexually transmitted infections.

D. Male victims rarely suffer psychological consequences following sexual assault.

2 Which step is appropriate when discharging a patient after a sexual assault evaluation?

A. Documenting the diagnosis as "alleged sexual assault" to avoid legal liability

B. Informing the patient that adult, competent patients must report the assault to law enforcement

C. Leaving evidence collected on the charge nurse's desk until picked up by law enforcement

D. Referring the patient to a rape crisis center

3 Which factor should be considered when evaluating a suspected victim of alcohol- and drug-facilitated sexual assault?

A. Urine and blood specimens are of no forensic value if collected more than 2 hours after the assault.

B. Urine and blood specimens should be sent to the in-hospital laboratory for testing.

C. Urine and blood tests are warranted for any victim with amnesia, dizziness, impaired motor skills, or other signs of acute intoxication.

D. Urine tests are likely to be contaminated and will be of little use in such cases.

4 Which statement accurately characterizes sexual assault?

A. Emotional sequelae of sexual assault are common.

B. Significant force is used in most sexual assaults, leading to serious injury.

C. The perpetrator is usually unknown to the victim.

D. The primary motive of sexual assault is the perpetrator's sexual gratification.

5 Which statement characterizes sexual assault in special populations?

A. Geriatric patients have no risk of being sexually assaulted.

B. Men are more likely than women to report sexual assault.

C. Patients with disabilities have a higher rate of sexual assault than the general population.

D. Women in the military are less likely than their male counterparts to report sexual assault.

6 What is the most common location of injury on women who have been sexually assaulted?

A. Clitoral hood

B. Hymen

C. Perineum

D. Posterior fourchette

7 A sexually assaulted patient's clothing is collected as evidence, but the clothing is wet. Which action demonstrates the best handling of the evidence?

A. Hanging it to dry in the staff lounge

B. Placing it in a labeled plastic bag and immediately notifying law enforcement that it needs to be dried before storage

C. Placing it in a labeled plastic bag and keeping it until it dries

D. Placing it in a labeled plastic bag and leaving it on the desk at the nursing station

8 What is the most common substance used in alcohol- and drug-facilitated sexual assault?

A. Alcohol

B. Fentanyl

C. Flunitrazepam

D. Gamma-hydroxybutyrate

9 Which statement is true regarding strangulation in sexual assault cases?

A. Patients always disclose strangulation without prompting.

B. Strangulation during sexual assault is less likely if the assault occurs in the context of an intimate relationship.

C. Strangulation may cause carotid artery dissection.

D. Strangulation never causes serious injury without obvious external signs.

10 **When should toluidine blue be applied?**
   A. After initial photographs
   B. After speculum examination
   C. Prior to initial photographs
   D. Toluidine blue should never be used

11 **When transferring a critically ill patient to another facility, what are sending physicians responsible for?**
   A. Considering the need for transfer to a receiving facility for a higher level of care or expert consultation
   B. Considering the risks and limitations of the transport environment and selecting the appropriate mode and level of transfer based on the patient's clinical condition and risk of deterioration
   C. Providing a medical screening examination and stabilizing the patient to the best of their capabilities, as per the Emergency Medical Treatment and Labor Act (EMTALA)
   D. All of these

12 **Which responsibility is not the role of the critical care transport team's medical director?**
   A. Dictating the mode of transport used during interfacility transports
   B. Helping dictate the configuration of the team in consultation with hospital, community, or corporate stakeholders
   C. Helping sending physicians understand the resources available in the community, including the modes of interfacility transport and scope of the crew members
   D. Training the team to care for critically ill patients in transport

13 **What types of responders most commonly comprise critical care transport teams?**
   A. EMT and nurse
   B. EMT and paramedic
   C. Paramedic and nurse
   D. Pharmacist and nurse

14 **Which EMS personnel can perform rapid sequence intubation in accordance with their scope of practice, if allowed by their medical director?**
   A. Advanced EMTs
   B. EMRs
   C. EMTs
   D. Paramedics

15 **Which statement about receiving physicians is correct?**
   A. They determine the configuration of critical care transport teams.
   B. They ensure bed availability and the required expertise at their facility prior to transfer.
   C. They should demand the fastest mode of transport to their facility.
   D. They should only accept interfacility transfer of critically ill patients by critical care transport organizations.

16 **Which factor is not a limitation of interfacility transport?**
   A. The devices and equipment available for transport
   B. The scope of practice of the transport personnel
   C. The type and quantity of medications available during transport
   D. Transport personnel with various levels of training and scope of practice

17 **Which group is an example of a specialty team?**
   A. Critical care transport team
   B. EMT-EMT team
   C. EMT-paramedic team
   D. Mobile extracorporeal membrane oxygenation cannulation and retrieval team

18 **Which action cannot be performed by critical care transport teams during transport?**
   A. Blood product administration
   B. Management of multiple infusion medications
   C. Mechanical ventilator titration
   D. Placement of central venous access

19 **Which organization is an accrediting body for critical care transport?**
   A. American Heart Association
   B. Commission on Accreditation of Ambulance Services
   C. Commission on Accreditation of Medical Transport Systems
   D. Joint Commission on Accreditation of Healthcare Organizations

20 **A 65-year-old patient who has chest pain but is hemodynamically stable and has no ST-elevation myocardial infarction on ECG requires transport to a hospital with a cardiac catheterization laboratory. What is the most appropriate mode of transportation?**
   A. Advanced life support
   B. Air medical transport
   C. Basic life support
   D. Critical care transport

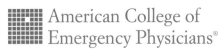

American College of
Emergency Physicians®

ADVANCING EMERGENCY CARE

Post Office Box 619911
Dallas, Texas 75261-9911

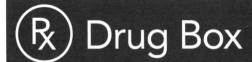

Tecovirimat

By Frank LoVecchio, DO, MPH, FACEP
Valleywise Health and ASU, Phoenix, Arizona

Objective
On completion of this column, you should be able to:
- Discuss the utilization of tecovirimat to treat monkeypox.

Antiviral medications to treat nonvariola *Orthopoxvirus* infections (eg, monkeypox) are limited. The FDA approved tecovirimat for symptomatic smallpox in July 2018. Tecovirimat became available to treat monkeypox through the CDC's expanded access investigational new drug (EA-IND) protocol in July 2022. There are no controlled human trials documenting tecovirimat's safety or efficacy in patients with monkeypox.

In an animal study, macaques were challenged with a lethal dose of monkeypox virus. Survival was 100% in animals that started treatment up to 5 days post challenge. In animals starting treatment 6, 7, or 8 days post challenge, survival was 67%, 100%, and 50%, respectively. Treatment initiation up to 4 days post challenge reduced the severity of clinical manifestations.

Infectious disease investigators at the University of California, Davis, described a case series in which tecovirimat was administered to and well tolerated by 25 patients with monkeypox.

Physicians and pharmacists can request tecovirimat for monkeypox through their health departments or the CDC Emergency Operations Center at 770-488-7100.

Adult Dosing
- Between 35 and <120 kg: 200 mg IV every 12 hours
- ≥120 kg: 300 mg IV every 12 hours **OR**
- Between 40 and <120 kg: 600 mg PO every 12 hours
- ≥120 kg: 600 mg PO every 8 hours
Duration of therapy: 14 days; may be longer (up to 90 days) or shorter depending on disease progression and the patient's clinical condition
Note: Initiate with oral therapy when possible. Patients unable to take oral therapy may start with IV therapy and switch as soon as possible. The first dose of the new form should be given at the same time and in place of the old form's next scheduled dose.

Adverse Effects
- *Common (>2%):* Nausea, abdominal pain, and vomiting
- *Less common:* Hives and allergic reactions (eg, breathing problems)
Pregnancy risk factor: Unknown, but limited systemic absorption may limit fetus drug levels

Contraindications
Hypersensitivity to tecovirimat or any component of the formulation is possible.
- *IV:* Severe renal impairment (creatinine clearance <30 mL/min)
- *Oral:* The manufacturer's US label lists no contraindications.

REFERENCES

Desai AN, Thompson GR III, Neumeister SM, Arutyunova AM, Trigg K, Cohen SH. Compassionate use of tecovirimat for the treatment of monkeypox infection. *JAMA.* 2022.
O'Laughlin K, Tobolowsky FA, Elmor R, et al. Clinical use of tecovirimat (Tpoxx) for treatment of monkeypox under an investigational new drug protocol — United States, May – August 2022. *MMWR Morb Mortal Wkly Rep.* 2022;71:1190-1195.
Russo AT, Grosenbach DW, Brasel TL, et al. Effects of treatment delay on efficacy of tecovirimat following lethal aerosol monkeypox virus challenge in cynomolgus macaques. *J Infect Dis.* 2018;218(9):1490-1499.

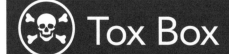

Dinitrophenol Overdose

By Christian A. Tomaszewski, MD, MS, MBA, FACEP
University of California San Diego Health

Objective
On completion of this column, you should be able to:
- Manage patients with DNP poisoning.

Dinitrophenol (DNP), a drug that blocks lipogenesis, was a weight-loss agent until banned by the FDA. Industrial DNP, in powder or tablet form, is still purchased online, mainly by body builders. DNP induces a hypermetabolic state that often results in death.

Mechanism of Action
- Uncouples oxidative phosphorylation with inhibition of ATP formation
- Increases cellular calcium with muscle contraction and heat production

Pharmacokinetics
- Rapidly absorbed after oral ingestion
- Can also be inhaled or dermally absorbed
- 1 to 3 mg/kg can cause toxicity
- Half-life is days, mainly hepatically metabolized

Clinical Manifestations
- *Temperature:* Hyperthermia
- *Cardiac:* Tachycardia
- *Pulmonary:* Tachypnea
- *Metabolic:* Acidosis
- *Hepatic:* Jaundice
- *Renal:* Failure
- *Muscular:* Spasms and rhabdomyolysis
- *Neurologic:* Confusion or agitation; seizures
- *Dermatologic:* Diaphoresis

Diagnostics
- Acetaminophen level in intentional ingestions
- Comprehensive metabolic panel in symptomatic cases to check for acidosis and hepatorenal function
- Creatine phosphokinase for rhabdomyolysis

Treatment
- Activated charcoal within 1 hour of massive ingestions if the patient is awake
- Benzodiazepines for agitation or seizure
- Fluid resuscitation
- External cooling
- Dantrolene, successful in case reports at approximately 2 mg/kg (can repeat dosing)

Disposition
- May medically clear if asymptomatic at 10 to 12 hours post ingestion
- Observe or admit symptomatic ingestions with hyperthermia or tachycardia

Critical decisions
in emergency medicine

Volume 36 Number 11: **November 2022**

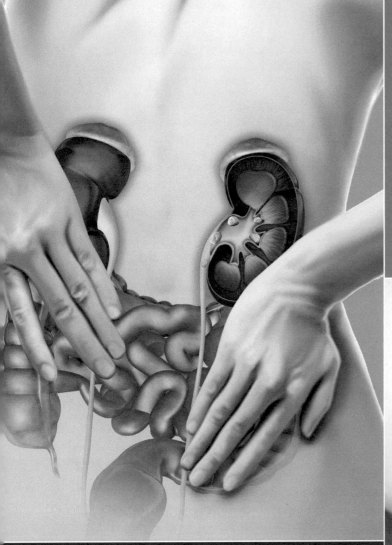

Hard Pass

Renal stone disease is a common diagnosis, with nearly 2% of emergency department visits related to ureteral colic. Despite the frequency of renal stones, the breadth of presentation, imaging options, and optimal treatments are moving targets. Emergency physicians should be versed in the latest literature to help optimize workup, diagnosis, and treatment of this common and painful disease.

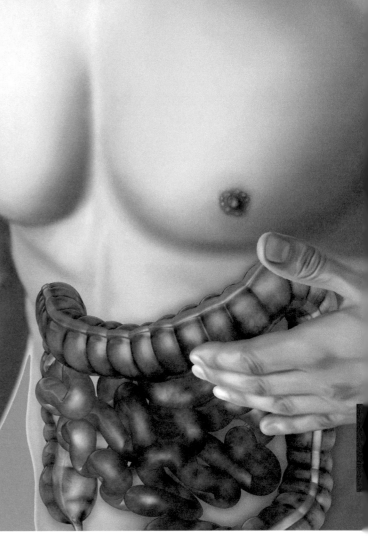

Gut Reaction

Mesenteric ischemia is an uncommon cause of abdominal pain, accounting for approximately 1 in 1,000 hospital admissions. Mesenteric ischemia can be challenging to diagnose and deadly if missed, with a 60% to 90% mortality rate. Emergency physicians must know the key features and tests to promptly diagnose and treat patients who present with this condition.

Individuals in Control of Content

1. Zach Burroughs, MD – Faculty
2. Joslin Gilley-Avramis, MD – Faculty
3. Robert Healy, MD, LT, MC, USN – Faculty
4. Joshua Kern, MD – Faculty
5. Shelby Marx, MD – Faculty
6. Daphne Morrison Ponce, MD, CDR, MC, USN – Faculty
7. Ryan Spangler, MD, FACEP – Faculty
8. Alvin Varghese, MD – Faculty
9. Joshua S. Broder, MD, FACEP – Faculty/Planner
10. Ann M. Dietrich, MD, FAAP, FACEP – Faculty/Planner
11. Andrew J. Eyre, MD, MS-HPEd – Faculty/Planner
12. Walter L. Green, MD, FACEP – Faculty/Planner
13. John Kiel, DO, MPH – Faculty/Planner
14. Frank LoVecchio, DO, MPH, FACEP – Faculty/Planner
15. Sharon E. Mace, MD, FACEP – Faculty/Planner
16. Amal Mattu, MD, FACEP – Faculty/Planner
17. Christian A. Tomaszewski, MD, MS, MBA, FACEP – Faculty/Planner
18. Steven J. Warrington, MD, MEd, MS – Faculty/Planner
19. Tareq Al-Salamah, MBBS, MPH, FACEP – Planner
20. Michael S. Beeson, MD, MBA, FACEP – Planner
21. Wan-Tsu Chang, MD – Planner
22. Kelsey Drake, MD, MPH, FACEP – Planner
23. John C. Greenwood, MD – Planner
24. Danya Khoujah, MBBS, MEHP, FACEP – Planner
25. Nathaniel Mann, MD – Planner
26. George Sternbach, MD, FACEP – Planner
27. Joy Carrico, JD – Planner/Reviewer

Contributor Disclosures. In accordance with the ACCME Standards for Integrity and Independence in Accredited Continuing Education, all relevant financial relationships, and the absence of relevant financial relationships, must be disclosed to learners for all individuals in control of content 1) before learners engage with the accredited education, and 2) in a format that can be verified at the time of accreditation. The following individuals have reported relationships with ineligible companies, as defined by the ACCME. These relationships, in the context of their involvement in the CME activity, could be perceived by some as a real or apparent conflict of interest. All relevant financial relationships have been mitigated to ensure that no commercial bias has been inserted into the educational content. Joshua S. Broder, MD, FACEP, is a founder and president of OmniSono Inc, an ultrasound technology company, and a consultant on the Bayer USA Cardiac Imaging Advisory Board. Sharon E. Mace, MD, FACEP, performs contracted research funded by Biofire Corporation, Genetesis, Quidel, and IBSA Pharma. All remaining individuals with control over content have no relevant financial relationships to disclose.

This educational activity consists of two lessons, eight feature articles, a post-test, and evaluation questions; as designed, the activity should take approximately 5 hours to complete. The participant should, in order, review the learning objectives for the lesson or article, read the lesson or article as published in the print or online version until all have been reviewed, and then complete the online post-test (a minimum score of 75% is required) and evaluation questions. Release date: November 1, 2022. Expiration date: October 31, 2025.

Accreditation Statement. The American College of Emergency Physicians is accredited by the Accreditation Council for Continuing Medical Education to provide continuing medical education for physicians.

The American College of Emergency Physicians designates this enduring material for a maximum of *5 AMA PRA Category 1 Credits™.* Physicians should claim only the credit commensurate with the extent of their participation in the activity.

Each issue of *Critical Decisions in Emergency Medicine* is approved by ACEP for 5 ACEP Category I credits. Approved by the AOA for 5 Category 2-B credits.

Commercial Support. There was no commercial support for this CME activity.

Target Audience. This educational activity has been developed for emergency physicians.

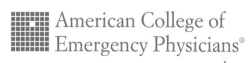
American College of Emergency Physicians®
ADVANCING EMERGENCY CARE

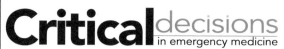
Criticaldecisions
in emergency medicine

Critical Decisions in Emergency Medicine is the official CME publication of the American College of Emergency Physicians. Additional volumes are available.

EDITOR-IN-CHIEF

Michael S. Beeson, MD, MBA, FACEP
Northeastern Ohio Universities, Rootstown, OH

SECTION EDITORS

Joshua S. Broder, MD, FACEP
Duke University, Durham, NC

Andrew J. Eyre, MD, MS-HPEd
Brigham and Women's Hospital/ Harvard Medical School, Boston, MA

John Kiel, DO, MPH, FACEP, CAQSM
University of Florida College of Medicine, Jacksonville, FL

Frank LoVecchio, DO, MPH, FACEP
Valleywise, Arizona State University, University of Arizona, and Creighton Colleges of Medicine, Phoenix, AZ

Sharon E. Mace, MD, FACEP
Cleveland Clinic Lerner College of Medicine/ Case Western Reserve University, Cleveland, OH

Amal Mattu, MD, FACEP
University of Maryland, Baltimore, MD

Christian A. Tomaszewski, MD, MS, MBA, FACEP
University of California Health Sciences, San Diego, CA

Steven J. Warrington, MD, MEd, MS
MercyOne Siouxland, Sioux City, IA

ASSOCIATE EDITORS

Tareq Al-Salamah, MBBS, MPH, FACEP
King Saud University, Riyadh, Saudi Arabia/ University of Maryland, Baltimore, MD

Wan-Tsu Chang, MD
University of Maryland, Baltimore, MD

Ann M. Dietrich, MD, FAAP, FACEP
University of South Carolina School of Medicine, Greenville, SC

Kelsey Drake, MD, MPH, FACEP
St. Anthony Hospital, Lakewood, CO

Walter L. Green, MD, FACEP
UT Southwestern Medical Center, Dallas, TX

John C. Greenwood, MD
University of Pennsylvania, Philadelphia, PA

Danya Khoujah, MBBS, MEHP, FACEP
University of Maryland, Baltimore, MD

Nathaniel Mann, MD
University of South Carolina School of Medicine, Greenville, SC

George Sternbach, MD, FACEP
Stanford University Medical Center, Stanford, CA

EDITORIAL STAFF

Suzannah Alexander, Editorial Director
salexander@acep.org

Joy Carrico, JD
Managing Editor

Alex Bass
Assistant Editor

Kel Morris
Assistant Editor

ISSN2325-0186 (Print)   ISSN2325-8365 (Online)

Contents

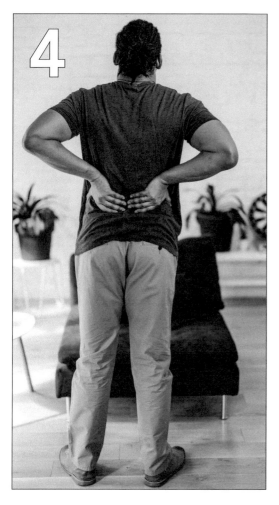

Lesson 21 4
Hard Pass
Kidney Stones in the Emergency Department
By Ryan Spangler, MD, FACEP; and Alvin Varghese, MD
Reviewed by Ann M. Dietrich, MD, FAAP, FACEP

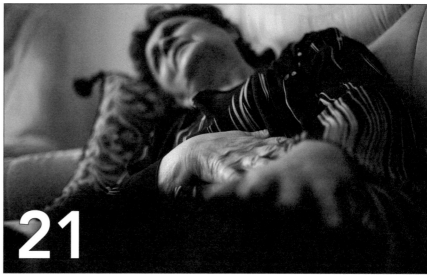

Lesson 22 21
Gut Reaction
Treating Mesenteric Ischemia
By Joshua Kern, MD; and Joslin Gilley-Avramis, MD
Reviewed by Walter L. Green, MD, FACEP

FEATURES

The Critical ECG — Hypokalemia Characteristics 11
    By Amal Mattu, MD, FACEP

Clinical Pediatrics   Monkeypox in the Pediatric Emergency Department 12
    By Shelby Marx, MD; Zach Burroughs, MD; and Ann M. Dietrich, MD, FAAP, FACEP
    Reviewed by Sharon E. Mace, MD, FACEP

The Literature Review — A Comparison of Ibuprofen Regimens for Acute Pain 14
    By Robert Healy, MD, LT, MC, USN; and Daphne Morrison Ponce, MD, CDR, MC, USN
    Reviewed by Andrew J. Eyre, MD, MS-HPEd

Critical Cases in Orthopedics and Trauma — An Atypical Presentation of Gout 16
    By John Kiel, DO, MPH

The Critical Image — An Adolescent With Knee Pain 18
    By Joshua S. Broder, MD, FACEP

The Critical Procedure — Management of Small, Bleeding Tongue Lacerations 20
    By Steven J. Warrington, MD, MEd, MS

CME Questions 30
    Reviewed by Ann M. Dietrich, MD, FAAP, FACEP; and Walter L. Green, MD, FACEP

Drug Box — Systemic Hydrocortisone 32
    By Frank LoVecchio, DO, MPH, FACEP

Tox Box — SGLT2-Inhibitor Toxicity 32
    By Christian A. Tomaszewski, MD, MS, MBA, FACEP

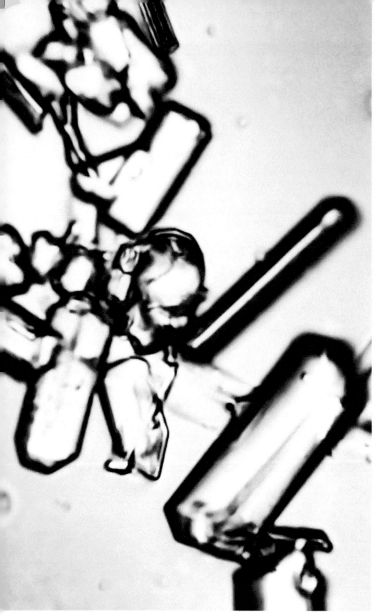

Hard Pass

Kidney Stones in the Emergency Department

LESSON 21

By Ryan Spangler, MD, FACEP; and Alvin Varghese, MD
Dr. Spangler is the director of undergraduate medical education in the Department of Emergency Medicine at the University of Maryland School of Medicine, and Dr. Varghese is a resident at the University of Maryland Medical Center in Baltimore.

Reviewed by Ann M. Dietrich, MD, FAAP, FACEP

Objectives

On completion of this lesson, you should be able to:

1. Describe risk factors and clinical manifestations of kidney stones.
2. Explain the imaging options for the diagnosis of kidney stones.
3. Discuss the predictive value of hematuria in kidney stones.
4. Summarize the medical management of kidney stones.
5. Identify admission criteria for a patient with kidney stones.

From the EM Model

15.0 Renal and Urogenital Disorders
    15.7 Structural Disorders
        15.7.1 Calculus of Urinary Tract

■ CRITICAL DECISIONS ■

- What diagnostic study should be ordered to assess patients with suspected kidney stones?
- How useful is hematuria as an indication of kidney stones?
- What is the best medical management for kidney stones?
- What is the prognosis in patients presenting with renal colic?
- Which patients require emergent surgical consultation?
- When should patients with kidney stones receive antibiotics?

Renal stone disease, and more specifically ureteral colic, is a bread-and-butter emergency medicine diagnosis; nearly 2% of emergency department visits are related to ureteral colic. Despite the frequency of renal stones, its breadth of presentation, imaging options, and optimal treatments are moving targets. Emergency physicians should be versed in the latest literature to help optimize workup, diagnosis, and treatment of this common and painful disease.

CASE ONE

A 59-year-old man presents complaining of right flank pain radiating to the right groin. The pain was insidious at first, progressed to 10 out of 10, and improved to 6 out of 10 with NSAIDs. He denies any medical history and takes no medications. His social history is positive for cigarette smoking. Initial vital signs include BP 140/86, P 82, R 18, and T 36.7°C (98.1°F).

The physical examination reveals an uncomfortable patient; his abdomen is soft with diffuse tenderness on palpation, which is greatest over the right lower quadrant. His genitourinary examination is unremarkable.

CASE TWO

A 34-year-old woman presents with 2 weeks of left flank pain that reminds her of a previous kidney stone. While she was waiting for the stone to pass, her pain worsened, and she started to have severe nausea and six episodes of nonbloody, nonbilious vomiting. The patient's initial vital signs include BP 133/76, P 101, R 16, and T 37.2°C (98.9°F). On physical examination, the patient has left lower quadrant pain and left costovertebral angle tenderness.

CASE THREE

A 63-year-old woman with a history of previous kidney stones presents with right flank pain, along with fever, nausea, vomiting, and difficulty urinating for the past day. The patient's vital signs include BP 150/74, P 112, R 14, and T 38.3°C (100.9°F). On physical examination, she has right costovertebral tenderness without abdominal tenderness, guarding, or rebound. Other than tachycardia, the cardiopulmonary examination is unremarkable. She is noted to have a capillary refill time of more than 3 seconds.

Introduction

Kidney stones (also known as urinary stone disease, renal stone disease, nephrolithiasis, or urolithiasis) is a general term used to describe the presence of stones within the urinary tract. Although stones are formed in the kidneys, they do not usually cause severe symptoms unless they drop into the collecting system and cause renal or ureteral colic. Nearly 2% of adult presentations are for suspected renal colic.[1] In the United States, approximately 13% of men and 7% of women are diagnosed with kidney stones.[2]

Clinical Manifestations

The classic presentation of kidney stones is severe flank pain with an acute onset that radiates to the ipsilateral groin; the pain often starts at night. Patients are typically writhing in distress and unable to find a comfortable position. The pain is usually episodic, lasting around 20 to 60 minutes. Patients may also complain of dysuria, urgency, and frequency.[3] Thirty percent of patients also complain of hematuria.[4] The renal capsule shares splanchnic innervation with the intestine; therefore, patients can also experience nausea and vomiting.[3] Fever is atypical, unless associated with an infection.

Risk Factors for Kidney Stones

Kidney stones are caused by certain biochemical abnormalities of urine composition. Risk factors are affected by modifiable and nonmodifiable factors, which vary in different populations. High urine calcium, high urine oxalate, low urine citrate, high urine uric acid, low urine volume, acidic urine below pH 5.5 (for uric acid stones), and alkaline urine above pH 6.5 (for calcium phosphate stones) are all factors that lead to stone formation.[5] In addition, lack of fluid intake and consumption of beverages containing sugar increase the risk of stone formation.[6] These modifiable factors account for more than 50% of kidney stones. Preventative measures can be taken to reduce these factors, such as eating a DASH diet (**D**ietary **A**pproaches to **S**top **H**ypertension) that is high in fruits and vegetables, moderate in low-fat dairy products, and low in animal protein.

A lower body mass index has also been shown to decrease the burden of kidney stones.[7]

In addition to modifiable risk factors, there are those that are nonmodifiable. Nonmodifiable risk factors that increase patients' chances of having kidney stones include a family history of the disease, male sex, White race, and certain medical conditions such as primary hyperparathyroidism, hypertension, diabetes, gout, obesity, and renal tubular acidosis.[8]

Differential Diagnosis for Acute Flank Pain

The differential diagnosis for acute flank pain is large, and physicians must differentiate acute flank pain caused by renal colic from other life-threatening pathologies. In a study that looked at 714 CT scans in patients who presented with acute flank pain, 63% of the patients were found to have kidney stones.[8] Some of the most common alternate diagnoses were cholelithiasis (5%), appendicitis (4%), pyelonephritis (3%), ovarian cyst (2%), renal mass (1.4%), and abdominal aortic aneurysm (AAA) with and without rupture (1.4%).[9] Renal colic is one of the most common misdiagnoses in patients with ruptured AAAs; therefore, care should be taken to rule out a AAA before diagnosing renal colic.[10] A complete differential for flank pain should always include vascular, pulmonary, and gastrointestinal systems, in addition to the urinary system (*Table 1*).[11]

Potentially Serious or Life-Threatening Causes	Benign Causes
• AAA	• Acute pyelonephritis
• Appendicitis	• Hepatitis
• Bowel obstruction	• Musculoskeletal pain
• Cholecystitis	• Ovarian cyst
• Ectopic pregnancy	• Peptic ulcer disease
• Pancreatitis	• Renal calculi
• Pulmonary embolism	• Renal cyst
• Renal vein thrombosis	• Varicella-zoster virus
• Renal malignancy and infarction	
• Testicular torsion	

TABLE 1. Differential diagnosis for acute flank pain

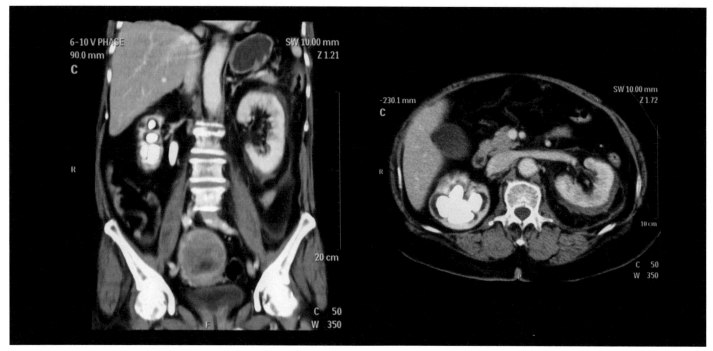

FIGURE 1. CT scan of kidney stones. *Credit:* Suttha Burawonk/Shutterstock.com.

STONE Score

The STONE score is a clinical assessment tool that helps predict the likelihood of ureteral stones in nontoxic-appearing patients with flank pain. The STONE score uses four objective criteria (ie, sex, timing, nausea or vomiting, and erythrocytes) to sort patients with suspected kidney stones into low-, moderate-, and high-risk groups.[12] The factors that increase the likelihood of a stone include male sex, less than 6 hours of pain prior to presentation, vomiting, and hematuria on a urine dipstick test.[13] High STONE scores (ie, 10-13) have an 87% specificity for a CT finding of a stone.[12] In patients with a high STONE score, it is often reasonable to forgo CT imaging for an ultrasound to evaluate for hydronephrosis, provided patients have no other complicating factors. A recent prospective study showed that patients with moderate STONE scores (6-9) can undergo a CT protocol with an 85% or more reduction in contrast without losing sensitivity.[14] If patients have a low STONE score, alternate diagnoses should be considered.[14]

CRITICAL DECISION

What diagnostic study should be ordered to assess patients with suspected kidney stones?

For patients who present with suspected renal colic, with or without hematuria, there is no consensus on whether imaging studies are necessary for a diagnosis. Imaging is currently used for two purposes. It is used to obtain information about the stone size and location and to confirm or rule out other diagnoses. If imaging is used, noncontrast CT of the abdomen and pelvis is the gold-standard imaging study because it has the highest diagnostic accuracy for renal and ureteral stones due to its high specificity and sensitivity (almost 100%) (*Figure 1*).[15-17] However, a retrospective cohort analysis that compared the negative predictive value of noncontrast CT versus contrast-enhanced CT showed that contrast-enhanced CT can safely exclude obstructing ureteral stones. This is particularly important

because of the benefit of intravenous contrast material in diagnosing other abdominopelvic pathology such as a ruptured AAA and appendicitis.[18]

Ultrasound is another imaging modality that can be used to evaluate for renal or ureteral stones. Ultrasound can identify hydronephrosis but is only sometimes successful at visualizing the presence of a ureteral stone; this is generally dependent on whether the stone is proximal or distal because the mid ureter is difficult to evaluate on ultrasound. However, ultrasound is quick, inexpensive, noninvasive, and does not expose patients to radiation.[19] In patients with high clinical suspicion for stone disease, using ultrasound as the primary imaging modality has shown to be both safe and effective without missing significant alternate pathologies (*Figure 2*).[20]

Although a stone that is distal to the renal pelvis or proximal to the ureterovesical junction (UVJ) is not likely to be seen with ultrasound, a visible stone can be identified as a hyperechoic structure with posterior shadowing.[21] Physicians can also look at the ureteral jets for asymmetry or absence and look for a color Doppler twinkling artifact (the focus of alternating colors behind a reflective object [such as calculus] on Doppler signal that gives the appearance of turbulent blood flow), both of which

✔ Pearls

- A UTI along with an obstructed stone is a urologic emergency.

- Poor outcomes are seen in patients with kidney stones combined with decreased renal function, previous urologic interventions, or symptoms of infections.

- Hematuria as an indicator of renal calculi has a cited accuracy of around only 60.9%, so its absence cannot exclude calculi.

can suggest a kidney stone diagnosis when the stone is not identified (*Figure 3*).[19,22] These findings, however, are not sensitive, and their absence does not rule out the presence of a stone. A prospective study that looked at ultrasound as the initial tool in 318 patients showed a sensitivity of 98.3% and specificity of 100% in identification of a stone.[23] Ultrasound is also unable to accurately size a stone.[24] In addition, the sensitivity and specificity vary depending on the equipment, performer's skill, and patient's body habitus.

Abdominal x-rays have historically been used as an imaging modality in the workup of flank pain. However, kidneys-ureter-bladder x-ray has poor sensitivity (45%-59%) and specificity (77%) for identifying stones and is unable to accurately size a stone. It is generally only used for follow-up in patients who already have a diagnosis of renal stones; x-rays have very limited utility in an emergency setting.[25]

CRITICAL DECISION

How useful is hematuria as an indication of kidney stones?

Hematuria is a common complaint or finding in patients with kidney stones. Macroscopic hematuria is obviously visible blood (ie, red or pink urine) and microscopic hematuria is visible only under the microscope. Hematuria often occurs because of glomerular basement membrane damage from injury, infection, or mass. Some drugs, calculi, and chemicals can also cause hematuria by eroding the mucosal surface of the urinary tract.[26] Macroscopic hematuria most frequently has a nonglomerular cause including renal or ureteral stones.

Hematuria has classically been used as an indicator of a kidney stone in patients presenting with flank pain. The accuracy of hematuria, however, as an indicator of renal calculi has been cited at around only 60.9%; therefore, its absence cannot exclude calculi.[27] Hematuria is most common during the first day of the disease, and 80% of patients experience either microscopic or macroscopic hematuria at some point during their disease course.[28] The size or location of the stone does not correlate with the presence or absence of hematuria.[27] A retrospective review showed that the absence of hematuria is associated with longer hospital stays.[29]

CRITICAL DECISION

What is the best medical management for kidney stones?

Generally, stone size and location determine the likelihood of stone passage.[30] Most stones 5 mm or smaller in diameter pass spontaneously. There is a progressive decrease in the likelihood of stone passage when they are larger than 4.5 mm in diameter

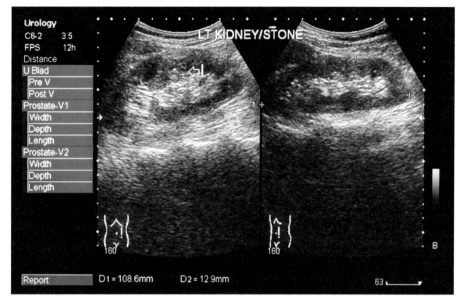

FIGURE 2. **Ultrasound of a kidney showing a left kidney stone.** *Credit:* Puwadol Jaturawutthichai/Shutterstock.com.

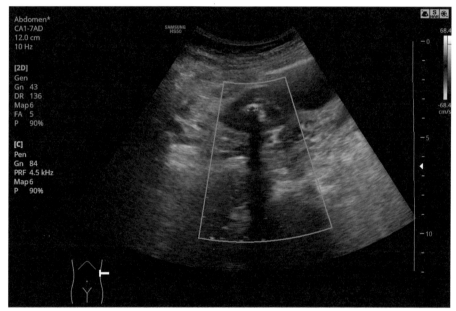

FIGURE 3. **Twinkling artifact.** *Credit:* Copyright 2022 Dr. Bálint Botz. Image courtesy of Dr Bálint Botz and Radiopaedia.org, rID: 84361. Used under license.

(87% passage versus 37% passage). Stones 10 mm or larger in diameter are very unlikely to pass.[31] Also, stones more distally located in the ureter have a greater likelihood of spontaneous passage (84% below the sacroiliac joint versus 52% above).[31]

When a patient presents with acute kidney stone–related pain, one of the main therapeutic goals is to get the pain under control. Prostaglandins are thought to play the biggest role in renal colic pain, which is caused by an increase in collecting-system pressure and ureteral spasm. Therefore, NSAIDs have been the preferred treatment for renal colic.[32] When compared to opioids, NSAIDs have fewer requirements for rescue analgesia, a lower rate of emesis, and fewer adverse effects.[32] Opioids, in comparison, do not inhibit prostaglandins, and, in some studies, are shown to increase ureteric muscle tone.[33] However, in patients with GI bleeds and impaired renal function, narcotics are helpful at treating renal colic pain. Studies have shown that patients' pain improves more when NSAIDs and opioids are given together, suggesting that multimodal pain management could be the appropriate therapy for patients presenting with severe renal colic.[34]

Intravenous hydration should be considered for individuals who are dehydrated from vomiting or have decreased their oral intake secondary to the pain.[35] A 2010 Cochrane review found that aggressive fluid resuscitation provides no added benefit for stone passage in acute ureteral colic.[35] However, improved hydration can prevent recurrences of stone formation.[36] In order to transition to oral fluids prior to discharge, some patients might need antiemetics.[37] A randomized controlled study showed that ondansetron is more effective than metoclopramide in preventing and improving vomiting in patients suffering from renal colic.[38]

In addition to analgesia and antiemetics, medical expulsive therapy (MET) initiation, such as tamsulosin 0.4 mg daily (an α-blocker) can be considered for stone passage; α-blockers inhibit smooth muscle contraction in the ureter, theoretically facilitating stone passage.[39] Two large multicenter, randomized controlled studies showed that MET with α-blockers such as tamsulosin is only beneficial for patients with 5- to 10-mm stones and not for patients whose stones measure less than 5 mm.[40] Another randomized controlled study showed that tamsulosin does not improve expulsion time for stones smaller than 7 mm but is associated with a signigcantly reduced need for analgesics when compared to the placebo group.[41] Although variability of the literature on this subject still exists, the American Urological Association (AUA) recommends α-blockers for MET. In many cases, few risks are associated with α-blockers, but careful consideration is warranted in patients at risk of hypotension and falls.

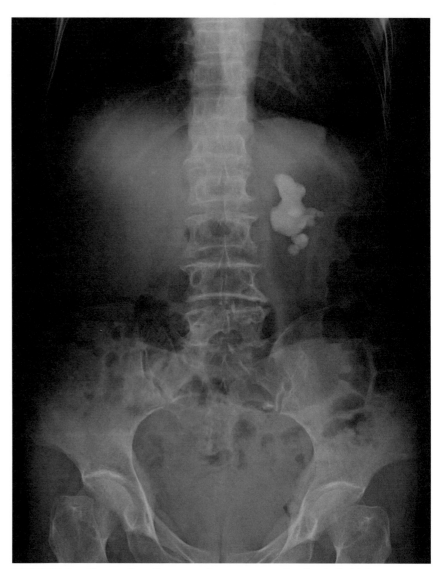

FIGURE 4. X-ray showing staghorn stones in the left kidney.
Credit: Suttha Burawonk/Shutterstock.com.

CRITICAL DECISION

What is the prognosis in patients presenting with renal colic?

Most patients who present with renal colic can be treated conservatively with pain management and oral hydration because the stones will pass spontaneously in most cases. Some factors that can affect spontaneous stone passage include stone size, location, and degree of obstruction.[33] Although specific measurements and location cutoffs vary by study, the larger the stone and the more proximally located it is in the ureter, the less likely it is to pass spontaneously.

Patients whose pain and nausea are controlled and who are without other complications should be discharged home with pain management, possible MET, and recommendations to continue oral hydration, decrease animal consumption, and decrease salt intake. Return precautions should include such things as intractable pain, nausea, vomiting, and fever.

CRITICAL DECISION

Which patients require emergent surgical consultation?

Although most patients can be conservatively managed, physicians must know how to recognize patients who need a urology consultation. Patients with acute renal failure, pyuria or bacteriuria, complete ureteral obstruction, or signs of sepsis should receive such a consultation.[42] Patients with intractable pain and vomiting may require inpatient admission for pain control or fluid resuscitation.[43]

Emergency surgical decompression is indicated for patients with obstructing stones and a urinary tract infection (UTI), bilateral obstruction and acute kidney injury, or unilateral obstruction with acute kidney injury in a solitary functioning kidney. The AUA and the Endourological Society recommend elective surgical management for ureteral stones larger than 10 mm; uncomplicated distal ureteral stones that are 10 mm or less in diameter and have not passed after 4 to 6 weeks of observation, with or without MET; or in pregnant patients with ureteral or kidney stones in whom observation has failed. Surgical management can be accomplished in various ways. For example, a urologist can perform a ureteroscopy and stenting or extraction, and an interventional radiologist can perform a decompressive percutaneous nephrostomy or lithotomy.[44]

Struvite stones (ie, stones composed of magnesium ammonium phosphate) make up 10% to 15% of kidney stones. These stones tend to make staghorn calculi that are associated with a much higher infection rate because they are often caused by bacterial urease production (*Figure 4*). Since antibiotic penetration in staghorn calculi is poor, the potential for urosepsis increases until the stone is removed. Staghorn calculi will not pass on their own, so surgical treatment is generally required.[45]

CRITICAL DECISION

When should patients with kidney stones receive antibiotics?

For patients with kidney stones who show evidence of a UTI based on urinalysis, antibiotics should be prescribed. Studies suggest that pyuria as low as 5 WBC/hpf has an 86% sensitivity and 79% specificity for a positive culture, and the likelihood increases as the concentration of WBCs increases.[46,47] To help guide antibiotic therapy, a urine culture should always be sent if there are signs of infection. Generally, antibiotics should target urinary pathogens including *Escherichia coli*, *Klebsiella*, and *Proteus*.[48] Patients can be started on a fluoroquinolone, such as ciprofloxacin or levofloxacin. If, however, there is concern for fluoroquinolone resistance, patients can get a dose of long-acting parenteral agents, such as intravenous ceftriaxone, and be sent home with oral trimethoprim-sulfamethoxazole, amoxicillin-clavulanate, or cefpodoxime.[49]

Patients who recently completed urologic procedures or were hospitalized should also get pseudomonal coverage such as intravenous carbapenem for admitted patients or oral fluoroquinolone for outpatient treatment.[50] Although most patients can be discharged home with oral antibiotics, admission for intravenous antibiotics should be considered if a patient has an obstructive stone or a UTI with systemic inflammatory response syndrome.

Summary

Kidney stone disease as a cause of flank pain frequently presents in a typical, predictable fashion. However, the risk of misdiagnosis exists due to similar presentations of other common, sometimes-deadly illnesses. Using a well-thought-out plan for imaging using ultrasound, CT without a contrast medium, or CT with a contrast medium in the appropriate situations can help expedite patient care and ensure safe evaluation. Knowledge of the complications of kidney stones, particularly infection and acute kidney injury, can help emergency physicians provide optimal treatment for patients with this condition.

✖ Pitfalls

- Delaying surgical consultation in patients with obstructing stones and a UTI.
- Failing to consider kidney stones in the absence of hematuria.
- Neglecting to consider cardiovascular and pulmonary catastrophes in acute flank pain.

REFERENCES

1. Westphalen AC, Hsia RY, Maselli JH, Wang R, Gonzales R. Radiological imaging of patients with suspected urinary tract stones: national trends, diagnoses, and predictors. *Acad Emerg Med*. 2011;18(7):99-707.
2. Stamatelou KK, Francis ME, Jones CA, Nyberg LM, Curhan GC. Time trends in reported prevalence of kidney stones in the United States: 1976-1994. *Kidney Int*. 2003;63(5):1817-1823.
3. Burrows PK, Hollander JE, Wolfson AB, et al. Design and challenges of a randomized clinical trial of medical expulsive therapy (tamsulosin) for urolithiasis in the emergency department. *Contemp Clin Trials*. 2017;52:91-94.
4. Moe OW. Kidney stones: pathophysiology and medical management. *Lancet*. 2006;367(9507):333-344.
5. Levy FL, Adams-Huet B, Pak CYC. Ambulatory evaluation of nephrolithiasis: an update of a 1980 protocol. *Am J Med*. 1995;98(1):50-59.
6. Ferraro PM, Taylor EN, Gambaro G, Curhan GC. Soda and other beverages and the risk of kidney stones. *Clin J Am Soc Nephrol*. 2013;8(8):1389-1395.
7. Ferraro PM, Taylor EN, Gambaro G, Curhan GC. Dietary and lifestyle risk factors associated with incident kidney stones in men and women. *J Urol*. 2017;198(4):858-863.
8. Fwu C-W, Eggers PW, Kimmel PL, Kusek JW, Kirkali Z. Emergency department visits, use of imaging, and drugs for urolithiasis have increased in the United States. *Kidney Int*. 2013;83(3):479-486.
9. Koroglu M, Wendel JD, Ernst RD, Oto A. Alternative diagnoses to stone disease on unenhanced CT to investigate acute flank pain. *Emerg Radiol*. 2004;10(6):327-333.
10. Marston WA, Ahlquist R, Johnson G Jr, Meyer AA. Misdiagnosis of ruptured abdominal aortic aneurysms. *J Vasc Surg*. 1992;16(1):17-22.
11. Carter MR, Green BR. Renal calculi: emergency department diagnosis and treatment. *Emerg Med Pract*. 2011;13(7):1-18.
12. Wang RC, Rodriguez RR, Moghadassi M, et al. External validation of the STONE score, a clinical prediction rule for ureteral stone: an observational multi-institutional study. *Ann Emerg Med*. 2016;67(4):423-432.e2.
13. Moore CL, Bomann S, Daniels B, et al. Derivation and validation of a clinical prediction rule for uncomplicated ureteral stone — the STONE score: retrospective and prospective observational cohort studies. *BMJ*. 2014;348:g2191.
14. Moore CL, Daniels B, Singh D, et al. Ureteral stones: implementation of a reduced-dose CT protocol in patients in the emergency department with moderate to high likelihood of calculi on the basis of STONE score. *Radiology*. 2016;280(3):743-751.
15. Smith RC, Verga M, McCarthy S, Rosenfield AT. Diagnosis of acute flank pain: value of unenhanced helical CT. *AJR Am J Roentgenol*. 1996;166(1):97-101.
16. Coursey CA, Casalino DD, Reimer EM, et al. ACR Appropriateness Criteria® acute onset flank pain — suspicion of stone disease. *Ultrasound Q*. 2012;28(3):227-233.
17. Varanelli MJ, Coll DM, Levine JA, Rosenfield AT, Smith RC. Relationship between duration of pain and secondary signs of obstruction of the urinary tract on unenhanced helical CT. *AJR Am J Roentgenol*. 2001;177(2):325-330.
18. Lei B, Harfouch N, Scheiner J, Demissie S, Hayim M. Can obstructive urolithiasis be safely excluded on contrast CT? A retrospective analysis of contrast-enhanced and noncontrast CT. *Am J Emerg Med*. 2021;47:70-73.
19. Nicolau C, Claudon M, Derchi LE, et al. Imaging patients with renal colic — consider ultrasound first. *Insights Imaging*. 2015;6(4):441-447.
20. Smith-Bindman R, Aubin C, Bailitz J, et al. Ultrasonography versus computed tomography for suspected nephrolithiasis. *N Engl J Med*. 2014;371(12):1100-1110.
21. Gaspari R, Horst K. Emergency ultrasound and urinalysis in the evaluation of flank pain. *Acad Emerg Med*. 2005;12(12):1180-1184.
22. Nagafuchi Y, Sumitomo S, Soroida Y, et al. The power Doppler twinkling artefact associated with periarticular calcification induced by intra-articular corticosteroid injection in patients with rheumatoid arthritis. *Ann Rheum Dis*. 2013;72(7):1267-1269.

CASE RESOLUTIONS

■ CASE ONE

The patient's urinalysis showed hematuria (3+), an increase in specific gravity (1.030), and trace protein. He had a STONE score of 10, ultrasound that showed mild hydronephrosis, and normal kidney function on his laboratory test results. He was given a small dose of oxycodone with resolution of his pain, so he was sent home with tamsulosin and the hope that he would pass the stone. The patient returned the next day with intractable pain. He received a CT scan that showed an 8-mm stone in the proximal ureter with hydronephrosis. Urology was consulted when analgesia could not be achieved in the emergency department. Urology recommended admission for stenting because the stone was unlikely to pass on its own.

■ CASE TWO

The patient had a urinalysis that showed positive leukocyte esterase as well as positive nitrate, a WBC count greater than 50×10^9/L, trace bacteria, and hematuria (2+). She had a CT that showed a left distal 4-mm ureteral stone at the UVJ without hydronephrosis. Ibuprofen and narcotics improved her pain. She was sent home with pain control and ciprofloxacin. Follow-up with a primary care physician and urology was recommended.

■ CASE THREE

The patient was noted to have a positive leukocyte esterase as well as a positive nitrate, a WBC count greater than 100×10^9/L, many bacteria, and 10 to 20 RBC/hpf. Her serum creatinine was 2.5 mg/dL (baseline around 1 mg/dL). Urine culture results revealed a *P. mirabilis* count of more than 100,000 CFU/mL. CT showed a stone extension into every calyx from the renal pelvis, indicating the presence of staghorn calculi. With concern for urosepsis, the patient was given amoxicillin-clavulanate, antiemetics, and a 30-mL/kg plasmacyte bolus. Blood pressure improved to a reading of 132/78 mm Hg. Urology was consulted, and the patient underwent a left percutaneous nephrolithotomy. Repeat CT showed complete clearance of the stone.

23. Park SJ, Yi BH, Lee HK, Kim YH, Kim GJ, Kim HC. Evaluation of patients with suspected ureteral calculi using sonography as an initial diagnostic tool: how can we improve diagnostic accuracy? *J Ultrasound Med.* 2008;27(10):1441-1450.

24. Vallone G, Napolitano G, Fonio P, et al. US detection of renal and ureteral calculi in patients with suspected renal colic. *Crit Ultrasound J.* 2013;5(suppl 1):S3.

25. Levine JA, Neitlich J, Verga M, Dalrymple N, Smith RC. Ureteral calculi in patients with flank pain: correlation of plain radiography with unenhanced helical CT. *Radiology.* 1997;204(1):27-31.

26. Saleem MO, Hamawy K. Hematuria. *StatPearls [Internet].* 2021.

27. Safriel Y, Malhotra A, Sclafani SJ. Hematuria as an indicator for the presence or absence of urinary calculi. *Am J Emerg Med.* 2003;21(6):492-493.

28. Lohr JA, Portilla MG, Geuder TG, Dunn ML, Dudley SM. Making a presumptive diagnosis of urinary tract infection by using a urinalysis performed in an on-site laboratory. *J Pediatr.* 1993;122(1):22-25.

29. Serinken M, Karcioglu O, Turkcuer I, Ozkan HI, Keysan MK, Bukiran A. Analysis of clinical and demographic characteristics of patients presenting with renal colic in the emergency department. *BMC Res Notes.* 2008;1:79.

30. Hübner WA, Irby P, Stoller ML. Natural history and current concepts for the treatment of small ureteral calculi. *Eur Urol.* 1993;24(2):172-176.

31. Jendeberg J, Geijer H, Alshamari M, Cierzniak B, Lidén M. Size matters: the width and location of a ureteral stone accurately predict the chance of spontaneous passage. *Eur Radiol.* 2017;27(11):4775-4785.

32. Pathan SA, Mitra B, Cameron PA. A systematic review and meta-analysis comparing the efficacy of nonsteroidal anti-inflammatory drugs, opioids, and paracetamol in the treatment of acute renal colic. *Eur Urol.* 2018;73(4):583-595.

33. Cole RS, Fry CH, Shuttleworth KU. The action of the prostaglandins on isolated human ureteric smooth muscle. *Br J Urol.* 1988;61(1):19-26.

34. Safdar B, Degutis LC, Landry K, Vedere S, Moscovitz H, D'Onofrio G. Intravenous morphine plus ketorolac is superior to either drug alone for treatment of acute renal colic. *Ann Emerg Med.* 2006;48(2):173-181.e1.

35. Worster AS, Supapol WB. Fluids and diuretics for acute ureteric colic. *Cochrane Database Syst Rev.* 2012;(2):CD004926.

36. Borghi L, Meschi T, Amato F, Briganti A, Novarini A, Giannini A. Urinary volume, water and recurrences of idiopathic calcium nephrolithiasis: a 5-year randomized prospective study. *J Urol.* 1996;155(3):839-843.

37. Raskolnikov D, Hall MK, Ngo SD, et al. Strategies to optimize nephrolithiasis emergency care (STONE): prospective evaluation of an emergency department clinical pathway. *Urology.* 2022;160:60-68.

38. Jokar A, Khademhosseini P, Ahmadi K, Sistani A, Amiri M, Sinaki AG. A comparison of metoclopramide and ondansetron efficacy for the prevention of nausea and vomiting in patients suffered from renal colic. *Open Access Maced J Med Sci.* 2018;6(10):1833-1838.

39. Sun Y, Lei GL, Yang L, Wei Q, Wei X. Is tamsulosin effective for the passage of symptomatic ureteral stones: a systematic review and meta-analysis. *Medicine (Baltimore).* 2019;98(10):e14796.

40. Ye Z, Zeng G, Yang H, et al. Efficacy and safety of tamsulosin in medical expulsive therapy for distal ureteral stones with renal colic: a multicenter, randomized, double blind, placebo controlled trial. *Eur Urol.* 2018;73(3):385-391.

41. Hermanns T, Sauermann P, Rufibach K, Frauenfelder T, Sulser T, Strebel RT. Is there a role for tamsulosin in the treatment of distal ureteral stones of 7 mm or less? Results of a randomised, double-blind, placebo-controlled trial. *Eur Urol.* 2009;56(3):407-412.

42. Teichman JM. Clinical practice. Acute renal colic from ureteral calculus. *N Engl J Med.* 2004;350(7):684-693.

43. Portis AJ, Sundaram CP. Diagnosis and initial management of kidney stones. *Am Fam Physician.* 2001;63(7):1329-1338.

44. Assimos D, Krambeck A, Miller NL, et al. Surgical management of stones: American Urological Association/Endourological Society guideline, part I. *J Urol.* 2016;196(4):1153-1160.

45. Kum F, Mahmalji W, Hale J, Thomas K, Bultitude M, Glass J. Do stones still kill? An analysis of death from stone disease 1999-2013 in England and Wales. *BJU Int.* 2016;118(1):140-144.

46. Abrahamian FM, Krishnadasan A, Mower WR, Moran GJ, Talan DA. Association of pyuria and clinical characteristics with the presence of urinary tract infection among patients with acute nephrolithiasis. *Ann Emerg Med.* 2013;62(5):526-533.

47. Dorfman M, Chan SB, Hayek K, Hill C. Pyuria and urine cultures in patients with acute renal colic. *J Emerg Med.* 51(4):358-364.

48. Jennings CA, Khan Z, Sidhu P, et al. Management and outcome of obstructive ureteral stones in the emergency department: emphasis on urine tests and antibiotics usage. *Am J Emerg Med.* 2019;37(10):1855-1859.

49. Singh KP, Li G, Mitrani-Gold FS, et al. Systematic review and meta-analysis of antimicrobial treatment effect estimation in complicated urinary tract infection. *Antimicrob Agents Chemother.* 2013;57(11):5284-5290.

50. Khusid JA, Hordines JC, Sadiq AS, Atallah WM, Gupta M. Prevention and management of infectious complications of retrograde intrarenal surgery. *Front Surg.* 2021;8:718583.

Hypokalemia Characteristics

By Amal Mattu, MD, FACEP
Dr. Mattu is a professor, vice chair, and director of the Emergency Cardiology Fellowship in the Department of Emergency Medicine at the University of Maryland School of Medicine in Baltimore.

Objective

On completion of this article, you should be able to:

■ Differentiate hypokalemia from diffuse ischemia on ECG.

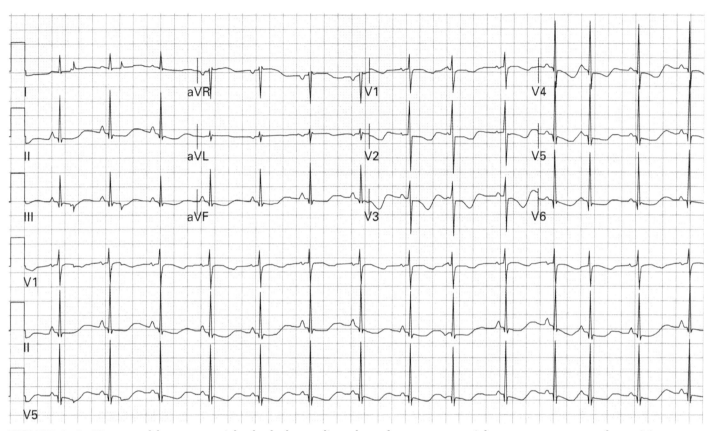

FIGURE 1. **A 63-year-old woman with alcohol use disorder who presents with severe nausea and vomiting**

Sinus rhythm, rate 84, occasional premature atrial contractions (PACs), T-wave abnormality, and prolonged QT interval consistent with diffuse ischemia versus hypokalemia. Hypokalemia can cause an assortment of ECG abnormalities, including atrial or ventricular ectopy, U waves, and T-wave flattening. Severe hypokalemia can also cause ST-segment sagging that mimics cardiac ischemia as well as a characteristic biphasic T-wave abnormality in which the initial portion of the T wave inverts and is followed by an upward deflection. The abnormality is most prominent in the precordial leads. The overall complex produces a prolonged QT interval. This complex is caused by the fusion of an inverted T wave with an upright U wave. This patient was suffering from alcoholic ketoacidosis and had profound hypokalemia (serum level 1.7 mEq/L; normal 3.5-5.3 mEq/L). Hypomagnesemia is another cause of QT-interval prolongation. The ninth and twelfth QRS complexes are PACs. The PACs, ST-segment depression, and T-wave abnormality resolved after correction of the electrolyte disturbance.

From Mattu A, Brady W. *ECGs for the Emergency Physician 2*. BMJ Publishing. Reprinted with permission.

Monkeypox in the Pediatric Emergency Department

By Shelby Marx, MD; Zach Burroughs, MD;
and Ann M. Dietrich, MD, FAAP, FACEP
University of South Carolina College of Medicine
and Prisma Health Children's Emergency Center, Greenville

Reviewed by Sharon E. Mace, MD, FACEP

Objective

On completion of this article, you should be able to:

■ Recognize monkeypox presentations and recall treatment options.

CASE PRESENTATION

A 17-year-old boy with a medical history significant for HIV presents after 4 days of nonbloody diarrhea and severe rectal pain. The patient reports that he has had exquisite pain when passing stool and wiping. He has not attempted to inspect his rectum, although he states that he has a history of hemorrhoids and a perirectal abscess. The patient assumes these to be the cause of his current discomfort. When questioned about his sexual history, the patient reports sexual intercourse with male partners; his most recent sexual exposure was receptive anal intercourse that occurred within the past month. He denies using protection during this sexual encounter.

The physical examination reveals an uncomfortable but nontoxic-appearing boy. Initial vitals include BP 134/87, P 123, and T 37.1°C (98.8°F). He has numerous well-circumscribed, white ulcerated perianal lesions (*Figure 1*). Although intensely painful, his rectal examination is otherwise unremarkable without evidence of internal abscess or gross blood. His initial laboratory workup reveals leukocytosis to 11.4×10^9/L and significantly elevated procalcitonin at 6.87 ng/mL. Perianal lesions are swabbed and evaluated for monkeypox using polymerase chain reaction (PCR) testing at the state public health department. Due to extreme tenderness on rectal examination, CT imaging is obtained. The CT scan reveals new and severe heterogeneous rectal wall thickening and enhancement with associated perirectal lymphadenopathy, consistent with infectious or inflammatory proctitis. Five days after the patient's presentation, the real-time PCR detects *Orthopoxvirus* DNA, confirming a monkeypox diagnosis.

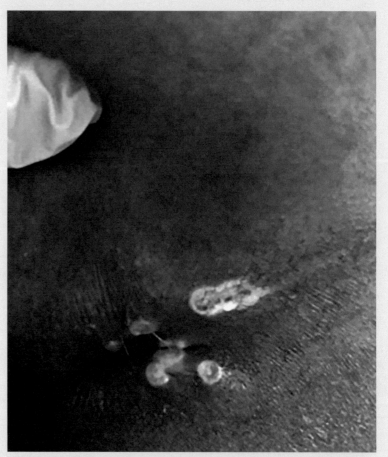

FIGURE 1. Physical examination showing numerous well-circumscribed, white ulcerated perianal lesions.
Credit: Shelby Marx, MD.

Discussion

Monkeypox, which belongs to the genus *Orthopoxvirus*, is a zoonotic viral infection. Monkeypox is not new. It was initially identified in monkeys in a Singapore laboratory in the 1950s; the first case in humans occurred in the Democratic Republic of the Congo in the 1970s.[1] In the spring of 2022, cases began appearing in nonendemic countries, including the United States and European countries. By the end of July 2022, the WHO proclaimed monkeypox a public health emergency due to its emergence in nonendemic countries.[1] As of October 26, 2022, there were 75,885 confirmed global cases, 28,087 of which occurred in the United States; 6 deaths have been reported in the United States.[2]

Transmission

The virus has multiple routes of transmission, although the specifics are currently under investigation. At this time, the most common routes are considered to be direct contact of mucous membranes or contact between bodily fluids from an infected person and breaks in the skin of a noninfected person. Less commonly, the virus transmits through respiratory secretions. Monkeypox's incubation period appears to be around 7 to 10 days.[2]

A case series published in the *New England Journal of Medicine* analyzed 528 cases of monkeypox that occurred between April 27 and June 24, 2022. Men who have sex with men accounted for 98% of these cases.[3] Although monkeypox is currently not considered a sexually transmitted disease under the classic definition, this case series found that transmission occurred during sexual relations in 95% of cases.[3] Transmission during sexual intercourse is hypothesized to occur from close contact with infected lesions rather than through semen or vaginal secretions, although additional research on this pathway is outstanding.[1]

Clinical Presentations

Although clinical presentations vary, there appear to be three mainstay components: systemic symptoms, rash, and either proctitis or tonsillitis. Many cases involve a prodrome of systemic flu-like symptoms followed by a rash; however, in some reported cases, the rash appears simultaneously with the systemic symptoms. Other reported cases have had a rash but no systemic symptoms.[4] There does not seem to be a single distinguishing rash in monkeypox; instead, lesions with varying characteristics are seen in infected individuals. The rash, described as both painful and pruritic, can include macules, papules, vesicles, umbilicated lesions, or pseudopustules. On average, lesions "scab over" within 1 to 2 weeks after their appearance. However, transmission can still occur after a lesion has scabbed over; lesions are considered noninfectious only once re-epithelialization has occurred.[2] Lesions commonly appear in the perioral and anogenital regions of infected individuals, although the rash can occur anywhere on the skin. In the most current monkeypox outbreak, many patients present with either proctitis or tonsillitis in addition to rash and systemic symptoms.[1]

Testing

Testing consists of directly swabbing the suspected monkeypox lesions and then performing an *Orthopoxvirus*-DNA PCR test.[1]

Treatment

Monkeypox treatment involves supportive care and antiviral treatment with a 14-day course of tecovirimat. Tecovirimat is an authorized treatment for smallpox, another member of the genus *Orthopoxvirus*; the CDC granted utilization of tecovirimat for monkeypox in the current outbreak.[5]

CASE RESOLUTION

The patient was admitted for pain control and managed symptomatically with lidocaine 4% cream for rectal pain; polyethylene glycol powder, sennosides, and docusate to soften stools; and oxycodone as needed for severe breakthrough pain. He spent 2 nights in the hospital and was discharged home with a 14-day course of tecovirimat. Upon discharge, the patient was instructed to complete the full course of tecovirimat and self-isolate until he was outside of the infectious stage of monkeypox.

REFERENCES

1. Isaacs SN, Mitja O. Epidemiology, clinical manifestations, and diagnosis of monkeypox. UpToDate. Updated September 16, 2022. https://www.uptodate.com/contents/epidemiology-clinical-manifestations-and-diagnosis-of-monkeypox
2. Monkeypox 2022 Outbreak Cases and Data. Centers for Disease Control and Prevention. Updated October 6, 2022. https://www.cdc.gov/poxvirus/monkeypox/response/2022/index.html
3. Thornhill JP, Barkati S, Walmsley S, et al. Monkeypox virus infection in humans across 16 countries — April–June 2022. *N Engl J Med.* 387(8):679-691.
4. Meyerowitz E, Baum S. Podcast 301: monkeypox — what to look for, how to treat. *NEJM Journal Watch.* Published August 19, 2022. https://podcasts.jwatch.org/index.php/podcast-301-monkeypox-what-to-look-for-how-to-treat/2022/00/19/
5. Isaacs S, Shenoy E, and Goldfarb I. Pre-exposure prophylaxis with orthopoxvirus vaccines. UpToDate. Updated September 16, 2022. https://www.uptodate.com/contents/treatment-and-prevention-of-monkeypox

A Comparison of Ibuprofen Regimens for Acute Pain

By Robert Healy, MD, LT, MC, USN; and
Daphne Morrison Ponce, MD, CDR, MC, USN
Navy Medical Center in Portsmouth, Virginia

Reviewed by Andrew J. Eyre, MD, MS-HPEd

Objective

On completion of this article, you should be able to:

- Restate recent findings regarding the effectiveness of ibuprofen in varying doses for the short-term relief of acute pain.

Motov S, Masoudi A, Drapkin J, et al. Comparison of oral ibuprofen at three single-dose regimens for treating acute pain in the emergency department: a randomized controlled trial. *Ann Emerg Med.* 2019 Oct;74(4):530-537.

KEY POINTS

- Ibuprofen is the most common analgesic used in emergency departments and is often dosed above the analgesic ceiling of 400 mg, 3 times daily.

- NSAIDs' adverse effect rates are dose and duration dependent.

- For short-term treatment of moderate-to-severe acute pain, ibuprofen doses above 400 mg PO do not appear to provide better analgesia.

Discussion

Ibuprofen is one of the most frequently used oral analgesics in emergency departments but is often dosed above the analgesic ceiling of 400 mg, 3 times daily. Ibuprofen, like other NSAIDs, has dose- and duration-dependent adverse effect rates. For short-term pain relief (up to 1 hour), ibuprofen doses at 400, 600, and 800 mg have similar analgesic efficacy.

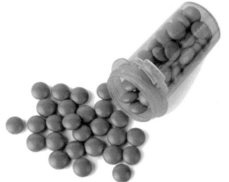

The authors conducted a randomized, double-blind equivalence trial that compared the analgesic efficacy of 400, 600, and 800 mg of oral ibuprofen for the treatment of acute pain in the emergency department. The study enrolled 225 adult patients who presented to a single-center, urban emergency department with acute pain and who were deemed appropriate for oral ibuprofen treatment. The study excluded women who were pregnant or breastfeeding and patients with peptic ulcer disease, renal or hepatic insufficiency, GI hemorrhage, allergies to NSAIDs, altered mental status, and opioid or NSAID use within 4 hours of arrival.

Study participants received a single dose of ibuprofen at either 400, 600, or 800 mg. Pain scores were obtained on a 0 to 10 rating scale prior to and 60 minutes after medication administration. A rescue analgesic selected by the treating physician was offered to participants who still wanted pain medication at 60 minutes. The primary outcome was the difference in mean pain scores at 60 minutes. Secondary outcomes included a comparison of mean pain score differences in each group from baseline to 60 minutes, the rate of adverse effects, and the need for rescue analgesia at 60 minutes.

Randomization was done by the research manager; the emergency pharmacist prepared all medications and maintained the randomization list. Emergency physicians, study participants, and data collectors were blinded to the medication allocation. The 400-, 600-, and 800-mg patient groups (each containing 75 participants) had similar baseline characteristics.

Study participants who were randomized to 400 mg of ibuprofen improved from a mean numeric pain rating scale of 6.48 to 4.36. The 600-mg group improved from 6.35 to 4.50. The 800-mg group improved from 6.46 to 4.50. Reductions in the mean numeric pain rating scale from baseline to 60 minutes were similar for all three groups, with no clinically meaningful differences. The difference in mean pain scores at 60 minutes was −0.14 between the 400- and 600-mg groups and −0.14 between the 400- and 800-mg groups. There was no difference between the 600- and 800-mg groups. Pain ratings across all three groups were similar at 60 minutes after ibuprofen administration. No clinically concerning adverse effects of ibuprofen occurred. Rescue analgesia was required for only one patient in the 600-mg group and four patients in both the 400- and 800-mg groups.

Study limitations include an enrollment limited to only a single center, possible selection bias, and a short study

Critical Decisions in Emergency Medicine's literature reviews feature articles recommended by the Academic Affairs Committee.
Available online at acep.org/moc/llsa.

14 *Critical Decisions in Emergency Medicine*

duration. Selection bias could have occurred if research and pharmacy teams enrolled participants based on convenience sampling; and convenience sampling could have underrepresented other patients who presented to the emergency department. The study's small sample size and short duration make it inadequate for comparing ibuprofen doses' downstream adverse effect profiles or analgesia beyond 60 minutes.

Disclosures

The views expressed in this article are those of the authors and do not necessarily reflect the official policy or position of the Department of the Navy, Department of Defense, or the United States Government.

This work was prepared as part of our official duties as military service members. Title 17 USC § 105 provides that "copyright protection under this title is not available for any work of the United States Government." A United States Government work is defined in 17 USC § 101 as a work prepared by a military service member or employee of the United States Government as part of that person's official duties.

An Atypical Presentation of Gout

By John Kiel, DO, MPH
Dr. Kiel is an assistant professor of emergency medicine and sports medicine at the University of Florida College of Medicine – Jacksonville

Objective

On completion of this article, you should be able to:

■ Discuss the diagnosis of and treatment for gout.

CASE PRESENTATION

A 46-year-old man presents with worsening right lower leg pain and swelling for the past week. He denies injury, inciting factors, or a history of leg problems. On examination, his vital signs are stable, and he appears uncomfortable. His right knee is notably effused, and his mid calf is markedly swollen compared to the unaffected limb. A CT is performed, and the scan shows a moderate knee effusion, a small Baker cyst, and a roughly 3 × 3 × 11-cm fluid collection in the medial calf (*Figures 1* and *2*). Ultrasound is used to evaluate the fluid collection and confirm the CT findings (*Figure 3*). Orthopedic surgery performs an arthrocentesis that identifies monosodium urate crystals.

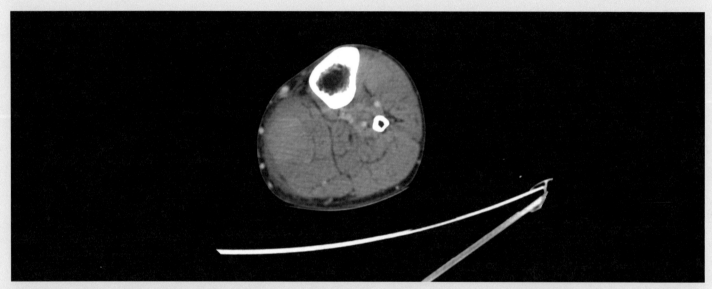

FIGURE 1. CT in axial view showing moderate joint effusion. *Credit:* John Kiel, DO, MPH.

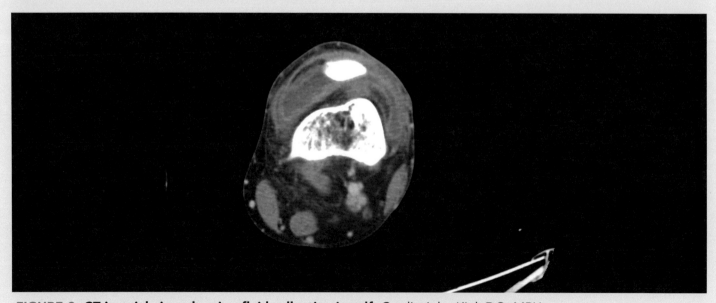

FIGURE 2. CT in axial view showing fluid collection in calf. *Credit:* John Kiel, DO, MPH.

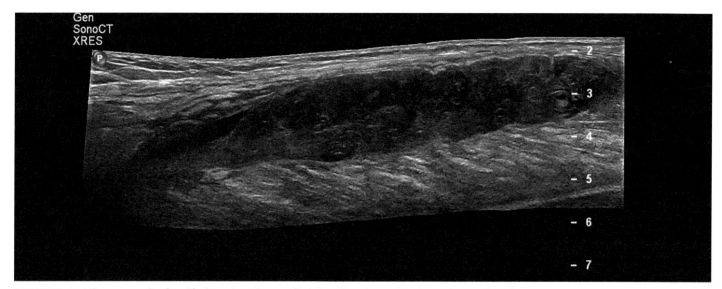

FIGURE 3. Ultrasound of calf showing large fluid collection. *Credit:* John Kiel, DO, MPH.

Discussion

Gout, a monosodium urate crystal arthropathy, is a relatively common condition that affects around 3% to 6% of men and 1% to 3% of women.[1] Gout is characterized by the accumulation of monosodium urate crystals in the synovial fluid of joints. Joints most affected by gout are the first metatarsophalangeal joint (in >50% of cases), midfoot, ankle, and knee. The risk of gout increases with alcohol and red meat consumption; the use of medications such as loop diuretics, tacrolimus, cyclosporine, niacin, and aspirin; and medical conditions including obesity, hypertension, chronic kidney disease, and diabetes.

Gout can be broken down into four general stages: asymptomatic, acute, intercritical, and chronic. An asymptomatic, hyperuricemia stage is common — about 20% of the US population has hyperuricemia; many people in this stage will never develop gout symptoms.[2] Acute gout is characterized by an abrupt onset of joint pain, erythema, warmth, swelling, or tenderness. The intercritical phase occurs between episodes of acute gout and is characterized by subclinical damage to the affected joints. Chronic gout is characterized by persistent arthralgias or repeated episodes of acute gout and is usually complicated by tophi formations.

Gout can be diagnosed clinically, although arthrocentesis is commonly performed to confirm the diagnosis and exclude septic arthritis. The American College of Rheumatology's diagnostic criteria for gout include characterizing symptom onset, location, and uric acid levels. There is no arthrocentesis requirement for diagnosis. If an arthrocentesis is performed, it classically demonstrates monosodium urate crystals in cases of gout. Notably, first metatarsophalangeal joint arthrocentesis can be challenging because of the small amount of fluid in the effused joint. Uric acid is typically elevated to about 6 mg/dL, although 14% of patients with acute gout have low or normal uric acid levels.[3] Radiology results may be normal, but in chronic cases, the results will show punched-out erosions, intraosseous tophi, and nonspecific soft-tissue swelling.[4] Ultrasound is a promising adjunct diagnostic imaging modality that is widely adopted by rheumatologists; emergency physicians have yet to adopt it.

Acute gout is typically managed with NSAIDs or, if NSAIDs are contraindicated, colchicine or oral corticosteroids. Depending on the clinical picture, patients may require more aggressive analgesia. The role of intra-articular corticosteroid injections is not well defined. As a long-term treatment, patients are advised to avoid alcohol, eat low purine foods, and increase exercise. Urate-lowering therapy is indicated if patients develop multiple episodes of acute gout.

CASE RESOLUTION

The patient was admitted to the hospital. Rheumatology agreed that the patient had gout but felt the patient was not experiencing an acute attack and discontinued indomethacin. The patient was known to suffer from alcohol use disorder, which was likely contributing to his symptoms; he was placed on the Clinical Institute Withdrawal Assessment for Alcohol protocol. Ultimately, there was no documentation that the calf fluid collection was ever addressed. The fluid collection contained synovial fluid and was thought to be a likely continuation of the Baker cyst. Following discharge, the patient did not follow up with orthopedic surgery or rheumatology.

REFERENCES

1. Dalbeth N, Merriman TR, Stamp LK. Gout. *Lancet.* 2016 Oct 22;388(10055):2039-2052.
2. Zhu Y, Pandya BJ, Choi HK. Prevalence of gout and hyperuricemia in the US general population: the National Health and Nutrition Examination Survey 2007-2008. *Arthritis Rheum.* 2011 Oct;63(10):3136-3141.
3. Schlesinger N, Norquist JM, Watson DJ. Serum urate during acute gout. *J Rheumatol.* 2009 Jun;36(6):1287-1289.
4. Perez-Ruiz F, Dalbeth N, Urresola A, de Miguel E, Schlesinger N. Imaging of gout: findings and utility. *Arthritis Res Ther.* 2009;11(3):232.

An Adolescent With Knee Pain

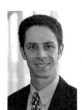

By Joshua S. Broder, MD, FACEP
Dr. Broder is a professor and the residency program director in the Department of Emergency Medicine at Duke University Medical Center in Durham, North Carolina.

Objectives

On completion of this article, you should be able to:

- Describe the clinical presentation of SCFE.
- Recognize the importance of early diagnosis and the risks of a missed or delayed diagnosis.
- Identify imaging findings of SCFE.

CASE PRESENTATION

A 14-year-old obese boy presents with right knee pain. For approximately 4 weeks, the patient has had right leg pain without any preceding trauma. He describes the pain as sharp and burning, centered on the right knee but radiating throughout the leg. He visited an outpatient orthopedic clinic where he underwent right knee, tibia, and ankle x-rays, all of which were normal. His pain worsened, and he has been walking with crutches for 2 weeks. He saw a physical therapist but reports no improvement. Worsening pain prompted his visit today. He has not had a fever. His parents report that the patient's left knee appears "bowlegged" and that this might have caused the patient to compensate and strain his right leg. The patient's vitals are BP 140/86, P 125, R 18, and T 36.7°C (98.1°F); SpO$_2$ is 98% on room air.

He is alert and in no distress while lying in bed. He complains of severe right knee and hip pain during any attempt to flex the right knee. He will not flex or extend the right hip because of the pain. His neurovascular examination is normal. No knee effusion or erythema is present. X-rays of the right hip are obtained (*Figure 1*).

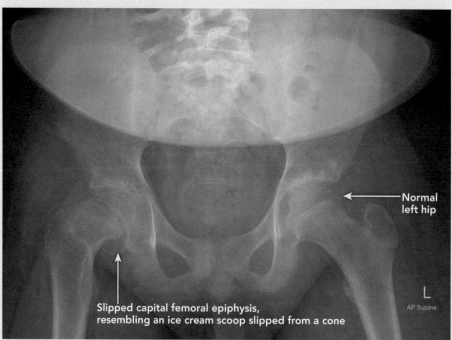

Normal left hip

Slipped capital femoral epiphysis, resembling an ice cream scoop slipped from a cone

L
AP Supine

FIGURE 1. Anteroposterior x-ray of the pelvis. By convention, displacement of distal anatomy is usually described with respect to more proximal anatomy. Using this nomenclature, the subcapital femoral neck is laterally displaced relative to the femoral epiphysis. Alternatively, the femoral epiphysis can be described as medially displaced. The magnitude of displacement is greater than one-third of the width of the femoral neck. *Credit:* Joshua S. Broder, MD, FACEP.

Discussion

Slipped capital femoral epiphysis (SCFE) is an injury through the growth plate of the femoral head that occurs in children. Clinical presentation includes extremity pain or abnormal gait, often without a specific preceding injury. Forty percent of patients with SCFE complain of pain in the knee or thigh rather than in the hip or groin. Although the mean age of onset is approximately 12 years, the reported range includes patients from ages 6 to 17 years.[1] Two-thirds of patients are boys, but importantly, one-third are girls. Physicians should not mistake SCFE as a condition unique to boys; doing so risks missing the diagnosis in female patients.[1] Symptoms of SCFE can be mild, so the condition should be suspected even when patients continue to engage in normal activities. Approximately half of

SCFE patients exceed the 95th percentile for weight, and 35% have bilateral hip involvement, often prompting prophylactic fixation of unaffected hips in those who do not yet have bilateral involvement.[1]

Imaging findings include variable degrees of displacement; in the most subtle slips, comparison with the contralateral side can be helpful. In a normal capital femoral epiphysis, a line drawn along the lateral femoral neck should intersect the femoral epiphysis; when the epiphysis is medially displaced, this intersection may not occur (*Figure 2*).

Diagnostic delay is common. One study of patients who presented to a children's hospital for surgical treatment of SCFE found that the mean duration of symptoms is 140 days and the mean diagnostic delay after a first primary care visit for

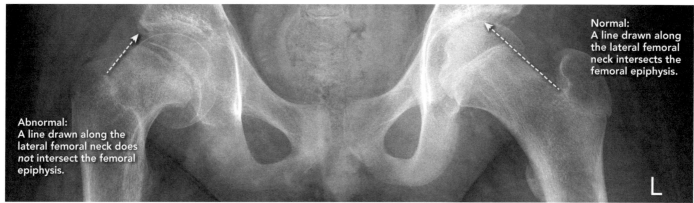

Normal:
A line drawn along the lateral femoral neck intersects the femoral epiphysis.

Abnormal:
A line drawn along the lateral femoral neck does *not* intersect the femoral epiphysis.

L

FIGURE 2. Anteroposterior x-ray of the pelvis. In subtle cases, comparison with the contralateral side may be helpful, although 35% of SCFE patients have bilateral abnormalities and, thus, the contralateral side may not be normal. In normal capital femoral epiphysis, a line drawn along the lateral femoral neck intersects the femoral epiphysis. *Credit:* Joshua S. Broder, MD, FACEP.

limb pain is 76 days.[1] Fifty-two percent of visits — including emergency department, urgent care, and office visits — before a referral to a children's hospital result in incorrect diagnoses. In general, two or more visits are common before an accurate diagnosis is made.[1] Initial diagnoses in patients ultimately found to have SCFE include knee pathology, Osgood-Schlatter disease, muscle strain, suspected tumor, and even appendicitis. Delay in diagnosis may be related to a lack of familiarity with SCFE and misdirection caused by the varied pain sites reported by patients. A more recent retrospective review found similar diagnostic delays.[2]

Making a diagnosis before significant displacement occurs is important for timely, effective treatment, and screw fixation is a successful treatment in approximately 90% of mild cases (ie, displacement <⅓ of the femoral neck width). In nearly 50% of patients who develop severe SCFE (ie, displacement >½ of the femoral neck width), avascular necrosis (AVN) occurs.[1] Some cases of AVN require total hip arthroplasty.

CASE RESOLUTION

The patient underwent surgical screw fixation. At a 3-month follow-up, no evidence of AVN or contralateral SCFE was present on x-ray (*Figure 3*).

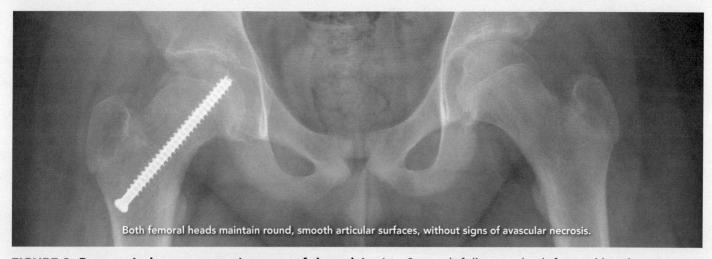

Both femoral heads maintain round, smooth articular surfaces, without signs of avascular necrosis.

FIGURE 3. Postsurgical anteroposterior x-ray of the pelvis. At a 3-month follow-up, both femoral heads maintain round, smooth articular surfaces without signs of AVN. The femoral epiphyses are both normally aligned. *Credit:* Joshua S. Broder, MD, FACEP.

Feature Editor: Joshua S. Broder, MD, FACEP. See also *Diagnostic Imaging for the Emergency Physician* (Winner of the 2011 Prose Award in Clinical Medicine, the American Publishers Award for Professional and Scholarly Excellence) and *Critical Images in Emergency Medicine* by Dr. Broder.

REFERENCES

1. Green DW, Reynolds RAK, Khan SN, Tolo V. The delay in diagnosis of slipped capital femoral epiphysis: a review of 102 patients. *HSS J.* 2005 Sep;1(1):103-106.
2. Schur MD, Andras LM, Broom AM, et al. Continuing delay in the diagnosis of slipped capital femoral epiphysis. *J Pediatr.* 2016 Oct;177:250-254.

The Critical Procedure

Management of Small, Bleeding Tongue Lacerations

By Steven J. Warrington, MD, MEd, MS
MercyOne Siouxland, Sioux City, Iowa

Objective
On completion of this article, you should be able to:
■ Treat small, bleeding tongue lacerations with less invasive methods.

Introduction
Tongue lacerations that are smaller than 2 cm often do not require repair unless they create a snake-tongue deformity. However, these wounds still need attention if there is ongoing bleeding. Although more severe complications like hemorrhage and airway compromise from such small tongue wounds are unlikely, patients may be distressed and uncomfortable when ongoing intraoral bleeding occurs.

Contraindications
■ An allergy to any treatment agent

Benefits and Risks
The primary benefit of treating bleeding tongue lacerations is the prevention of hemorrhage and airway compromise. A secondary benefit of treatment is easing the distress that often occurs when patients or family members see even a slow ooze of blood coming from the tongue. Teaching patients treatment methods that can be used at home such as the ice and tea bag techniques, should tongue bleeding recur, is also beneficial.

The risks of treatment include failure to control the bleeding, a recurrence of bleeding after it has been controlled, or an allergic reaction to treatment substances.

Alternatives
Tongue bleeding can be treated using multiple methods in a stepwise fashion depending on how quickly bleeding resolves. Techniques for controlling tongue bleeding, other than those listed below, include cautery, laceration repair, and intravenous therapy using various products.

Reducing Side Effects
Minimal side effects are expected when using these treatment techniques, unless a patient is allergic to one of the substances. With the tea bag technique, the tea bag does not need to be steeped in hot water before attempting treatment; if it is steeped in hot water, it should be cooled before being applied to the site of bleeding to avoid scalding the patient.

Special Considerations
Considering certain points when using the tea bag technique can make it more effective at managing tongue bleeding. Although steeping the tea bag is unnecessary prior to application, steeping can release tannins that help stop the bleeding. Tea type also affects tannin concentration. Black tea is the best choice, if available. Even a teabag of unknown type steeped briefly in cool water can successfully control a small, bleeding tongue laceration. Squeezing the tea bag can release additional tannins, so applying pressure to the tea bag on the site of bleeding is recommended.

TECHNIQUE

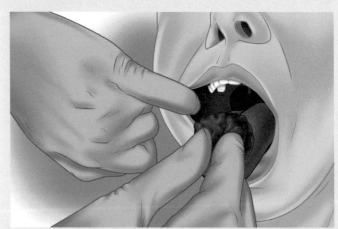

FIGURE 1. Using a teabag to stop a bleeding tongue laceration. *Credit:* ACEP.

1. **Discuss** the treatment steps and timeline with the patient and explain that multiple attempts may be made to control the bleeding. Make sure the patient understands and is willing to cooperate.

2. **Direct** the patient to apply ice to the affected area and swish and spit ice water while a tea bag is obtained.

3. **Moisten** the tea bag (preferably black tea) and apply it directly to the bleeding area. Have the patient press the teabag against the wound for 15 minutes without removing it. If the bleeding is improved but still unresolved, attempt another 15-minute trial.

4. **Soak** a 4 x 4 inch gauze in tranexamic acid (or distribute the powder of a crushed 500-mg tranexamic acid tablet onto a damp gauze) if there is still ongoing bleeding. Have the patient hold and apply pressure to the saturated gauze over the bleeding site for 30 minutes.

5. **Use** topical thrombin on the laceration if there is still bleeding.

6. **Inject** lidocaine with epinephrine into the laceration if bleeding is still ongoing. Depending on the laceration's location, an inferior alveolar nerve block may help the patient tolerate an injection into the tongue.

7. **Consider** treatment with intravenous products, cauterization, repair of the laceration, or referral to a specialist if bleeding persists beyond these treatment techniques.

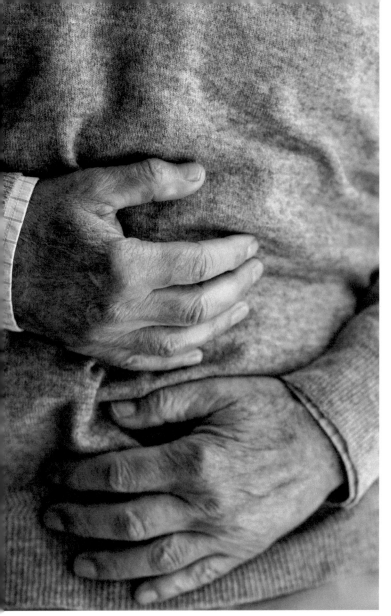

Gut Reaction

Treating Mesenteric Ischemia

LESSON 22

By Joshua Kern, MD; and Joslin Gilley-Avramis, MD
Drs. Kern and Gilley-Avramis are assistant professors in the Department of Emergency Medicine at the University of Texas Southwestern Medical Center in Dallas.

Reviewed by Walter L. Green, MD, FACEP

Objectives

On completion of this lesson, you should be able to:

1. Describe patient history characteristics associated with mesenteric ischemia.
2. Discuss the physical examination findings in patients with mesenteric ischemia.
3. List and explain the different laboratory values found in mesenteric ischemia.
4. Identify the imaging modalities used to evaluate for mesenteric ischemia.
5. Recall the treatment and management of patients with mesenteric ischemia.

From the EM Model

2.0 Abdominal and Gastrointestinal Disorders
    2.8 Small Bowel
        2.8.6 Vascular Insufficiency

■ **CRITICAL DECISIONS** ■

- What are the types of mesenteric ischemia and their underlying causes?

- What patient history characteristics should increase suspicion for mesenteric ischemia?

- What physical examination findings are seen with mesenteric ischemia?

- What diagnostic laboratory values should be ordered to assess for mesenteric ischemia?

- What diagnostic imaging should be used to evaluate for mesenteric ischemia?

- What is the treatment and management of mesenteric ischemia?

Mesenteric ischemia is an uncommon cause of abdominal pain, accounting for approximately 1 in 1,000 hospital admissions. Mesenteric ischemia can be challenging to diagnose and deadly if missed, with a 60% to 90% mortality rate. Emergency physicians must know the key features and tests to promptly diagnose and treat patients who present with mesenteric ischemia.

■ CASE ONE

A 72-year-old woman with a history of diabetes, hypertension, atrial fibrillation, and coronary artery disease presents via EMS with abdominal pain as her chief complaint. She is currently taking warfarin. The patient states her pain started in the morning about 20 minutes after eating breakfast. She has not experienced this abdominal pain in the past; it is associated with nausea and nonbloody vomiting. Her pain is constant, diffuse, severe (at 10/10), and worsening. She has never had abdominal surgery. She has not had a fever, diarrhea, chest pain, shortness of breath, upper respiratory symptoms, COVID-19 exposures, or urinary symptoms. Her vital signs are BP 110/82, P 126, R 16, and T 37.2°C (98.9°F); SpO_2 is 100% on room air. During examination, she has a soft, nondistended abdomen, minimal abdominal pain on palpation, and no lower extremity edema. On auscultation, no abdominal bruit is heard, and she has clear breath sounds and an irregular heart rate with tachycardia.

■ CASE TWO

A 69-year-old man with a history of hypertension, stroke, and myocardial infarction presents with severe and worsening diffuse abdominal pain that began approximately 15 minutes to 1 hour after eating. He reports being on aspirin and antihypertensives. The patient states this pain has been ongoing for at least 1 year and occurs after each meal. He states that he sometimes has severe nausea and nonbloody vomiting after eating and no longer has an appetite. He states, "I feel so bad after eating that I don't eat anymore. I'm losing lots of weight, probably 40 pounds over the past few months." He denies a history of cancer, HIV, melena, hematemesis, alcohol use, pancreatitis, cholelithiasis, peptic ulcer disease, fever, or any other symptoms. The patient's vitals are BP 160/92, P 98, R 14, and T 37°C (98.6°F); SpO_2 is 100% on room air. On examination, the patient appears slightly cachectic and malnourished. He has a regular heart rate and rhythm with no murmurs, rubs, or gallops. His lungs are clear, and he has no lower extremity edema. His abdomen is mildly tender to palpation, mostly in the midepigastric area; abdominal bruit is heard on auscultation.

Introduction

Acute mesenteric ischemia (AMI) is a sudden interruption of the blood supply to a segment of the small intestine that ultimately leads to ischemia, intestinal necrosis, and, if left untreated, death (*Figure 1*). Despite advances in treating mesenteric ischemia, the most critical factors that influence outcomes are the speed of diagnosis and intervention. Although mesenteric ischemia is an uncommon cause of abdominal pain, an inaccurate or delayed diagnosis can result in catastrophic complications with mortality rates as high as 60% to 90%.[1]

CRITICAL DECISION

What are the types of mesenteric ischemia and their underlying causes?

There are several types of mesenteric ischemia that vary by their underlying causes (*Table 1*). Mesenteric arterial embolism is the most common type, accounting for approximately 50% of cases. Mesenteric arterial embolism usually has cardiac origins, most typically atrial dysrhythmias (atrial fibrillation, specifically), endocarditis, myocardial ischemia,

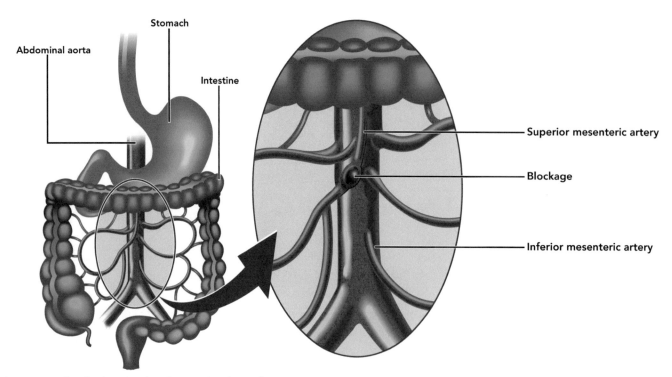

FIGURE 1. Occlusion in the SMA. *Credit:* Rob3000/Dreamstime.com.

Type	Cause	Prevalence
Mesenteric arterial embolism	Embolic occlusion usually originating in the heart due to atrial dysrhythmias, endocarditis, myocardial ischemia, or cardiomyopathy	50% of cases
Mesenteric arterial thrombosis	Thrombotic occlusion of already stenotic vessels due to atherosclerotic disease progression	20% to 35% of cases
Nonocclusive mesenteric ischemia	Mesenteric vasospasm and vasoconstriction due to sepsis, hemorrhagic shock, dehydration, vasopressors, or cardiogenic shock	20% of cases
Mesenteric venous thrombosis	Ischemia often due to inherited hypercoagulable diseases, acquired thrombophilia, and localized intra-abdominal inflammatory processes such as trauma, sepsis, pancreatitis, and inflammatory bowel disease	10% of cases

TABLE 1. Types of mesenteric ischemia

and cardiomyopathy. The superior mesenteric artery (SMA) is the most frequently affected blood vessel because of its large diameter and narrow takeoff from the aorta. The majority of emboli lodge 3 to 10 cm distal to the origin of the SMA, classically sparing the colon and jejunum.[2]

Mesenteric arterial thrombosis often occurs when atherosclerotic disease progresses in the mesenteric vasculature. Thrombotic occlusion of already stenotic vessels accounts for 20% to 35% of mesenteric ischemia cases. Unlike embolic occlusions, thrombosis usually occurs at the proximal SMA. Many patients with mesenteric arterial thrombosis have a history consistent with chronic mesenteric ischemia that includes postprandial abdominal pain, weight loss, and "food fear."

Nonocclusive mesenteric ischemia occurs in the absence of arterial obstruction; instead, it is due to mesenteric vasospasm and vasoconstriction. It accounts for approximately 20% of cases of mesenteric ischemia. Vasospasm and vasoconstriction are the result of mesenteric hypoperfusion caused by a variety of conditions such as sepsis, hemorrhagic shock, dehydration, vasopressors, and cardiogenic shock.[2] The bowel is adaptable. By increasing oxygen extraction (up to 90%), autoregulating arterial resistance, and instigating capillary recruitment, it can tolerate a 75% reduction in blood flow for up to 12 hours.[3] Its adaptability, however, is limited.

Mesenteric venous thrombosis, the least common cause of mesenteric ischemia, accounts for approximately 10% of all mesenteric ischemic events. It most commonly affects the superior mesenteric vein and its branches. It causes increased bowel wall edema and increased vascular resistance that reduce arterial blood and lead to bowel ischemia. Inherited hypercoagulable diseases are the most common

cause, but acquired thrombophilia from oral contraceptive use, malignancies, and hematologic disorders can cause mesenteric venous thrombosis.[2] Localized intra-abdominal inflammatory processes such as trauma, sepsis, pancreatitis, and inflammatory bowel disease can also lead to mesenteric venous thrombosis (see *Table 1*).

CRITICAL DECISION

What patient history characteristics should increase suspicion for mesenteric ischemia?

Patients' medical history can provide clues that suggest mesenteric ischemia. For instance, mesenteric ischemia is more common in patients in their 60s and 70s. Women are three times more likely than men to have AMI.[4] Mesenteric ischemia is also more frequently associated with comorbidities such as diabetes, hypertension, renal insufficiency, coronary artery disease, and atrial fibrillation.[5] Atherosclerosis is a well-known risk factor for mesenteric ischemia. In patients with atherosclerosis, emboli can dislodge from the aorta, travel downstream, and become lodged in the narrower portion of the SMA, leading to an occlusion. Atherosclerosis can also directly narrow portions of the SMA over time and cause critical stenosis and chronic mesenteric ischemia. Fifty percent of all AMI patients have an acute embolism to the SMA, and nearly 50% of those patients have a history of atrial fibrillation.[6,7]

A diagnosis of atrial fibrillation in patients with abdominal pain should alert emergency physicians to consider mesenteric ischemia. In patients with atrial fibrillation, AMI can occur when clots from the left atrium become dislodged. Other red flags for mesenteric ischemia are valvular heart disease and intravenous drug use because they put patients at risk for endocarditis. Decreased ejection fraction is a risk factor for nonocclusive mesenteric ischemia because it can cause splanchnic vasoconstriction.[8] Less common mesenteric ischemia risk factors include mesenteric artery dissection, mycotic aneurysm, and vasculitis.[9]

Mesenteric venous thrombosis can be caused by any hypercoagulable medical condition. Particular hypercoagulable medical conditions that should raise alarm for mesenteric ischemia are factor V Leiden, protein C and S deficiencies, an antithrombin deficiency, a prothrombin gene mutation, antiphospholipid antibody syndrome, and a COVID-19 infection. Patients with a COVID-19 infection are at an increased risk of thrombosis in venous, arterial, and small vessels. Acquired thrombophilia from a malignancy or oral contraceptive use should also increase suspicion for mesenteric ischemia.[10,11]

The classic presentation of mesenteric ischemia is acute-onset, generalized postprandial abdominal pain that typically starts 10 to 30 minutes after a meal, with or without nausea, vomiting, or bloody stools. Some symptoms of mesenteric ischemia are more common than others:

- 95% of patients with mesenteric ischemia have abdominal pain;
- 44% have nausea;
- 35% have vomiting;
- 35% have diarrhea; and
- 10% to 16% have bloody stools or describe rectal bleeding.[7]

Roughly 33% of patients with mesenteric ischemia have a triad of symptoms (ie, fever, hemoccult-positive stools, and abdominal pain) that occurs once an infarction develops.[7,12] Chronic mesenteric ischemia normally presents with food avoidance, weight loss, and malnutrition.

CRITICAL DECISION

What physical examination findings are seen with mesenteric ischemia?

The most common examination finding in mesenteric ischemia is abdominal pain out of proportion to findings in the physical examination. Mesenteric ischemia patients typically state they have severe (10/10) pain, but their abdomen may be minimally tender to nontender. However, 20% to 25% of patients may have an acute abdomen on examination, and 17% to 87% may have an abdominal bruit.[13-16] Peritoneal irritation happens only after an infarction and full-thickness necrosis. Once necrosis occurs, patients may look ill and become hypotensive. On rectal examination, 10% to 16% of patients may have rectal bleeding.

CRITICAL DECISION

What diagnostic laboratory values should be ordered to assess for mesenteric ischemia?

Laboratory values in AMI are nonspecific and generally unreliable. No serum laboratory marker is sensitive or specific enough to establish or exclude a diagnosis of AMI. However, in patients suspected to have AMI, a broad workup should be initiated, including a CBC with differential, comprehensive metabolic panel, lipase test, urinalysis, lactate test, blood gas test, and ECG to assess for atrial dysrhythmia. Many patients present with elevated hematocrit levels due to hemoconcentration and metabolic acidosis from dehydration and poor oral intake.

Inflammatory and Infection Markers

The onset of intestinal ischemia often produces a profound leukocytosis with a WBC elevation of more than $20 \times 10^9/L$. Any patient with abdominal pain and a WBC count greater than $20 \times 10^9/L$ should have AMI in their differential diagnosis. Leukocytosis may not be present in patients who are immunocompromised. However, leukocytosis has low diagnostic specificity for intestinal ischemia and does not differentiate between AMI and other intestinal and intra-abdominal disorders.[17] C-reactive protein level, which can also be elevated in intestinal ischemia, is nonspecific and does not differentiate between nonspecific abdominal pain and conditions that need definitive surgical management.[18] Procalcitonin has been suggested as a marker for intestinal ischemia. In a meta-analysis of 659 patients, the study found that procalcitonin's sensitivity for mesenteric ischemia ranges from 72% to 100% and its specificity from 68% to 91%.[19]

Serum Lactate

Lactate levels (L-lactate) have traditionally been the laboratory test that most emergency physicians use to rule out AMI. A meta-analysis determined that elevated L-lactate has a sensitivity of 86% but a specificity of only 44% for mesenteric ischemia.[20] Many times, an elevated L-lactate indicates at least segmental, severe ischemia or irreversible bowel injury, but it is not helpful to wait for evidence of an increasing lactate before proceeding with further testing. Intervention should, ideally, take place before lactic acidosis develops to minimize the risk of further bowel ischemia. These limitations aside, the serum lactic acid level is currently the most useful laboratory test when considering mesenteric ischemia as a diagnosis. The serum lactic acid test is widely available, has a rapid turnaround time, and has a short half-life (approximately 20 minutes) that makes it useful for serial measurements, especially early in the course of suspected AMI.

D-dimer

Traditionally, emergency physicians have used a D-dimer test to rule out deep vein thrombosis or pulmonary embolism. D-dimer tests may also help with ruling out AMI. A prospective study found that in a group of patients older than 50 years who were admitted for acute abdominal pain, no patients with a negative D-dimer test had acute intestinal ischemia.[21] A meta-analysis found that the D-dimer test in AMI has a pooled sensitivity of 96% but a specificity of only 40%.[20] Elevated D-dimer levels may be present in a variety of other conditions; therefore, elevated D-dimer levels may be less useful in diagnosing AMI, and a normal D-dimer may only be helpful in excluding this diagnosis.

Future Laboratory Implications

While serum tests for L-lactate are commonly used in emergency departments, D-lactate, a stereoisomer of L-lactate, shows some promise with diagnosing AMI. The D-lactate enzyme increases in the blood when there is bacterial overgrowth due to infection, increased intestinal permeability, or mesenteric infarction. A recent meta-analysis demonstrated a pooled sensitivity of 71.7% and specificity of 74.2% for D-lactate in mesenteric ischemia.[18] However, just like L-lactate, D-lactate may not be elevated until late in AMI's presentation.

✔ Pearls

- A diagnosis of mesenteric ischemia should always be considered in older patients with abdominal pain, especially when they have cardiovascular or thromboembolic risk factors.

- CTA of the abdomen is the imaging modality of choice for diagnosing AMI.

- Early surgical consultation is usually necessary for managing AMI.

- Interventional radiology may be needed for endovascular thrombectomy or catheter-directed thrombolysis in cases of mesenteric ischemia.

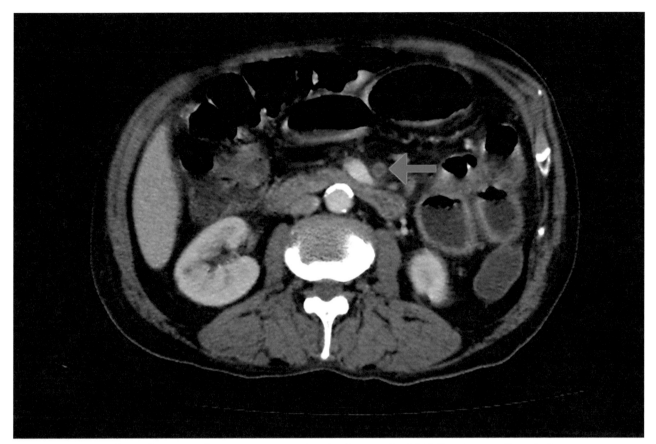

FIGURE 2. CT of an obstructed SMA (*arrow*). *Credit:* Copyright 2022 Dr. Ameen Rageh. Image courtesy of Dr. Ameen Rageh and Radiopaedia.org, rID:57530. Used under license.

Intestinal fatty acid–binding protein (I-FABP), a plasma marker released by enterocytes of the intestinal mucosal villi, also exhibits promise in diagnosing AMI. When intestinal ischemia occurs, an elevated I-FABP can diagnose mucosal damage at high-tissue specificity. A meta-analysis demonstrated a pooled sensitivity of 80% and a specificity of 86% for I-FABP.[18] Unfortunately, neither of these assays is readily available in most emergency departments. Ultimately, emergency physicians should use laboratory studies to investigate for other causes of acute abdominal pain but cannot exclude the diagnosis of AMI from laboratory results alone.

CRITICAL DECISION

What diagnostic imaging should be used to evaluate for mesenteric ischemia?

Diagnostic imaging is the most reliable method to diagnose AMI. A variety of imaging modalities can be used, including CT angiogram of the abdomen, doppler ultrasound, and MRI angiogram.

Plain X-rays

Plain x-rays of the abdomen (eg, kidney, ureter, and bladder x-ray) are usually nonspecific. Later in the disease course, plain x-rays may demonstrate multiple round, smooth soft-tissue densities in the intestinal lumen, called "thumbprinting," once mucosal and submucosal edema and hemorrhage set in. Late plain x-ray findings that indicate intestinal infarction and are more specific for intestinal ischemia are pneumatosis intestinalis and portal venous gas. Because plain x-rays are nonspecific and only demonstrate findings late in AMI, they should not be used for diagnosis.

Doppler Ultrasound

Ultrasonography is an effective, low-cost tool to diagnose AMI, but it is more accurate for assessing proximal rather than distal vasculature. For AMI, ultrasonography has a high degree of reliability and reproducibility with a sensitivity and specificity of 80% to 90%.[22] A diagnosis of AMI with ultrasound depends on measuring a significantly elevated peak systolic velocity. A more recent prospective study demonstrated that elevated peak systolic velocity on ultrasound has an 80% sensitivity for SMA occlusion and a negative predictive value of 100%.[23] However, ultrasound's diagnostic value depends on the skill of the technician, and quality images can be difficult to obtain in cases of obesity, bowel gas, and heavy calcification of the vessels. Ultrasound is better reserved for patients with chronic mesenteric ischemia.

CT Angiography

Abdominal CT is routinely used to screen hemodynamically stable patients with acute abdominal pain. However, for patients with a high index of suspicion for AMI, multidetector CT angiography (CTA) drastically increases the ability to detect AMI (*Figure 2*). CTA is preferred over abdominal CT because it can exclude other causes of acute abdominal pain and assess bowel perfusion. CTA should be performed with thin axial images of 1 to 3 mm and without oral contrast agents.

Oral contrast agents could delay an AMI diagnosis because they can obscure the mesenteric vessels and prevent bowel wall enhancement. CTA can also detect atherosclerotic changes to the SMA and celiac axis as a cause of mesenteric ischemia. Findings on CTA that are consistent with AMI are focal or segmental bowel wall thickening, mesenteric stranding, bowel dilation, intestinal pneumatosis, portomesenteric venous thrombosis, and solid organ infarction. A meta-analysis of 23 studies demonstrated a pooled sensitivity of 94% and specificity of 95% for CTA in diagnosing AMI.[20] Although CTA is the best test in the emergency department for diagnosing AMI, CTA's sensitivity is not as high for acute mesenteric venous thrombosis. This can be improved, however, by using two-phase imaging to enhance visceral venous drainage. In patients with nonocclusive mesenteric ischemia, CTA can detect areas of segmental narrowing in major arteries and decreased blood flow in smaller vessels.

MR Angiography

MR angiography (MRA) of the mesenteric vessels is a rapidly evolving imaging modality. Theoretically, it is appealing because it is noninvasive and avoids the risk of allergic reactions and nephrotoxicity from iodinated contrast agents. Unfortunately, MRA has several limitations. It is less available and requires much more time to perform than CTA. MRA also has poor spatial resolution that makes it difficult to identify distal emboli, limiting MRA primarily to evaluating the proximal celiac artery and SMA. Furthermore, MRA can overestimate the degree of arterial stenosis. Secondary signs of AMI, such as bowel wall thickening and indurated fat, are more difficult to assess on MRA than on CTA.[24] Although CTA is the more optimal test for acute mesenteric arterial embolus or thrombosis, MRA can be more sensitive for diagnosing acute mesenteric venous thrombosis and should be used in patients with an iodine contrast allergy.

Of all the possible imaging techniques in the emergency department, CTA is the best for diagnosing AMI. In patients with renal failure, CTA should still be performed because the risks of a delayed or missed AMI diagnosis far outweigh the risks of exposing the kidneys to iodinated contrast agents.

CRITICAL DECISION

What is the treatment and management of mesenteric ischemia?

Once AMI is diagnosed, the goals of treatment are to restore mesenteric blood flow as soon as possible, manage underlying conditions, treat persistent mesenteric vasospasm, and mitigate the risk of further clot propagation. Aggressive fluid resuscitation with crystalloid fluids and blood products is essential to properly manage AMI. Early hemodynamic monitoring should be initiated to guide fluid resuscitation. Electrolyte and acid-base levels should be serially monitored because bowel infarction and reperfusion can cause hyperkalemia and severe metabolic acidosis, and acidosis is a univariant marker of mortality. Vasopressors should be used with caution and only when trying to avoid volume overload or abdominal compartment syndrome. Dobutamine, low-dose dopamine, and milrinone are shown to improve cardiac function and have less vasoconstriction on the mesenteric vasculature.[9]

Early loss of the mucosal barrier in AMI puts patients at a high risk of sepsis by facilitating bacterial translocation. Broad-spectrum antibiotics are associated with improved outcomes in critically ill patients and should be promptly administered. Metronidazole and ceftriaxone or piperacillin and tazobactam are antibiotics of choice for AMI. Heparin should also be initiated as soon as possible for patients with acute ischemia or an exacerbation of chronic ischemia.

In all cases of mesenteric ischemia, a vascular surgeon should be emergently consulted, and if unavailable, the patient should be transferred to a facility where one is available. If there are peritoneal signs, such as intestinal infarction, perforation with peritonitis, and gastrointestinal bleeding, prompt surgical consultation for an emergent exploratory laparotomy is warranted.

Surgical Approaches to AMI

There are two different surgical approaches to managing AMI, open repair and endovascular repair. The goals of open surgical therapy are to revascularize the occluded vessel, assess the viability of the bowel, and resect the necrotic bowel. Emboli that occlude the proximal SMA generally respond well to surgical embolectomy. During hospitalization, up to 57% of patients managed with open repair require a "second look" for further bowel resection.[7,25,26] Short-term mortality after open revascularization ranges from 26% to 65% and is higher among patients with advanced age, renal insufficiency, metabolic acidosis, and a longer duration of symptoms.[7,25-27] Open repair of AMI is associated with longer hospital stays and recovery periods than endovascular repair.[28]

Endovascular repair has become more common over the last 10 years. Theoretically, endovascular strategies can restore perfusion more rapidly than open repair and may prevent the progression of mesenteric ischemia to bowel ischemia. The largest review comparing endovascular and open repair outcomes for AMI showed a lower in-hospital mortality of 25% when endovascular repair is performed compared to 40% when open repair is performed. Furthermore, endovascular repair is successful in 87% of cases.[28] Endovascular repair is usually accomplished by mechanical thrombectomy or angioplasty and stenting. Data from studies suggest endovascular repair may be the appropriate strategy for patients who have severe comorbidities that place them at a high risk of death and other complications from open repair.

Nonocclusive Mesenteric Ischemia

Patient outcomes with nonocclusive mesenteric ischemia depend on managing the underlying cause; overall mortality is 50% to 83% in these patients.[1] The main goals in managing nonocclusive mesenteric ischemia include addressing hemodynamic instability and minimizing the use of vasoconstrictors such as vasopressors. Additional treatment includes systemic anticoagulation and vasodilator use in patients without bowel infarction. Interventional radiology may need to be consulted for catheter-directed vasodilatory and antispasmodic agents, most commonly papaverine.

Mesenteric Venous Thrombosis

The treatment for mesenteric venous thrombosis is unique in that nonoperative management may be adequate in the absence of peritoneal findings. Unless a contraindication exists, heparin is the first-line treatment for mesenteric venous thrombosis and is associated with improved survival if started early. Patients should be admitted to the hospital in coordination with a vascular surgery consultation, and a hypercoagulable workup should be undertaken. Generally, patients are transitioned to oral anticoagulation, which is associated with lower rates of recurrence and death compared to no anticoagulation use.[22]

Chronic Mesenteric Ischemia

Revascularization is indicated for all patients with chronic mesenteric ischemia who develop symptoms; endovascular repair is preferred over open repair for revascularization. Angioplasty with stenting versus angioplasty alone during endovascular repair is used more frequently because angioplasty alone results in poor patency and is associated with poor long-term symptom relief.[2] Endovascular repair is a successful, minimally invasive approach that provides initial symptom relief in up to 95% of patients and has a lower rate of complications than open repair.[29] However, endovascular techniques are associated with lower rates of long-term patency, meaning restenosis occurs in up to 40% of patients, with 20% to 50% of these patients requiring another intervention.[30-34] Choosing the most appropriate approach requires weighing patients' state of health against the short- and long-term benefits and risks of each procedure. In most hospitals, endovascular repair is the first-line therapy, but in lower-risk younger patients with longer life expectancies, open repair may be the preferable option.

✖ Pitfalls

- Misinterpreting a normal serum lactate result as ruling out AMI. Serum lactate level cannot diagnose or rule out AMI.

- Believing a normal D-dimer result rules out AMI. Although a normal D-dimer level makes AMI less likely, it does not rule it out.

- Forgetting that vasopressors should be used cautiously in patients with AMI. Vasopressor use should be limited to patients with fluid overload or abdominal compartment syndrome. When used, the best options are dobutamine, low-dose dopamine, and milrinone.

- Failing to consider the diagnosis of chronic mesenteric ischemia in patients with chronic abdominal pain. Chronic mesenteric ischemia generally occurs in older patients; the most common symptoms are postprandial pain, food avoidance, and weight loss.

Summary

Mesenteric ischemia is a diagnostic challenge for emergency physicians. It is one of the least common causes of abdominal pain but one of the deadliest, having an extremely high morbidity and mortality rate. Diagnosis is difficult because mesenteric ischemia often presents with variable and nonspecific findings in the history, physical examination, and laboratory tests. Early consideration of mesenteric ischemia in patients with risk factors is critical to timely diagnosis and improved outcomes. CTA is the diagnostic modality of choice, and early consultation with a vascular surgeon and interventional radiologist is key to preventing further patient decompensation. Depending on the cause of mesenteric ischemia, management strategies in the emergency department may include aggressive fluid resuscitation to correct electrolyte and acid-base disorders, broad-spectrum antibiotics, and anticoagulation.

REFERENCES

1. Schoots IG, Koffeman GI, Legemate DA, Levi M, van Gulik TM. Systematic review of survival after acute mesenteric ischaemia according to disease aetiology. *Br J Surg*. 2004 Jan;91(1):17-27.

2. Oldenburg WA, Lau LL, Rodenberg TJ, Edmonds HJ, Burger CD. Acute mesenteric ischemia: a clinical review. *Arch Intern Med*. 2004 May 24;164(10):1054-1062.

3. Al-Diery H, Phillips A, Evennett N, Pandanaboyana S, Gilham M, Windsor JA. The pathogenesis of nonocclusive mesenteric ischemia: implications for research and clinical practice. *J Intensive Care Med*. 2019 Oct;34(10):771-781.

4. Wyers MC. Acute mesenteric ischemia: diagnostic approach and surgical treatment. *Semin Vasc Surg*. 2010 Mar;23(1):9-20.

5. Vokurka J, Olejnik J, Jedlicka V, Vesely M, Ciernik J, Paseka T. Acute mesenteric ischemia. *Hepatogastroenterology*. 2008 Jul-Aug;55(85):1349-1352.

6. Acosta S. Mesenteric ischemia. *Curr Opin Crit Care*. 2015;21(2):171-178.

7. Park WM, Gloviczki P, Cherry KJ Jr, et al. Contemporary management of acute mesenteric ischemia: factors associated with survival. *J Vasc Surg*. 2002 Mar;35(3):445-452.

8. Boley SJ, Brandt LJ, Sammartano RJ. History of mesenteric ischemia. The evolution of a diagnosis and management. *Surg Clin North Am*. 1997 Apr;77(2):275-288.

9. Bala M, Kashuk J, Moore EE, et al. Acute mesenteric ischemia: guidelines of the World Society of Emergency Surgery. *World J Emerg Surg*. 2017 Aug 7;12:38.

10. Cohn DM, Roshani S, Middeldorp S. Thrombophilia and venous thromboembolism: implications for testing. *Semin Thromb Hemost*. 2007 Sep;33(6):573-581.

11. Fan BE, Chang CCR, Teo CHY, Yap ES. COVID-19 coagulopathy with superior mesenteric vein thrombosis complicated by an ischaemic bowel. *Hamostaseologie*. 2020 Dec;40(5):592-593.

12. Terlouw LG, Moelker A, Abrahamsen J, et al. European guidelines on chronic mesenteric ischaemia - joint United European Gastroenterology, European Association for Gastroenterology, Endoscopy and Nutrition, European Society of Gastrointestinal and Abdominal Radiology, Netherlands Association of Hepatogastroenterologists, Hellenic Society of Gastroenterology, Cardiovascular and Interventional Radiological Society of Europe, and Dutch Mesenteric Ischemia Study group clinical guidelines on the diagnosis and treatment of patients with chronic mesenteric ischaemia. *United European Gastroenterol J*. 2020 May;8(4):371-395.

13. Berland T, Oldenburg WA. Acute mesenteric ischemia. *Curr Gastroenterol Rep*. 2008;10(3):341-346.

CASE RESOLUTIONS

■ CASE ONE

The patient's abdominal pain differential was broad, and both abdominal pain and cardiac workups were necessary. She was given intravenous pain medication and intravenous antiemetics. An ECG was obtained and showed atrial fibrillation with rapid ventricular response without ST elevation or depression. Her chest x-ray was significant for cardiomegaly that was unchanged compared to prior x-rays. Her cardiac enzymes were normal, but CBC was abnormal with leukocytosis of 22×10^9/L with a left shift and a slightly hemoconcentrated hemoglobin. Her urinalysis, liver function, and lipase results were unremarkable. Her serum lactate level was elevated at 2.4 mEq/L, and she had metabolic acidosis with a high anion gap. Her INR was subtherapeutic at 1.2. A CTA of the mesenteric vessels was ordered and demonstrated an occlusion of the SMA with a thrombus, pneumatosis intestinalis, and bowel wall thickening with abnormal enhancement of the bowel wall. A diagnosis of AMI was made, and the physician started a second large-bore intravenous line. A fluid bolus, a heparin drip, and broad-spectrum antibiotics were given. Both vascular and general surgery were consulted. The patient went to the operating room for a bowel resection and continues to recover in the surgical ICU.

■ CASE TWO

A peripheral intravenous line was started, an ECG was completed, and laboratory tests for liver function, lipase, urinalysis, INR, PTT, lactate, and HIV were sent. The patient was given 4 mg of intravenous ondansetron and 4 mg of intravenous morphine. His ECG demonstrated left ventricular hypertrophy but was otherwise unremarkable. His laboratory results were also unremarkable except for a newly elevated creatinine level of 1.8 mg/dL. His lipase, urinalysis, and liver function results were all normal. CTA of the mesenteric vessels showed diffuse occlusive disease of the SMA with more than 70% stenosis and severe narrowing of multiple vessels from atherosclerosis. The patient had no pneumatosis intestinalis and a normal appendix, pancreas, and gallbladder. He was admitted to the hospitalist service on a heparin drip and was followed by vascular surgery, interventional radiology, and gastroenterology. The patient went on to have endovascular revascularization of the SMA.

14. Martin MC, Wyers MC. Mesenteric vascular disease. In: Cronenwett JL, Johnson W, eds. *Rutherford's Vascular Surgery*. 8th ed. Elsevier; 2014:2398-2413.

15. Moawad J, Gewertz BL. Chronic mesenteric ischemia. Clinical presentation and diagnosis. *Surg Clin North Am*. 1997 Apr;77(2):357-369.

16. Mensink PB, van Petersen AS, Geelkerken RH, Otte JA, Huisman AB, Kolkman JJ. Clinical significance of splanchnic artery stenosis. *Br J Surg*. 2006 Nov;93(11):1377-1382.

17. van den Heijkant TC, Aerts BAC, Teijink JA, Buurman WA, Luyer MDP. Challenges in diagnosing mesenteric ischemia. *World J Gastroenterol*. 2013 Mar 7;19(9):1338-1341.

18. Montagnana M, Danese E, Lippi G. Biochemical markers of acute intestinal ischemia: possibilities and limitations. *Ann Transl Med*. 2018 Sep;6(17):341.

19. Cosse C, Sabbagh C, Kamel S, Galmiche A, Regimbeau J-M. Procalcitonin and intestinal ischemia: a review of the literature. *World J Gastroenterol*. 2014;20(47):17773-17778.

20. Cudnik MT, Darbha S, Jones J, Macedo J, Stockton SW, Hiestand BC. The diagnosis of acute mesenteric ischemia: a systematic review and meta-analysis. *Acad Emerg Med*. 2013 Nov;20(11):1087-1100.

21. Block T, Nilsson TK, Björck M, Acosta S. Diagnostic accuracy of plasma biomarkers for intestinal ischaemia. *Scand J Clin Lab Invest*. 2008;68(3):242-248.

22. Clair DG, Beach JM. Mesenteric ischemia. *N Engl J Med*. 2016 Mar 10;374(10):959-968.

23. Sartini S, Calosi G, Granai C, Harris T, Bruni F, Pastorelli M. Duplex ultrasound in the early diagnosis of acute mesenteric ischemia: a longitudinal cohort multicentric study. *Eur J Emerg Med*. 2017 Dec;24(6):e21-e26.

24. Carlos RC, Stanley JC, Stafford-Johnson D, Prince MR. Interobserver variability in the evaluation of chronic mesenteric ischemia with gadolinium-enhanced MR angiography. *Acad Radiol*. 2001 Sep;8(9):879-887.

25. Arthurs ZM, Titus J, Bannazadeh M, et al. A comparison of endovascular revascularization with traditional therapy for the treatment of acute mesenteric ischemia. *J Vasc Surg*. 2011 Mar;53(3):698-704.

26. Kougias P, Lau D, El Sayed HF, Zhou W, Huynh TT, Lin PH. Determinants of mortality and treatment outcome following surgical interventions for acute mesenteric ischemia. *J Vasc Surg*. 2007 Sep;46(3):467-474.

27. Acosta-Merida MA, Marchena-Gomez J, Hemmersbach-Miller M, Roque-Castellano C, Hernandez-Romero JM. Identification of risk factors for perioperative mortality in acute mesenteric ischemia. *World J Surg*. 2006 Aug;30(8):1579-1585.

28. Beaulieu RJ, Arnaoutakis KD, Abularrage CJ, Efron DT, Schneider E, Black JH III. Comparison of open and endovascular treatment of acute mesenteric ischemia. *J Vasc Surg*. 2014 Jan;59(1):159-164.

29. Oderich GS, Malgor RD, Ricotta JJ II. Open and endovascular revascularization for chronic mesenteric ischemia: tabular review of the literature. *Ann Vasc Surg*. 2009 Sep-Oct;23(5):700-712.

30. Oderich GS, Bower TC, Sullivan TM, Bjarnason H, Cha S, Gloviczki P. Open versus endovascular revascularization for chronic mesenteric ischemia: risk-stratified outcomes. *J Vasc Surg*. 2009 Jun;49(6):1472-1479.e3.

31. Cai W, Li X, Shu C, et al. Comparison of clinical outcomes of endovascular versus open revascularization for chronic mesenteric ischemia: a meta-analysis. *Ann Vasc Surg*. 2015 Jul;29(5):934-940.

32. Atkins MD, Kwolek CJ, LaMuraglia GM, Brewster DC, Chung TK, Cambria RP. Surgical revascularization versus endovascular therapy for chronic mesenteric ischemia: a comparative experience. *J Vasc Surg*. 2007 Jun;45(6):1162-1171.

33. van Petersen AS, Kolkman JJ, Beuk RJ, Huisman AB, Doelman CJ, Geelkerken RH; Multidisciplinary Study Group of Splanchnic Ischemia. Open or percutaneous revascularization for chronic splanchnic syndrome. *J Vasc Surg*. 2010 May;51(5):1309-1316.

34. Tallarita T, Oderich GS, Macedo TA, et al. Reinterventions for stent restenosis in patients treated for atherosclerotic mesenteric artery disease. *J Vasc Surg*. 2011 Nov;54(5):1422-1429.e1.

CME Questions

Reviewed by Ann M. Dietrich, MD, FAAP, FACEP; and Walter L. Green, MD, FACEP

Qualified, paid subscribers to *Critical Decisions in Emergency Medicine* may receive CME certificates for up to 5 ACEP Category I credits, 5 *AMA PRA Category 1 Credits*™, and 5 AOA Category 2-B credits for completing this activity in its entirety. Submit your answers online at acep.org/cdem; a score of 75% or better is required. You may receive credit for completing the CME activity any time within 3 years of its publication date. Answers to this month's questions will be published in next month's issue.

1 A 35-year-old man presents with left flank pain, nausea, and vomiting for 2 days. He is tender in the left lower quadrant. CT of the abdomen and pelvis shows a 4-mm stone. He does not have evidence of a urinary tract infection on his urinalysis. Which therapy should be prescribed?

- A. Antiemetics and oral fluids
- B. Antiemetics, pain control, and oral fluids
- C. Antiemetics, pain control, tamsulosin, and oral fluids
- D. Antiemetics, pain control, tamsulosin, antibiotics, and oral fluids

2 Which finding is a risk factor for the formation of kidney stones?

- A. High urine citrate
- B. High urine oxalate
- C. Low urine calcium
- D. Low urine uric acid

3 What is the current gold-standard imaging study for the diagnosis of kidney stones?

- A. CT abdomen and pelvis with contrast
- B. CT abdomen and pelvis without contrast
- C. Kidneys-ureter-bladder x-ray
- D. Ultrasound

4 What is the preferred option for pain control due to renal colic?

- A. Acetaminophen
- B. NSAIDs
- C. Opioids
- D. Tramadol

5 Which patient does not require admission to the hospital with ureteral stones?

- A. Acute kidney injury in someone with a single kidney
- B. Acute renal failure
- C. No obstructive stone but intractable vomiting
- D. No obstructive stone but with evidence of urinary tract infection

6 What is the size threshold for elective surgical management as recommended by the American Urological Association/Endourological Society?

- A. 7 mm
- B. 8 mm
- C. 9 mm
- D. 10 mm

7 In patients with ureteral colic and chronic kidney disease, what is the recommended choice of pain medication?

- A. Acetaminophen
- B. NSAIDs
- C. Opioids
- D. Tramadol

8 Ultrasound is an excellent tool to evaluate stone disease. What can ultrasound be used to identify?

- A. Hydronephrosis
- B. Signs of infection
- C. Stone location
- D. Stone size

9 What stone type almost always requires surgical management?

- A. Calcium oxalate
- B. Calcium phosphate
- C. Struvite
- D. Uric acid

10 What patients need pseudomonal coverage for a urinary tract infection in the setting of renal calculi?

- A. Patients older than 65 years
- B. Patients who have been recently hospitalized
- C. Patients with a previous history of urinary tract infections
- D. Patients with uric acid stones

11 Which laboratory value is the most helpful in excluding early acute mesenteric ischemia?

- A. Complete blood count
- B. D-dimer
- C. Serum electrolytes
- D. Serum lactate

12 A 58-year-old man presents with acute abdominal pain, nausea, and vomiting for the past 3 days. On examination, he has peritoneal signs. A CT angiogram of the abdomen demonstrates an acute superior mesenteric artery embolism with pneumatosis intestinalis. What is the best next step in management?

A. Administer heparin
B. Administer vasopressors
C. Consult interventional radiology for endovascular revascularization
D. Consult surgery for an exploratory laparotomy

13 An 82-year-old woman presents with a 1-year history of postprandial abdominal pain and weight loss. Her abdomen is soft and nontender. Her laboratory values are normal. A CT angiogram of the abdomen demonstrates an acute thrombosis of the superior mesenteric artery. What would be the best therapeutic option for this patient?

A. Administer broad-spectrum antibiotics
B. Administer vasopressors
C. Consult interventional radiology for endovascular revascularization
D. Consult surgery for an exploratory laparotomy

14 What clinical history should increase suspicion for acute mesenteric ischemia?

A. Acute onset of severe generalized postprandial pain that is out of proportion to the abdominal examination, with associated nausea and vomiting
B. Burning mild intermittent pain that is not associated with anything in particular
C. Dull pain that improves after eating
D. Fever and flank and lower abdominal pain

15 A 70-year-old man with a history of atrial fibrillation, hypertension, and stroke presents with acute abdominal pain. He has no peritoneal signs on examination. CT angiogram of his abdomen demonstrates an acute mesenteric occlusion. What is the most likely site of the acute mesenteric occlusion?

A. Celiac trunk
B. Inferior mesenteric artery
C. Left colic artery
D. Superior mesenteric artery

16 What is the imaging modality of choice to diagnose acute mesenteric ischemia?

A. CT angiogram of the abdomen and mesenteric vessels
B. Duplex ultrasonography
C. MRI angiogram of the abdomen and mesenteric vessels
D. Plain x-rays

17 What risk factor increases a person's chance of mesenteric ischemia?

A. Atrial fibrillation
B. Cirrhosis
C. Diabetes
D. Hypothyroidism

18 Vasopressors should be used infrequently and cautiously. In the event one is needed, which ones are best?

A. Isoproterenol, vasopressin, and milrinone
B. Low-dose dopamine, dobutamine, and milrinone
C. Norepinephrine, epinephrine, and milrinone
D. Vasopressin, norepinephrine, and milrinone

19 Which findings are frequent signs and symptoms of chronic mesenteric ischemia?

A. Elevated liver function tests, weight loss, and pancreatitis
B. Leukocytosis, fever, and weight gain
C. Weight gain, lower abdominal pain, and fever
D. Weight loss, food avoidance, abdominal bruit, and malnutrition

20 A 55-year-old woman with a history of end-stage renal disease on hemodialysis 3 times per week and congestive heart failure with an ejection fraction of 20% presented with hypotension, shortness of breath, and fever. The patient remained hypotensive for several hours despite aggressive fluid resuscitation. She was diagnosed with septic shock from pneumonia and was then placed on norepinephrine. She remained in emergency department boarding for 2 days. Suddenly, she had abdominal distention and an episode of bloody diarrhea. What is the etiology of this patient's ischemic bowel?

A. Acute superior mesenteric embolus
B. Hypotension, norepinephrine, and septic shock
C. Mesenteric venous thrombosis
D. Vasculitis

ANSWER KEY FOR OCTOBER 2022, VOLUME 36, NUMBER 10

1	2	3	4	5	6	7	8	9	10	11	12	13	14	15	16	17	18	19	20
A	D	C	A	C	D	B	A	C	A	D	A	C	D	B	D	D	D	C	A

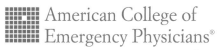

American College of
Emergency Physicians®

ADVANCING EMERGENCY CARE

Post Office Box 619911
Dallas, Texas 75261-9911

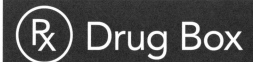 Drug Box

Systemic Hydrocortisone

By Frank LoVecchio, DO, MPH, FACEP
Valleywise Health and ASU, Phoenix, Arizona

Objective
On completion of this column, you should be able to:
- Recognize hydrocortisone's general uses and adverse effects.

Hydrocortisone, also called cortisone, is a steroidal anti-inflammatory drug that chemically differs from other steroids like methylprednisolone. Hydrocortisone reduces symptoms of rash, swelling, asthma attacks, and certain types of pain typically within an hour.

Hydrocortisone is the preferred replacement therapy for patients with adrenocortical insufficiency because it has both glucocorticoid and mineralocorticoid properties. Concomitant administration of a more potent mineralocorticoid (eg, fludrocortisone) may be necessary in some patients. In suspected or known adrenal insufficiency, parenteral hydrocortisone therapy can be used preoperatively or during serious trauma, illness, or shock if patients are unresponsive to conventional therapy. Along with other treatments, intravenous therapy, preferably with hydrocortisone, is essential in cases of shock.

Adult and Pediatric Dosing
- Dose adjustment based on the condition treated and patients' response
- No dosing change for hepatic and renal impairment

Indications
Allergic states; dermatologic and respiratory diseases
Endocrine disorders: Acute adrenocortical insufficiency and other adrenal issues; shock in cases of suspected or known adrenal insufficiency if unresponsive to conventional therapy
GI diseases: Ulcerative colitis and regional enteritis during early, critical phases
Hematologic disorders: Acquired (autoimmune) hemolytic anemia; immune thrombocytopenia (formerly idiopathic thrombocytopenic purpura) in adults
Neoplastic diseases: Leukemias and lymphomas (adults), acute leukemia (children) for palliative care
Ophthalmic diseases: Severe, acute, and chronic allergic and inflammatory eye processes
Rheumatic disorders: Acute and subacute joint pathologies, lupus, and rheumatoid arthritis as short-term adjunctive therapy

Warnings and Precautions
Myopathic
Adrenal: Hypercortisolism or suppression of the hypothalamic-pituitary-adrenal (HPA) axis, particularly in young children or any patient receiving high doses for prolonged periods; adrenal crisis from HPA-axis suppression; when corticosteroids are taken longer than a week, doses should be tapered slowly before discontinuing
Immunologic: Kaposi sarcoma from immunosuppression of prolonged corticosteroid treatment
Psychiatric: Euphoria, insomnia, mood swings, personality changes, severe depression, psychotic manifestations

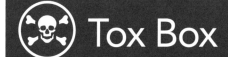 Tox Box

SGLT2-Inhibitor Toxicity

By Christian A. Tomaszewski, MD, MS, MBA, FACEP
University of California San Diego Health

Objective
On completion of this column, you should be able to:
- Manage patients with SGLT2-inhibitor toxicity.

Sodium-glucose cotransporter-2 (SGLT2) inhibitors are approved to lower glucose levels in patients with type 2 diabetes. SGLT2 inhibitors include ertugliflozin, dapagliflozin, canagliflozin, and empagliflozin. Chronic ingestion of these inhibitors can precipitate euglycemic diabetic ketoacidosis (eDKA), especially after a recent illness or surgery. Most SGLT2-inhibitor overdoses do not cause hypoglycemia.

Mechanism of Action
- Inhibits glucose reabsorption in the proximal tubule
- Results in osmotic diuresis

Pharmacokinetics
- 2-hour peak, 3- to 6-hour half-life (with a normal GFR)
- Negligible metabolism
- Mainly renal excretion (90%)
- Toxic dose >5 g in adults, >100 mg/kg in children

Clinical Manifestations
- *Cardiac:* Tachycardia and hypotension (secondary to dehydration)
- *GI:* Nausea and vomiting
- *Metabolic:* Anion-gap acidosis, hyponatremia, eDKA
- *Infectious:* Increased risk of urinary tract and genital mycotic infections

Diagnostics
- Finger-stick glucose (SGLT2 inhibitors usually do not cause hypoglycemia)
- Basic metabolic panel
- Ketones (urine or blood levels)
- Venous blood gas analysis
- Acetaminophen levels in intentional overdoses

Treatment
- Fluids for hypotension
- Dextrose (add to fluids, especially for eDKA)

Disposition
- Home management for children with small, unintentional ingestions
- Observation for several hours for intentional overdoses
- Assessment of mental status and polyuria or tachypnea prior to discharge

Critical decisions
in emergency medicine

Volume 36 Number 12: **December 2022**

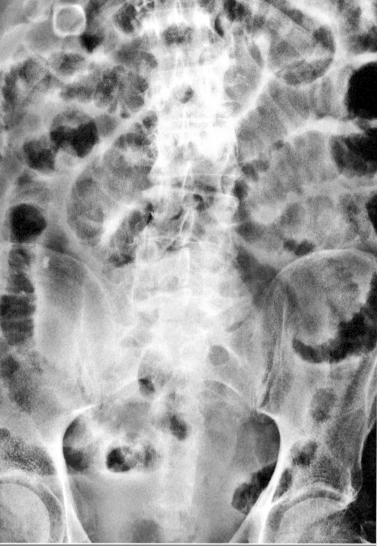

Holding Up the Show

Ileus and small bowel obstruction are common presentations in emergency departments, with small bowel obstruction responsible for 20% of emergent operations for abdominal pain. If left untreated, these conditions can lead to bowel ischemia, necrosis, and perforation. Emergency physicians must promptly recognize and treat these GI motor abnormalities to prevent more serious, life-threatening complications.

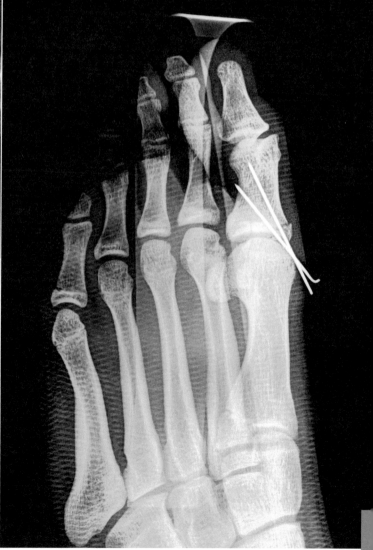

Casing the Joint

The cause of a painful, swollen joint can be particularly challenging to determine because it can range from aseptic causes, such as simple osteoarthritis or gout, to an acutely septic joint. Identification of promulgating factors is essential in reaching a successful diagnosis and preventing significant complications, such as joint destruction, disseminated disease, and even mortality.

THE OFFICIAL CME PUBLICATION OF THE AMERICAN COLLEGE OF EMERGENCY PHYSICIANS

Individuals in Control of Content

1. Colin Danko, MD – Faculty
2. Anthony Han, MD – Faculty
3. Matthew P. Hanley, MD – Faculty
4. Adeola A. Kosoko, MD, FACEP – Faculty
5. Nicholas G. Maldonado, MD, FACEP – Faculty
6. Faroukh Mehkri, DO – Faculty
7. Joan Papp, MD – Faculty
8. Jordan L. Thomas – Faculty
9. Joshua S. Broder, MD, FACEP – Faculty/Planner
10. Andrew J. Eyre, MD, MS-HPEd – Faculty/Planner
11. Walter L. Green, MD, FACEP – Faculty/Planner
12. John C. Greenwood, MD – Faculty/Planner
13. John Kiel, DO, MPH – Faculty/Planner
14. Frank LoVecchio, DO, MPH, FACEP – Faculty/Planner
15. Sharon E. Mace, MD, FACEP – Faculty/Planner
16. Nathaniel Mann, MD – Faculty/Planner
17. Amal Mattu, MD, FACEP – Faculty/Planner
18. Christian A. Tomaszewski, MD, MS, MBA, FACEP – Faculty/Planner
19. Steven J. Warrington, MD, MEd, MS – Faculty/Planner
20. Tareq Al-Salamah, MBBS, MPH, FACEP – Planner
21. Michael S. Beeson, MD, MBA, FACEP – Planner
22. Wan-Tsu Chang, MD – Planner
23. Ann M. Dietrich, MD, FAAP, FACEP – Planner
24. Kelsey Drake, MD, MPH, FACEP – Planner
25. Danya Khoujah, MBBS, MEHP, FACEP – Planner
26. George Sternbach, MD, FACEP – Planner
27. Joy Carrico, JD – Planner/Reviewer

Contributor Disclosures. In accordance with the ACCME Standards for Integrity and Independence in Accredited Continuing Education, all relevant financial relationships, and the absence of relevant financial relationships, must be disclosed to learners for all individuals in control of content 1) before learners engage with the accredited education, and 2) in a format that can be verified at the time of accreditation. The following individuals have reported relationships with ineligible companies, as defined by the ACCME. These relationships, in the context of their involvement in the CME activity, could be perceived by some as a real or apparent conflict of interest. All relevant financial relationships have been mitigated to ensure that no commercial bias has been inserted into the educational content. Joshua S. Broder, MD, FACEP, is a founder and president of OmniSono Inc, an ultrasound technology company, and a consultant on the Bayer USA Cardiac Imaging Advisory Board. Sharon E. Mace, MD, FACEP, performs contracted research funded by Biofire Corporation, Genetesis, Quidel, and IBSA Pharma. All remaining individuals with control over content have no relevant financial relationships to disclose.

This educational activity consists of two lessons, eight feature articles, a post-test, and evaluation questions; as designed, the activity should take approximately 5 hours to complete. The participant should, in order, review the learning objectives for the lesson or article, read the lesson or article as published in the print or online version until all have been reviewed, and then complete the online post-test (a minimum score of 75% is required) and evaluation questions. Release date: December 1, 2022. Expiration date: November 30, 2025.

Accreditation Statement. The American College of Emergency Physicians is accredited by the Accreditation Council for Continuing Medical Education to provide continuing medical education for physicians.

The American College of Emergency Physicians designates this enduring material for a maximum of 5 *AMA PRA Category 1 Credits™*. Physicians should claim only the credit commensurate with the extent of their participation in the activity.

Each issue of *Critical Decisions in Emergency Medicine* is approved by ACEP for 5 ACEP Category I credits. Approved by the AOA for 5 Category 2-B credits.

Commercial Support. There was no commercial support for this CME activity.

Target Audience. This educational activity has been developed for emergency physicians.

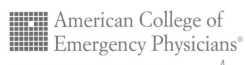

American College of Emergency Physicians®

ADVANCING EMERGENCY CARE

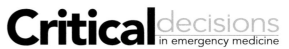
Critical decisions in emergency medicine

Critical Decisions in Emergency Medicine is the official CME publication of the American College of Emergency Physicians. Additional volumes are available.

EDITOR-IN-CHIEF
Michael S. Beeson, MD, MBA, FACEP
Northeastern Ohio Universities, Rootstown, OH

SECTION EDITORS
Joshua S. Broder, MD, FACEP
Duke University, Durham, NC

Andrew J. Eyre, MD, MS-HPEd
Brigham and Women's Hospital/ Harvard Medical School, Boston, MA

John Kiel, DO, MPH, FACEP, CAQSM
University of Florida College of Medicine, Jacksonville, FL

Frank LoVecchio, DO, MPH, FACEP
Valleywise, Arizona State University, University of Arizona, and Creighton Colleges of Medicine, Phoenix, AZ

Sharon E. Mace, MD, FACEP
Cleveland Clinic Lerner College of Medicine/ Case Western Reserve University, Cleveland, OH

Amal Mattu, MD, FACEP
University of Maryland, Baltimore, MD

Christian A. Tomaszewski, MD, MS, MBA, FACEP
University of California Health Sciences, San Diego, CA

Steven J. Warrington, MD, MEd, MS
MercyOne Siouxland, Sioux City, IA

ASSOCIATE EDITORS
Tareq Al-Salamah, MBBS, MPH, FACEP
King Saud University, Riyadh, Saudi Arabia/ University of Maryland, Baltimore, MD

Wan-Tsu Chang, MD
University of Maryland, Baltimore, MD

Ann M. Dietrich, MD, FAAP, FACEP
University of South Carolina School of Medicine, Greenville, SC

Kelsey Drake, MD, MPH, FACEP
St. Anthony Hospital, Lakewood, CO

Walter L. Green, MD, FACEP
UT Southwestern Medical Center, Dallas, TX

John C. Greenwood, MD
University of Pennsylvania, Philadelphia, PA

Danya Khoujah, MBBS, MEHP, FACEP
University of Maryland, Baltimore, MD

Nathaniel Mann, MD
University of South Carolina School of Medicine, Greenville, SC

George Sternbach, MD, FACEP
Stanford University Medical Center, Stanford, CA

EDITORIAL STAFF
Suzannah Alexander, Editorial Director
salexander@acep.org

Joy Carrico, JD
Managing Editor

Alex Bass
Assistant Editor

Kel Morris
Assistant Editor

ISSN2325-0186 (Print)   ISSN2325-8365 (Online)

Contents

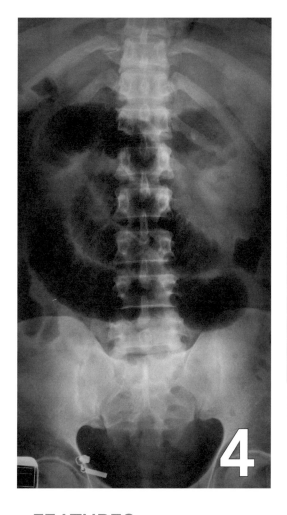

Lesson 23 4
Holding Up the Show
Small Bowel Obstruction and Ileus
By Anthony Han, MD; Faroukh Mehkri, DO; and Colin Danko, MD
Reviewed by Walter L. Green, MD, FACEP

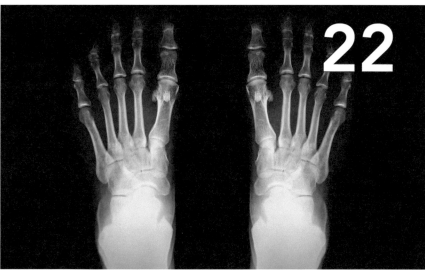

Lesson 24 22
Casing the Joint
Septic Arthritis and Gout
By Nathaniel Mann, MD; and Joan Papp, MD
Reviewed by John C. Greenwood, MD

FEATURES

The Critical ECG — Second-Degree AV Blocks: Mobitz Type I 11
  By Amal Mattu, MD, FACEP

Clinical Pediatrics — Acute Otitis Media 12
  By Jordan L. Thomas; and Adeola A. Kosoko, MD, FACEP
  Reviewed by Sharon E. Mace, MD, FACEP

The Literature Review — Outpatient Stress Testing for Suspected Acute Coronary Syndrome After
  a Negative Workup 14
  By Matthew P. Hanley, MD; and Nicholas G. Maldonado, MD, FACEP
  Reviewed by Andrew J. Eyre, MD, MS-HPEd

The Critical Procedure — Dix-Hallpike Maneuver 16
  By Steven J. Warrington, MD, MEd, MS

Critical Cases in Orthopedics and Trauma — Chronic Shoulder Dislocation 18
  By John Kiel, DO, MPH

The Critical Image — A Toddler With Bloody Stool 20
  By Joshua S. Broder, MD, FACEP

CME Questions 30
  Reviewed by Walter L. Green, MD, FACEP; and John C. Greenwood, MD

Drug Box — Tenecteplase for Acute Stroke 32
  By Frank LoVecchio, DO, MPH, FACEP

Tox Box — Sodium Fluoroacetate Poisoning 32
  By Christian A. Tomaszewski, MD, MS, MBA, FACEP

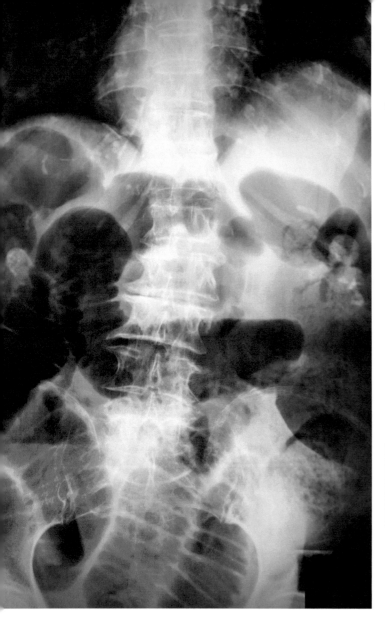

Holding Up the Show

Small Bowel Obstruction and Ileus

LESSON 23

By Anthony Han, MD; Faroukh Mehkri, DO; and Colin Danko, MD
Dr. Han is a resident and Dr. Mehkri and Dr. Danko are assistant professors in the Department of Emergency Medicine at UT Southwestern Medical Center in Dallas, Texas. Dr. Mehkri is also the deputy medical director at the Dallas Fire-Rescue Department.
Reviewed by Walter L. Green, MD, FACEP

Objectives
On completion of this lesson, you should be able to:

1. Distinguish the difference between the pathophysiology of SBO and ileus.
2. Describe common clinical presentations of and risk factors for SBO and ileus.
3. Recall diseases that can present similarly to SBO and ileus.
4. Discuss the different imaging modalities used to diagnose SBO and ileus.
5. Explain the critical steps in treating SBO and ileus.

From the EM Model
2.0   Abdominal and Gastrointestinal Disorders
    2.8   Small Bowel
        2.8.3   Motor Abnormalities
            2.8.3.1   Obstruction
            2.8.3.2   Paralytic Ileus

▬ CRITICAL DECISIONS ▬

- What are the symptoms of SBO and ileus, and why do they occur?
- What patient populations are most at risk of SBO and ileus?
- What is the differential diagnosis of patients with suspected SBO or ileus?
- What physical examination findings suggest SBO?
- How are SBO and ileus diagnosed?
- What are the treatment modalities for SBO versus ileus?

Ileus and small bowel obstruction (SBO) are common presentations in emergency departments, with SBO responsible for 20% of emergent operations for abdominal pain. If left untreated, these conditions can lead to bowel ischemia, necrosis, and perforation. Emergency physicians must promptly recognize and treat these GI motor abnormalities to prevent more serious, life-threatening complications.

CASE ONE

A 72-year-old man presents with altered mental status from a nursing home. The nursing home staff is concerned that he may have a GI bleed and reports that the patient's history includes hypertension, cirrhosis complicated by esophageal varices, metastatic hepatocellular carcinoma, and mild dementia. The patient reportedly had nonbloody emesis for 2 days that the staff believed to be self-limiting. However, this morning he appeared more agitated and began vomiting foul-smelling, dark material. On arrival, the patient is confused, mildly combative, and unable to provide his case history. His abdomen is distended, and during deep palpation, he guards and attempts to push the physician away. The patient has had no previous surgeries. He takes an extensive medication regimen, including scheduled narcotic medications.

CASE TWO

A 47-year-old woman presents with diffuse abdominal pain that has persisted for 2 days. She developed nausea with several episodes of nonbloody emesis this morning and reports she has not had a bowel movement in 5 days. She is unsure if she has passed flatus during this time. She denies fever, dysuria, or other genitourinary complaints. Upon further review of her records, her past surgical history includes a cholecystectomy, an appendectomy, and two cesarean deliveries. On examination, she has a distended, mildly tender abdomen without rebound and multiple, well-healed surgical scars.

CASE THREE

A 35-year-old woman presents with abdominal pain. She reports that the pain started as intermittent left groin pain a few months ago but became constant and severe 2 days ago. Despite her initial reluctance to come to the emergency department due to a lack of insurance, she was convinced to seek help when the pain spread to her whole abdomen. She also reports noticing a mass in her left groin that is painful to the touch. She has not had a bowel movement for the past 2 days and has not been able to pass flatus today. She denies any medical problems or previous surgeries. On examination, her abdomen is mildly distended and tender to palpation, without guarding or rebound. The mass located inferior to her left inguinal crease is warm and firm.

Introduction

SBO and ileus are GI motor abnormalities that disrupt the normal coordinated, propulsive activity of the intestines. SBOs are mechanical obstructions caused by a blockage in the small intestines (*Figure 1*). These obstructions can be partial or complete and can cause acute abdominal pain, nausea, vomiting, and difficulty defecating and passing gas. Ileus is often a temporary dysfunction of the intestines caused by nonmechanical factors; that is, the disruption in movement is not caused by a physical blockage. Ileus leads to obstipation and intolerance of oral intake and often occurs after abdominal and nonabdominal surgeries.[1] SBO accounts for 2% to 4% of abdominal pain complaints in the emergency department and 20% of emergent surgical operations for abdominal pain.[2,3] SBO's incidence is similar for men and women, and the average age of onset is 64 years.[4] However, SBO and ileus can affect patients of any age and can be triggered by a wide variety of comorbidities.

CRITICAL DECISION

What are the symptoms of SBO and ileus, and why do they occur?

SBO

SBO is associated with obstipation, crampy and progressive abdominal pain and tenderness, nausea, and emesis. SBO is a blockage, typically acute, of the normal mechanical movement of material through the small intestines. Bowels that are functioning normally contain gastric, biliary, and pancreatic secretions as well as air and food. If an obstruction develops, these secretions and bowel contents are unable to progress down the GI tract. Even if patients are not eating, emesis and abdominal distension occur because secretions continue to accumulate in the

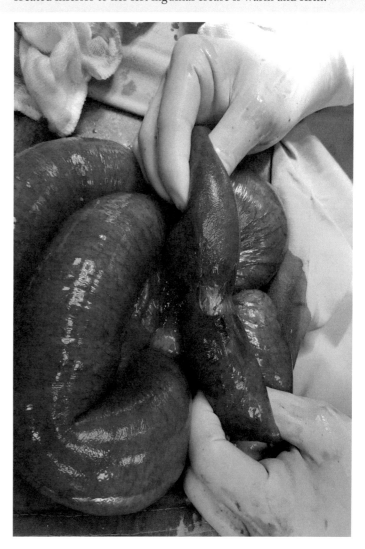

FIGURE 1. Acute obstruction. *Credit:* dr_Shweta/Shutterstock.com.

X-ray Findings of SBO

Upright or Lateral Decubitus	Supine or Prone
• Multiple air-fluid levels • String-of-beads sign • Air-fluid level >2.5 cm • Air-fluid levels of unequal heights in the same small bowel loop	• Dilated small bowel >2.5-3 cm • Dilated stomach • Gasless abdomen • Paucity of colorectal gas • Stretch sign

TABLE 1. SBO signs on x-rays

bowel. Emesis, poor oral intake, and decreased absorption of fluid from the bowels can cause dehydration and electrolyte imbalances over time. Ultimately, dehydration in patients with SBO puts stress on the kidneys and can lead to renal failure. If an obstruction is left untreated, other complications can also occur. An obstruction can cause an increase in intraluminal pressure to the point that bowel ischemia occurs. Subsequently, bowel necrosis and perforation become serious concerns. Patients can ultimately develop septic shock and decline rapidly.[5]

SBOs are generally categorized as partial or complete and, in some cases, can occur at two separate points along the bowel, known as closed loop obstructions. In closed loop obstructions, there are no proximal or distal outlets for the obstruction. Closed loop obstructions can occur when there is an incarcerated hernia or a complete colon obstruction in the presence of a closed ileocecal valve. A careful history, physical examination, and workup are necessary for these patients because this type of obstruction is sometimes missed on x-rays.

Ileus

Ileus, like SBO, presents with obstipation, crampy and progressive abdominal pain and tenderness, nausea, and emesis. Ileus, also known as a pseudo-obstruction, occurs when intestinal contents stop flowing because of intestinal paralysis, or a nonmechanical stoppage. Although patients with ileus can present similarly to patients with SBO, disease pathophysiology and management differ greatly. Ileus can occur anywhere in the GI tract, while SBO occurs in the small intestines. Additionally, ileus usually presents in the first 3 to 5 days after an operation and is usually transient, with the small bowel typically returning to normal function within 24 hours, the stomach within 48 hours, and the colon within 72 hours.[6-8]

CRITICAL DECISION

What patient populations are most at risk of SBO and ileus?

SBO

SBOs are typically caused by processes external to the bowel. Adhesions are the most common cause (*Figure 2*). They can form after abdominal surgery to cause adhesive SBOs. Hernias are another common cause.[9,10] Case reports exist of SBO in patients with Crohn disease, where the SBO is thought to be secondary to swelling and scar tissue from the chronic disease.[11,12] Areas of swelling in the small intestine can also lead to strictures, which can further

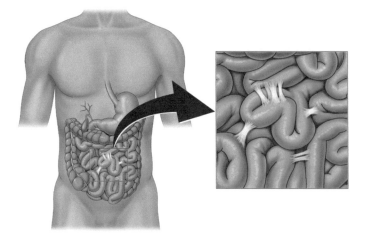

FIGURE 2. Adhesion causing obstruction.
Credit: ACEP.

increase the risk of SBO. After years of disease, patients with ulcerative colitis often undergo a colectomy, and 10% of these patients develop SBO within 3 years of the procedure. In the case of a restorative proctocolectomy, up to 25% of these patients develop SBO.[13,14]

The risk of SBO is increased in patients with intra-abdominal cancers, specifically patients with peritoneal metastases and those with prior radiation treatment to the abdomen. Patients who have undergone Roux-en-Y gastric bypass surgery also have an increased risk of SBO because of their increased risk of internal hernias and their complicated GI anatomy.[5]

Intraluminal causes of SBO are rarer and include small bowel lesions such as polyps, lymphomas, or adenocarcinomas; gallstone ileus; and bezoars from fibrous vegetables or other indigestible materials. Patients with a known history of these conditions who present with abdominal pain should always be evaluated for a possible SBO.

In children with SBO, physicians should consider intussusception and congenital abnormalities as potential causes. Intussusception is generally associated with episodic abdominal pain with vomiting, a sausage-shaped mass in the abdomen, "currant jelly" stool, and a target sign on ultrasound.[15] Careful history taking should also include questions about foreign body ingestion, which can cause a bowel obstruction. In older patients, sigmoid volvulus is a potential cause of obstruction, especially in patients who take anticholinergic medications. X-rays may show the "coffee bean" sign when sigmoid volvulus is present. In pregnant patients, physicians must also consider cecal volvulus.[5]

Ileus

Ileus has fewer causes than SBO. The overwhelming majority of cases are of functional or paralytic ileus secondary to recent abdominal surgery. Those most at risk of ileus are geriatric patients, bedridden patients, and patients taking anticholinergic medications or tricyclic antidepressants. A single-center study of 356 patients found that postoperative ileus is more likely when specific risk factors are present, including male sex, poor performance status, and high intraoperative in-out balance (ie, the volume of fluid intake is greater than the volume of fluid loss) per body weight.[16] When none of these three factors were present, the incidence of postoperative ileus was 2.5%; with two factors present, the incidence increased to 36.1%; and with all three, it was 75%.[16]

Ogilvie syndrome, also known as acute colonic pseudo-obstruction, is a rare, specific type of large bowel ileus that is managed with supportive care. The exact cause and underlying mechanism for Ogilvie syndrome are not well understood, but the three most common conditions associated with it are nonoperative trauma, infection, and heart disease, particularly myocardial infarction and congestive heart failure.[17]

CRITICAL DECISION

What is the differential diagnosis of patients with suspected SBO or ileus?

The differential diagnosis for patients suspected of having SBO or ileus includes gastroenteritis, constipation, dyspepsia, appendicitis, pancreatitis, cholecystitis, diverticulitis, mesenteric ischemia, large bowel obstruction, and Ogilvie syndrome. Although most obstructions occur in the small bowel, roughly 20% to 25% occur in the large bowel, such as Ogilvie syndrome and sigmoid volvulus.[18] Because the differential diagnosis for SBO or ileus is long and includes life-threatening conditions, physicians must carefully gather the history and complete a thorough physical examination and workup for proper diagnosis and management.

CRITICAL DECISION

What physical examination findings suggest SBO?

Physical examination findings in SBO can vary. On inspection, patients with SBO can have abdominal distension, surgical scars from prior operations, or a hernia.

On auscultation, active, high-pitched bowel sounds may be heard when SBO is developing, but sounds may be diminished or absent if SBO has been present for more than a few hours.[5] On palpation, presentations range from localized or general tenderness to signs of peritonitis. On percussion, patients may have a tympanitic abdomen. If a concomitant large bowel or rectal obstruction is present, a rectal examination may demonstrate a mass or fecal impaction. Physicians should remember that stool present in the rectal vault does not rule out SBO.[5]

Nausea with emesis is a common finding in patients with SBO. In more severe cases, emesis can become bilious or even feculent if the obstruction is distal enough. Systemically, patients can appear dehydrated or have vital signs consistent with an infection or shock, raising concern for infection, bowel ischemia, or perforation.

Patients should be asked when their last bowel movement was and if they have been able to pass flatus. However, the ability to pass flatus when a patient's history is otherwise consistent with SBO does not rule out the condition; it could be a sign of a partial or developing SBO.

CRITICAL DECISION

How are SBO and ileus diagnosed?

Imaging

Upright abdominal x-rays can be used to evaluate SBO or ileus and may show diagnostic signs (*Table 1*). The characteristic findings of SBO on plain x-rays are small bowel dilation (diameter >2.5-3 cm), lack of colonic dilation (colon diameter <6 cm and cecum diameter <9 cm), and a relative paucity of colonic gas.[19,20] When present, the "string-of-beads" sign on x-ray is diagnostic of SBO and results from

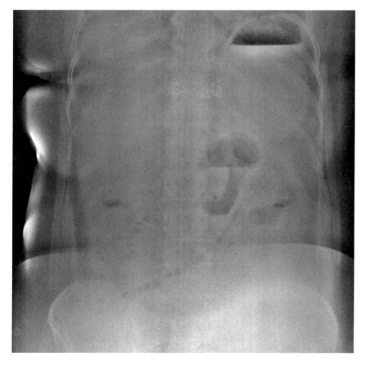

FIGURE 3. String-of-beads sign. *Credit:* Copyright 2022 Dr. Maulik S. Patel. Image courtesy of Dr. Maulik S. Patel, Radiopaedia.org, rID: 13853. Used under license.

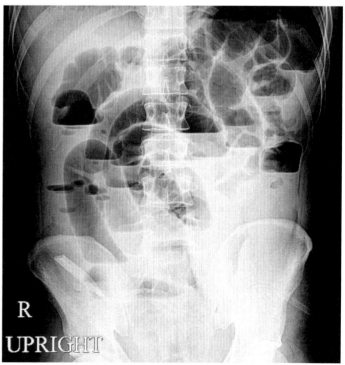

FIGURE 4. Classic air-fluid levels with dilated loops of bowel. *Credit:* Tomatheart/Shutterstock.com.

small pockets of gas getting trapped in the superior wall of the small bowel (*Figure 3*). If patients cannot be placed in an upright position, a lateral decubitus abdominal x-ray may still show free air and air-fluid levels (*Figure 4*). The characteristic x-ray finding for ileus is dilated loops of the small bowel. However, x-rays can be normal when ileus is present, so a normal x-ray does not exclude ileus. One study found that in diagnosing SBO, x-rays have low sensitivity (77%), specificity (50%), and accuracy (75%).[21] X-ray for SBO and ileus is most useful for ruling out free air in the abdomen, which would necessitate emergent surgical intervention.

Some sources, such as the Appropriateness Criteria Suspected Small-Bowel Obstruction published by the American College of Radiology (ACR), rate x-ray as "may be appropriate (disagreement)" and CT as "usually appropriate" for diagnosing an obstruction. Unlike x-ray, CT can demonstrate the precise location, extent, and cause of the obstruction. CT of the abdomen and pelvis with intravenous contrast should be obtained and has a 93% sensitivity and a 100% specificity for diagnosing an obstruction.[21] Although the use of intravenous contrast is not shown to increase sensitivity for detecting an obstruction, it is shown to increase sensitivity for detecting ischemia.[22] Enteric contrast can be considered during evaluation for SBO. However, for high-grade obstructions with significant distension, oral contrast may be unnecessary; fluid in the bowel acts as a natural, neutral contrast agent and provides the same diagnostic accuracy as oral contrast.[22] Additionally, oral contrast administration takes time, which is problematic in patients with high-grade disease at risk of ischemia or perforation. In low-grade cases of SBO, however, oral contrast is shown to increase diagnostic accuracy.[23]

Ultrasound and MRI are alternative imaging options for suspected SBO or ileus. Ultrasound has a sensitivity of 83% and a specificity of 100%.[21] One of ultrasound's disadvantages, however, is that its quality depends on the skill of the technician conducting it. Ultrasound is also poor at detecting the level and cause of an obstruction as well as bowel ischemia and perforation. Ultrasound is better reserved for patients who are too medically unstable for or have a contraindication to CT (eg, very young patients, pregnant patients, patients with an allergy to contrast agents, or patients who have received high doses of radiation in the past). MRI with or without intravenous contrast is another option for patients with contraindications to CT. However, MRI is not always available in the emergency department, and obtaining images through MRI requires much more time than CT, x-ray, or ultrasound.

Laboratory Tests

Blood work such as a CBC and basic metabolic panel can be ordered to assess for leukocytosis, dehydration, and metabolic derangements. A leukocyte count greater than 20×10^9/L raises concern for an abscess, gangrene, or peritonitis.[5] However, a lack of leukocytosis and a normal metabolic panel do not rule out SBO or ileus. Elevations in lactate levels also raise concern for advanced disease and the development of bowel ischemia. Other tests such as a lipase test, coagulation profile, type and screen blood test, and urinalysis are of little use in SBO but are often obtained in

patients with undifferentiated abdominal pain to investigate other potential causes from the differential diagnosis.

CRITICAL DECISION

What are the treatment modalities for SBO versus ileus?

Initial and Conservative Management of SBO

Physicians should always consider the ABCs (ie, airway, breathing, and circulation) in the initial management of SBO and ileus in sick-appearing patients. Because these patients are likely to be volume depleted, fluid resuscitation and electrolyte correction may be necessary. If patients exhibit signs of peritonitis or shock on examination, emergent surgical intervention is required. All patients with an obstruction should be admitted, but not all of them will need operative management. Patients who are stable and without complications (eg, ischemia or perforation) can be observed, although guidelines vary on the length of observation. Patients with an obstruction who are awaiting admission should be further stabilized and treated in the emergency department. Food and drinks should be witheld (ie, patients should be designated as nothing by mouth, or NPO), but medications for pain and nausea should be administered. A nasogastric (NG) tube can decompress the abdomen, especially in patients with severe distension and vomiting.[5] This more conservative management of obstructions is estimated to be successful in 65% to 83% of cases.[24-26]

When obstructions are caused by adhesions that form after surgery, hypertonic, water-soluble GI contrast agents, such as diatrizoate meglumine and diatrizoate sodium solution, are a good treatment option. Diatrizoate meglumine and diatrizoate sodium solution is contraindicated in pregnant patients and not well studied for other causes of obstruction and; for SBO unrelated to adhesions, the underlying cause should be treated. Once the stomach is well decompressed from the NG tube, a one-time dose of 100 mL of undiluted diatrizoate meglumine and diatrizoate sodium solution is given, and the NG tube is clamped for the next 2 to 4 hours. A follow-up kidneys, ureter, and bladder x-ray should be obtained 6 to 24 hours later to see if the contrast agent is

✔ Pearls

- Because numerous risk factors exist for SBO and ileus, physicians must perform a careful history, physical examination, and review of medications.

- For SBO, upright abdominal x-rays can be considered for first-line imaging, but CT of the abdomen and pelvis with intravenous contrast is more sensitive and specific.

- Although many SBOs can be managed conservatively, surgical consultation is typically required if normal bowel function does not return or if complications such as bowel ischemia or perforation develop.

progressing through the GI tract. Progression of the contrast agent to the colon is highly predictive of SBO resolution from conservative management.[27] If the contrast agent does not reach the colon within 24 hours, operative management should be considered.

Surgical Management

Bowel ischemia, necrosis, perforation, and closed loop obstructions cannot be managed conservatively and require immediate surgery. Complications can arise from surgery, and that risk should be factored in when deciding how to manage the obstruction. Prior to surgery, treatment in the emergency department is usually necessary. For example, bowel ischemia, which can occur in 7% to 42% of obstructions, requires broad-spectrum antibiotic treatment in the emergency department.[18] For patients without complications and whose symptoms do not resolve within 3 to 5 days of admission, operative intervention is indicated. In these cases, the decision to operate should always be based on the individual patient's health status and comorbidities as well as the etiology, severity, and location of the obstruction. For example, if the obstruction occurs within 6 weeks of an abdominal surgery, some evidence suggests it is safe to conservatively manage patients for up to 6 more weeks.[28] However, older adults tend to show higher rates of mortality with delayed surgical management.[29]

Management of Ileus

Treatment of ileus in the emergency department is supportive, but the comorbidities in patients with ileus often warrant inpatient admission for observation and vigorous intravenous fluid resuscitation. Any medications that inhibit bowel motility should be temporarily discontinued to encourage the return of normal bowel function.

Summary

SBO and ileus are serious conditions that can lead to life-threatening complications if not properly identified and managed by emergency physicians. Both conditions lead to high rates of hospital admissions and, in the case of SBO, can require surgery. Diagnosis is aided by a thorough history that identifies risk factors because many comorbidities are strongly tied to SBO and ileus. Classic symptoms of SBO include abdominal pain and distention, nausea with vomiting, and obstipation. A broad differential diagnosis should be considered because many conditions present with similar abdominal pain. As with any patient in the emergency department, the extent of workup depends on the patient's clinical status. Ill-appearing patients who present with unstable vital signs or peritonitis on examination can be taken to the operating room for surgical exploration without waiting for imaging studies. For patients stable enough to undergo imaging studies, upright or lateral decubitus x-rays can be considered, but their utility is debated. CT of the abdomen and pelvis with intravenous contrast has a higher sensitivity and specificity for SBO and ileus and can reveal the obstruction's location and signs of ischemia. Ultrasound and MRI can be considered for special populations but have disadvantages compared to other imaging. Management of the obstruction consists of providing medication for pain and nausea and decompressing the stomach with an NG tube. Fluid resuscitation is frequently required because patients are usually dehydrated. If SBO is diagnosed, patients should be admitted for conservative management or operative intervention. Surgery is typically indicated if conservative measures fail or patients develop complications. If ileus is diagnosed, patients should be managed conservatively with bowel rest and the reversal of contributing factors, such as medications that inhibit bowel motility.

REFERENCES

1. Townsend CM Jr, Beauchamp RD, Evers BM, Mattox KL, eds. *Sabiston Textbook of Surgery: The Biological Basis of Modern Surgical Practice.* 21st ed. Elsevier; 2022.
2. Cappell MS, Batke M. Mechanical obstruction of the small bowel and colon. *Med Clin North Am.* 2008 May;92(3):575-597, viii.
3. Gore RM, Silvers RI, Thakrar KH, et al. Bowel obstruction. *Radiol Clin North Am.* 2015 Nov;53(6):1225-1240.
4. Drożdż W, Budzyński P. Change in mechanical bowel obstruction demographic and etiological patterns during the past century: observations from one health care institution. *Arch Surg.* 2012 Feb;147(2):175-180.
5. Tintinalli JE, Ma OJ, Yealy DM, et al, eds. *Tintinalli's Emergency Medicine: A Comprehensive Study Guide.* 9th ed. McGraw Hill Education; 2020.
6. Holte K, Kehlet H. Postoperative ileus: a preventable event. *Br J Surg.* 2000 Nov;87(11):1480-1493.
7. Livingston EH, Passaro EP Jr. Postoperative ileus. *Dig Dis Sci.* 1990 Jan;35(1):121-132.
8. Vilz TO, Stoffels B, Strassburg C, Schild HH, Kalff JC. Ileus in adults. *Dtsch Arztebl Int.* 2017 Jul 24;114(29-30):508-518.
9. Menzies D, Ellis H. Intestinal obstruction from adhesions — how big is the problem? *Ann R Coll Surg Engl.* 1990 Jan;72(1):60-63.
10. ten Broek RPG, Issa Y, van Santbrink EJP, et al. Burden of adhesions in abdominal and pelvic surgery: systematic review and met-analysis. *BMJ.* 2013 Oct;347:f5588.
11. Shah J, Etienne D, Reddy M, Kothadia JP, Shahidullah A, Baqui AAMA. Crohn's disease manifesting as a duodenal obstruction: an unusual case. *Gastroenterology Res.* 2018 Dec;11(6):436-440.
12. Qureshi A, Aziz A, Jehangir Q, Jehangir A. S2308 Small bowel obstruction in a Crohn's disease patient with chronic pillcam retention. *Am J Gastroenterol.* 2020 Oct;115(suppl 1):S1222.

✖ Pitfalls

- Ruling out SBO or ileus based on a normal upright abdominal x-ray.
- Failing to recognize life-threatening complications (eg, ischemia, necrosis, and perforation) and expedite the workup in patients with suspected SBO or ileus.
- Failing to recognize a closed loop obstruction, which requires immediate surgical intervention and cannot be managed by conservative measures.
- Forgetting that patients with a complete SBO do not need oral contrast in addition to intravenous contrast during CT. Oral contrast can harm patients with a complete SBO.

CASE RESOLUTIONS

■ CASE ONE

An upright abdominal x-ray demonstrated multiple air-fluid levels and dilated loops of the small bowel. CT of the abdomen and pelvis with intravenous contrast was obtained for further evaluation and showed a primary liver lesion consistent with hepatocellular carcinoma and multiple abdominal metastases; it also showed large amounts of stool throughout the ileum and bowel wall thickening with intramural bowel gas, raising concern for SBO with possible ischemia and necrosis of the bowel wall. The patient had elevated lactate levels at 4.8 mmol/L and leukocytosis with a WBC count greater than 20×10^9/L. He was given intravenous fluids and medication for pain and nausea. Intravenous antibiotics were started, and general surgery was consulted. General surgery recommended taking the patient to the operating room for emergent surgery. The patient's son, who holds medical power of attorney, was contacted and agreed to the plan. The patient underwent an exploratory laparotomy and had a significant portion of his ischemic small bowel resected. He briefly stayed in the surgical ICU, was downgraded to the surgical ward, and was discharged 2 weeks later.

■ CASE TWO

An upright abdominal x-ray demonstrated no free air under the diaphragm but showed multiple dilated loops of the small bowel as well as a string-of-beads sign. CT of the abdomen and pelvis with intravenous contrast showed a mechanical obstruction of the small bowel without signs of ischemia or perforation. Surgery was consulted and, after a discussion with the patient, recommended admission for monitoring and conservative management. An NG tube was placed for abdominal decompression. The patient was given fluids and pain and nausea medications intravenously. She was admitted to the surgical ward for an adhesive SBO, where she was given the contrast agent diatrizoate meglumine and diatrizoate sodium solution by NG tube. A follow-up abdominal x-ray 6 hours later showed the contrast agent in the colon. Normal bowel function returned within the next 8 hours. She was able to go home on hospital day 2 with primary care follow-up.

■ CASE THREE

The patient's laboratory results were unremarkable. However, CT of the abdomen and pelvis with intravenous contrast demonstrated an incarcerated femoral hernia. Despite the patient being well appearing, the general surgery consultant agreed that the patient's obstipation, lack of flatus, and incarcerated femoral hernia indicated a closed loop bowel obstruction that needed surgical intervention. The patient went to the operating room for a hernia repair. No adhesions or mesenteric twisting was seen. The hernia was reduced, and the defect was repaired. She had an uncomplicated postoperative course and, after the return of normal bowel function, was discharged 2 days later with a scheduled follow-up.

13. Parikh JA, Ko CY, Maggard MA, Zingmond DS. What is the rate of small bowel obstruction after colectomy? *Am Surg.* 2008 Oct;74(10):1001-1005.

14. Aberg H, Påhlman L, Karlbom U. Small-bowel obstruction after restorative proctocolectomy in patients with ulcerative colitis. *Int J Colorectal Dis.* 2007 Jun;22(6):637-642.

15. Intussusception. Children's Hospital of Philadelphia. Published March 31, 2014. https://www.chop.edu/conditions-diseases/intussusception

16. Namba Y, Hirata Y, Mukai S, et al. Clinical indicators for the incidence of postoperative ileus after elective surgery for colorectal cancer. *BMC Surg.* 2021 Feb;21(1):80.

17. Ogilvie syndrome. National Organization for Rare Disorders. Published 2012. https://rarediseases.org/rare-diseases/ogilvie-syndrome/

18. Markogiannakis H, Messaris E, Dardamanis D, et al. Acute mechanical bowel obstruction: clinical presentation, etiology, management and outcome. *World J Gastroenterol.* 2007 Jan;13(3):432-437.

19. Nelms DW, Kann BR. Imaging modalities for evaluation of intestinal obstruction. *Clin Colon Rectal Surg.* 2021 Jul;34(4):205-218.

20. Paulson EK, Thompson WM. Review of small-bowel obstruction: the diagnosis and when to worry. *Radiology.* 2015 May;275(2):332-342.

21. Suri S, Gupta S, Sudhakar PJ, Venkataramu NK, Sood B, Wig JD. Comparative evaluation of plain films, ultrasound and CT in the diagnosis of intestinal obstruction. *Acta Radiol.* 1999 Jul;40(4):422-428.

22. Atri M, McGregor C, McInnes M, et al. Multidetector helical CT in the evaluation of acute small bowel obstruction: comparison of non-enhanced (no oral, rectal or IV contrast) and IV enhanced CT. *Eur J Radiol.* 2009 Jul;71(1):135-140.

23. Ros PR, Huprich JE. ACR Appropriateness Criteria on suspected small-bowel obstruction. *J Am Coll Radiol.* 2006 Nov;3(11):838-841.

24. Cox MR, Gunn IF, Eastman MC, Hunt RF, Heinz AW. The safety and duration of non-operative treatment for adhesive small bowel obstruction. *Aust N Z J Surg.* 1993 May;63(5):367-371.

25. Jeong WK, Lim S-B, Choi HS, Jeong S-Y. Conservative management of adhesive small bowel obstructions in patients previously operated on for primary colorectal cancer. *J Gastrointest Surg.* 2008 May;12(5):926-932.

26. Seror D, Feigin E, Szold A, et al. How conservatively can postoperative small bowel obstruction be treated? *Am J Surg.* 1993 Jan;165(1):121-126.

27. Ceresoli M, Coccolini F, Catena F, et al. Water-soluble contrast agent in adhesive small bowel obstruction: a systematic review and meta-analysis of diagnostic and therapeutic value. *Am J Surg.* 2016 Jun;211(6):1114-1125.

28. Bower KL, Lollar DI, Williams SL, Adkins FC, Luyimbazi DT, Bower CE. Small bowel obstruction. *Surg Clin North Am.* 2018 Oct;98(5):945-971.

29. Springer JE, Bailey JG, Davis PJB, Johnson PM. Management and outcomes of small bowel obstruction in older adult patients: a prospective cohort study. *Can J Surg.* 2014 Dec;57(6):379-384.

Second-Degree AV Blocks: Mobitz Type I

By Amal Mattu, MD, FACEP

Dr. Mattu is a professor, vice chair, and director of the Emergency Cardiology Fellowship in the Department of Emergency Medicine at the University of Maryland School of Medicine in Baltimore.

Objective

On completion of this article, you should be able to:

- Recognize the signs of Mobitz type I atrioventricular block on ECG.

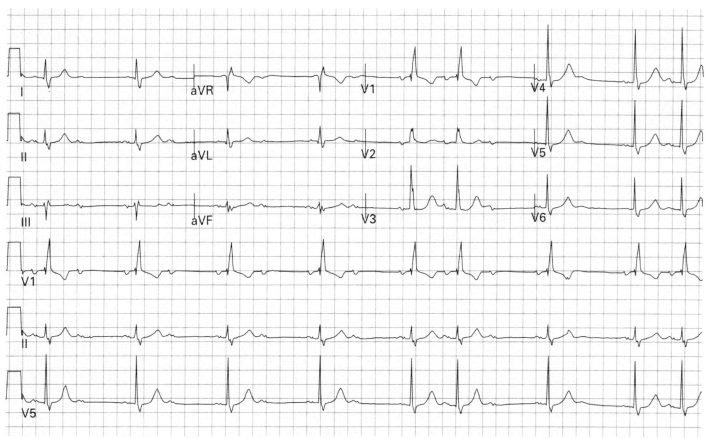

FIGURE 1. A 74-year-old man presents after a syncopal episode. *Credit:* BMJ Publishing.

Sinus rhythm with second-degree atrioventricular (AV) block type 1 (Mobitz type I or Wenckebach), rate 50, right bundle branch block (*Figure 1*). The atrial rate is approximately 88, and there are frequent nonconducted P waves that result in an overall ventricular rate of 50. A second-degree AV block is present mostly with a 2:1 conduction ratio (two P waves for every one QRS). When 2:1 conduction occurs, whether the rhythm is Mobitz type I or Mobitz type II cannot be determined with certainty. In this case, however, 3:2 conduction occurs in two portions of the rhythm strip, in the fifth and sixth and in the eighth and ninth ventricular beats. In these two areas, the PR interval increases, confirming the diagnosis of Mobitz type I.

From Mattu A, Brady W. *ECGs for the Emergency Physician 2.* BMJ Publishing. Reprinted with permission.

Acute Otitis Media

By Jordan L. Thomas; and
Adeola A. Kosoko, MD, FACEP
McGovern Medical School at The University of
Texas Health Science Center at Houston

Reviewed by Sharon E. Mace, MD, FACEP

Objective

On completion of this article, you should be able to:

■ Recognize examination findings of AOM and manage accordingly.

CASE PRESENTATION

A 24-month-old girl without a significant medical history is brought in by her parents who report the patient has had a fever. She started attending day care last month. Her parents state that for the past 2 days, she has had a cold with a runny nose. They became concerned by her 39.4°C (103°F) fever. Otherwise, the patient has had normal behavior and normal intake and output during her illness. Other vital signs include BP 107/68, P 122, and R 18; SpO_2 is 98% on room air.

The patient appears well and has clear nasal discharge. She cries when approached but is easily consoled by her mother. The patient's left ear shows a dull, bulging, erythematous tympanic membrane (TM) by otoscopy and a normal ear canal and external ear by visual inspection. She has two small, mobile, palpable lymph nodes at the left anterior cervical region.

History and Physical Examination

Children with acute otitis media (AOM) often present with complaints of fever and symptoms of an upper respiratory infection. Most cases occur in children younger than 2 years, so caregivers are often the ones to provide key historical information. Otalgia, or ear pain, is the only symptom associated with an increased probability of AOM. Because ear pain is present in only about half of patients with AOM, however, the absence of ear pain does not rule out the diagnosis. Other symptoms such as fever and headache and signs of upper respiratory infection are nonspecific and do not increase the likelihood of AOM.[1] Changes in eating patterns can also help establish a diagnosis because AOM can diminish appetite when inflammation and purulent collection in the middle ear cause swallowing discomfort. Pneumatic otoscopy is the hallmark physical examination method for AOM and visually assesses the appearance and mobility of the TM (*Figure 1*).

Diagnosis

Children younger than 5 years are most likely to develop AOM because their eustachian tubes are shorter and more easily obstructed compared to those of older children and adults. AOM is diagnosed clinically based on three criteria: acute onset of symptoms, inflammation of the middle ear, and middle ear effusion (*Figure 2*).[2,3] When using pneumatic otoscopy during a physical examination, physicians should use the largest speculum that will fit in the ear canal to obtain a better view and for better pneumatic functionality. Pneumatic otoscopy that shows a cloudy, bulging, or nonmobile TM is effectively diagnostic for AOM. An erythematous TM is also predictive of disease but is less accurate than other otoscopic findings. Redness likely occurs because crying can cause blood vessel engorgement in the middle ear. Patients with TMs of normal color and mobility are unlikely to have AOM.[1,4]

Management

Most cases of AOM are caused by viral and bacterial infections (20%-70% of patients), although allergic and other inflammatory processes can also cause AOM.[5] The

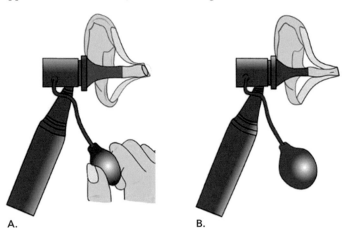

FIGURE 1. Pneumatic otoscopy. Pneumatic otoscopy visualizes movement of the TM in response to pressure changes in the ear canal. The speculum is meant to have a tight seal. Lack of TM movement highly suggests AOM. **A.** Positive pressure is applied by squeezing the bulb. **B.** Negative pressure is applied by releasing the bulb. *Credit:* Adeola A. Kosoko, MD, FACEP.

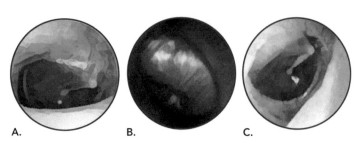

A.   B.   C.

FIGURE 2. Animated otoscopy findings of the TM.
A. An injected, erythematous, transparent TM without effusion is shown. The malleus is well demarcated, and findings are nonspecific. **B.** A bulging, erythematous, dull, and opaque TM with loss of landmarks highly suggests AOM. **C.** Middle ear effusion with normal light reflex and landmarks is shown. Findings are nonspecific. *Credit:* Adeola A. Kosoko, MD, FACEP.

most common bacterial sources of AOM are *Streptococcus pneumoniae*, *Haemophilus influenzae*, and *Moraxella catarrhalis* (50%-92% of patients).[5] Distinguishing viral from bacterial causes is quite difficult. Regardless of the causal organism, many cases resolve spontaneously.[6,7] To combat antibiotic resistance, physicians should consider which patients with AOM are likely to benefit from their use. Instead of being prescribed antibiotics, healthy children with mild illness can be observed for symptom resolution and given supportive management on an outpatient basis.[7] Antibiotics, however, should be prescribed to patients when they have bilateral AOM, they have otorrhea or another severe illness, or they are 2 years old or younger.[2,8,9]

As initial antibiotic therapy, patients should receive high-dose amoxicillin (80-90 mg/kg/day) for 10 days. If the infection returns after a completed course of amoxicillin, patients should receive a 10-day course of a similarly high dose of amoxicillin and clavulanate for broader coverage of *H. influenzae* and *M. catarrhalis*. In cases of penicillin allergy or microbial resistance, physicians should consider macrolides, clindamycin, and cephalosporins (eg, cefdinir).[2]

Patients with AOM commonly complain of pain. Limited data suggest that acetaminophen and ibuprofen may be effective at reducing pain associated with AOM.[10]

Some lifestyle factors increase the risk of AOM. These include breastfeeding, exposure to secondhand smoke, and the use of pacifiers. Modifying these factors could reduce the incidence of AOM in young children.[11]

Differential Diagnosis of AOM

Complications of AOM generally occur idiopathically rather than from prolonged undertreatment. Mastoiditis occurs when chronic inflammation causes a blockage in mastoid air cells that allows purulent cysts to form in the mastoid bone. Examination reveals a classic area of swelling, tenderness, and possibly, fluctuance at the mastoid process behind the ear. Antibiotic use can mask these symptoms, so all patients with AOM should be assessed for mastoiditis.[12]

Cases of middle ear effusion can overlap with cases of AOM. Even after an episode of AOM has resolved, effusion can persist in the middle ear. Other noninfectious mechanisms can also cause this fluid buildup. If middle ear effusion persists, tympanostomy tubes can be placed to help drain the middle ear and prevent future antibiotic use.[13]

Otalgia in patients with a normal ear examination necessitates further workup to find a cause outside of the ear. Possible causes include temporomandibular joint syndrome, pharyngitis, and dental caries.

Other Considerations

Spontaneous TM perforation due to AOM is rare; it presents with a relief of pain and perhaps drainage of fluid from the affected middle ear. If perforation occurs due to AOM, topical antibiotics *may* be useful to directly combat the source of infection. Topical ciprofloxacin has the potential to damage the inner ear, but topical ofloxacin is safe in cases of perforation. Whether or not topical antibiotics are prescribed, patients should receive oral antibiotics when TM perforation occurs during AOM. Additionally, patients' caregivers should be instructed to keep water and other moisture out of the middle ear.

Recurrent cases of AOM indicate eustachian tube dysfunction. Recurrent AOM is defined as three or more episodes of AOM in 6 months *or* at least four episodes in 12 months (with one episode in the past 6 months).[14] If recurrent cases are associated with middle ear effusions, patients should be referred to outpatient otolaryngology for possible tympanostomy tube placement. Patients who have AOM despite tympanostomy tube placement should be treated with topical antibiotics; they may not necessarily need oral antibiotics.[14]

CASE RESOLUTION

The child remained playful and tolerated food and drink in the emergency department. There were no signs of AOM complications. The pneumatic otoscopy was difficult because the patient's parents had to restrain her. After receiving education on and treatment options for AOM, the parents helped determine the preferred treatment course. They were given a prescription for antibiotics but stated that they would first watch the child for clinical improvement over the next 2 days. If symptoms persist, they will fill the prescription and treat their child at home with high-dose amoxicillin.

REFERENCES

1. Rothman R, Owens T, Simel DL. Does this child have acute otitis media? *JAMA.* 2003 Sep 24;290(12):1633-1640.
2. Ramakrishnan K, Sparks RA, Berryhill WE. Diagnosis and treatment of otitis media. *Am Fam Physician.* 2007 Dec 1;76(11):1650-1658.
3. Coker TR, Chan LS, Newberry SJ, et al. Diagnosis, microbial epidemiology, and antibiotic treatment of acute otitis media in children: a systematic review. *JAMA.* 2010 Nov 17;304(19):2161-2169.
4. Karma PH, Penttilä MA, Sipilä MM, Kataja MJ. Otoscopic diagnosis of middle ear effusion in acute and non-acute otitis media. I. The value of different otoscopic findings. *Int J Pediatr Otorhinolaryngol.* 1989 Feb;17(1):37-49.
5. Ruohola A, Meurman O, Nikkari S, et al. Microbiology of acute otitis media in children with tympanostomy tubes: prevalences of bacteria and viruses. *Clin Infect Dis.* 2006 Dec 1;43(11):1417-1422.
6. Rosenfeld RM, Kay D. Natural history of untreated otitis media. *Laryngoscope.* 2003 Oct;113(10):1645-1657.
7. Spiro DM, Tay KY, Arnold DH, Dziura JD, Baker MD, Shapiro ED. Wait-and-see prescription for the treatment of acute otitis media: a randomized controlled trial. *JAMA.* 2006 Sep 13;296(10):1235-1241.
8. Eskin B. Evidence-based emergency medicine/systematic review abstract. Should children with otitis media be treated with antibiotics? *Ann Emerg Med.* 2004 Nov;44(5):537-539.
9. Rawof S, Upadhye S. Antibiotics for acute otitis media: which children are likely to benefit? *CJEM.* 2009;11(6):553-557.
10. Sjoukes A, Venekamp RP, van de Pol AC, et al. Paracetamol (acetaminophen) or non-steroidal anti-inflammatory drugs, alone or combined, for pain relief in acute otitis media in children. *Cochrane Database of Syst Rev.* 2016 Dec 15;12(12):CD011534.
11. Marchisio P, Nazzari E, Torretta S, Esposito S, Principi N. Medical prevention of recurrent acute otitis media: an updated overview. *Expert Rev Anti Infect Ther.* 2014 May;12(5):611-620.
12. Kynion R. Mastoiditis. *Pediatr Rev.* 2018 May;39(5):267-269.
13. Isaacson G, Griswold S. Differentiating acute otitis media from otitis media with effusion. *Vis J Emerg Med.* 2020 Oct;21:100891.
14. Rosenfeld RM, Schwartz SR, Pynnonen MA, et al. Clinical practice guideline: tympanostomy tubes in children. *Otolaryngol Head Neck Surg.* 2013 Jul;149(suppl 1):S1-S35.

Outpatient Stress Testing for Suspected Acute Coronary Syndrome After a Negative Workup

By Matthew P. Hanley, MD;
and Nicholas G. Maldonado, MD, FACEP
University of Florida College of Medicine,
Department of Emergency Medicine, Gainesville
Reviewed by Andrew J. Eyre, MD, MS-HPEd

Objective

On completion of this article, you should be able to:

- Manage patients with suspected ACS and a negative workup in the emergency department.

Natsui S, Sun BC, Shen E, et al. Evaluation of outpatient cardiac stress testing after emergency department encounters for suspected acute coronary syndrome. *Ann Emerg Med.* 2019 Aug;74(2):216-223.

KEY POINTS

- For patients who present with CP and suspected ACS and are discharged after a negative workup, guidelines recommend outpatient stress testing within 72 hours as a further diagnostic strategy.

- A large, multicenter study at an integrated health system showed that only one-third of patients obtained outpatient stress testing post discharge within the recommended time frame.

- MACE rates were low for all patients in the cohort, with no difference between those who received stress testing within 72 hours and those who did not.

- The study suggests that early outpatient stress testing does not benefit low-risk patients with suspected ACS and a negative initial emergency department workup.

Chest pain (CP) is one of the most common presentations, with causes ranging from benign to life-threatening. One cardiac etiology for CP is acute coronary syndrome (ACS). The emergency department approach to patients with CP and suspected ACS includes history taking for cardiac risk factors and typical anginal or anginal-equivalent symptoms, a physical examination, ECG, cardiac biomarkers testing, and risk stratification. If the workup is negative, physicians must decide if patients' pretest probability and overall risk of ACS warrant further diagnostic testing. If so, physicians must then decide how to assess for biomarker-negative, unstable angina and risk stratify patients for major adverse cardiac events (MACE). In some cases, stress testing to assess for inducible ischemia or imaging to assess for anatomic coronary artery disease may be appropriate. To shorten the emergency department length of stay and avoid hospital admission, stress testing can be conducted at an outpatient clinic.

For patients in whom this is appropriate, the American Heart Association and American College of Cardiology recommend outpatient cardiac stress testing within 72 hours of discharge (ie, early noninvasive cardiac stress testing). However, previous reports have produced varied results on how often patients follow through with this testing and the outcomes associated with it. A multicenter, retrospective study from an integrated health system investigated rates of completion of early noninvasive cardiac stress testing and the 30-day incidence of MACE in patients who were discharged after a negative workup for suspected ACS.

The study included 13 Kaiser Permanente emergency departments in Southern California where emergency physicians were able to order noninvasive cardiac stress testing as part of patients' discharge and follow-up plans. The study population included patients who were at least 18 years old and had been discharged after an initial evaluation for CP (including a troponin test) with an order for outpatient cardiac stress testing. Patients with a do-not-resuscitate order or hospice status, an acute myocardial infarction (AMI) diagnosis, and a troponin level greater than 0.5 ng/mL were excluded. Other exclusion factors included those who died in the emergency department, transferred from another hospital, or completed a stress test before discharge.

The primary determination was the proportion of patients who completed an early outpatient stress test within 72 hours from emergency department discharge, who completed it between 4 and 30 days, or who failed to complete it within 30 days. Secondary outcomes included the 30-day incidence of MACE, defined as all-cause death, AMI, and revascularization by percutaneous coronary intervention or coronary artery bypass grafting. Separate and composite 30-day MACE rates for patients completing noninvasive cardiac stress testing within 72 hours were compared with the other patient groups (*Figure 1*). Mortality data were obtained from administrative records and supplemented with data from the State of California and Social Security Administration. Patient characteristics (ie, demographics, clinical data, comorbidities), time of the emergency department visit (ie, day of the week and hour of discharge), physician details (ie, group physician, per diem, and other employee type), and name of the facility were obtained from the electronic health and administrative records and incorporated into the study's analysis.

The study found that no patient or physician characteristic was significantly associated with completion of the 72-hour test; instead, system-level and nonclinical factors had stronger associations with its completion. Specifically, the day of the week had a large effect — Thursday to Friday discharges had much lower rates of 72-hour test completion than Saturday to Wednesday

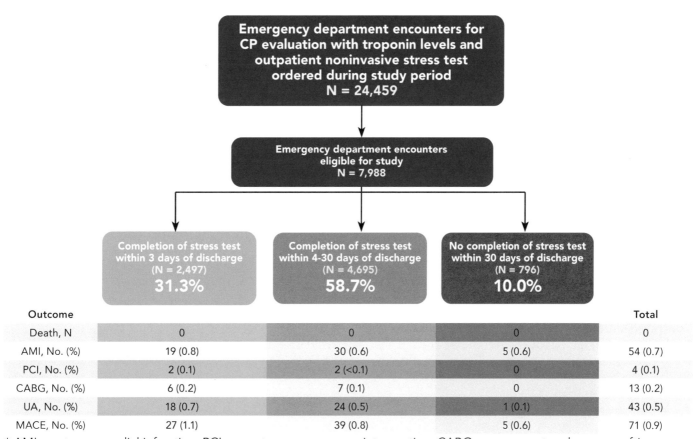

Outcome	Completion of stress test within 3 days of discharge (N = 2,497) 31.3%	Completion of stress test within 4-30 days of discharge (N = 4,695) 58.7%	No completion of stress test within 30 days of discharge (N = 796) 10.0%	Total
Death, N	0	0	0	0
AMI, No. (%)	19 (0.8)	30 (0.6)	5 (0.6)	54 (0.7)
PCI, No. (%)	2 (0.1)	2 (<0.1)	0	4 (0.1)
CABG, No. (%)	6 (0.2)	7 (0.1)	0	13 (0.2)
UA, No. (%)	18 (0.7)	24 (0.5)	1 (0.1)	43 (0.5)
MACE, No. (%)	27 (1.1)	39 (0.8)	5 (0.6)	71 (0.9)

* AMI, acute myocardial infarction; PCI, percutaneous coronary intervention; CABG, coronary artery bypass grafting; UA, unstable angina; MACE, major adverse cardiac events (includes death, AMI, PCI, and CABG)

FIGURE 1. Comparison of patients with CP, suspected ACS, and a negative workup.
Credit: Matthew P. Hanley, MD; and Nicholas G. Maldonado, MD, FACEP.

discharges (15.7% versus 84.3%). In addition, test completion varied quite a bit by medical center, from less than 10% to nearly 70% completion, even after adjustment for relevant patient, visit, and facility characteristics. Subgroup analysis of emergency department encounters with documented HEART scores showed no effect of different risk pools — low (0-3), moderate (4-6), or high risk (7-10) — on the timing of follow-up stress testing.

Overall, this study supports previous literature that suggested a low compliance rate of outpatient stress testing within 72 hours for patients presenting with CP, suspected ACS, and a negative initial workup. Even in an integrated health system, only one-third of patients obtained outpatient stress testing within 72 hours post discharge. Regardless, MACE rates were low for all patients, with no difference between those who completed stress testing within 72 hours and those who did not. This suggests no identifiable benefit to early outpatient noninvasive stress testing for this population. If future guidelines maintain this recommendation, institutional efforts are needed to improve adherence, with particular attention to system-level and nonclinical factors to reduce variability. In systems where consistent guideline adherence is low or unfeasible, alternative methods of further cardiac risk stratification should be considered. However, in the era of high-sensitivity cardiac troponin and increases in downstream invasive testing, cardiac risk stratification for patients with CP, suspected ACS, and a negative initial workup may not be required at all.

Critical Decisions in Emergency Medicine's literature reviews features articles recommended by the Academic Affairs Committee. Available online at acep.org/moc/llsa.

The Critical Procedure

Dix-Hallpike Maneuver

By Steven J. Warrington, MD, MEd, MS
MercyOne Siouxland, Sioux City, Iowa

Objective

On completion of this article, you should be able to:
- Perform and interpret the Dix-Hallpike maneuver to evaluate for BPPV.

Introduction

Dizziness can be a challenging complaint to assess because it is associated with many pathologies of varying severity. Along with the case history and neurologic examination, the Dix-Hallpike maneuver can help evaluate for anterior (superior) and posterior canal benign paroxysmal positional vertigo (BPPV) as a potential cause of a patient's dizziness.

Contraindications
- Severe cervical spine disease;
- Unstable spinal injury;
- Unstable heart condition;
- Carotid stenosis (high grade); and
- Unprovoked nystagmus (ie, nystagmus that occurs at rest).

Benefits and Risks

The Dix-Hallpike maneuver is a quick physical examination tool that can help diagnose specific causes of vertigo (*Figure 1*). Its risks include misinterpretation of results and diagnostic delay of more urgent conditions, such as ischemic strokes, oncologic pathologies, and demyelination syndromes.

Alternatives

Other physical examination techniques can also help determine the cause of vertigo, although they are not exactly alternatives to the Dix-Hallpike maneuver. The HINTS examination, which consists of a head impulse test, nystagmus test, and test of skew, can help in the differentiation of vertigo causes.

TECHNIQUE

1. **Discuss** with the patient what to expect and that some symptoms may worsen during the procedure.
2. **Instruct** the patient to sit on the examination table.
3. **Rotate** and hold the patient's head to one side at 30° to 45° and instruct them to keep their eyes opened and focused.
4. **Lay** the patient flat quickly with their head slightly extended over the edge of the examination table.
5. **Ask** if the patient is experiencing vertigo and watch the patient's eyes for nystagmus.
6. **Repeat** the maneuver on the other side.
7. **Interpret** the results to determine the location of the issue (ie, left or right ear, superior or posterior canal).

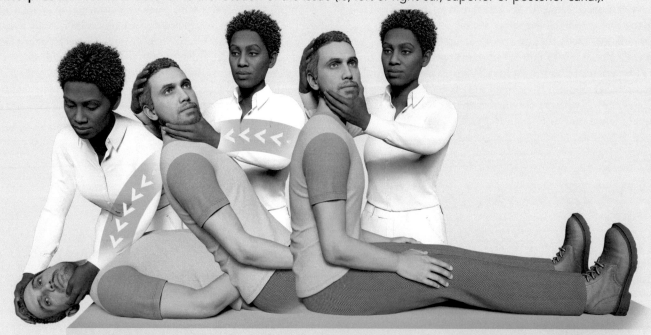

FIGURE 1. Dix-Hallpike maneuver. *Credit:* ACEP.

Reducing Side Effects

During the Dix-Hallpike manuever, some patients experience sudden worsening of their symptoms, including nausea to the point of vomiting. Being aware of this side effect can help physicians avoid exposure to patients' bodily fluids and reduce the risk of patients aspirating their vomit.

Special Considerations

Central nervous system conditions can mimic BPPV, including strokes, demyelination syndromes, neoplasms, and Chiari malformations. Findings that should point physicians to one of these other conditions, and that are not seen in patients with BPPV, include headache, diplopia, abnormal cranial nerve or cerebellar examinations, nystagmus without dizziness, and other neurologic symptoms that do not resolve with therapeutic maneuvers.

Importantly, downbeat nystagmus can be seen in anterior canal BPPV and central causes of vertigo; a finding of downbeat nystagmus generally warrants a consultation and imaging.

The Dix-Hallpike maneuver evaluates both the anterior (superior) and posterior canals of the inner ear for BPPV. A positive test reveals vertigo and nystagmus, lasting up to a minute, after a brief delay (1-10 seconds) at the end of the maneuver. Whichever ear is facing down when symptoms are most severe is likely the affected ear. For patients with posterior canal involvement, upbeat and torsional nystagmuses (from the patient's perspective) are expected. Patients with anterior (superior) canal involvement are expected to have downbeat nystagmus. The horizontal canal is not tested by performing the Dix-Hallpike maneuver and, instead, would be tested by following with a supine roll test.

Chronic Shoulder Dislocation

By John Kiel DO, MPH

Dr. Kiel is an assistant professor of emergency medicine and sports medicine at the University of Florida College of Medicine – Jacksonville

Objective

On completion of this article, you should be able to:
■ Recognize and manage a chronically dislocated shoulder.

CASE PRESENTATION

A 58-year-old man presents with impaired use of his left shoulder for the past 6 weeks. He states that the pain and swelling suddenly started in his shoulder after he fell backward and landed on it; however, at that time, he did not seek medical evaluation. On arrival, he reports left shoulder pain and loss of range of motion, with an inability to lift his arm. He denies neurologic complaints. On examination, the shoulder has a gross deformity with generalized bony tenderness. He is unable to passively or actively flex, extend, or abduct his left shoulder. The skin is intact. Radial pulse is 2+. Motor examination is normal from the elbow to the wrist. X-rays identify an anterior shoulder dislocation (*Figure 1*). Orthopedic surgery is consulted and does not recommend reduction at this time because of the long duration of the dislocation. Outpatient follow-up at the orthopedic clinic is recommended.

Discussion

Although debated in the literature, the most accepted definition of a chronic shoulder dislocation is a joint that remains dislocated for at least 3 weeks.[1] Many shoulder dislocations, the most common of which is anterior dislocation, are emergently reduced within hours of the injury. Therefore, chronic shoulder dislocations are relatively rare, and their epidemiology is not well defined. One study estimated their prevalence to be 0.10% to 0.18%.[2] Chronic shoulder dislocations occur most commonly in geriatric patients with lax or weakened soft tissues and degenerative joint disease. Other risk factors for chronic dislocations include alcoholism, epilepsy, and repetitive trauma.

A chronically dislocated shoulder has a significant effect on function.[3] Patients often report severe pain and limited ability to accomplish functional activities. Chronic shoulder dislocations are also associated with other injuries, including Bankart lesions, Hill-Sachs lesions, glenoid bone loss, acromion fractures, and proximal humerus fractures. Neurovascular injuries are rarely reported. Disuse of the shoulder in chronic dislocations can lead to rapid atrophy of the rotator cuff muscles. In some cases, underlying chronic rotator cuff tearing facilitates the dislocation.

Management of chronically dislocated shoulders is controversial and not well defined in the orthopedic surgery literature. Conservative management has a high failure rate, and closed reduction is typically not possible because of fibrous capsular contracture. Publications are limited to case reports, with no large trials that evaluate the various surgical methods. Surgical techniques that are discussed in the literature include closed reduction, open reduction, Bankart repair, the Latarjet procedure, hemiarthroplasty, reverse shoulder hemiarthroplasty, and reverse total shoulder arthroplasty. Determining the appropriate surgical intervention involves the consideration of many factors, including the duration of the dislocation, associated injuries, status of the rotator cuff, hand dominance, previous operative and nonoperative management, and the functional demands of the patient.

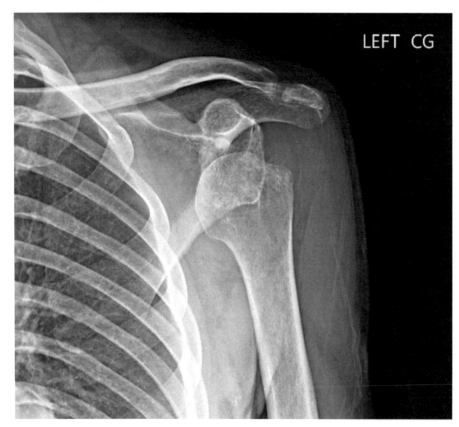

LEFT CG

FIGURE 1. Anterior-posterior x-ray of the shoulder that demonstrates an anterior shoulder dislocation. *Credit:* John Kiel DO, MPH.

During orthopedic follow-up, the patient still had an anteroinferior shoulder dislocation. He reported continued pain and loss of range of motion without numbness or tingling. An MRI was obtained and demonstrated an anterior shoulder dislocation with both a Hill-Sachs lesion and bony Bankart lesion, along with complex labrum tearing, atrophy, myositis, and tendinosis of the supraspinatus and infraspinatus (*Figures 2* and *3*). At the last orthopedic visit, he was scheduled for a reverse total shoulder arthroplasty because of significant atrophy of the rotator cuff musculature; however, he was later lost to follow-up.

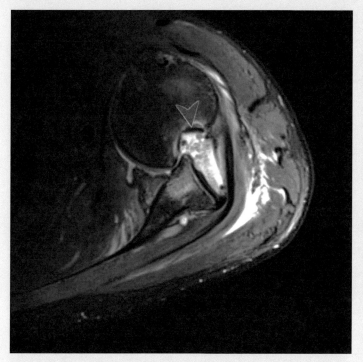

FIGURE 2. **Axial view of a shoulder MRI that shows anterior dislocation and large Hill-Sachs lesions (*red arrow*).** *Credit:* John Kiel DO, MPH.

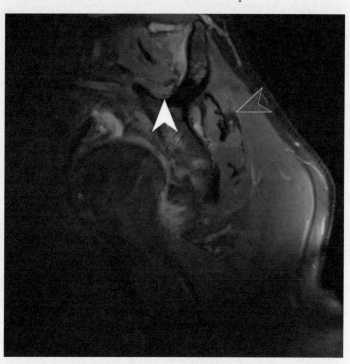

FIGURE 3. Sagittal view of a shoulder MRI that shows atrophy of the supraspinatus (*yellow arrow*) and infraspinatus (*red arrow*). *Credit:* John Kiel DO, MPH.

REFERENCES

1. Micic ID, Mitkovic MB, Mladenovic DS. Unreduced chronic dislocation of the humeral head with ipsilateral humeral shaft fracture: a case report. *J Orthop Trauma*. 2005 Sep;19(8):578-581.
2. Rai AK, Bandebuche AR, Bansal D, Gupta D, Naidu A. Chronic unreduced anterior shoulder dislocation managed by Latarjet procedure: a prospective study. *Cureus*. 2022 Jan 31;14(1):e21769.
3. Rowe CR, Zarins B. Chronic unreduced dislocations of the shoulder. *J Bone Joint Surg Am*. 1982 Apr;64(4):494-505.

The Critical Image
A Toddler With Bloody Stool

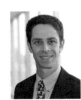

By Joshua S. Broder, MD, FACEP
Dr. Broder is a professor and the residency program director in the Department of Emergency Medicine at Duke University Medical Center in Durham, North Carolina.

Objective

On completion of this article, you should be able to:
- Describe the differential diagnosis and select the appropriate diagnostic imaging for GI bleeding in young children.

CASE PRESENTATION

A 21-month-old boy presents after having a bloody stool. He was born at term and is fully immunized for his age. The patient's mother reports that he had a single large stool of mixed fecal matter and blood after having no bowel movement in the preceding 2 days. She presents a diaper full of what appears to be bloody stool (*Figure 1*). She does not believe he has had much pain, although he has been a little fussy. He is still drinking milk but not eating much. The patient's mother denies that he had any fever or vomiting. She states that 6 months ago, he had another episode of bloody, bright red stools. He was seen at an urgent care, but no further diagnostic workup was undertaken. There is no history of abdominal or perineal injury, and the patient has not been witnessed to ingest any foreign bodies. He has not had any known recent exposures to infectious diseases, well water, or unpasteurized dairy products. There is also no family history of inflammatory bowel disease.

The patient's vital signs are BP 140/86, P 100, R 20, and T 36.6°C (97.9°F); SpO_2 is 99% on room air. On examination, he is in no apparent distress and has no abdominal tenderness or palpable masses. He has some dried blood around his rectum but no apparent injuries. X-rays of the chest, abdomen, and pelvis are negative for radiopaque foreign bodies such as button batteries (*Figure 2*). An ultrasound does not show any evidence of intussusception. A nuclear medicine scan is ordered to assess for Meckel diverticulum.

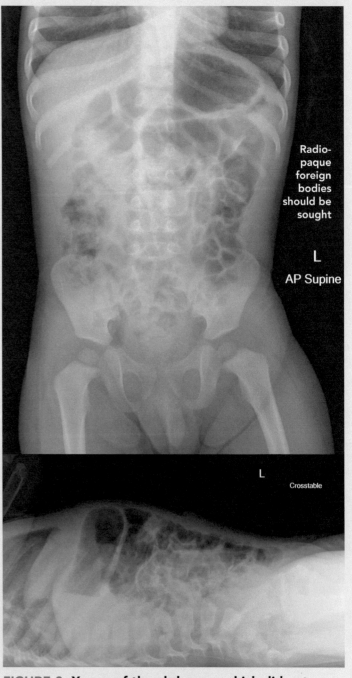

Radio-paque foreign bodies should be sought

L

AP Supine

L

Crosstable

FIGURE 2. X-rays of the abdomen, which did not demonstrate radiopaque foreign bodies.
The upright chest x-ray (*not shown*) did not reveal free air.

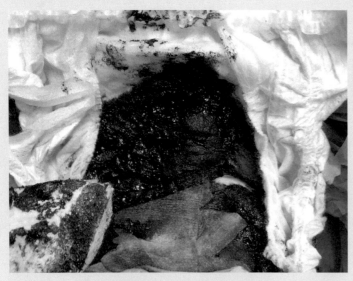

FIGURE 1. The patient's stool, which appeared bloody and tested guaiac positive

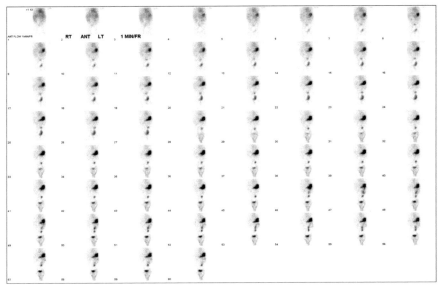
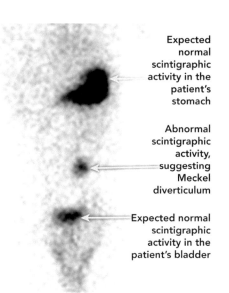

Expected normal scintigraphic activity in the patient's stomach

Abnormal scintigraphic activity, suggesting Meckel diverticulum

Expected normal scintigraphic activity in the patient's bladder

FIGURE 3. A nuclear medicine scan demonstrating abnormal scintigraphic activity (where the radiotracer is taken up by specialized gastric mucosal cells) outside of the expected locations of the stomach and urinary bladder. The area of abnormal activity suggests Meckel diverticulum. *At left,* images were taken over 60 minutes after radioisotope injection, with an exposure of 1 minute per frame. *At right* is an enlarged view of the frame taken at 45 minutes after radioisotope injection.

Discussion

The most common congenital abnormality of the GI tract is Meckel diverticulum. Autopsy data reveal that the condition occurs in 2% of the population.[1] Meckel diverticula contain ectopic gastric or pancreatic mucosal tissue, and most occur within 100 cm of the ileocecal valve. Complications include hemorrhage from ulceration, small bowel obstruction, diverticulitis, and intussusception.[1]

The selected imaging approaches should be based on the age-appropriate differential diagnosis; in pediatric patients, this includes foreign body ingestion, malrotation, intussusception, and arteriovenous malformation. Meckel diverticulum can present as nonspecific abdominal pain. Consequently, initial imaging modalities commonly include plain x-rays (to identify foreign bodies), ultrasound (for suspected appendicitis or intussuseption), and CT (for bowel obstruction and appendicitis). Meckel diverticulum may appear on ultrasound or CT as a blind-ended tubular structure attached to the small bowel, but the diagnosis is not always clear from these modalities. Complications of Meckel diverticulum along with calcified enteroliths may also be seen with these modalities.

When Meckel diverticulum is suspected, nuclear scintigraphy with ^{99m}Tc sodium pertechnetate can identify ectopic gastric mucosa because pertechnetate localizes to gastric mucosal tissue (*Figure 3*). Its sensitivity in pediatric patients is 85% to 90%. The technique may require sedation in young children to prevent motion artifact because exposures are made over a period of 1 hour and each frame is acquired over 1 minute.[1]

CASE RESOLUTION

The patient underwent surgery, and a small bowel diverticulum lined with gastric mucosa was resected. Pathology identified gastric mucosal cells, confirming the diagnosis of Meckel diverticulum.

REFERENCE
1. Elsayes KM, Menias CO, Harvin HJ, Francis IR. Imaging manifestations of Meckel's diverticulum. *AJR Am J Roentgenol.* 2007 Jul;189:81-88.

Feature Editor: Joshua S. Broder, MD, FACEP. See also *Diagnostic Imaging for the Emergency Physician* (Winner of the 2011 Prose Award in Clinical Medicine, the American Publishers Award for Professional and Scholarly Excellence) and *Critical Images in Emergency Medicine* by Dr. Broder.

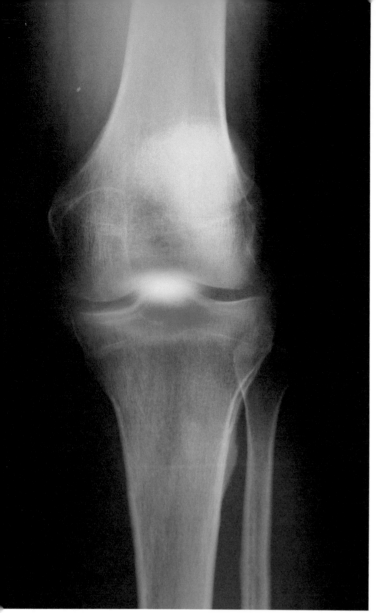

Casing the Joint

Septic Arthritis and Gout

LESSON 24

By Nathaniel Mann, MD; and Joan Papp, MD

Dr. Mann is an assistant professor at the University of South Carolina School of Medicine Greenville and an attending physician at Prisma Health Upstate. Dr. Papp is an associate professor in the Department of Emergency Medicine at Case Western Reserve University School of Medicine and an attending physician at MetroHealth Medical Center in Cleveland, Ohio.

Reviewed by John C. Greenwood, MD

Objectives

On completion of this lesson, you should be able to:

1. Recognize red flags in the history and physical examination that can indicate a life-threatening swollen joint.
2. Identify various risk factors and treatments for the common etiologies of a swollen joint.
3. Discuss which diagnostic tests can aid in the evaluation of an undifferentiated swollen joint.
4. Differentiate a septic joint from a noninfected joint.
5. Explain the diagnosis and management of gout and pseudogout.

From the EM Model

11.0   Musculoskeletal Disorders (Nontraumatic)
    11.3   Joint Abnormalities
        11.3.1   Arthritis
            11.3.1.1 Septic
            11.3.1.2 Crystal Arthropathies

■ CRITICAL DECISIONS ■

- How should the initial assessment of a swollen joint be approached?

- What clinical findings should raise suspicion for septic arthritis?

- What laboratory tests are most valuable for differentiating infection from inflammation?

- What treatments for septic arthritis should be initiated in the emergency department?

- What other diagnoses should be considered in a patient who presents with a swollen joint?

A painful, swollen joint is a symptom, not a diagnosis. Its cause can be particularly challenging because of the broad spectrum of etiologies that must be considered, ranging from aseptic causes, such as simple osteoarthritis or gout, to an acutely septic joint. Septic arthritis is an uncommon condition but has a high mortality rate of 5% to 20%. Identification of the promulgating factors is essential to reaching a successful diagnosis and preventing significant complications, such as joint destruction, disseminated disease, and even mortality.

CASE ONE

A 17-year-old boy presents with 4 days of increasingly painful swelling in his left knee. He reports that he was treated for an abscess on his right thigh 2 weeks ago; treatment included incision and drainage, intravenous antibiotics, and a brief hospital stay. All symptoms related to that episode have since resolved.

The patient has no other significant medical history and takes no medications. His immunizations are current, and he denies any sexual activity or illicit drug use. He is afebrile and his other vital signs are also normal. He appears to be physically fit and generally healthy.

The teenager is holding his left knee in slight flexion and will not allow passive range of motion due to significant discomfort. The joint is diffusely swollen, warm, erythematous, and tender; the rest of his examination is unremarkable.

CASE TWO

A 64-year-old man presents with pain, swelling, and redness in his left ankle that began 2 days ago. He states that he had similar symptoms in the past that resolved with NSAIDs. He has a history of diabetes, hyperlipidemia, chronic renal insufficiency, and hypertension. He takes metformin,

hydrochlorothiazide, metoprolol, and a daily baby aspirin. He smokes about 10 cigarettes per day and drinks alcohol on the weekends; he has never used illicit drugs.

The patient is afebrile, and his other vital signs are also normal, with the exception of a mildly elevated blood pressure (142/70 mm Hg). He complains of significant discomfort with the slightest movement of the joint, which is warm, erythematous, swollen, and tender. Other than moderate obesity, the rest of his examination is unrevealing.

CASE THREE

A 79-year-old woman with a history of hypertension, rheumatoid arthritis, and class II heart failure presents for an erythematous, swollen, and painful right wrist. The pain has worsened over the last 2 days. She denies any trauma, injury, recent infections, fevers, or similar joint pain in the past. She takes lisinopril, metoprolol, furosemide, and methotrexate; rarely uses alcohol; and denies any illicit substance use. Her capillary refill and vital signs are normal. Her right wrist is warm, swollen, and painful to palpation throughout the joint, and she has limited range of motion. No other joints, including the elbow, are painful or swollen.

Introduction

A swollen joint has a range of etiologies (*Table 1*). Each patient presents with a variable set of signs and symptoms, and from these clues, emergency physicians must initiate relevant diagnostic tests, identify the underlying disease, and recommend appropriate treatment. The most potentially destructive of these etiologies is septic arthritis — a joint infection caused by pyogenic bacteria — which must be considered in any patient who presents with a warm, swollen, and painful joint.[1-4]

CRITICAL DECISION

How should the initial assessment of a swollen joint be approached?

It can be difficult to distinguish between an infected joint and a joint swollen from an inflammatory process, such as gout or rheumatoid arthritis. A thorough history should be focused on eliciting details related to symptom onset; the presence of fevers; previous joint disease, surgeries, or systemic illnesses; medications; recent infections (including sexually transmitted diseases); and any history of blunt or penetrating trauma to the affected joint.

Information should also be gathered about past episodes of joint inflammation, including any history of monoarticular or polyarticular joint involvement. Common etiologies of polyarticular arthritis, which affects five or more joints, include rheumatoid arthritis, systemic diseases, and spondyloarthropathy. Monoarticular joint disease is more likely to be caused by infection, trauma, or crystalline diseases, such as gout or pseudogout (see *Table 1*).[5-7]

The physical examination should include an attempt to move the affected joint through its full range of motion. Pain severe enough to impede any attempt at movement is a critical examination finding that is highly suspicious for septic arthritis; if this diagnosis cannot be excluded, a joint aspiration should follow.[5-7]

Possible Causes of a Swollen Joint	
Infectious	• Bacteria • Viruses • Spirochetes (eg, Lyme disease, syphilis) • Fungi
Crystalline	• Gout (ie, monosodium urate) • Pseudogout (ie, calcium pyrophosphate dehydrate) • Basic calcium phosphate (ie, BCP, hydroxyapatite)
Traumatic	• Occult fracture, hemarthrosis, meniscal tear, or ligamentous injury • Foreign body • Iatrogenic causes (eg, injections)
Systemic	• Autoimmune conditions (eg, rheumatoid arthritis, juvenile rheumatoid arthritis, sarcoidosis, Behçet disease, systemic lupus erythematosus) • Spondyloarthropathy (eg, reactive arthritis, psoriatic arthritis, ankylosing spondyloarthritis)
Endocrine	• Hypothyroidism • Hypoparathyroidism
Other	• Osteonecrosis • Osteoarthritis • Vasculitis • Malignancy • Coagulopathy

TABLE 1. Etiologies of an acutely swollen joint[5-7]

An examination of the joint bursa (*Figure 1*) and overlying skin and soft tissue can also provide clues about the cause of patients' symptoms. Special attention should be paid to determine if the symptoms are localized or generalized. Swelling, erythema, or tenderness overlying a bursa indicates bursitis, whereas generalized swelling and tenderness suggest joint inflammation.[7]

What clinical findings should raise suspicion for septic arthritis?

The term *arthritis* refers to inflammation within a joint and is not to be confused with *arthralgia*, or joint pain *without* inflammation. Septic arthritis is a true emergency. It can lead to rapid joint destruction and loss of function, systemic infection, and even death. Although the disease itself is uncommon (2-5 patients/100,000/year), overall mortality in adults is high, ranging from 5% to 20%, with higher rates of death among older patients, immunocompromised patients, and patients with disseminated disease.[1,8-14] Septic arthritis is far more common in patients with a history of preexisting joint disease, which can make the initial diagnosis challenging.[1-3,14] The incidence demonstrates a bimodal pattern; peaks occur in patients younger than 15 years and older than 55 years.[3]

The classic presentation of septic arthritis is a single acutely painful, warm, swollen joint with restricted movement.[1-3] Despite the common assumption that these patients will be febrile, fewer than 60% present with an elevated temperature; however, the presence of a fever should raise clinical suspicion for septic arthritis.[1,2] Clinical examination findings can be subtle but generally include a reduction in joint mobility and function and, occasionally, an extra-articular site of infection or toxic appearance.[1-3,14]

Septic arthritis is typically a monoarticular disease of large joints, most commonly the knee, which is seen in 45% to 50% of adult cases.[1,2] Other frequently affected sites are the hip (15%), ankle (9%), elbow (8%), wrist (6%), and shoulder (5%). This disease rarely affects the axial skeleton in patients who do not use illicit intravenous drugs.[2] A polyarticular pattern is seen in 10% to 20% of septic arthritis cases.[3]

Pathogenesis and Bacteriology

Bacterial arthritis is usually the result of occult bacteremia.[1-3] The synovial tissue is highly vascular and has no basement membrane protection; therefore, bacteria in the bloodstream can spread to the joint space quite easily (*Figure 2*). Within hours of entering the sterile joint space, these bacteria trigger an acute inflammatory cell response, which results in the purulent joint effusion that is characteristic of this disease process.[1-3]

Common sources of occult bacteremia include pneumonia, pyelonephritis, and skin and soft tissue infections. The presence of these conditions in patients' histories increases the likelihood that they are the source of septic arthritis.

In some cases, joints may be directly inoculated by trauma or illicit intravenous drug use. Iatrogenic infections due to arthroscopy and steroid injections are less common.[1-3]

Staphylococcus and *streptococcus* are the most frequent microbial isolates, with *Staphylococcus aureus* predominating; however, any pathogenic microorganism can lead to septic arthritis.[1-3,5-7,10] Methicillin-resistant *S. aureus* (MRSA) is an increasingly common and important pathogen to consider in patients with suspected septic arthritis.[2,15] Patients with MRSA are at greater risk of developing a more severe infection or subperiosteal abscess that requires surgical intervention.[15]

Neisseria gonorrhoeae is the pathogen responsible for most cases of septic arthritis in young adults; however, the rate of gonococcal arthritis has been decreasing since the 1980s.[2] Gonococcal arthritis is a relatively benign disease that presents most commonly as a single purulent monoarticular arthritis but can manifest as disseminated asymmetric aseptic polyarthritis. Gonorrhea should remain a consideration, especially in sexually active young adult patients without previous disease.[16]

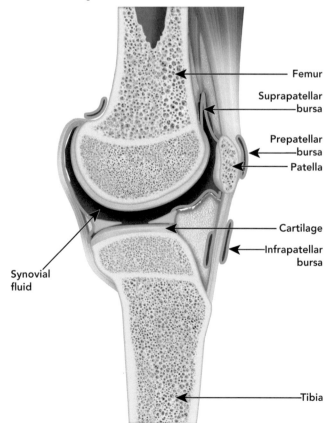

FIGURE 1. Synovial joint of the knee. *Credit:* ACEP.

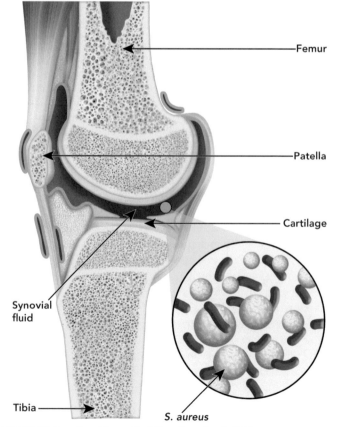

FIGURE 2. Septic arthritis. *Credit:* ACEP.

Risk Factors

Disorders that can predispose patients to septic arthritis include diabetes mellitus, HIV, dermatitis or loss of skin integrity, illicit intravenous drug use, and previous joint disease or replacement.[1-3,14] However, an estimated 22% of patients present with no identifiable risk factor.

As many as 47% of patients ultimately diagnosed with septic arthritis have a history of prior joint disease. Of these, 14% report a history of rheumatoid arthritis, the most common type of inflammatory arthritis (present in 1% of the population).[2,14] Patients with rheumatoid arthritis are at a particularly high risk of septic arthritis because their joints are already damaged and they take long-term immunosuppressing steroids and tumor necrosis factor inhibitors.[2,3,14] This latter class of medications has been associated with fatalities from joint sepsis triggered by uncommon organisms, such as *Salmonella*, *Actinobacillus,* and *Listeria*.[2,3] Occupational exposure to animals or recent emigration from developing nations can predispose patients to infection with *Brucella* or *Mycobacterium tuberculosis,* respectively.[3]

CRITICAL DECISION

What laboratory tests are most valuable for differentiating infection from inflammation?

The only definitive way to confirm septic arthritis is an analysis of the synovial fluid, which can be obtained in the emergency department by aspirating the joint. The collected fluid should be cultured, Gram stained, and evaluated for crystals. Although a positive Gram stain can confirm septic arthritis, the test may be negative in 20% to 40% of patients with the disease.[2,3] The presence of crystals likely indicates an acute inflammatory process (eg, gout or pseudogout), an autoimmune disorder, or a chronic degenerative disease, such as osteoarthritis.

Collected fluid yields the best results when inoculated into a blood culture medium — a technique that is more effective and less prone to contamination than standard solid plating.[2,3,14] Culture bottles can dilute bacterial inhibitors (such as complement) and contain lytic agents (such as saponin) that aid in the release of intracellular bacteria.

Current guidelines for interpreting synovial fluid WBC counts are as follows:[17,18]
- Noninflammatory: 200 to 2,000 cells/μL;
- Inflammatory: 200 to 50,000 cells/μL; and
- Infectious: more than 50,000 cells/μL.

Despite these commonly accepted guidelines, other data suggest that hard numbers may be unreliable and insensitive for diagnosing septic arthritis.[19] Although an elevated synovial WBC count may increase the probability of a septic joint, a normal WBC count should not be used to decrease the pretest probability of septic arthritis.[20] Physicians should use patient history, clinical suspicion, and examination findings to guide their decisions (*Figure 3*).[1]

Other recommended tests include blood cultures, complete blood count (CBC), erythrocyte sedimentation rate (ESR), and C-reactive protein (CRP) measurements. When used in conjunction with other diagnostic tools, including synovial analysis and examination findings, these tests can help confirm a diagnosis of septic arthritis. None of them should be used alone to rule it out, however. Although most septic arthritis patients have elevated ESR and CRP levels, some will have normal test results.[1]

Blood cultures are of particular importance because associated bacteremia is present in as many as one-third of patients with septic arthritis.[2] Urea, liver function, and electrolyte measurements can also be helpful by providing information regarding end-organ damage in severe cases. Patients' level of renal function needs to be known prior to initiating antibiotic therapy.[7]

Gonococcal arthritis can be more difficult to diagnose with laboratory tests because synovial fluid cultures are positive in only 50% of such cases.[2] Bacteremia is uncommon, even in cases of polyarticular disease. If clinical suspicion is high for gonorrhea, all mucosal surfaces, including the oropharynx, cervix, urethra, and rectum, should be cultured.

CRITICAL DECISION

What treatments for septic arthritis should be initiated in the emergency department?

Antibiotics and joint drainage are the mainstays of therapy for septic arthritis. Initial treatment should be aimed at *Staphylococcus* and *Streptococcus* until available culture results indicate otherwise. In most cases, empiric vancomycin is the antibiotic of choice because it covers most of the organisms responsible for septic arthritis in the absence of implanted hardware.[2,21-23] Ceftriaxone is a reasonable choice if the patient's Gram stain is negative; if a *Pseudomonas* infection is suspected, cefepime or piperacillin-tazobactam should be added until culture results are obtained. Aggressive treatment is warranted in all cases of suspected septic arthritis due to its destructive nature and potential for high morbidity and mortality.[3]

In the past, physicians were instructed to start intravenous antibiotics as soon as possible because of the risk of morbidity and mortality from an untreated joint infection. However, many orthopedic specialists now rely on data that suggests antibiotics should be withheld until after a culture is obtained in patients without disseminated infection, sepsis, or septic shock.[1,2] Empiric antibiotic administration prior to culturing the joint fluid appears to decrease culture sensitivity.[24,25] As a result, for patients going directly into an operation, many orthopedists prefer to culture the joint in the operating suite and recommend starting antibiotics post procedure.[26-28]

An orthopedic consultation for definitive management is mandatory in all cases of septic arthritis. Drainage of the joint can be accomplished operatively with arthroscopy, arthrotomy, or serial arthrocentesis.[3] Open surgical drainage is often required, although arthroscopy may be preferred for shoulder and knee infections due to its improved visualization, ease of irrigation, and reduction of postprocedure morbidity.[2,3]

Antimicrobial therapy is more complex in patients with prosthetic joints. Treatment typically involves both prolonged species-specific antibiotics and rifampin. An additional operation and, sometimes, hardware removal may be required.[21]

Joint aspiration (ie, arthrocentesis) is the definitive means of collecting potentially infected fluid and should be performed on any patient with suspected septic arthritis. Fluid analysis can also help clarify the diagnosis when the etiology of the joint swelling is unclear. The procedure has the added benefit of potentially relieving pain and pressure in a tense joint in the setting of an inflammatory effusion or traumatic hemarthrosis.

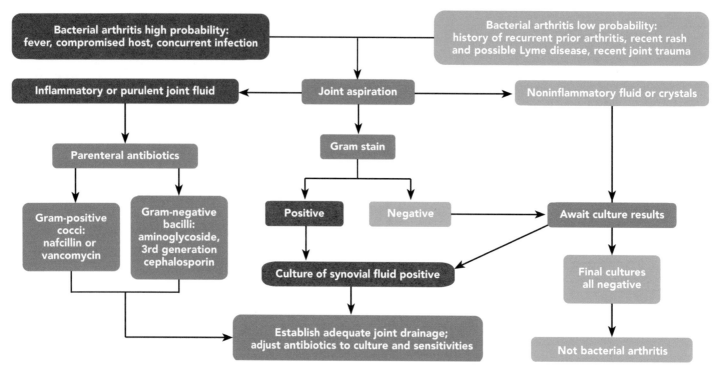

FIGURE 3. Algorithm for evaluating a hot, swollen joint. *Credit*: ACEP.

CRITICAL DECISION

What other diagnoses should be considered in a patient who presents with a swollen joint?

If an acute septic joint remains an unlikely diagnosis after a thorough assessment and workup, other causes of joint swelling should be entertained. Outside the scope of this lesson are other potential etiologies, including autoimmune disorders, spondyloarthropathies, reactive arthritis, and trauma (see *Table 1*).

Gout and Pseudogout

Gout, a common presentation in the emergency department, often manifests as flares of pain, erythema, and swelling in one or more of the lower-extremity joints, most often the first metatarsophalangeal joint (ie, podagra).[29-31] Most patients experience a peak onset of symptoms within the first 24 hours.[30,31] The disease classically affects men (1-3 patients/1,000/year), most commonly in their 40s. In women, the incidence of gout increases with advancing age.[29]

Gout and pseudogout are characterized by the deposition of monosodium urate (MSU) and calcium pyrophosphate dihydrate, respectively. When deposited in synovial fluid, these crystals cause a reactive arthritis. When they collect in the soft tissues, by contrast, they result in tophi. Deposition of MSU crystals in the kidneys can also lead to nephrolithiasis and urate nephropathy. Acute gouty attacks are typically preceded by periods of asymptomatic hyperuricemia; however, elevated serum uric acid levels are common and usually do not progress to acute symptoms.

Uric acid, a chemical byproduct created when the body breaks down purines, is catalyzed by the oxidation of urate oxidase or uricase enzymes.[30,31] The etiologies of hyperuricemia are multifactorial and can include a combination of defective enzymes, a high purine diet, alcohol consumption, or diuretic use.[29-32] An isolated serum uric acid test is unlikely to be helpful in confirming a gout diagnosis because uric acid levels can remain normal in an acute flare.[33]

Gout can be confirmed by the presence of negatively birefringent urate crystals in the patient's synovial fluid, which can be aspirated and examined using polarized light microscopy (*Figure 4*). If this definitive test is unavailable, physicians should adhere to the diagnostic criteria set forth by the American College of Rheumatology (*Table 2*).[34] Treatment should be initiated if suspicion for gout is high and septic arthritis has been excluded.

Although a history of prior flares raises suspicion for gout, there may be more to the story. Patients can present with concomitant septic and gouty arthritis, a diagnosis that should not be missed. In patients with concomitant septic and gouty arthritis, the most commonly affected joint is the knee, followed by the ankle, shoulder, and wrist.[4] The most likely mode of infection is a rupture of subcutaneous tophi and secondary wound infection in patients with long-standing disease.[4]

✔ Pearls

- Limited range of motion in a patient with a swollen joint is the hallmark sign of septic arthritis. Always perform a joint aspiration in this setting to prevent permanent damage to cartilage and significant morbidity and mortality.

- A blood culture medium is preferred over standard solid medium to inoculate synovial fluid.

- Consult orthopedics immediately if there is any suspicion for septic arthritis, which can be fatal if not managed properly.

- In patients with an isolated septic joint without evidence of disseminated infection, sepsis, or septic shock, antibiotics should be withheld until a culture is obtained.

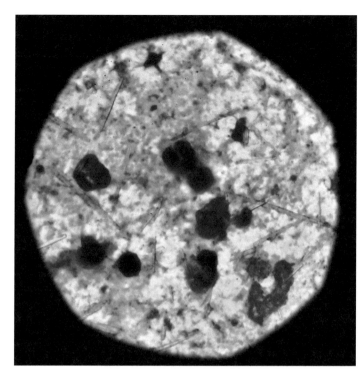

FIGURE 4. Uric acid crystals in synovial fluid indicating gout. *Credit:* toeytoey2530/Getty Images Plus.

Symptom Control

Treatment for an acute gouty attack should be aimed at symptom control; drug therapy and long-term modification of risk factors can help reduce the frequency of future flares and permanent joint destruction. NSAIDs and corticosteroids are the first-line therapies for acute episiodes.[31] Colchicine is an effective second-line therapy; in higher doses, however, it may cause significant adverse effects, such as nausea, vomiting, and abdominal pain. In addition, colchicine must be reserved for patients without significant renal impairment. These medications can also be supplemented with opioids, including oxycodone and hydrocodone.[31]

Summary

Septic arthritis must be considered in any patient with joint swelling and restricted motion. The disease can cause

✖ Pitfalls

- Failing to consider a diagnosis of septic arthritis based on standard guidelines (WBC count of 50,000 cells/μL on synovial fluid analysis) — an oversight that can lead to devastating consequences.

- Assuming that all gout exacerbations are benign. Septic arthritis can develop in the setting of an acute gout attack. If fever and restricted motion are present, the joint should be aspirated for synovial fluid analysis.

- Neglecting to check baseline renal functioning in a patient at risk of chronic kidney failure before starting colchicine or NSAIDs for acute gout. Steroids may be a safer first-line choice in these patients.

Gout May Be Diagnosed if *One* of the Following Criteria Is Present:

Monosodium urate crystals in synovial fluid

OR

Tophi confirmed with crystal examination

OR

At least *six* of the following findings are present:
- Asymmetric swelling within a joint on x-ray
- First metatarsophalangeal joint is tender or swollen (ie, podagra)
- Hyperuricemia
- Maximal inflammation developed within 1 day
- Monoarthritis attack
- More than one acute arthritis attack
- Redness observed over joints
- Subcortical cysts without erosions on an x-ray
- Suspected tophi
- Synovial fluid culture negative for organisms during an acute attack
- Unilateral first metatarsophalangeal joint attack
- Unilateral tarsal joint attack

TABLE 2. American College of Rheumatology preliminary criteria for gout[34]

the rapid destruction of cartilage, and a diagnostic delay may lead to permanent joint damage and significant morbidity and mortality. Joint aspiration, the only means of ruling out this disease, is mandatory in patients with a suspected infection.

Gout and pseudogout, other commonly encountered etiologies for joint swelling, can be diagnosed either by the detection of crystals within the synovial fluid or based on specific clinical criteria. Treatment should be aimed at symptom control with NSAIDs or steroids. Emergency physicians must be vigilant in considering concomitant septic and gouty arthritis because this process can have a misleading presentation but can be devastating if missed.

REFERENCES

1. Margaretten ME, Kohlwes J, Moore D, Bent S. Does this adult patient have septic arthritis? *JAMA*. 2007 Apr 4;297(13):1478-1488.

2. Ross JJ. Septic arthritis. *Infect Dis Clin N Am*. 2005 Dec;19(4):799-817.

3. Garcia-De La Torre I. Advances in the management of septic arthritis. *Infect Dis Clin N Am*. 2006 Dec;20(4):773-788.

4. Yu KH, Luo SF, Liou LB, et al. Concomitant septic and gouty arthritis — an analysis of 30 cases. *Rheumatology*. 2003;42(9):1062-1066.

5. Fagan HB. Approach to the patient with acute swollen/painful joint. *Clinics Fam Prac*. 2005;7(2):305-319.

6. Maury EE, Flores RH. Acute monoarthritis: diagnosis and management. *Prim Care*. 2006;33(3):779-793.

7. Coakley G, Mathews C, Field M, et al; British Society for Rheumatology Standards, Guidelines and Audit Working Group. BSR & BHPR, BOA, RCGP and BSAC guidelines for management of the hot swollen joint in adults. *Rheumatology (Oxford)*. 2006 Aug;45(8):1039-1041.

8. Shirtliff ME, Mader JT. Acute septic arthritis. *Clin Microbiol Rev*. 2002 Oct;15(4):527-544.

9. Andersen K, Bennebaek FN, Hansen BL. Septic arthritis. *Ugeskr Laeger*. 1994 Jun 27;156(26):3871-3875.

10. Kaandorp CJ, Dinant HJ, van de Laar MA, Moens HJ, Prins AP, Dijkmans BA. Incidence and sources of native and prosthetic joint infection: a community based prospective survey. *Ann Rheum Dis*. 1997 Aug;56(8):470-475.

CASE RESOLUTIONS

■ CASE ONE

Suspecting septic arthritis, the physician immediately performed a joint aspiration on the teenage boy's swollen knee. Laboratory test results revealed elevated levels of serum WBC, ESR, and CRP. The synovial WBC count was 56,000 cells/μL, and a Gram stain showed a number of polymorphonuclear leukocytes (PMNs), but no crystals or other organisms were seen.

An orthopedic consultation was obtained; the patient was admitted to the operating room for surgical drainage and irrigation and was started on vancomycin. Several days later, intraoperative synovial fluid cultures grew *S. aureus* sensitive to vancomycin, clindamycin, and sulfamethoxazole.

The patient's previous abscess was suspected to be the culprit behind his infection. He had an uneventful postoperative course and was discharged home 4 days later.

■ CASE TWO

The older man's swollen ankle was suspicious for concomitant gouty and septic arthritis. The diagnosis was confirmed by an analysis of the patient's synovial fluid, which revealed a WBC count of 62,000 cells/μL. A Gram stain was positive for PMNs and clustered gram-positive cocci; a blood culture revealed negatively birefringent urate crystals. Empiric treatment with vancomycin was initiated, and an orthopedics consultation was requested.

The patient was admitted to the hospital for serial needle joint aspirations and intravenous antibiotics. Synovial cultures were positive for *S. aureus* on day 2 in the hospital and were sensitive to oxacillin, cefazolin, and vancomycin. Vancomycin was continued, and the joint fluid was confirmed to be sterile in a repeat culture 1 week later. The patient was discharged home with oral cephalexin and a short course of oral narcotics; he was also advised to decrease his alcohol intake and counseled on a low-purine diet.

■ CASE THREE

The patient consented to arthrocentesis for her atraumatic swollen and painful joint. Approximately 3 mL of turbid, thick, yellow fluid was drawn from her right wrist. Afterward, she had improved range of motion, although the joint pain continued. Basic laboratory tests revealed a normal WBC count and kidney function but an ESR of 60 mm/h and a CRP level of 179 mg/L. An x-ray of the wrist was unremarkable. Her synovial fluid analysis demonstrated positively birefringent crystals and a WBC count of 19,000 cells/μL. A diagnosis of pseudogout was made, with age, diuretic use, and occasional alcohol use as the most likely contributing factors. She was started on NSAIDs and steroids and discharged from the emergency department with instructions on diet and alcohol adjustment. Follow-up with her primary care physician was encouraged.

11. Kaandorp CJ, Krijnen P, Moens HJ, Habbema JD, van Schaardenburg D. The outcome of bacterial arthritis: a prospective community-based study. *Arthritis Rheum*. 1997 May;40(5):844-892.

12. Kaandorp CJ, Van Schaardenburg D, Krijnen P, Habbema JD, van de Laar MA. Risk factors for septic arthritis in patients with joint disease. A prospective study. *Arthritis Rheum*. 1995;38(12):1819-1825.

13. Klein RS. Joint infection, with consideration of underlying disease and sources of bacteremia in hematogenous infection. *Clin Geriatr Med*. 1998 May;4(2):375-394.

14. Kherani RB, Shojania K. Septic arthritis in patients with pre-existing inflammatory arthritis. *CMAJ*. 2007 May 22;176(11):1605-1608.

15. Arnold SR, Elias D, Buckingham SC, et al. Changing patterns of acute hematogenous osteomyelitis and septic arthritis: emergence of community-associated methicillin-resistant *Staphylococcus aureus*. *J Pediatr Othop*. 2006 Nov-Dec;26(6):703-708.

16. Dalla Vestra M, Rettore C, Sartore P, et al. Acute septic arthritis: remember gonorrhea. *Rheumatol Int*. 2008;29(1):81-85.

17. El-Gabalawy HS, Tanner S. Synovial fluid analyses, synovial biopsy, and synovial pathology. In: Firestein GS, Budd, RC, Gabriel SE, Koretzky GA, McInnes IB, O'Dell JR, eds. *Firestein & Kelley's Textbook of Rheumatology*. 11th ed. Elsevier; 2021; 841-585.

18. Sanford SO. Arthrocentesis. In: Roberts JR, Custalow CB, Thomsen TW, eds. *Roberts and Hedges' Clinical Procedures in Emergency Medicine and Acute Care*. 7th ed. Elsevier; 2019; 1105-1124.

19. McGillicuddy DC, Shah KH, Friedberg RP, Nathanson LA, Edlow JA. How sensitive is the synovial fluid white blood cell count in diagnosing septic arthritis? *Am J Emerg Med*. 2007 Sep;25(7):749-752.

20. Carpenter CR, Schuur JD, Everett WW, Pines JM. Evidence-based diagnostics: adult septic arthritis. *Acad Emerg Med*. 2011 Aug;18(8):781-796.

21. Osmon DR, Berbari EF, Berendt AR, et al; Infectious Diseases of America. Diagnosis and management of prosthetic joint infection: clinical practice guidelines by the Infectious Disease Society of America. *Clin Infect Dis*. 2013 Jan;56(1):e1-e25.

22. Zimmerli W, Trampuz A, Ochsner PE. Prosthetic-joint infections. *N Engl J Med*. 2004 Oct 14;351(16):1645-1654.

23. Workowski KA, Berman SM; Centers for Disease Control and Prevention. Sexually transmitted diseases treatment guidelines, 2006. *MMWR Recomm Rep*. 2006;55(RR-11):1-94.

24. Hindle P, Davidson E, Biant LC. Septic arthritis of the knee: the use and effect of antibiotics prior to diagnostic aspiration. *Ann R Coll Surg Engl*. 2012;94(5):351-355.

25. Morgan DS, Fisher D, Merianos A, Currie BJ. An 18 year clinical review of septic arthritis from tropical Australia. *Epidemiol Infect*. 1996 Dec;117(3):423-428.

26. Matthews PC, Berendt AR, McNally MA, Byren I. Diagnosis and management of prosthetic joint infection. *BMJ*. 2009 May 29;338:b1773.

27. Mathews CJ, Weston VC, Jones A, Field M, Coakley G. Bacterial septic arthritis in adults. *Lancet*. 2010;375(9717):846-855.

28. Goldenberg DL. Septic arthritis. *Lancet*. 1998 Jan 17;351(9097):197-202.

29. Wise CM. Crystal-associated arthritis in the elderly. *Clin Geriatr Med*. 2005;21(3):491-511.

30. Keith MP, Gilliland WR. Updates in the management of gout. *Am J Med*. 2007;120(3):221-224.

31. Eggebeen AT. Gout: an update. *Am Fam Physician*. 2007;76(6):801-808.

32. Lioté F, Ea HK. Gout: update on some pathogenic and clinical aspects. *Rheum Dis Clin North Am*. 2006 May;32(2):295-311.

33. Schlesinger N, Norquist JM, Watson DJ. Serum urate during acute gout. *J Rheumatol* 2009 Jun;36(6):1287-1289.

34. Wallace SL, Robinson H, Masi AT, Decker JL, McCarty DJ, Yü TF. Preliminary criteria for the classification of the acute arthritis of primary gout. *Arthritis Rheum*. 01977;20(3):895-900.

CME Questions

Reviewed by Walter L. Green, MD, FACEP; and John C. Greenwood, MD

Qualified, paid subscribers to *Critical Decisions in Emergency Medicine* may receive CME certificates for up to 5 ACEP Category I credits, 5 *AMA PRA Category 1 Credits*™, and 5 AOA Category 2-B credits for completing this activity in its entirety. Submit your answers online at acep.org/cdem; a score of 75% or better is required. You may receive credit for completing the CME activity any time within 3 years of its publication date. Answers to this month's questions will be published in next month's issue.

1 What is the most common cause of small bowel obstruction?

A. Adhesions
B. Bezoars
C. Crohn disease
D. Primary lymphoma

2 Ogilvie syndrome is a rare type of ileus. What is it associated with?

A. Gallstones
B. Mesenteric ischemia
C. Nonoperative trauma, infection, and heart disease
D. Small bowel dilatation

3 A patient presents with a high-grade bowel obstruction. What is a likely finding?

A. Elevated blood urea nitrogen level
B. Elevated hematocrit level
C. Leukocytosis
D. All of these

4 In a nonpregnant adult patient with stable vital signs and a suspected high-grade bowel obstruction, what imaging study is most appropriate?

A. Abdominal ultrasound
B. CT of the abdomen and pelvis with intravenous contrast
C. CT of the abdomen and pelvis with intravenous and oral contrast
D. Plain x-ray

5 Which section of the GI tract tends to return to normal function first in the setting of a postoperative ileus?

A. Colon
B. Small bowel
C. Stomach
D. All sections tend to return at the same time

6 A 75-year-old patient presents with severe abdominal pain, distention, and altered mental status. An upright abdominal x-ray shows free air under the diaphragm, indicating a hollow viscus perforation. What is the next step in management?

A. An emergent surgical consultation
B. An evaluation for an incarcerated hernia
C. A repeat abdominal x-ray in the lateral decubitus view
D. An urgent CT of the abdomen and pelvis with intravenous contrast

7 Which patient with a small bowel obstruction would be an appropriate candidate for a diatrizoate meglumine and diatrizoate sodium solution challenge?

A. A 22-month-old child with colicky abdominal pain, a sausage-shaped mass in the belly, and a target-sign finding of the intestine on ultrasound
B. A 41-year-old woman at 18 weeks' gestation (gravidity 4, parity 3) with a history of two cesarean deliveries and a cholecystectomy
C. A 50-year-old obese man with a history of appendectomy, cholecystectomy, and hernia repair surgery
D. A 67-year-old woman with abdominal pain who develops fever and peritonitis while in the emergency department

8 Compared to other causes of small bowel obstructions, what is an additional concern that should be addressed in a patient with a small bowel obstruction secondary to an incarcerated hernia?

A. A careful history to evaluate for diabetes and smoking status
B. Increased future likelihood of bowel malignancy
C. Ischemia and necrosis, if the cause of obstruction goes untreated
D. The possibility of a closed loop obstruction

9 A 19-month-old girl with no past medical history is brought into the emergency department by her parents. She is reported to have had episodic colicky abdominal pain for the past 2 days, causing her to draw her knees to her chest. Also, she has had no bowel movements in the last 24 hours. Which of the following is not a classic finding of the suspected condition?

A. "Currant jelly" stools
B. Olive-shaped mass in the epigastrium
C. Sausage-shaped mass in the abdomen
D. Target sign on ultrasound

10 A 64-year-old man presents with a painful mass to the umbilicus that has been hurting and is associated with emesis and constipation for the last 2 days. He reports he has had the mass for years and can typically "push it back in" but has not been able to for the last 2 days. His pain acutely worsened 1 hour prior to arrival. He is ill-appearing and has significant abdominal tenderness with rebound and guarding. Vital signs are significant for BP 95/58, P 135, and T 38.1°C (100.6°F). What is the most appropriate next step?

A. Obtain a CT of the abdomen and pelvis with intravenous contrast
B. Obtain an emergent surgical consultation
C. Obtain intravenous access and start intravenous fluid resuscitation and broad-spectrum antibiotics
D. Obtain upright abdominal x-rays

11 **Which test is most specific for ruling in a septic joint?**

A. C-reactive protein
B. Erythrocyte sedimentation rate
C. Serum leukocyte count
D. Synovial leukocyte count

12 **What is not included in the American College of Rheumatology's preliminary criteria for gout?**

A. Hyperuricemia
B. Polyarticular disease
C. Presence of podagra
D. Suspected tophi

13 **What can be used to rule out a septic joint?**

A. A history of osteoarthritis
B. Known previous diagnosis of gout
C. Polyarticular disease
D. None of these

14 **Which joint is least likely to be affected by septic arthritis?**

A. Ankle
B. Hip
C. Shoulder
D. Wrist

15 **A 50-year-old man with a history of a recent perirectal abscess presents for an acutely swollen, tender, and erythematous left knee. It is extremely painful with any movement, and he cannot bear weight on it. He is afebrile, has a serum WBC count of 9,900 cells/μL, and a C-reactive protein level of 221 mg/L. What is an appropriate management strategy for this patient?**

A. Admission to the hospital for intravenous vancomycin administration and trending of C-reactive protein level, WBC count, and temperature
B. Diagnostic arthrocentesis and consultation with orthopedics for a potential operational washout
C. Therapeutic arthrocentesis, NSAIDs, steroids, and outpatient follow-up with an orthopedist
D. X-ray of the knee, discharge with NSAIDs, and primary care follow-up, if negative

16 **Which statement about gonococcal arthritis is true?**

A. Blood cultures are often useful in making the diagnosis
B. Gonococcal arthritis commonly presents in a polyarticular pattern
C. Incidence of gonococcal arthritis decreases with age
D. Synovial cultures will likely yield the diagnosis

17 **Which option would be an inappropriate management strategy for a patient with diagnosed septic arthritis?**

A. Arthroscopy
B. Open arthrotomy
C. Serial arthrocentesis
D. Systemic antibiotics only

18 **A 76-year-old woman with a history of osteoarthritis, hypertension, stage IV kidney disease, and previous left hip replacements presents with an acutely swollen and tender right ankle. She is afebrile. Arthrocentesis reveals a synovial WBC count of 2,100 cells/μL, negatively birefringent crystals, and a negative Gram stain. What would be the best treatment strategy?**

A. Colchicine and therapeutic arthrocentesis
B. Open arthrotomy with washout
C. Oxycodone and cefalexin
D. Prednisone and acetaminophen

19 **Which bacterium genus in septic arthritis has been linked to the use of tumor necrosis factor inhibitors?**

A. *Actinobacillus*
B. *Neisseria*
C. *Staphylococcus*
D. *Streptococcus*

20 **Which antimicrobial agent should not be routinely used as a first-line therapy in cases of suspected septic arthritis?**

A. Cefepime
B. Ceftriaxone
C. Doxycycline
D. Vancomycin

ANSWER KEY FOR NOVEMBER 2022, VOLUME 36, NUMBER 11

1	2	3	4	5	6	7	8	9	10	11	12	13	14	15	16	17	18	19	20
B	B	B	B	D	D	C	A	C	B	B	D	C	A	D	A	A	B	D	B

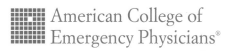
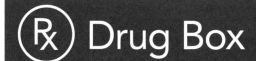

Drug Box

Tenecteplase for Acute Stroke

By Frank LoVecchio, DO, MPH, FACEP
Valleywise Health and ASU, Phoenix, Arizona

Objective
On completion of this column, you should be able to:
- Recall the latest research on tenecteplase for acute ischemic stroke.

Background
Tenecteplase is a modified tissue plasminogen activator with presumed pharmacologic and practical advantages over alteplase. Alteplase is currently the only FDA-approved thrombolytic drug for ischemic stroke. IV tenecteplase has shown similar efficacy and safety outcomes to alteplase in previous acute stroke trials, but the optimal dose remains uncertain.

Research
The Norwegian Tenecteplase Stroke Trial 2 (NOR-TEST 2) was a randomized, open-label, blinded-endpoint, noninferiority phase 3 trial conducted to compare tenecteplase and alteplase at specific dosages for acute stroke. The study included 216 patients who had an NIH Stroke Scale score of ≥6, qualified for thrombolysis, and were admitted within 4-5 hours of symptom onset. Patients were randomly assigned IV tenecteplase (0.4 mg/kg) or standard-dose alteplase (0.9 mg/kg).

In June 2022, the NOR-TEST 2 found higher rates of symptomatic intracranial hemorrhage (ICH) with tenecteplase 0.4 mg/kg compared to alteplase 0.9 mg/kg (6/100 patients [6%] versus 1/104 patients [1%]; unadjusted odds ratio, 6.57 [95% CI, 0.78-55.62]; $P = 0.061$). Furthermore, any type of ICH was significantly more frequent with tenecteplase (21/100 patients [21%] versus 7/104 patients [7%]; unadjusted odds ratio, 3.68 [95% CI, 1.49-9.11]; $P = 0.0031$). The tenecteplase group had significantly fewer positive functional outcomes (31/96 patients [32%] versus 52/101 patients [51%]; unadjusted odds ratio, 0.45 [95% CI, 0.25-0.80]; $P = 0.0064$) and a significantly higher mortality rate (15/96 patients [16%] versus 5/101 patients [5%]; unadjusted odds ratio, 3.56 [95% CI, 1.24-10.21]; $P = 0.013$). The trial was terminated early because tenecteplase was thought to be more harmful and less efficacious than alteplase. Although no single trial is definitive, the study's authors warn that tenecteplase 0.4 mg/kg should not be utilized for IV thrombolysis until further studied. Ongoing stroke trials are evaluating the efficacy and safety of lower-dose tenecteplase (0.25 mg/kg).

REFERENCE
Kvistad CE, Næss H, Helleberg BH. Tenecteplase versus alteplase for the management of acute ischaemic stroke in Norway (NOR-TEST 2, part A): a phase 3, randomised, open-label, blinded endpoint, non-inferiority trial. *Lancet Neurol.* 2022 Jun;21(6):511-519.

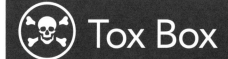

Tox Box

Sodium Fluoroacetate Poisoning

By Christian A. Tomaszewski, MD, MS, MBA, FACEP
University of California San Diego Health

Objective
On completion of this column, you should be able to:
- Recognize and treat sodium fluoroacetate poisoning.

Sodium fluoroacetate (compound 1080) is a metabolic poison that was previously used in the United States as a rodenticide and is now only used in livestock collars as a predacide. This white powder is an extremely hazardous pesticide. All exposures should be considered potentially deleterious.

Toxicokinetics
- Rapid oral absorption; >2 mg/kg is potentially fatal
- Inhalation or absorption through broken skin can be toxic
- Operates by halting the tricarboxylic acid cycle by substituting for acetate

Clinical Manifestations
- ***GI:*** Nausea, vomiting, abdominal pain
- ***Cardiac:*** QT prolongation, hypotension, ventricular tachycardia or fibrillation
- ***Neurologic:*** Agitation, cerebellar dysfunction, seizure, coma
- ***Pulmonary:*** Respiratory depression
- ***Metabolic:*** Acidosis
- ***Electrolytes:*** Hypocalcemia and hypomagnesemia

Diagnostics
- ECG
- Comprehensive metabolic panel
- Calcium, magnesium levels

Treatment
- Oral activated charcoal or gastric aspiration, if early
- Supplemental oxygen as needed
- IV fluids for hypotension; norepinephrine if refractory
- IV benzodiazepines, propofol, or barbiturates for seizures
- Calcium repletion as needed
- IV lipid emulsion therapy and methylene blue are hypothetically beneficial

Disposition
- Discharge if asymptomatic after approximately 4 hours.
- Admit for hypotension, dysrhythmias, or GI, respiratory, or neurologic symptoms.

Made in United States
Troutdale, OR
11/26/2023

14992963R00224